Administrative Medical Assisting

Foundations and Practices

Second Edition

Administrative Medical Assisting

Foundations and Practices

Christine Malone

MBA, MHA, CMPE, CPHRM, FACHE

Contributors:
Lorraine M. Papazian-Boyce

MS, CPC
AHIMA-Approved ICD-10-CM/PCS Trainer
President, PB Resources

Kristiana D. Routh

RMA

PEARSON

Boston   Columbus   Indianapolis   New York   San Francisco   Upper Saddle River
Amsterdam   Cape Town   Dubai   London   Madrid   Milan   Munich   Paris   Montréal   Toronto
Delhi   Mexico City   São Paulo   Sydney   Hong Kong   Seoul   Singapore   Taipei   Tokyo

Publisher: Julie Levin Alexander
Publisher's Assistant: Regina Bruno
Acquisitions Editor: Marlene Pratt
Program Manager: Faye Gemmellaro
Editorial Assistant: Lauren Bonilla
Development Editor: Alexis Ferraro, iD8-TripleSSS Media
    Development, LLC
Marketing Manager: Brittany Hammond
Senior Marketing Coordinator: Alicia Wozniak
Marketing Specialist: Michael Sirinides
Project Management, Team Lead: Cindy Zonneveld
Project Manager: Yagnesh Jani
Full-Service Project Management: Peggy Kellar/Aptara®, Inc.
Senior Operations Specialist: Mary Ann Gloriande
Digital Program Manager: Amy Peltier
Media Project Manager: Lorena Cerisano
Creative Director: Andrea Nix
Art Director: Maria Guglielmo Walsh
Cover and Interior Designer: Ilze Lemesis
Cover Image: manaemedia/shutterstock
Composition: Aptara®, Inc
Printing and Binding: RR Donnelley/Willard
Cover Printer: Phoenix Color/Hagerstown
Text Font: Minion Pro Regular

Credits and acknowledgments borrowed from other sources and reproduced, with permission, in this textbook appear on appropriate page within text.

Library of Congress Cataloging-in-Publication Data

Malone, Christine, author.
    Administrative medical assisting: foundations and practices / Christine Malone; contributors,
Lorraine M. Papazian-Boyce, Kristiana D. Routh.—2e.
        p. ; cm.
    Includes bibliographical references and index.
    ISBN-13: 978-0-13-343065-3
    ISBN-10: 0-13-343065-0
    I. Papazian-Boyce, Lorraine.   II. Routh, Kristiana D.   III. Title.
    [DNLM: 1. Practice Management, Medical.   2. Allied Health Personnel. W 80]
    R728.8
    610.73'7092—dc23

                                                                    2014001208

10 9 8 7 6 5 4 3 2

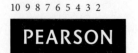

ISBN 13: 978-0-13-343065-3
ISBN 10:   0-13-343065-0

Dedication

To my Ian, whose life was a constant battle to improve the health care system for those who would come after him.

Brief Contents

Contents

SECTION IV Practice Finances and Management of the Medical Office   293

17 Insurance Billing   294

18 Diagnostic Coding   353

19 Procedural Coding   378

LIST OF PROCEDURES

Preface

The Development of This Text

I was first inspired to write this textbook after reviewing countless administrative medical assisting textbooks and finding numerous inaccuracies and dated material in those texts. I found myself adopting texts currently available on the market, yet having to supplement the material with numerous handouts and case studies in order to ensure my students were fully competent in the administrative areas. As an instructor who has spent over 30 years in medical office management, I felt a textbook needed to be written by someone with extensive experience in the field of administrative medical office work.

This text stands out from others on the market in that it includes all needed materials, with examples for instructors to use to help clarify the concepts. Without excess bulk in the material, instructors are able to concentrate on the materials students need to know to successfully complete their medical-assisting program.

In developing this text, it was my desire to complete a textbook that would fully address the administrative competencies of both the Accrediting Bureau of Health Education Schools (ABHES), and the Commission on Accreditation of Allied Health Education Programs (CAAHEP) for medical assisting programs. In addition, at the beginning of relevant chapters, a Certification Exam Coverage feature is included that lists the certification exam topics of the American Association of Medical Assistants (CMA), American Medical Technologists (CMAS and RMA), and the National Center for Competency Testing (NCMA). Note that at the time this text went to press, the NHA was in the process of revising its test plan. For the most up-to-date information regarding the NHA test plan and certification exam topics, please visit their website at www.nhanow.com.

How to Use This Text

The information in this textbook can be used by both ABHES- and CAAHEP-accredited schools or those schools applying for accreditation, and by students studying for the AAMA (CMA), AMT (CMAS), AMT (RMA), or NCCT (NCMA) exams. This textbook meets both content and competency requirements in the administrative area.

The material in this text is divided into five sections. Section I is an introduction to the history of medicine and health care and the administrative medical assistant profession; Section II delves into the administrative responsibilities of the medical assistant; Section III focuses on responding to emergencies in the medical office; Section IV highlights the area of medical practice finances and the management of the medical office; and Section V outlines the practicum experience and career strategies for the medical assistant.

Section I: Introduction to the Administrative Medical Assisting Profession

Section I begins with Chapter 1 and the history of medicine and health care, providing the medical assisting student with knowledge of how health care began, the history of the profession, and milestones we've seen along the way. Chapter 2 provides the medical assisting student with detailed information on the educational requirements of the medical assistant; the benefits of certifying or registering as a medical assistant; the professional organizations that certify or register medical assistants; MA scope of practice; and professional associations that certify other allied health professionals. Chapter 3 provides detailed coverage of the professional qualities of the medical assistant as well as career opportunities available. This chapter also discusses the roles, responsibilities, and educational requirements of various members of the health care team, including physicians, nurses, pharmacists, and others. Chapter 4 provides the student with an understanding of medical law from the medical assistant's point of view. This chapter begins with an overview of the American legal system and works through medical malpractice, HIPAA legislation, and mandatory reporting requirements. Chapter 5, which is new to this second edition, provides students with information pertaining to ethical issues they may face in the medical office, and how those issues affect the medical assistant's job. Specific examples of ethical issues, as well as information on what makes those issues ethical in nature, are clearly spelled out. Chapter 6 focuses on interpersonal communication skills for the medical assistant. This chapter highlights areas such as the communication process, verbal communication, nonverbal communication, and communicating with patients who may present special challenges, such as the hearing impaired, or communicating with patients via interpreters. Section I ends with Chapter 7 on written communication. This chapter relays information on writing professional correspondence, how to chart in the patient's medical chart, how to correct errors in charting, and using email in a professional manner to communicate with patients.

Section II: Administrative Responsibilities of the Medical Assistant

Section II begins with Chapter 8 on telephone procedures. This chapter covers this topic in depth, including how to call in prescriptions and refill requests, taking emergency telephone calls, and documenting calls from patients. Chapter 9 focuses on the front desk and reception duties. This chapter covers preparing patient files, escorting patients, and maintaining the reception room in the medical office. Chapter 10 outlines various methods of patient appointment scheduling. It includes information on both manual and computerized scheduling; scheduling patients for in- and outpatient procedures; and managing the physician's professional schedule. Chapter 11 presents detailed information on medical records management and stresses the important role these records play in health care delivery. The various forms of charting (narrative style, SOAP, POMR, source-oriented, CHEDDAR); using flow charts; common medical abbreviations; charting patient communication; managing paper medical records; filing systems used in the medical office; correcting errors in the medical chart, and the legalities of retaining patient medical records are discussed. Chapter 12 presents information on electronic health records and conducting research with medical records. This chapter includes information on converting paper medical records to electronic format, as well as how HIPAA legislation pertains to electronic health records. Chapter 13 focuses on computers in the medical office. This chapter begins with the basics of computer hardware and software and discusses the use of various computer peripherals, electronic pads, tablets, PDAs, and smart phones; maintaining equipment; computer security; and the use of Internet search engines for conducting research. Computer ergonomics and personal computer use in the medical office are also discussed. Chapter 14 discusses equipment, maintenance, and supply inventory in the medical office. This chapter presents an in-depth look at working with medical equipment, documenting maintenance of equipment, and all aspects of inventorying, ordering, and stocking supplies. Chapter 15 outlines the need for office policies and procedures, including instructions on writing office policies, how to write a mission statement, as well as creating a personnel manual. This chapter gives information regarding documentation of infection control procedures as well as creating a quality-improvement and risk-management procedure manual.

Section III: Responding to Emergencies in the Medical Office

Section III comprises Chapter 16: Handling Medical Office Emergencies. This chapter presents the student with information on how to prevent accidents and injuries in the medical office. It presents the competencies medical assistants must have when performing life-saving procedures such as adult rescue breathing or cardiopulmonary resuscitation, and when aiding patients in shock. It also presents information on the medical assistant's role in emergency preparedness and developing an environmental exposure plan.

Section IV: Practice Finances and Management of the Medical Office

Section IV begins with Chapter 17: Insurance Billing. Streamlined for this edition, this chapter is an up-to-date and accurate view of how insurance billing and authorizations are handled in the medical office. The chapter covers topics from health insurance plans to all aspects of Medicare and Medicaid coverage, to completing insurance claim forms both manually and electronically. The use of COBRA coverage, flexible spending accounts, and health savings accounts are also covered. Chapter 18, which is new to this edition, provides the specifics of ICD-10-CM diagnostic coding. Written by an AHIMA-approved ICD-10-CM/PCS trainer and respected author, this chapter presents instructions for using the ICD-10-CM coding book and its various volumes, and educates students on how to avoid fraud in medical coding (Appendix A includes coverage of ICD-9-CM for those programs that require this content). Chapter 19, Procedural Coding, describes the layout of the CPT coding book; provides steps for accurate CPT coding, including determining correct codes; and explains the relationship between accurate documentation and reimbursement. This chapter includes in-depth coverage of the use of modifiers in proper coding as well as the steps to follow to determine the proper evaluation and management (E&M) code. Exercises and examples are provided throughout. Chapter 20 focuses on billing, collections, and credit, and includes information on how to discuss fees with patients and collecting on patient accounts. Chapter 20 ends with a discussion of the use of collection agencies and small claims court. Chapter 21 focuses on payroll, accounts payable, and banking procedures. In this chapter, students are introduced to handling payroll in the medical office, reconciling bank statements, paying office invoices, and working with petty cash. Chapter 22 discusses the role of the medical office manager, including how to conduct an effective staff meeting, how to conduct interviews, and how to perform employee evaluations. Chapter 22 also discusses the topic of risk management in the medical office, including filing an incident report and ensuring employee safety. Chapter 23, Marketing the Medical Office, is new to this edition, and introduces the medical assistant to the function of marketing in the practice and the role of the medical office manager in creating and executing the business's marketing initiative.

Section V: The Practicum Experience and Career Strategies

Section V consists of Chapter 24: The Practicum Experience and Competing in the Job Market. This chapter presents invaluable information not only on the student's practicum experience, but also on the tasks necessary to successfully compete in the job market. Writing an effective résumé and cover letter, identifying places to look for employment, completing job applications, preparing for the interview, presenting the right image, following-up after an interview, and changing jobs are discussed.

New to This Edition

- New photos and tables appear throughout the text to illustrate and expand upon key concepts.
- A new feature, Certification Exam Coverage, appears at the beginning of each relevant chapter. This feature provides students with a list of exam topics that are covered in the chapter.
- New and updated content appears throughout the text, covering such topics as medical ethics, the Patient Affordable Care Act, electronic health records, meaningful use, ICD-10-CM, marketing the medical office, and more.
- Chapter 5, Medicine and Ethics, has been added to provide the student with a clear understanding of what society and the medical assisting profession expect with regard to ethical practice, as well as the ethical concepts medical assistants may encounter in the field. Ethics in medicine, ethical considerations of the medical assistant, performing within the scope of practice, ethical issues in the management of care, and bioethics are all addressed.
- The insurance, procedural coding, and diagnostic coding chapters have been updated and streamlined for ease of use and understanding, and an entire chapter, written by Lorraine Papazian-Boyce, an AHIMA-approved ICD-10-CM/PCS trainer, is dedicated to ICD-10-CM diagnostic coding. A new appendix (Appendix A) includes coverage of ICD-9-CM coding for those schools that require this content. Examples and exercises throughout the coding chapters help to clarify important concepts and provide opportunities for students to apply what they have learned.
- Chapter 23, Marketing the Medical Office, introduces the student to the function of marketing in the medical office and the medical office manager's role in executing the marketing imitative.
- An icon appears next to those procedures that require students to complete and submit products that prove their mastery of the competency.

Pedagogical Features in This Textbook

The following special features appear throughout the text:

- **Learning Objectives:** Specific learning objectives appear at the beginning of each chapter, stating what is to be achieved upon successful completion of the chapter.
- **Certification Exam Coverage:** Each chapter lists AAMA (CMA), AMT (CMAS), AMT (RMA), and NCCT (NCMA) certification exam topics that are covered in the specific chapter.

- **Competency Skills Performance:** This feature lists all of the procedures presented in the chapter.
- **Key Terminology and Abbreviations:** Terms and their definitions appear at the beginning of each chapter as well as in the narrative and the comprehensive glossary.
- **Medical Terminology:** In addition to medical terminology and abbreviations presented at the beginning of each chapter, the text also features a separate appendix of Medical Terminology Word Parts, designed to help students analyze medical terms, understand word parts and word-part guidelines, and define basic medical terms and terms used to describe major body systems, body direction, and diseases and disease conditions.
- **Case Study:** A thought-provoking case study is presented at the beginning of each chapter, with critical thinking questions interspersed throughout the chapter. Students must rely on the content in the text and their own critical thinking skills to answer the questions.
- **Pulse Points:** Each chapter contains brief, helpful tips containing practice advice for succeeding in the health care setting.
- **Informational Charts and Tables:** Informative charts and tables appear throughout the text and summarize pertinent information for the reader. They provide students with visuals and comparisons to reinforce the lesson.
- **Color Photos:** Color photos help to illustrate and reinforce the concepts presented in the text.
- **HIPAA Compliance:** This feature contains helpful advice on how to apply the concepts presented in the text to create a HIPAA-compliant atmosphere in the health care setting.
- **In-Practice:** These real-world scenarios with critical thinking questions present opportunities for readers to think about and apply the concepts presented in the text.
- **Procedures:** For each competency, theory and rationale are discussed, required materials are listed, and the procedure is presented.
- **Chapter Summary:** The chapter summary is an excellent review of the chapter content, often used for certification exams.
- **Chapter Review Questions:** End-of-chapter questions are provided in Multiple-Choice, True/False, Short Answer, and Research format, and help reinforce learning. The review questions measure the student's understanding of the material presented in the chapter. These tools are available for use by the student or by the instructor as an outcome assessment.
- **Practicum Application Experience:** This end-of-chapter feature places the student in a simulated situation he or she might encounter at a practicum site.
- **Resource Guide:** This list provides additional resources for the reader to consult for further information on the topics contained within the chapter.

About the Author

Christine Malone, BS, MBA, MHA, CMPE, CPHRM, FACHE studied management practice and theory at Henry Cogswell College, receiving her BS in Professional Management. She continued her education at the University of Washington, obtaining her Master's Degree in Health Administration. Christine went on to earn her MBA from Northcentral University, with a health care focus, and is currently pursuing her doctorate in education from City University of Seattle. Christine has earned the status of a Certified Medical Practice Executive (CMPE) with the Medical Group Management Association, a Certified Professional in Healthcare Risk Management (CPHRM) from the American Society of Healthcare Risk Managers, and she is a Fellow in the American College of Healthcare Executives (FACHE) with the American College of Healthcare Executives.

Christine has over 30 years' experience in the health care field, having spent time working as a dental assistant, a medical receptionist, an X-ray technician, medical clinic director, and as a consultant to health care providers, focusing on strategic management, efficient office flow, and human resource management. Since 2004, Christine has been teaching in the Health Professions Department at Everett Community College in Washington State. There she is a tenured instructor teaching Medical Office Management, Computer Applications in the Medical Office, Medical Practice Finances, Intercultural Communications in Healthcare, and Medical Law and Ethics. In 2006 Christine researched and developed a certificate program in Healthcare Risk Management. This series of three courses is offered via distance learning and provides the student who successfully completes the three courses a Certificate in Healthcare Risk Management. In 2013, Christine accepted a position as the Program Director for the BS in Healthcare Administration Program at City University of Seattle. She teaches for both Everett Community College and City University of Seattle.

Christine was elected to the Snohomish County Charter Review Commission, a one-year position from 2005–2006. She is the past co-chair of the Young Careerists Group in the Business and Professional Women's Association of Greater Everett, a member of the American College of Healthcare Executives (ACHE), a member of the Washington State Healthcare Executive Forum (WSHEF), a member of the American Society for Healthcare Risk Management (ASHRM), a member of the American College of Medical Practice Executives (ACMPE), and is active in health care politics on both a local and national level. Christine has been the guest speaker at various events on health care issues and in continuing-education meetings across Washington State and has received her certification in vocational teaching as well as in pediatric palliative care training. Christine sits on the board of directors of the Big Brothers Big Sisters Association of Snohomish County as well as on the Board of the Snohomish County Palliative Care Council. She volunteers with Planned Parenthood of the Great Northwest, and serves on several committees with health care organizations and training programs geared toward patient safety.

Christine has five children and lives in a 105-year-old home in Everett, Washington. In 1999, her third child, Ian, was injured due to medical negligence during his birth. Ian lived four and a half years before succumbing to his injuries in 2004. This was the genesis of Christine's work toward improving patient safety in health care. Her input has been sought by legislative committees, editorial boards, and many policymakers. Legislation that was coauthored by Christine has been enacted into law at both the state and federal levels. A nationally recognized health care reform advocate, Christine has appeared on the *Today Show*, *NBC Nightly News*, *ABC Nightly News*, the CBC's *The National*, in *The New York Times*, *The Los Angeles Times*, and on *Salon.com*.

Acknowledgments

The author would like to extend a thank-you to Alexis Breen Ferraro, Developmental Editor, for her experienced management and oversight of this project.

In addition, I'd like to thank my children Corey, Mallory, Molly and Riley—thank you for your patience while this project was completed.

Last, but far from least, thank you to my colleagues at Everett Community College—Beth Adolphsen, CMA (AAMA); and Karla Pouillon, RN, MEd. You are a team clearly dedicated to providing outstanding education to future medical assistants.

Reviewers

The author and publisher wish to thank the following reviewers, all of whom provided valuable feedback and helped to shape the final text:

Amy Semenchuk, BSN, RN
Dean of Academics
Rockford Career College
Rockford, IL

Barb Westrick, AAS, CMA (AAMA), CPC
Program Chair - Medical Assisting and Medical Billing
Ross Medical Education Center
Ann Arbor, MI

Cheri Goretti, CMA (AAMA), MA, MT (ASCP)
Professor, Coordinator - Medical Assisting and Allied Health Programs
Quinebaug Valley Community College
Danielson, CT

David O. Martinez, MHSA, RMA
Professor – Medical Assisting
University of Phoenix
El Paso, TX

Dawn Eitel, BAS, CMA (AAMA)
Program Director, Instructor - Medical Assisting
Kirkwood Community College
Cedar Rapids, IA

Jeff Turner, EMT-P, MA, MSM
Director of Education
Southern Careers Institute
Corpus Christi, TX

Johnicka L. Byrd, AAS, BA, CMA (AAMA)
Instructor - Allied Health
Virginia College
Greenville, SC

Lisa Graese, CMT
Instructor - Medical Assisting
Spokane Community College
Spokane, WA

Lucinda Hunsberger, AAS, BS, CMA (AAMA)
Instructor – Medical Assisting
YTI Career Institute Lancaster
Lancaster, PA

Lynnae Lockett, CMRS, MSN, RN, RMA
Ohio Market Program Director – Medical Assisting and Medical Administrative Assisting
Bryant & Stratton College
Parma, OH

Michaelann M. Allen, CMA (AAMA), MA.Ed
Program Instructor - Medical Assisting
North Seattle College
Seattle, WA

Mindy Brown, AAS, BA, MS, RMA
Instructor - Medical Assisting/Administrative Assisting
Pima Medical Institute
Colorado Springs, CO

Pamela J. Edwards, MA, BA, BA, CBCS, NRCMA
Adjunct Professor, Medical Office Administration
Lone Star College System-Montgomery Campus
Conroe, TX

The Learning Package

The Student Package

- Textbook
- Student Workbook that contains Chapter Outlines; Chapter Reviews; Learning Activities; Terminology Review; Critical Thinking Questions; Chapter Review Test, with Multiple Choice questions and additional True/False and Short Answer Questions; and Competency Check-Off Skill Sheets.

The Instructional Package

- Instructor's Resource Manual with lesson plans, teaching tips, concepts for lecture, PowerPoint lecture slides, suggestions for classroom activities and homework assignments, and answers to all textbook and workbook questions.
- Transition Guides to help make text implementation easy.
- PowerPoint slides
- MyTest test bank

Chapter Opener Features

Objectives

Each chapter opens with a list of learning objectives that can be used to identify the material and skills the student should know upon successful completion of the chapter.

Case Study

Thought-provoking case studies provide scenarios that help students understand how the material presented in the chapter relates to the medical assisting profession.

4

Medicine and the Law

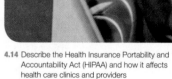

Case Study

Read the following case study and answer the critical thinking questions presented throughout the chapter.

Victoria Mason is a registered medical assistant in Dr. Kozlowski's office. Victoria takes a telephone call from a man named Bart. He tells Victoria that one of his employees is a patient of Dr. Kozlowski's and asks her to tell him when his employee was last in the office and what treatment she received.

Objectives

After completing this chapter, you should be able to:

4.1 Define and spell the key terminology in this chapter.
4.2 Explain the sources of law.
4.3 Classify varied laws as they apply to health care.
4.4 Understand and classify types of consent.
4.5 Define the types of malpractice, and describe the types of malpractice insurance policies available.
4.6 Describe how medical malpractice is proven.
4.7 Describe how to prevent and defend against medical malpractice claims.
4.8 Describe the concept of tort reform and how it applies to malpractice cases.
4.9 Outline the physician's public duties and describe causes for disciplinary action.
4.10 Compare the duties of the physician and the

4.14 Describe the Health Insurance Portability and Accountability Act (HIPAA) and how it affects health care clinics and providers
4.15 List and describe various types of advance directives.
4.16 Discuss employment laws and their impact on health care.
4.17 Outline important information contained in the patients' bill of rights.
4.18 Identify the monitoring agencies that address ambulatory health care.
4.19 Define the Controlled Substances Act and discuss the rules of compliance.

Certification Exam Coverage

This feature provides students with a list of topics in the chapter that are covered on the respective exams (AAMA [CMA], AMT [CMAS], AMT [RMA], and NCCT [NCMA]).

Certification Exam Coverage

AAMA (CMA) Exam Coverage:
- Patient interviewing techniques
  - Legal restrictions
- Medicolegal guidelines and restrictions
  - Medical practice acts
  - Revocation/suspension of license
    1) Criminal/unprofessional conduct
    2) Professional/personal incapacity
- Legislation
  - Advance directives
  - Occupational Safety and Health Act (OSHA)
  - Food and Drug Administration (FDA)
  - Clinical Laboratory Improvement Act (CLIA '88)
  - Americans with Disabilities Act (ADA)
  - Health Insurance Portability and Accountability Act (HIPAA)
- Documentation/reporting
  - Sources of information
  - Drug Enforcement Administration (DEA)

- Physician–patient relationship
  - Contract
    1) Legal obligations
    2) Consequences for noncompliance
  - Responsibility and rights
    1) Patient
    2) Physician
    3) Medical assistant
  - Professional liability
    1) Current standard of care
    2) Current legal standards
    3) Informed consent
  - Arbitration agreements
  - Affirmative defenses
    1) Statute of limitations
    2) Comparative/contributory negligence
    3) Assumption of risk
  - Termination of medical care
    1) Establishing policy
    2) Elements for withdrawal

Critical Thinking Questions

Critical thinking questions are interspersed in the body of the chapter, and students must rely on the content in the text and their own critical thinking skills to answer the questions.

Critical Thinking Question 4-6

Refer back to the case study at the beginning of the chapter. Assume that the patient was fired after the medical office gave her employer her private health information without her permission. How should the patient go about filing a complaint with HIPAA authorities?

Medical Terminology and Abbreviations

The Medical Terminology and Abbreviations sections appear at the beginning of each chapter. The terms are listed in alphabetical order, a definition is provided, and the terminology appears in boldface on first introduction in the text. All terms are defined in the comprehensive glossary that appears at the back of the book, and phonetic pronunciations for difficult medical terminology are also provided.

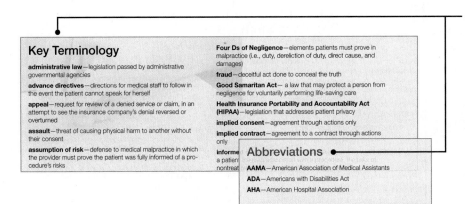

Key Terminology

administrative law—legislation passed by administrative governmental agencies

advance directives—directions for medical staff to follow in the event the patient cannot speak for herself

appeal—request for review of a denied service or claim, in an attempt to see the insurance company's denial reversed or overturned

assault—threat of causing physical harm to another without their consent

assumption of risk—defense to medical malpractice in which the provider must prove the patient was fully informed of a procedure's risks

Four Ds of Negligence—elements patients must prove in malpractice (i.e., duty, dereliction of duty, direct cause, and damages)

fraud—deceitful act done to conceal the truth

Good Samaritan Act— a law that may protect a person from negligence for voluntarily performing life-saving care

Health Insurance Portability and Accountability Act (HIPAA)—legislation that addresses patient privacy

implied consent—agreement through actions only

implied contract—agreement to a contract through actions only

informe
a patien
nontreat

Abbreviations

AAMA—American Association of Medical Assistants

ADA—Americans with Disabilities Act

AHA—American Hospital Association

Appendix of Medical Terminology Word Parts

The text also features a separate appendix of Medical Terminology Word Parts, designed to help students analyze medical terms, understand word parts and word part guidelines, and define basic medical terms and terms used to describe major body systems, body direction, and diseases and disease conditions.

Analyzing a Medical Term

You can often decipher the meaning of a medical term by breaking it down into its separate parts. Consider the following examples:

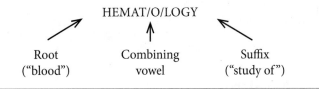

HEMAT/O/LOGY

Root ("blood")   Combining vowel   Suffix ("study of")

A list of competencies appears at the beginning of each chapter in which procedures are presented. For each competency, Theory and Rationale are discussed, Required Materials are listed, and the procedure is presented.

Competency Skills Performance

1. Prepare an informed consent for treatment form.
2. Obtain authorization for the release of patient medical records.
3. Respond to a request for copies of a patient's medical record.

Competency Skills Performance/ Procedures

This unique text meets the highest standards outlined by CAAHEP and ABHES and provides all of the tools needed for student success. This comprehensive text can be used by both ABHES-and CAAHEP-accredited schools or those applying for accreditation to meet both content and competency requirements in the administrative and clinical areas.

PROCEDURE 4-1 Prepare an Informed Consent for Treatment Form

Theory and Rationale

While the task of explaining the procedures, risks, and alternatives falls to the physician, the medical assistant is often the person who discusses the paperwork with the patient and obtains the patient's signature.

Materials

- Informed consent for treatment form
- Blue or black ink pen
- Copy machine

Competency

1. As the physician goes over the details of the upcoming procedure with the patient, fill in the informed consent form. The form must include:
   - The name of the procedure or treatment to be performed
   - The expected benefits of the procedure
   - Any possible risks of the procedure
   - Any accepted alternatives to the procedure and the risks or benefits associated with each

- The fact that the patient may choose to forego the procedure and the possible risks or benefits associated with that choice
2. Be certain the form lists the patient's name, birth date, and the place the procedure is to be performed (in office, hospital, etc.).
3. Show the consent form to the physician for him or her to verify that all information is correct.
4. After the physician has left the room, go over the form with the patient. If the patient has further questions about the procedure, have the patient wait in the treatment room while you ask the physician to return to answer the questions. If the patient has no further questions about the procedure, have the patient sign the consent form.
5. Sign the consent form as a witness to the patient's signature.
6. Go over any specifics with the patient about the procedure day, such as any restrictions to eating or drinking on the day of the surgery, or where the patient should park her car.
7. Make a copy of the consent form for the patient. Place the original form in the patient's file.

▶▶▶ Pulse Points

The Value of Signed Consent Forms

Lack of a valid, signed informed consent form has been cause for malpractice claims to be filed against health care providers. Without a signed consent form prior to a procedure, for example, the patient may sue the provider for performing that procedure without proper consent.

Pulse Points

Helpful tips for career success are interspersed throughout the text to highlight the importance of professionalism.

In Practice

These real-life scenarios require students to pause and apply the knowledge presented in the chapter to answer critical thinking questions.

In Practice

Sharon is the administrative medical assistant who completes billing work in the office. One day when she receives a patient file for billing, Sharon notices that the fee slip the physician completed indicates that he drained a cyst on the patient's wrist. When Sharon reviews the chart notes to assign a diagnosis code, she finds that the physician has written nothing in the chart about the cyst or the procedure. In situations like these, Sharon usually just "jots something" in the chart. What might be wrong with this scenario?

HIPAA Compliance

These feature boxes highlight the need-to-know law.

HIPAA Compliance

Patients can give anyone verbal access to their medical information by notifying the medical office in writing. Permission for verbal access is restricted solely to giving verbal information about a patient's medical care; providing copies, either on paper or electronically, is not permitted with verbal access permission. Such information becomes part of the patients' permanent medical records. For example, if Julius Reiman gives written permission for his wife, Ruth, to have knowledge of his care, the physician can talk to Ruth about Julius's care or condition.

Electronic Health Records

An entire chapter of this text is devoted to the important topic of electronic health records.

- Maintain an active medication allergy list
- Vital signs
- Smoking status
- Implement one clinical decision support rule and the ability to track the patient's compliance with that rule
- Calculate and transmit Centers for Medicare and Medicaid Services (**CMS**) quality measure
- Electronic copy of health information
- Clinical summaries
- Exchange key clinical information
- Privacy and security

Additional criteria exist for Stages 2 and 3 and can be found at the following sites:

http://www.cms.gov/Regulations-and-Guidance/Legislation/EHRIncentivePrograms/Meaningful_Use.html

http://www.healthit.gov/providers-professionals/how-attain-meaningful-use

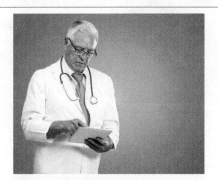

Figure 12-8 ■ A physician uses a handheld electronic notepad to make notes in a patient's medical record.
Source: Shutterstock © Aaron Amat.

▶▶ Pulse Points

Protecting Electronic Health Records

Electronic health records must be protected—both the information and the computer systems. Computers must be password-protected and safeguards must be in place to limit access to protected information.

Benefits of Electronic Health Records

Depending on the program, electronic records are available via keyboard connected to a computer system or stylus tapped on a notebook computer, or on a personal digital assistant (PDA). These devices have many of the same functions as a full-size computer and have the added benefit of being small enough for physicians to carry with them from patient to patient. Some of these devices use a stylus pen to make choices on the screen; others are used simply with one's fingertip. Most electronic health records systems can be configured to work according to an office's specific needs. The following is a list of the functions many of these systems provide:

- Time-stamp recordings in the EHR
- Prescriptions printed or faxed to the pharmacy
- Printed patient education information that directly relates to the patient's care
- Search for a certain type of condition or certain age or geographic location of a group of patients
- Digital photos or X-rays attached in the patient's EHR
- Electronically ordered lab results, imaging items, or medical tests
- Electronic graphs of lab results of height, weight, or blood pressure data

- Letters to patients
- Electronic data transmission to other health care providers

One of the many benefits of such systems is the ability to access medical record information from many locations in the health care facility and to quickly search for and retrieve information in the patient's medical record (**Figure 12-8** ■). These devices are often helpful for physicians who see patients in different settings, such as in the hospital, a skilled nursing facility, or even in the patient's home. Using the handheld electronic device, the physician can access and document in the patient's electronic health record, even when she is nowhere near a desktop computer.

● In Practice

Dr. Jonas runs a private practice and makes rounds in two local hospitals. He uses one type of electronic health records software in his private office and two other packages in the two hospitals. Not only must Dr. Jonas learn three software systems, he may at times be unable to move patient information between those systems due to incompatibility. What might Dr. Jonas do to address these issues?

There are additional benefits to using electronic health records, which are discussed in the following sections.

Electronic Signatures

An office that uses electronic health records may use an **electronic signature**. In offices where medical notes are dictated and printed for patient files, an electronic signature or rubber-stamp signature may replace handwritten signatures. In these offices, there must be a permanent record of the signer, as well as an original version of the signature on file.

Emergency Preparedness

This text includes the latest information on emergency preparedness and the medical assistant's role in protective practices.

TABLE 16-1 Emergency Intervention

Life-Threatening Condition	Not Life-Threatening: Immediate Intervention	Not Life-Threatening: Intervention as Soon as Possible
• Extreme shortness of breath (airway or breathing problems) • Cardiac arrest • Severe, uncontrolled bleeding • Head injuries • Poisoning • Open chest or abdominal wounds • Shock • Severe burns, including face, hands, feet, and genitals • Potential neck injuries	• Decreased levels of consciousness • Chest pain • Seizures • Major or multiple fractures • Neck injuries • Severe eye injuries • Burns not on face, hands, feet, or genitals	• Severe vomiting and diarrhea, especially in the very young and the elderly • Minor injuries • Sprains • Strains • Simple fractures

Managing Medical Emergencies

When emergencies arise in the medical office, medical assistants must remember to stay calm so they can direct patients as needed. Patients look to medical assistants as authority figures.

Understanding and Classifying Consent

Before patients are accepted for care in a medical office, they must give their consent to be examined and/or treated by the physician or health care provider and sign a consent form. Before asking the patient or parent/guardian to consent for any examination or treatment, it is the responsibility of the provider to explain the suggested care. Part of this explanation must be to outline the benefits and risks, if any, as well as any accepted alternative to the treatment. Once that information has been explained to the patient and the patient has been given the opportunity to ask any questions, the patient should be asked to sign a consent form. This is the process of obtaining informed consent from the patient. The following information must be included on a consent form:

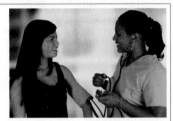

Figure 4-1 ■ This patient has given implied consent to have her blood pressure taken.
Source: Shutterstock © Rob Marmion.

- Being seen for information regarding birth control or abortion
- Being seen for treatment regarding drug or alcohol abuse

Consent forms must be written in the languages patients speak. Most facilities that treat patients from other cultures

Medical Ethics

With a growing number of medical ethical issues facing medical assistants today, this chapter provides in-depth information on how those ethical issues play out in the real practice of the medical assistant's duties.

Medical Law

Medical assistants face many situations that involve the law; therefore, a comprehensive chapter is provided to highlight the need-to-know law and to present scenarios that could have a legal impact on patients. Informational tables and charts summarize key concepts.

Ethical Model

An unethical physician might ask the medical assistant to break the law. Medical assistants are legally bound by law and scope of practice to treat patients lawfully and ethically and to document correctly in patients' charts. If medical assistants wonder whether actions cross ethical or legal boundaries, they should consider the following questions based on the Blanchard and Peale Ethical Model:

1. Is the action legal?
2. Is the action ethical?
3. How will the action make me feel?
4. How would I feel if the action, and my involvement, was published in the local newspaper? If I had to explain my actions to my child/spouse/parent?

If the medical assistant is uncomfortable with any of the answers to these four questions, the action likely crosses an ethical or legal boundary and the medical assistant should decline to participate. Any local Association of Medical Assistants chapter is a good place to call when in doubt about an action. Bad actions can hinder future employment. Prospective employers must believe new staff are ethical and will practice within their legal scopes of practice. Medical assistants who are associated with a medical practice or a physician who is practicing unethically or illegally will unfortunately gain that same reputation (**Figure 5-3** ■).

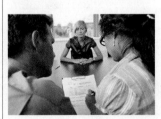

Figure 5-3 ■ The medical assistant might find it difficult to gain future employment if a negative work history becomes known.
Source: Shutterstock © StockLite.

In Practice

Jan has been working as an administrative medical assistant for Dr. Borse for seven years. Dr. Borse frequently asks Jan to add charges to a patient account for services he did not perform.

Jan is paid well and feels she is harming no patients by complying with the doctor's requests. Dr. Borse says he only submits the false claims to make up for the money he loses by treating Medicare and Medicaid patients. One day, Dr. Borse is arrested for insurance fraud; he eventually serves two years in prison and loses his license to practice medicine. Jan is originally arrested too, as a participant in the crime. Because she testifies against her employer, she is not charged with a crime. In the months after this event, Jan has a very hard time getting a new job. Dr. Borse's story has been in all the local papers, and employers do not want to work with unethical staff.

How could Jan have changed the course of events? What advice would have helped Jan while she was working with Dr. Borse?

Raising Ethical Issues in Health Care

The American Medical Association (AMA) has outlined several areas surrounding ethics in the management of patient care, some of which include:

- With regard to organ transplantation, physicians must not consider age in the decision of who gets the organ. Priority must be given to the patient who has the strongest chance of obtaining long term benefit; a person's individual worth to society must not be considered.
- With regard to clinical research, physicians must fully inform any patient involved in research and must give that patients the highest of level of respect and care. The goal of any research program must be to obtain some type of scientific data.
- With regard to obstetrics, physicians must perform abortions within the boundaries of state and federal laws. If physicians do not wish to perform abortions, they must

Informational Tables

These appear throughout the text and summarize pertinent information for the reader. They provide students with visuals and comparisons to reinforce the lesson.

TABLE 4-2 Intentional Torts	
Assault	Threat of causing physical harm to another without their consent. *Example:* Telling a patient their temperature will be taken whether they want it to be or not after they refuse to allow it.
Battery	Act of harming another person without the person's consent. *Example:* Taking a patient's temperature against the patient's will.
Defamation of character	Intentional false or negative statements about a person that causes damages. *Example:* Telling patients they should not see the cardiologist across the street because that cardiologist has a drinking problem.
Duress	Act of coercing someone into an act. *Example:* Telling patients they must have a tetanus vaccine or they will develop a life-threatening infection. The patients feel they have no choice but to comply, even though they do not want the vaccine.
Fraud	Deceitful act made to conceal the truth. *Example:* Falsifying a patient's medical record to conceal a medical mistake.
Invasion of privacy	The intentional prying or intruding into another person's confidential information or matters. *Example:* Releasing a patient's medical records without the patient's consent or a court order.
Undue influence	Intentionally persuading people to do things they do not want to do. *Example:* Convincing single mothers that they should give their children up for adoption when they clearly do not want to.

PEARSON GENERAL HOSPITAL

COMPLETE ORIGINAL IN INK FOR HOSPITAL CHART
PATIENT MUST BE AWAKE, ALERT AND ORIENTED WHEN SIGNING
DATE: _____ TIME: _____ ☐ AM ☐ PM

I AUTHORIZE THE PERFORMANCE UPON_____
OF THE FOLLOWING OPERATION (state nature and extent):_____

TO BE PERFORMED UNDER THE DIRECTION OF DR. _____

1. I HAVE BEEN ADVISED THAT THERE IS A FAVORABLE LIKELIHOOD OF SUCCESS, BUT I UNDERSTAND THAT A COMPLETELY SUCCESSFUL OUTCOME MAY NOT BE ACHIEVABLE, AND THERE ARE NO GUARANTEES REGARDING THE OUTCOME. I ALSO UNDERSTAND THAT CERTAIN ADVERSE EVENTS COULD OCCUR AS A RESULT OF THE PERFORMANCE OF THE PROCEDURE OR TREATMENT, INCLUDING PAIN, INFECTION, LACERATION OR PUNCTURE OF INTERNAL ORGANS, BLEEDING, NERVE DAMAGE OR EVEN IN RARE CASES, DEATH. I UNDERSTAND THAT HOSPITALIZATION OR OTHER INSTITUTIONAL CARE, HOME CARE OR CARE BY HEALTH PROFESSIONALS MAY BE NEEDED FOLLOWING THE PROCEDURE OR TREATMENT, RELATED TO FULL RECOVERY, RECUPERATION OR CONVALESCENCE. I UNDERSTAND THE ALTERNATIVES TO THIS PROCEDURE, INCLUDING MY RIGHT TO REFUSE TO CONSENT TO IT, AND I NEVERTHELESS HAVE DECIDED TO CONSENT TO PERFORMANCE OF THE PROCEDURE OR TREATMENT.

2. I CONSENT TO THE PERFORMANCE OF OPERATIONS AND PROCEDURES IN ADDITION TO OR DIFFERENT FROM THOSE NOW CONTEMPLATED, WHETHER OR NOT ARISING FROM PRESENTLY UNFORESEEN CONDITIONS WHICH THE ABOVE NAMED DOCTOR OR HIS/HER ASSOCIATES OR ASSISTANTS MAY CONSIDER NECESSARY OR ADVISABLE IN THE COURSE OF THE OPERATION.

3. I CONSENT TO THE DISPOSAL BY HOSPITAL AUTHORITIES OF ANY TISSUES OR PARTS WHICH MAY BE REMOVED.

4. THE NATURE AND PURPOSE OF THE OPERATION/PROCEDURE, POSSIBLE ALTERNATIVE METHODS OF TREATMENT, THE RISK AND BENEF THE COURSE OF RECUPERATION HAVE BEEN FULLY EXPLAINED TO ME. NO GUARANTEE OR ASSURANCE HAS BEEN GIVEN BY ANYONE A THAT MAY BE OBTAINED.

5. I UNDERSTAND AND AGREE WITH THE ABOVE INFORMATION. I HAVE NO QUESTIONS WHICH HAVE NOT BEEN ANSWERED TO MY FULL SAT UNDERSTAND THAT I HAVE THE RIGHT TO ASK FOR FURTHER INFORMATION BEFORE SIGNING THIS CONSENT.

I have crossed out any paragraph above which does not apply or to which I do not give consent.

PATIENT SIGNATURE: _____   WITNESS SIGNATURE: _____
(OR PARENT OR GUARDIAN IF PATIENT IS UNDER 18 YEARS OF AGE)   *(OF PATIENT, PARENT OR GUARDIAN SIGNATURE)*

RELATIONSHIP: _____   WITNESS SIGNATURE: _____
                                 ☐ **TELEPHONE CONSENT** *(2ND WITNESS NEEDED FOR T*

Figure 4-2 ■ Sample informed consent form.

Color Photos and Illustrations

New color photos and illustrations appear throughout the book to support the text and reinforce key concepts.

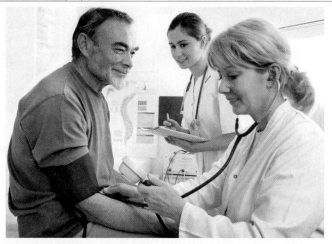

Figure 4-3 ■ The physician and medical assistant work closely together to maintain safe care for their patients.
Source: Shutterstock © Alexander Raths.

Chapter Summary

Each chapter summary is an excellent review of the chapter content.

REVIEW

Chapter Summary

- U.S. laws arise from varying sources to achieve varying legal purposes.
- Obtaining consent from patients is done both for the release of that patient's information to another source, as well as for consent to the performance of a procedure.
- Malpractice is a serious, wide-ranging issue in health care that the medical assistant can address both individually and as a member of the health care team.
- Tort reform is a concept that has been addressed in many states in the United States. Most legislation in this area is aimed at reducing the amount of money an injured victim may recover after a malpractice incident.
- Physicians have a number of public duties to perform to ensure patient safety and confidentiality are upheld.
- Both physicians and patients have duties they should uphold in the physician–patient relationship. Many of these are dictated by law, especially the physician's responsibilities.
- Contracts in health care encompass the consent for care and payment for services rendered.
- Medical assistants play a crucial role in patient confidentiality procedures.

- The Health Insurance Portability and Accountability Act (HIPAA) is a law that outlines how patient personal information is to be kept confidential.
- The Good Samaritan Act mandates that a person who provides emergency assistance while outside his normal job duties in the health care setting cannot be sued for additional injuries sustained by the victim.
- The various federal and state organizations driving current health care practices demand compliance from all members of the medical staff.
- Health care professionals must be vigilant about all relevant legislation, including the patients' bill of rights.
- Various advance directives exist to provide legal means for an individual to express her health care wishes in the event she cannot speak for herself.
- The patients' bill of rights is a list of rights patients have upon entering a particular health care facility.
- Various monitoring agencies such as The Joint Commission and OSHA provide rules and regulations that protect the safety of patients and employees in the health care setting.
- The Controlled Substances Act defines the ways in which controlled substances are to be monitored, recorded, and prescribed.

Chapter Review Questions

End-of-chapter questions are provided in Multiple-Choice, True/False, Short Answer, and Research formats, and help reinforce learning. The review questions measure the student's understanding of the material presented in the chapter. These tools are available for use by the student or by the instructor as an outcome assessment.

Practicum Application Experience

This feature places the student in a practicum site with a simulated situation the student might encounter. Critical thinking questions appear at the end of each brief scenario, and students must rely on the knowledge acquired in the chapter and on their own critical thinking skills to answer each question.

Resource Guide

This list provides additional information (organization contact information, Web sites, etc.) related to chapter content.

Chapter Review

Multiple Choice

1. *Res judicata* is Latin for:
   a. The physician is responsible
   b. The thing speaks for itself
   c. Let the master answer
   d. The thing has been decided
   e. There is a master–servant relationship in place
2. Which of the following is the threat of causing harm to another without their consent?
   a. Assault
   b. Battery
   c. Duress
   d. Invasion of privacy
   e. Coercion
3. Which of the following refers to the release of private information about another person without the person's consent?
   a. Assault
   b. Battery
   c. Duress
   d. Invasion of privacy
   e. Coercion
4. Which of the following refers to the actual physical touching of another person without the person's consent (includes physical abuse)?
   a. Assault
   b. Battery
   c. Duress
   d. Invasion of privacy
   e. Coercion
5. Which of the following is the act of coercing someone into an act?
   a. Assault
   b. Battery
   c. Duress
   d. Invasion of privacy
   e. Violation

True/False

T F 1. In most states, children under age 18 may receive medical attention for a sexually transmitted infection without parental consent.

T F 2. Patients win most medical malpractice cases.

T F 3. Patients may refuse treatment for any reason.

T F 4. Hospitals that receive federal funding, such as Medicare and Medicaid, are required to be Joint Commission certified.

T F 5. The statute of limitations for medical malpractice cases is the same in every state.

T F 6. Classes of felony crimes are the same in every state.

T F 7. The physician must report any vaccine injuries.

Short Answer

1. In addition to the examples provided in the text, what other type of persons would the medical office need to have an HIPAA Business Associate Agreement for?
2. What is the Good Samaritan Act?
3. What are the Four Ds of Negligence?
4. Differentiate "implied consent" from "expressed consent."
5. Explain what is meant by "informed consent."
6. Describe the steps the physician must take to legally terminate the physician–patient relationship.
7. Explain the function of the HIPAA Privacy Officer in the medical office.

Research

1. Are there caps on the medical malpractice awards allowed in your state? If so, what are they?
2. Search the Internet for a medical malpractice case. What were the specifics of the case?

Practicum Application Experience

Joe Rutigliano is a patient of Dr. Mallory's. As Joe is leaving the office after his appointment, he overhears Dr. Mallory and her medical assistant discussing his treatment plan in the hallway. He believes other patients also overhear their conversation, and he is upset. What should the medical assistant do?

Resource Guide

American Association of Medical Assistants
20 N. Wacker Dr., Suite 1575
Chicago, IL 60606
Phone: (312) 899-1500
Fax: (312) 899-1259
http://www.aama-ntl.org/

Health Care Providers Service Organization
159 E. County Line Road
Hatboro, PA 19040-1218
Phone: (800) 982-9491
Fax: (800) 739-8818
www.hpso.com

Public Citizen
1600 20th St. NW
Washington, DC. 20009
Phone: (202) 588-1000
www.citizen.org

Sorry Works
P.O. Box 531
Glen Carbon, IL 62034
Phone: (618) 559-8168
http://www.sorryworks.net

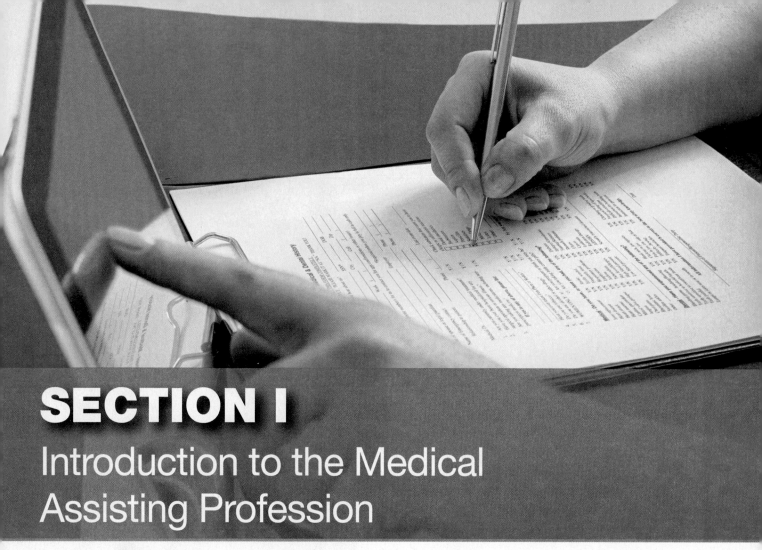

SECTION I
Introduction to the Medical Assisting Profession

My name is Harris Anderson, and I recently graduated from a medical assisting program with a focus on administrative medical assisting. During my education, practicum experience, and on-the-job training, I learned the importance of patient confidentiality and how it impacts all aspects of patient care.

As an administrative medical assistant now working in a large family medical practice, I am responsible for charting in the patient's electronic health record, calling patients, communicating with patients' relatives, faxing messages, and working with insurance companies. In performing these tasks, I must ensure that all patient health information is kept private and confidential in order to protect the physician and the patient's privacy. Understanding and complying with HIPAA privacy laws is an integral part of my duties as an administrative medical assistant.

1

The History of Medicine and Health Care

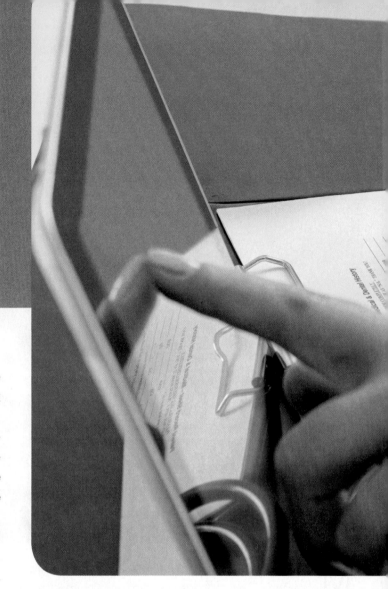

Case Study

Read the following case study and answer the critical thinking questions presented throughout the chapter.

Dr. Kenyon will be giving a presentation on the history of medicine to a local community group. She has asked her medical assistant to prepare some background materials for this event. Because Dr. Kenyon is a surgeon, she wants her medical assistant to find information about early medical practices, including how patients were anesthetized and operated on in early days. Dr. Kenyon asks her medical assistant to prepare an outline of the presentation, including tables and charts showing milestones in the history of medicine.

Objectives

After completing this chapter, you should be able to:

1.1 Define and spell the key terminology in this chapter.

1.2 Identify and discuss early medical practices.

1.3 Describe the major turning points of modern medicine.

1.4 List and describe the role of important organizations in medical history.

1.5 Identify important women in health care and discuss their contributions to medicine.

1.6 Discuss advances in medical care today.

1.7 Describe the history of the medical assisting profession.

Key Terminology

American Association of Medical Assistants (AAMA)— national-level professional association for medical assistants

American Red Cross—humanitarian organization that provides emergency assistance

anatomy—study of the structure and organization of animals and plants

anesthesia—general or local loss of sensation induced by interventions or drugs to permit the performance of an otherwise painful procedure

antisepsis—destruction of the microorganisms that produce sepsis or septic disease

astrology—study of how the planets and stars influence events and the lives and behaviors of individuals

autopsy—examination of a body after death to determine the cause of death

caduceus—emblem of the medical profession

chiropractic—a system of complementary therapy that corrects misalignments of the joints, especially those of the spinal column

chloroform—early method of general anesthesia used to render a patient unconscious

ether—anesthetic used in the mid-19th century to alleviate pain during surgical procedures

evidence-based medicine—the practice of integrating the best, current clinical evidence from systematic research with individual clinical expertise

faith healer—practitioner who uses prayer or faith rather than medicine to heal patients

Hippocrates—an ancient Greek physician who is known as the "Father of Medicine"; considered one of the most outstanding figures in the history of medicine

Human Genome Project—a scientific project designed to study and identify all human genes

pharmaceuticals—drugs, medicines, and chemical compounds

physiology—study of the mechanical, physical, and biochemical functions of living organisms

public health—all health services designed to improve and protect community health

radiocarbon dating—a radiometric dating procedure that measures a substance's decay of carbon to determine its age

shaman—a religious or spiritual figure that acts as an intermediary between the natural and supernatural worlds; someone who is believed to use magic to cure illness

ultrasound—method of using sound waves to create three-dimensional images for diagnostic or therapeutic purposes

Abbreviations

AAMA—American Association for Medical Assistants

AHA—American Hospital Association

AMA—American Medical Association

CT—computed tomography

DNA—deoxyribonucleic acid

ECG—electrocardiograph

FAA—Federal Aviation Administration

JAMA—Journal of the American Medical Association

MRI—magnetic resonance imaging

TB—tuberculosis

WHO—World Health Organization

Introduction

Medicine has been practiced for a long time, but many of its advancements, including X-rays, medications, and anesthesia, are relatively new. Until the mid- to late 1800s, surgery was performed without anesthesia, and penicillin was not commonly used until the 1940s. Today, it would be hard to imagine health care without the advancements of the past century alone. Many of today's vaccinations were discovered in the 20th century, as were nearly all currently prescribed medications.

The profession of medical assisting has seen many advances since its introduction to the medical professions. Medical assistants were once trained on the job; however, today most are trained in accredited medical assisting programs. As the scope of practice for medical assistants expands, so will the need for continuing education in the field.

The Earliest Medical Practices

The history of medical treatment is rooted in ancient times. Cave paintings discovered in the Lascaux caves in France depict people using plants and herbs to treat illness. Using **radiocarbon dating**, these paintings have been estimated to date from 13,000 to 25,000 B.C. Even the emblem of the medical profession, the **caduceus**, derives from ancient times. This emblem, which depicts two snakes wrapped around a healing

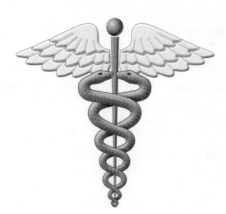

Figure 1-1 ■ The caduceus is the emblem of the medical profession.

staff (**Figure 1-1** ■), reflects the early Greeks' use of nonpoisonous snakes to treat patients' wounds.

Ancient practitioners used nonpoisonous snakes and the roots, leaves, and flowers of plants to treat patients, but early medical treatments were often painful and sometimes fatal. In fact, the earliest medical treatments are thought to have killed patients nearly as often as diseases. Back then, most cultures believed demons or gods caused diseases and illnesses. As a result, most early medical practitioners were **faith healers** or **shamans** who were well versed in the superstitions of the day (**Figure 1-2** ■).

Critical Thinking Question 1-1

Referring back to the case study presented at the beginning of this chapter, what are the historical roots of modern medicine? How would Dr. Kenyon's medical assistant find additional information about what to include in this part of the presentation?

Early Egyptian Medicine

As far back as 3000 B.C., there is evidence that the Egyptians provided medical care for such conditions as tuberculosis and pneumonia. Other records suggest that they were performing surgery as well. Fossils from this era indicate that an Egyptian patient underwent brain surgery and survived. The patient's skull bones had healed long before the patient died.

A practitioner named Imhotep, who lived from 2667 to 2648 B.C., is credited as founding Egyptian medicine in the Third Dynasty (**Figure 1-3** ■). He authored some of the original material on which the world's earliest known medical document, the *Edwin Smith Papyrus*, is based. Written around 1600 B.C., the *Papyrus* details the known cures, examination findings, and prognoses of the time and is thought to be a compilation of multiple authors.

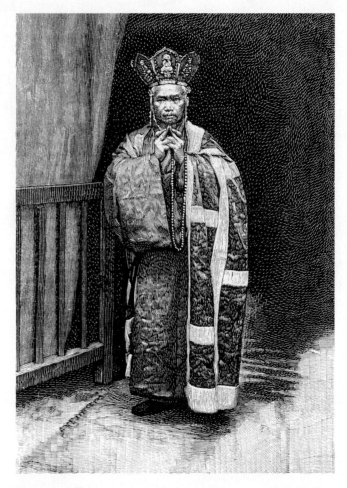

Figure 1-2 ■ Most early medical practitioners were faith healers or shamans.
Source: Fotolia/Erica Guilane-Nachez.

Early Chinese Medicine

Classical Chinese medicine has been traced as far back as 2700 B.C. Much of it reflects the culture's beliefs that everything, including humans, is interconnected and that optimal health comes from living harmoniously in the world. Classical Chinese practitioners believed the following five methods helped patients achieve good health:

1. Cure the patient's spirit.
2. Nourish the patient's body.
3. Give medications as needed.
4. Treat the entire body, not just the illness.
5. Use acupuncture.

The Chinese also developed a list of the medical uses for many plants and herbs.

In the 1950s, the Chinese government commissioned 10 Western physicians to add scientific theory to classical Chinese medicine. The result, called traditional Chinese medicine, is taught in Chinese medical schools today. Today, traditional Chinese medicine is considered a broad range of medical practices that include various forms of herbal medicine. Approximately

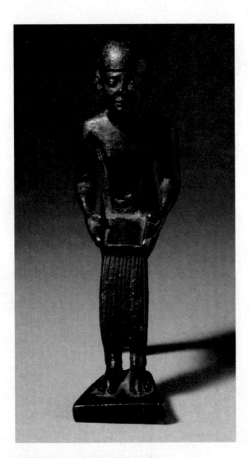

Figure 1-3 ■ Imhotep (332–330 B.C.)
Source: Ancient Art & Architecture/DanitaDelimont.com.

I swear by Apollo the physician, and Asclepius, and Hygieia and Panacea and all the gods and goddesses as my witnesses, that, according to my ability and judgement, I will keep this Oath and this contract:

To hold him who taught me this art equally dear to me as my parents, to be a partner in life with him, and to fulfill his needs when required; to look upon his offspring as equals to my own siblings, and to teach them this art, if they shall wish to learn it, without fee or contract; and that by the set rules, lectures, and every other mode of instruction, I will impart a knowledge of the art to my own sons, and those of my teachers, and to students bound by this contract and having sworn this Oath to the law of medicine, but to no others.

I will use those dietary regimens which will benefit my patients according to my greatest ability and judgement, and I will do no harm or injustice to them.

I will not give a lethal drug to anyone if I am asked, nor will I advise such a plan; and similarly I will not give a woman a pessary to cause an abortion.

Figure 1-4 ■ The Hippocratic Oath.
Source: http://www.nlm.nih.gov/hmd/greek/greek_oath.html. Translated by Michael North, National Library of Medicine, 2002.

13,000 medicinals are used in China; over 100,000 medicinal recipes have been recorded in China's ancient literature.

Early Native American Medicine

Native Americans were among the earliest and most effective medical practitioners. Native American healers, whose practices date as far back as 40,000 years in the United States, believed they must always honor the patient's wishes and never force treatment. Though medical treatments varied among the Native American tribes, suicide was considered one of the highest forms of bravery. The elderly and sick of many tribes traditionally committed suicide during periods of famine.

When treatment was an option, some Native American tribes used herbs and such comfort measures as natural pain relievers. Patients who recovered were often thought to have supernatural powers. Because tribes lacked written language at the time, early Native American healers used oral means to pass their medical knowledge to younger tribe members.

The Father of Medicine

Hippocrates, known as the "Father of Medicine," helped shift medical care from a religious and superstitious practice to a

scientific one by basing his practice of medicine on the belief that illness was the result of a physical condition. He believed that the body, rather than just one ailment, should be treated, and he was the first physician to note that some individuals recovered faster from their illnesses than others. Hippocrates, who lived from 460 B.C. to 377 B.C., founded a medical school on the island of Cos, Greece, where he taught his ideas. Around the fourth century B.C. he wrote *Ancient Medicine*, a book that described his medical theories, as well as the Hippocratic Oath, which is physicians' promise to treat their patients to the best of their abilities (**Figure 1-4** ■). Contemporary medical schools still recite the Hippocratic Oath at graduation.

Critical Thinking Question 1-2

Why was Hippocrates called "The Father of Medicine"? Referring to the case study at the beginning of this chapter, why would Dr. Kenyon want to include information about this historical figure in her presentation?

Early European Medicine

The Greek physician Galen, who lived from 129 to 200 C.E. (**Figure 1-5** ■), is credited with advancing Hippocrates's work. As was common practice at the time, Galen advocated bloodletting as a form of treatment. This treatment consisted of cutting into the patient's veins and allowing the patient to bleed. The belief was that patients might be ill because they had too

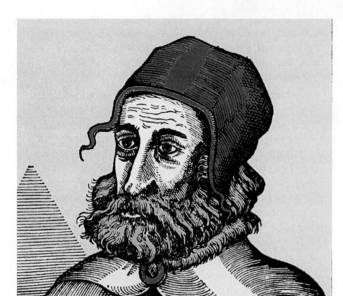

Figure 1-5 ■ Galen (129–200 C.E.)
Source: Photo Researchers, Inc./Sheila Terry.

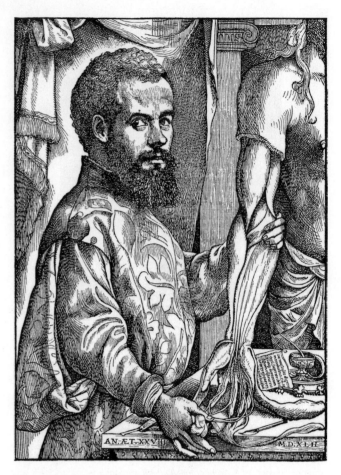

Figure 1-6 ■ Andreas Vesalius (1514–1564).
Source: Dorling Kindersley.

much blood in their systems. Galen was the first physician to record a patient's pulse, although he failed to realize the pulse was related to the heart's action. He was also the first to document many parts of the human body. Since human **autopsies** were illegal during Galen's time, many of his findings were inaccurate because he studied dead animals.

In addition to studying deceased animals, Galen experimented with live ones. He once publicly dissected a living pig to show that severing the laryngeal nerve stopped the pig from squealing. In other public experiments, Galen tied the ureters of living animals to show that urine comes from the kidneys, and he severed spinal cords to cause paralysis. Galen also performed many operations, including cataract surgeries, on living human patients. To remove a cataract, he inserted a needle into the eye behind the lens and pulled back slightly.

Although Galen died in 200 C.E., his work was considered the authority on **anatomy** and **physiology** until the 16th century, when Andreas Vesalius corrected many of Galen's anatomy errors and wrote the first roughly correct anatomy textbook. Vesalius fared better than Galen because Vesalius was able to perform autopsies on human bodies (the ban was lifted during Vesalius's time). He autopsied the bodies of executed criminals and commissioned artists to create drawings for his textbook (**Figure 1-6** ■).

In the first century, a Roman named Varro suggested that all disease was caused by tiny animals. His theory was that these tiny animals were carried through the air and entered the body through the mouth and nose. With no microscopes available at that time, Varro's theory could not be tested.

During the first two centuries, the Romans evolved into skilled engineers, creating the first public health system. After noticing that the citizens who lived in close proximity to swamps were more often victims of malaria than those people who did not live near the swamps, the Romans drained the swamps. They did not, however, realize that it was the mosquitoes in the swamps that carried malaria. With an understanding that cleanliness was one way to discourage disease, the Romans built aqueducts to bring clean water into the towns. In order to keep sewage from mixing with the water from the aqueducts, the Romans built public lavatories with streams running beneath to carry the sewage away.

In the fourth century, the western half of the Roman Empire was invaded and much of the medical and surgical skill was lost. The Roman system of public health was dissolved, and towns and streets were once again filled with filth and the ensuing disease. The eastern half of the Roman Empire continued to thrive and the medical skills were passed on to the Muslims by the ninth century.

In the ninth century, an Arabic physician was the first to distinguish between smallpox and measles. The Arabic physician Ibn-Sina wrote many books in the ninth century; these books were translated into Latin and were the dominant source of medical information in Europe for several centuries. Muslims established many hospitals in the ninth and tenth centuries. It was a Muslim physician who first wrote about hemophilia and invented a system for purifying substances via distillation.

In the 11th century, the Italians began building schools of medicine. By the 13th century, schools of medicine were formed in several locations throughout Europe. Because the average person at this time could not afford to pay to see a physician, folk remedies were still more widely sought than Western medicine.

During the Middle Ages, doctors believed in the curative practices of bloodletting. It was believed that regular bleeding maintained good health, so doctors would cut the patients and allow them to bleed into a bowl. Doctors at this time also believed in the curative powers of purging the system via laxatives. Patients were regularly given enemas via a greased tube attached to a pig's bladder. Doctors during this era also believed that the urine of the patient was important to examine in order to determine the need for medicines. The color, smell, and taste of the patient's urine all pointed to various treatments prescribed by the attending doctor.

During the Middle Ages, much of the spiritual world was still intertwined with medical practice. **Astrology** was an important part of medical practice of this time. Doctors believed that people born under certain zodiacal signs were more likely to be stricken with illness than those born under other, more favorable, signs. During this time, the church ran the only hospitals. In many outlying towns, monks and nuns provided for the sick and injured.

In the 13th century, the barber-surgeon became very popular throughout Europe. Individuals could see this person, either male or female, for a haircut, to have teeth pulled, or for simple operations such as amputations or the setting of broken bones. The red and white pole hanging outside the barber-surgeon's shop indicated to illiterate people the trade that was practiced within. The colors red and white symbolized blood and bandages.

Syphilis was common during the 16th and 17th centuries. The standard treatment consisted of mercury administered via a syringe into the urethra. Syringes were also used to irrigate wounds with wine during this time.

The Turning Points of Modern Medicine

Medical practice changed dramatically in the 18th century. Chemistry knowledge advanced, and people began to believe that sickness and bacteria, rather than superstitions and religious beliefs, caused disease. A number of tools and discoveries helped advance medical study.

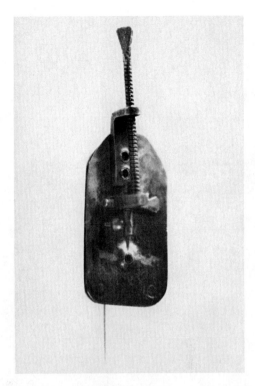

Figure 1-7 ■ Anton Van Leeuwenhoek's prototype microscope. *Source:* © Bettmann/CORBIS.

Medical Discoveries

A Dutch lens maker named Anton van Leeuwenhoek helped advance medical understanding by introducing the microscope in 1674 (**Figure 1-7** ■). German physicist Daniel Fahrenheit invented the mercury thermometer in 1714.

Surgeon John Hunter, who lived from 1728 to 1793, developed many of the surgical techniques that are still used today. In 1796, English physician Edward Jenner discovered the smallpox vaccine. This discovery was made when he noticed that milkmaids who contracted cowpox were immune from contracting smallpox. Jenner's theory was that the body built up a resistance to the smallpox virus after fighting off the cowpox virus. He found that injecting patients with small amounts of material from smallpox blisters gave those patients immunity from the disease (**Figure 1-8** ■).

Jenner's smallpox discovery shifted the focus of medicine from cures to prevention. **Public health** and nutrition improvements, as well as pivotal medical discoveries that continued into the 19th century, caused the decline of many diseases of the time. In 1816, French physician René Laënnec invented the stethoscope (**Figure 1-9** ■). At the time, Laënnec was well known for extensively researching tuberculosis (**TB**) and for being the first physician to recognize cirrhosis of the liver as a disease.

American physician and pharmacist Crawford W. Long was the first to employ modern **anesthesia** in 1842 when he used an **ether**-based anesthesia to remove a tumor from a patient's neck (**Figure 1-10** ■). Long went on to use his

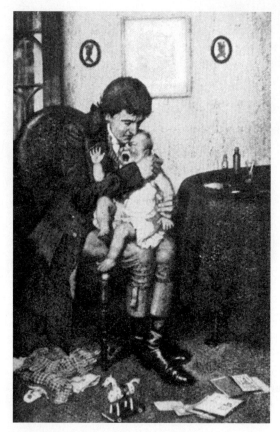

Figure 1-8 ■ Dr. Edward Jenner administering vaccination against smallpox (to his son), 1789.
Source: Getty/Photolibrary/Peter Arnold, Inc.

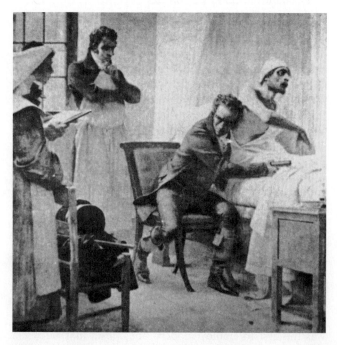

Figure 1-9 ■ René Laënnec using a stethoscope.
Source: Photo Researchers, Inc./SPL.

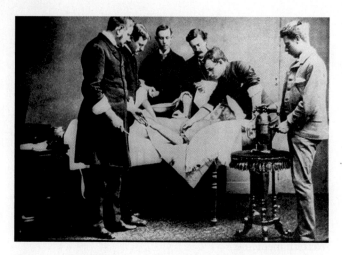

Figure 1-10 ■ A patient receives anesthesia during surgery.
Source: Photo Researchers. Inc./Science Photo Library.

anesthesia technique in amputations and childbirth events. In 1846, American dentist William Morton also used an ether-based anesthesia on a patient before removing a neck tumor. Morton tried to keep his compound secret, however, and later had it patented. Despite Morton's efforts, the compound's ingredients were quickly identified, and anesthesia use spread throughout Europe by the end of 1846.

Because ether had many side effects, **chloroform** replaced it as an anesthetic agent in 1853. Chloroform also had drawbacks, however: many patients died when untrained practitioners used it improperly. Therefore, physicians reverted to the use of ether to anesthetize patients. The first effective topical anesthetic was used in 1859 for an ophthalmic surgery. The substance, a form of cocaine, replaced salt and ice for numbing a small area.

In 1853, Scottish physician Alexander Wood invented the hypodermic needle, which allowed physicians to inject and extract liquids into and from patients' bodies. In 1903, Willem Einthoven, a physician in the Netherlands, invented the electrocardiograph (**ECG**) (**Figure 1-11** ■). This invention enabled physicians to record the electrical activity of a patient's heart.

Critical Thinking Question 1-3

Referring to the case study at the beginning of the chapter, what information would Dr. Kenyon want to include in her presentation about why chloroform replaced ether in anesthesia use?

The Beginning of Hand Washing in Health Care

In 1847, Hungarian physician Ignaz Semmelweiss (**Figure 1-12** ■) noticed a dramatic difference in the death rate of new mothers from childbed fever when the women delivered

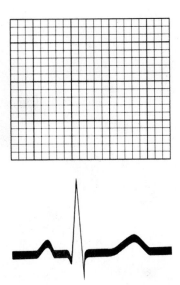

Figure 1-11 ■ An ECG strip.

Source: DK Images/Photographer: Tony Graham.

their babies at home with the help of midwives rather than in hospitals with surgeons. Childbed fever was a condition caused by a severe vaginal or uterine infection. Women who delivered at home were far more likely to survive. Because he suspected poor hospital hygiene as the cause, Dr. Semmelweiss began an experiment that required physicians to wash their hands before treating women in childbirth. At the time, physicians failed to wash their hands between patients, often attending to women in childbirth after working with recently deceased patients. The data from Semmelweiss's experiment showed that hand washing markedly reduced the death rate of women who delivered in hospitals.

Antisepsis Use in Health Care

Despite his landmark discovery, Semmelweiss received little respect from his colleagues. As a result, hand washing by doctors as they moved between patients began to enjoy widespread use in hospitals only after British surgeon Joseph Lister discovered in 1867 that an **antiseptic** on wounds helped prevent infection. Lister based his study of **antisepsis** on the discoveries of French biologist Louis Pasteur.

While Pasteur is best known for inventing pasteurization in 1862, a process that uses heat to destroy bacteria, he also worked to prevent anthrax transmission and discovered the vaccine for rabies in 1885. Pasteur's pasteurization findings led to the use of heat in surgical-instrument sterilization. For all his work, Pasteur earned the title "Father of Preventive Medicine."

Figure 1-13 ■ shows a late 19th century sterilization device.

Critical Thinking Question 1-4

Refer to the case study at the beginning of the chapter. What might Dr. Kenyon say about Dr. Semmelweiss and why his colleagues were skeptical of the benefits of hand washing?

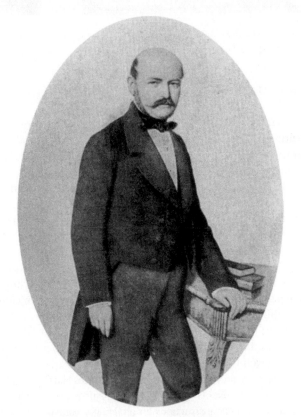

Figure 1-12 ■ Ignaz Semmelweiss (1818–1865).

Source: The Bridgeman Art Library International/Wenck, (20th Century).

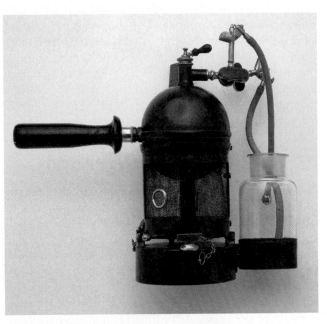

Figure 1-13 ■ Late 19th century sterilization device.

Source: DK Images/Photographer: Mike King.

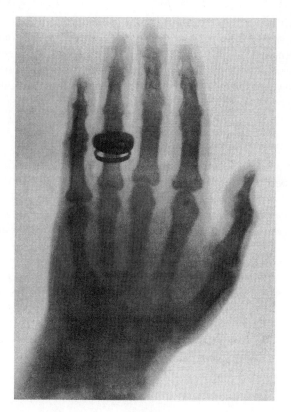

Figure 1-14 ■ X-ray image of Roentgen's wife's hand, January 1896.

Source: International Museum of Surgical Science/Brian Warling.

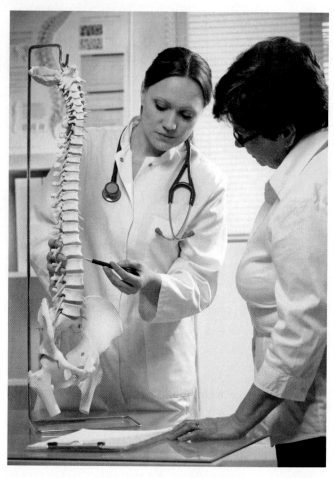

Figure 1-15 ■ A chiropractor shows a model spine to a patient.

Source: Fotolia/© Alexander Raths.

The Medical Value of X-rays

Wilhelm Roentgen revolutionized medical diagnosis in 1895 when he discovered X-rays while experimenting with vacuum tubes. His first X-ray image was of his wife's hand (**Figure 1-14** ■). Roentgen called the radiation rays he used "X" to indicate that they were unknown, but many of his colleagues called them Roentgen rays, a name that is still used in many languages today. In 1901, Roentgen received the Nobel Prize in Physics for his discovery.

Chiropractic Practices in Medicine

In 1895, a man named D. D. Palmer started **chiropractic** practices when he found he could restore a man's hearing by correcting the man's spinal misalignment. Chiropractic is the study of disorders of the musculoskeletal system and how a misalignment in that system can cause a host of problems for the patient. Chiropractors practice holistic medicine; they treat the patient without using medicines. Chiropractors are trained to recognize a variety of ailments, to prescribe exercises and nutritional therapy, and to recommend herbal supplements as part of a patient's treatment plan (**Figure 1-15** ■).

Medicine in the 20th Century

For many reasons, the 20th century is a notable era in medical treatment. Immunizations, a powerful weapon in disease prevention, are just one important 20th-century advancement. Table 1-1 reviews the history of vaccines.

In 1901, biologist and physician Karl Landsteiner contributed to the development of modern medicine by creating the contemporary system of blood-group classification. For his discovery, Landsteiner won the Nobel Prize in Physiology in 1930.

In 1928, Scottish scientist Alexander Fleming noticed circles of nongrowth around certain areas of mold in petri dishes. He believed the mold was releasing a substance that was inhibiting bacterial growth, and he named that substance penicillin. Penicillin was first used successfully in patient treatment in 1930 and came into popular use during World War II, when it was used to save the lives and limbs of wounded soldiers. Fleming won the Nobel Prize in 1945 for his discovery.

Scientists James Dewey Watson and Frances Harry Compton Crick also won a Nobel Prize. In 1953, the pair became the first to identify the genetic instructions for all living organisms: deoxyribonucleic acid (**DNA**). Their groundbreaking work became the foundation for today's medical research (**Figure 1-16** ■).

TABLE 1-1 Vaccine History

Vaccine	Year
Diphtheria	1923
Pertussis	1926
Tuberculosis	1927
Tetanus	1927
Yellow fever	1935
Typhus	1937
Influenza	1945
Rabies	1946
Polio (Salk)	1952
Anthrax	1954
Polio (oral)	1962
Measles	1964
Mumps	1967
Rubella	1970
Chicken pox	1974
Swine flu	1976
Pneumonia	1977
Meningitis	1978
Hepatitis B	1981
Haemophilus influenzae type B (HiB)	1985
Hepatitis A	1992
Lyme disease	1998
Rotavirus	1998
Human papillomavirus	2006
Shingles	2006
Nasal influenza mist	2007
H1N1 influenza	2009
Tdap recommended for adults	2011

Source: Centers for Disease Control and Prevention: www.cdc.gov.

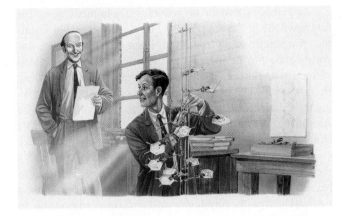

Figure 1-16 ■ Scientists Watson and Crick working on their DNA model.
Source: DK Images/Peter Dennis.

first artificial heart was implanted in patient Barney Clark. Clark survived for 112 days.

In 1990, the U.S. Department of Energy's Health and Environmental Research Program launched the **Human Genome Project**, an initiative aimed at identifying all the genes in human DNA. As the project progressed, several companies began using its research to determine if people had predispositions to such conditions as cancer, blood-clotting disorders, cystic fibrosis, and liver disease. Companies also began researching medicines that could be linked to a person's genetic makeup.

The Human Genome Project reached its goal in 2003, and its findings were made available to scientists worldwide. Scientists hope to use this information to learn how diseases work from the molecular level and thereby find cures for many diseases (**Figure 1-17** ■).

Other critical medical inventions and discoveries followed. For example, John Hopps invented the first heart pacemaker in 1950, though this early device was large and painful and was mounted externally. Smaller external pacemakers were invented throughout the 1950s, but they relied on external electrodes and had to be plugged into outlets. The first pacemaker was implanted into a patient in 1958 in Sweden, but it lasted only three hours. A second one was implanted into the same patient and lasted two days. That patient lived until 2001, having received 22 pacemakers in his lifetime.

The 1950s continued to be a decade of medical advances. During that time, the first open-heart surgery was performed successfully, the first heart–lung machine was used in surgery, and the first kidney was transplanted into a patient. A heart was first transplanted into a human by Dr. Christiaan Barnard in South Africa in 1967.

The 1970s ushered in the computed tomography (**CT**) scan and the advent of **ultrasound** technology. In 1982, the

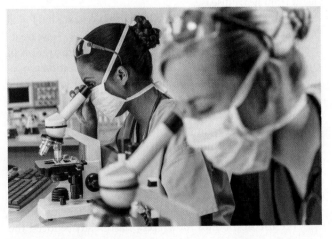

Figure 1-17 ■ Scientists use information from the Human Genome Project to learn how diseases work and to find cures for many diseases.
Source: Fotolia/© Darren Baker.

Scientists believe the biggest advances in medicine in the future will be in the area of prevention of disease. For example, using information from the Human Genome Project, scientists expect to develop a genetic test for a gene associated with prostate cancer. Scientists have already developed a drug that greatly lowers the risk of this type of cancer. By identifying those individuals who are at risk, this medication could be administered, and the hope is that prostate cancer could be eliminated.

Information technology has created advancements in medical care over the past decade. Where physicians used to have to go to a library to research medical conditions or use a medical textbook, physicians today have ready access to numerous electronic sources where this information can be accessed immediately. With information technology, physicians can quickly look up a medication, determine if the patient's insurance carrier will pay for that medication, discover if the patient is on any medications that may counteract with the needed prescription, and check the proper dosage. This technology has dramatically reduced the amount of time physicians spend looking up this information in other formats and has allowed physicians to quickly access the newest information on diseases, treatments, and medications.

Critical Thinking Question 1-5

Referring to the case study at the beginning of the chapter, what might Dr. Kenyon include in her presentation about how research from the Human Genome Project improves the delivery of contemporary health care?

With the passage of some sort of smoking ban in 27 states, the Institute of Medicine reports that the public smoking bans have lessened the amount of exposure to secondhand smoke, which has contributed to a reduction in heart attacks and death from heart disease.

The American Heart Association set a decade-long goal in 2000 to reduce coronary heart disease by 25%. New treatment preventions, such as the immediate administration of clot-busting drugs and quick access to a catheterization procedure, have reduced the number of deaths due to coronary heart disease by 40% since 2000, far overachieving the original goal set by the American Heart Association.

Antiretroviral treatments for viruses such as acquired immune deficiency syndrome (AIDS) have dramatically lengthened the life span of persons diagnosed with this illness. Whereas a 20-year-old diagnosed with AIDS in 1996 would have an expected life span of 3 to 5 years, today that patient has an expected life span of 69 years of age, with proper medications.

The use of robotics for surgery has greatly reduced the complications, scarring, and time away from work for patients needing surgical procedures. In the late 1990s, a patient having a kidney removed would incur a 10-inch scar. Using robotics, the same surgery can now be performed with a single incision through the patient's navel.

Important Organizations in Medical History

Throughout the years, a number of entities have been formed to advance various facets of the medical profession.

The History of American Hospitals

Early American hospitals bore little resemblance to the hospitals of today, in large part because people preferred to receive medical care in their own homes in the country's early days.

Benjamin Franklin built the first American hospital in Philadelphia in 1751. By 1910, that hospital and others like it had begun to run like today's scientific institutions. They used antiseptics, focused on cleanliness, and relieved pain with medications. In 1921, National Hospital Day was first celebrated on May 12, the birthday of famous nurse Florence Nightingale (see the following section on important female figures in medicine). National Hospital Day continues to be recognized during the week of Nightingale's birth every year.

According to the American Hospital Association (**AHA**), by 2005 the United States had 5,756 hospitals with staffed beds totaling near 1 million. Hospitals today fall into the four following categories:

1. **General or community**—Range from 10 beds to several hundred. Hospitals in this category, found in nearly every U.S. community, account for nearly 5,000 of the hospitals documented by the AHA in 2005.
2. **Teaching**—Found near university medical schools and have medical students, interns, and residents treating patients under the supervision of licensed physicians. In general, these facilities offer the same services as general hospitals (see preceding).
3. **Specialty**—Offer care to a certain patient type (e.g., children, burn victims, psychiatric patients, or patients undergoing drug or alcohol rehabilitation).
4. **Research**—Treat patients while researching certain disease types. Examples of these hospitals include cancer research facilities and Shriners hospitals that care for children with spinal cord injuries, cleft palate, burns, or orthopedic conditions.

Note: Some hospitals are a combination of hospital types. For example, a teaching hospital may also be a research hospital.

The History of the American Medical Association

The American Medical Association (**AMA**) was founded in 1847 at the University of Pennsylvania with the goals of "scientific advancement, standards for medical education, launching a program of medical ethics, and improved public health" (www.ama-assn.org). It began organizing state and local associations in 1901, and its first meeting included 250 delegates from 28 states. Physician membership in the group went from 8,000 in 1900 to over 70,000 by 1910. At that point, the AMA counted fully half of licensed U.S. physicians among its membership.

The growth of the AMA marked the beginning of organized medicine. Table 1-2 lists AMA milestones.

TABLE 1-2 AMA Milestones

Year	Event
1847	The organization is founded.
1848	Makes dangers of "secretive remedies" the focus of education to the public.
1858	Establishes Committee of Ethics.
1873	Sets up AMA Judicial Council.
1883	Launches *Journal of the American Medical Association* (**JAMA**).
1884	Supports experimentation on animals.
1897	Incorporates the organization.
1898	Starts Committee on Scientific Research to provide medical research grants.
1899	Sets up Committee on National Legislation to represent group's interests in U.S. government.
1905	Launches Council on Pharmacy and Chemistry to set drug manufacturing and advertising standards.
1912	Establishes Federation of State Medical Boards to deem group's rating of medical schools authoritative.
1948	Hires public relations firm to defeat government-run universal health care coverage.
1960	States that a blood alcohol level of 0.1% should be evidence of alcohol intoxication.
1970	Encourages the Federal Aviation Administration (**FAA**) to require all airlines to separate nonsmokers and smokers.
1974	Makes recommendations to ensure adequate protection of individuals used in human medical experimentation.
1982	Urges each state medical society to support laws to raise the legal drinking age to 21.
1988	Creates the Office of HIV/AIDS.
1995	Starts a campaign for liability reform.
2000	Supports Patients' Bill of Rights legislation in Congress.
2001	Provides a list of 3,500 volunteer physicians to aid in treatment of patients after September 11 terrorist attacks.
2005	Drives the successful effort to pass the Patient Safety and Quality Improvement Act.
2009	Launches a Facebook and Twitter presence for social media.
2010	Supports the passage of the Patient Protection and Affordable Care Act.
2011	Launches Weigh What Matters program to combat obesity.

Source: American Medical Association: www.ama-assn.org.

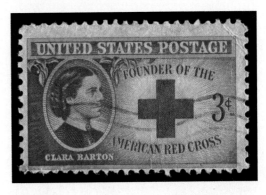

Figure 1-18 ■ As shown on this commemorative postage stamp, Clara Burton, founder of the American Red Cross. *Source: Fotolia/© rook76.*

The Start of the American Red Cross

Clara Barton, born in 1821, is one of the most honored women in American history (**Figure 1-18** ■). Barton was a teacher, nurse, and humanitarian. She served as a nurse during the Civil War, and later, while visiting Europe, worked with a relief organization known as the International Red Cross. When she returned home, she focused on educating the public and lobbied for an American branch of this organization. On May 21, 1881, Clara Barton formed and served as president of the **American Red Cross**, now one of the largest humanitarian organizations in the world. Local chapters were later formed throughout the country to help citizens during natural disasters. In 1882, the United States joined the International Red Cross.

During her life, Barton received the Iron Cross, the Cross of Imperial Russia, and the International Red Cross Medal. In 1904, at age 83, Barton founded the National First Aid Society.

The World Health Organization (WHO)

In 1945, when diplomats met to form the United Nations, one of the items they discussed was the setting up of a global health organization. The World Health Organization (**WHO**) was launched on April 17, 1948, a date celebrated today as World Health Day.

The WHO is the world's leading health organization and is responsible for providing leadership on many global health issues. The policies and programs of the World Health Organization impact international public health. Some of the stated goals of the WHO are to shape the health research agenda, set the norms and standards for health issues worldwide, articulate evidence-based policy options, provide technical support to countries, and monitor and assess health trends around the globe.

Important Women in Health Care

Women like Clara Barton have featured prominently in medical history throughout the years.

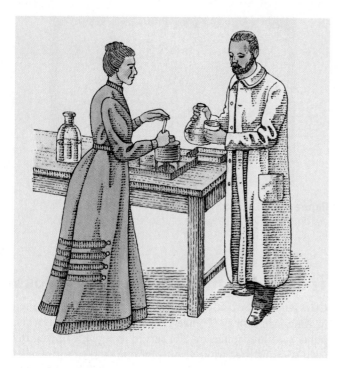

Figure 1-19 ■ Marie Curie (1864–1934), Polish-born French physicist, and her husband at work in the laboratory.
Source: DK Images/Rodney Shackell.

The Work of Marie Curie

Born in Warsaw, Poland, in 1867, Marie Curie was a physicist famous for her work on radioactivity. She made history when she became the first female instructor at the Sorbonne in France, and, in 1903, the first woman in France to complete her doctorate. Curie was the first person to win two Nobel Prizes in two different fields, physics and chemistry, and to this day she remains the only woman to have done so.

Marie Curie and her scientist husband, Pierre Curie, were honored for their work on radioactivity and their discoveries of the radioactive elements polonium and radium (**Figure 1-19** ■). After her husband's death, she continued her work in radioactivity. When World War I broke out in 1914, Curie advocated the use of X-ray machines in the field, and after the war, she used her notoriety to advance her research and raise money to establish a radium research facility in Warsaw.

Curie's work with radium eventually caused her death from radiation poisoning in 1934.

The Role of Florence Nightingale

Born in Florence, Italy, in 1820, Florence Nightingale is known as the founder of nursing. In the 1850s, nursing had a poor reputation and was not a respected profession. Nurses followed armies around, providing care and cooking meals. During the Crimean War, Nightingale worked with a team of nurses to improve unsanitary conditions at a British base hospital; their work reduced the death count by two-thirds. Nightingale's writings influenced worldwide health care

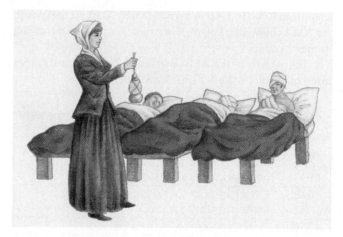

Figure 1-20 ■ Florence Nightingale with patients.
Source: DK Images/Peter Visscher.

reform; she helped advance the care of the poor, advocating improved medical care and commitment to the nursing profession (**Figure 1-20** ■). In 1860, she opened the St. Thomas' Hospital and the Nightingale Training School for Nurses. The school of nursing is still training nurses today.

The Contributions of the Blackwell Sisters

In 1869, Nightingale opened the first women's medical school with Elizabeth Blackwell, the first woman in the United States to practice medicine with a degree. Given prejudices against women at the time, Blackwell herself had to apply to several medical schools before she was finally accepted by Geneva College in New York. She graduated at the top of her class. Although she was originally barred from practice in most hospitals because of her gender, Blackwell founded her own hospital in 1857, the New York Infirmary for Indigent Women and Children.

Blackwell's sister, Emily, was the third woman to earn a medical degree in the United States. The sisters worked together at the New York Infirmary for Indigent Women and Children for over 40 years. In 1868, they founded the Women's Medical College in New York. By 1899, the college had graduated nearly 400 women doctors.

In 1970, 8 percent of all U.S. physicians were women. By 1980, that number had exceeded 12 percent. As of 2003, the number of applicants to medical school was just over 50 percent female. Since then, that percentage has declined, and, as of 2012, just over 47 percent of applicants to medical school are women.

Critical Thinking Question 1-6

Refer to the case study presented at the beginning of the chapter. What could Dr. Kenyon comment on about why the number of women attending medical school in the United States has increased so dramatically since 1970?

Medical Care Today

From the 1950s to the 1980s, medical care advanced rapidly with the discovery of numerous **pharmaceuticals**, **CT** scans, and magnetic resonance imaging (**MRI**).

Health care will likely continue to yield critical discoveries. Among the promising areas of research are stem cell research, transplants, and chemistry in the area of pharmacology. However, ongoing challenges remain. From 1950 to 1960, the cost of a hospital stay doubled, causing many Americans, especially the elderly, to have difficulty affording care. Since 1990, health care costs in the United States have risen at double the rate of inflation. By 2011, just under 16 percent of all Americans, or 44 million people, were uninsured (United States Census Bureau, 2011).

The Patient Protection and Affordable Care Act, also known as Obamacare, was signed into law in March 2010. This law mandates a system that provides and offers health care coverage for all Americans. The goal of this law is to reduce the costs of health care for individuals as well as the government, and to expand Medicaid coverage to individuals and families that would previously not qualify.

Part of the Affordable Care Act mandates that insurance companies may no longer deny coverage to individuals for pre-existing conditions. Another mandate includes the rule that insurance companies cannot force higher premiums on individuals based on age and gender. With the Affordable Care Act, all Americans must either be covered by some form of health care coverage or face a fine. Each state must have an exchange program in place where individuals and companies can purchase health care coverage at an affordable premium, based on the level of coverage desired.

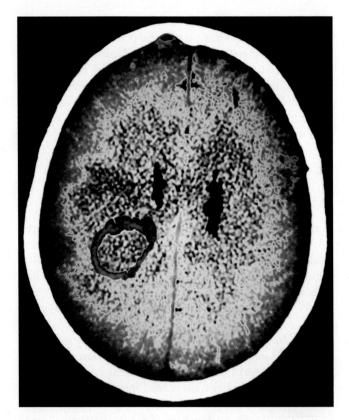

Figure 1-21 ■ This computed tomography (CT) scan shows the brain of a 41-year-old patient with a cerebral abscess.
Source: © Zephyr/Science Photo Library/Corbis

▶▶▶Pulse Points

CT Scans and MRIs

CT scans use X-rays to take three-dimensional images of the insides of objects (**Figure 1-21** ■).

MRI uses a large magnet to visualize the inside of an object (**Figure 1-22** ■).

Evidence-based Medicine

With health care costs in the United States rising far faster than inflation, eliminating costly and ineffective treatments is one way for the medical community to bring those costs under control. Evidence-based medicine has arisen as one solution to the problem.

Evidence-based medicine uses scientific findings, randomized controlled trials, and medical literature to find the most effective ways to treat disease. According to the Centre for Evidence-Based Medicine, "Evidence-based medicine is the conscientious, explicit, and judicious use of current best evidence in making decisions and the care of individual patients" (Centre for Evidence-Based Medicine). In essence, this form of

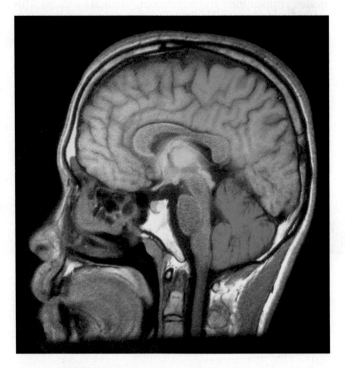

Figure 1-22 ■ MRI of head showing brain structures.
Source: © Callista Images/Cultura/Corbis.

medicine is based on the idea that medical practice has a scientific method and that many traditional practices have no scientific basis and therefore can be costly and ineffective.

Physicians who practice evidence-based medicine are dedicated to treating patients with the most current, scientifically valid treatments. To keep abreast of drug trials and scientific studies, those providers must keep current with constant review of the medical literature.

The History of the Medical Assisting Profession

Traditionally, physicians hired nurses to work in their offices. With a shortage of nurses, physicians began to seek other qualified staff who could fulfill administrative and clinical duties. As a result, the demand for formally trained medical assistants began to rise.

When medical assisting began in the early 1950s, the Kansas Medical Assistants Society formed a professional organization for those in the field. A year later, the organization voted to rename itself the **American Association of Medical Assistants (AAMA)**. At the time, medical assistants lacked formal education; physicians trained most of their assistants on the job, and the AAMA held educational sessions designed to increase the professionalism of medical assisting. Since 1957, the AAMA has kept its national headquarters in Chicago, Illinois.

The first AAMA president was Maxine Williams. Williams was a strong advocate for medical assisting. In 1959, she donated $200 of her own money to begin a fund to help needy students pursue their goal of becoming medical assistants. This fund, which still exists today, is called the Maxine Williams Scholarship Fund.

In 1978, the U.S. Department of Education followed the example of the AAMA and recognized medical assisting as a profession. In 1991, the AAMA approved the current definition of medical assisting as, "… an allied health profession whose practitioners function as members of the health care delivery team and perform administrative and clinical procedures" (AAMA, 2007). Table 1-3 lists other AAMA milestones.

Today, medical assistants are well-trained, valuable members of the health care team.

In Practice

In coming years, the scope of practice for the medical assistant will expand to meet the needs of an aging population and the evolving field of patient care. As it does, new graduates will acquire new skills. How will current medical assistants keep their skills up to date? What resources can assistants use to further their training?

TABLE 1-3 History of the American Association of Medical Assistants (AAMA)

Year	Event
1961	Establishes certifying board.
1962	Offers sample exam.
1963	Holds first exams.
1977	Engages National Board of Medical Examiners as a test consultant.
1978	Gives exam in January and June at nationwide centers.
1980	Allows medical assistants to recertify via continuing education or exam.
1998	Requires exam candidates to complete medical-assisting programs accredited by the Commission on Accreditation of Allied Health Education Programs (CAAHEP).
1999	Makes graduates of medical assisting programs accredited by the Accrediting Bureau of Health Education Schools eligible for the exam.
2002	Places certified medical assistant pin in space aboard a NASA shuttle.
2003	Renders recertification mandatory for certified medical assisting credential; adds October exam.
2005	Makes health care provider-level cardiopulmonary resuscitation mandatory to maintain medical-assisting certification.
2008	The credential designation changed from Certified Medical Assistant (CMA) to either Certified Medical Assistant (AAMA) or CMA (AAMA).
2009	Computer-based testing for the CMA (AAMA) began.

Source: American Association of Medical Assistants: www.aama-ntl.org.

REVIEW

Chapter Summary

- The world's earliest medical practices have left a significant imprint on contemporary medical practices.
- Each century, dating back to ancient times, has contributed notable medical inventions and discoveries.

- A number of longstanding, pivotal organizations have formed throughout the years to further the advances of medical knowledge and achievement. These include but are not limited to the American Hospital Association (AHA), the American Medical

Association (AMA), and the World Health Organization (WHO).

● Women including Clara Barton, Marie Curie, Florence Nightingale, Elizabeth Blackwell, and Emily Blackwell have played a significant role in medicine throughout history.

● Modern medical practices have built on the achievements of the past.

● Health care will likely continue to yield critical discoveries. Among the promising areas of research are stem cell research, transplants, and chemistry in the area of pharmacology.

● The medical assisting profession has a long history of advocating for the patient in the medical office.

Chapter Review

Multiple Choice

1. Penicillin became commonly used during which of the following decades?
   a. 1920s
   b. 1930s
   c. 1940s
   d. 1950s
   e. 1960s

2. Who was known as "The Father of Medicine"?
   a. Hippocrates
   b. Galen
   c. Vesalius
   d. Blackwell
   e. Curie

3. Which early physician performed public displays of anatomy by cutting open live animals?
   a. Hippocrates
   b. Galen
   c. Vesalius
   d. Blackwell
   e. Curie

4. Which health care professional was the first to advocate that physicians wash their hands between patients?
   a. Fleming
   b. Pasteur
   c. Jenner
   d. Semmelweiss
   e. Galen

5. Who discovered penicillin?
   a. Fleming
   b. Pasteur
   c. Jenner
   d. Semmelweiss
   e. Galen

6. Who founded modern nursing?
   a. Clara Barton
   b. Florence Nightingale
   c. Marie Curie
   d. Elizabeth Blackwell
   e. Emily Blackwell

7. Who was the first woman to graduate from medical school in the United States?
   a. Clara Barton
   b. Florence Nightingale
   c. Marie Curie
   d. Elizabeth Blackwell
   e. Emily Blackwell

True/False

T F 1. Emily Blackwell founded the American Red Cross.

T F 2. One of the first physicians to use an ether-based compound as an anesthetic was given a U.S. patent for his concoction.

T F 3. The Human Genome Project has not yet been completed.

T F 4. The cost of health care in the United States is rising faster than the rate of inflation.

T F 5. Penicillin use became widespread during World War I.

T F 6. The Patient Protection and Affordable Care Act mandates a system that provides and offers health care coverage for all Americans.

T F 7. Marie Curie is the only woman to have won two Nobel prizes.

Short Answer

1. What is evidence-based medicine?
2. Why were Galen's anatomy findings only partially accurate?
3. Why was the letter *x* used in the word *X-ray*?
4. Who discovered the rabies vaccine?
5. How many pacemakers did the first internal-pacemaker patient receive, and how long did the patient live?

Research

1. Using the Internet as a resource, research the history of a commonly used medical instrument.
2. What is the history of the medical assistants' association in the state where you live?

3. Take one of the topics on the history of medicine covered in this chapter. Research this topic further to provide more details about how this innovation or invention has changed the way medicine is practiced.

Practicum Application Experience

A patient asks the medical assistant to help identify resources for researching a physician-recommended vaccine. What should the medical assistant tell the patient? Which types of resources would help?

Resource Guide

American Hospital Association
One North Franklin
Chicago, IL 60606-3421
Phone: (312) 422-3000
http://www.aha.org

American Medical Association
AMA Plaza
330 N. Wabash Avenue
Chicago, IL 60611-5885
Phone: (800) 621-8335
www.ama-assn.org

Centers for Disease Control and Prevention
1600 Clifton Road
Atlanta, GA 30333
Phone: (404) 639-3311 / (404) 639-3534 / (800) 311-3435
http://www.cdc.gov/

Centre for Evidence-Based Medicine
Department of Primary Care
Old Road Campus
Headington, Oxford, OX3 7LF, United Kingdom
Phone: +44 (0)1865 226991
Fax: +44 (0)1865 226845
http://www.cebm.net/

Duke University Library
Introduction to Evidence-Based Medicine:
http://www.hsl.unc.edu/services/tutorials/ebm/

Fisher, L. E. (1980). *The hospitals.* New York: Holiday House.

Holland, A. (2000). *Voices of Qi: An introductory guide to traditional Chinese medicine.* Berkeley, CA: North Atlantic Books, Northwest Institute of Acupuncture and Oriental Medicine.

Human Genome Project
U.S. Department of Energy
1000 Independence Ave., SW
Washington, D.C. 20585
Phone: (800) 342-5363
Fax: (202) 586-4403
http://www.ornl.gov/sci/techresources/Human_Genome/home.shtml

Maciocia, G. (2005). *The foundations of Chinese medicine: A comprehensive text for acupuncturists and herbalists.* New York: Churchill Livingstone.

PBS's Health Care Crisis: Health Care Timeline
Issues TV
18 Twin Ponds Drive
Bedford Hills, NY 10507-1208
Phone: (800) 752-9727
e-mail: issuestv@aol.com
http://www.pbs.org/healthcarecrisis/history.htm

Porter, R. (1999). *The greatest benefit to mankind: A medical history of humanity from antiquity to the present.* New York: W.W. Norton and Company.

Shriners Hospital for Children
2900 Rocky Point Drive
Tampa, FL 33607
Phone: (800) 237-5055
http://www.shrinershq.org/Hospitals/_Hospitals_for_Children/

Vallejo-Manzur, F. et al. (2003). The resuscitation greats. Andreas Vesalius: The concept of an artificial airway. *Resuscitation, 56:*3–7.

Wells, S. (2001). *Out of the dead house: Nineteenth-century women physicians and the writing of medicine.* Madison, WI: University of Wisconsin Press.

2

Medical Assisting Certification and Scope of Practice

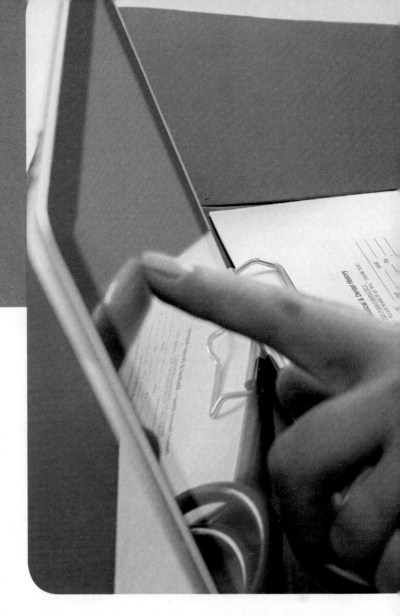

Case Study

Read the following case study and answer the critical thinking questions presented throughout the chapter.

Karla Wilkins and Carrie Smith, a medical assistant, were friends in high school. By the time the two unexpectedly met again at the local grocery store, they had not been in touch for several months. Carrie told Karla about becoming certified as a medical assistant and included such details as course load and topics. Looking confused, Karla asked, "If medical assistants don't *have* to be certified, why waste the time going to school? Why not just find a job and learn on the job?"

Objectives

After completing this chapter, you should be able to:

2.1 Define and spell the key terminology in this chapter.

2.2 List the educational requirements of the medical assistant.

2.3 Discuss the benefits of certifying or registering as a medical assistant.

2.4 List the professional organizations that certify or register medical assistants.

2.5 Name the benefits of membership in professional organizations.

2.6 Define the scope of practice for medical assisting.

2.7 List the professional associations that certify other allied health professionals.

Competency Skills Performance

1. Adapt to change.

Key Terminology

accredited—endorsed by a reputable overseeing agency

Accrediting Bureau of Health Education Schools (ABHES)—agency that helps support the certification of medical assistants through program endorsement; accredits private and postsecondary institutions offering allied health education programs in medical assisting, medical laboratory technicians, and surgical technology programs

administrative—pertaining to office functions (e.g., computer operation, medical records management, coding, and billing)

American Medical Technologists (AMT)—national, professional association for medical technologists

associate degree—degree awarded by community colleges after a roughly 2-year course of study

certified medical assistant (CMA)—graduate of an accredited medical assisting program who has passed the certification examination of the American Association of Medical Assistants (AAMA)

clinical—pertaining to direct patient care (e.g., drawing blood samples, taking vital signs, assisting with surgery)

Commission of Accreditation of Allied Health Education Programs (CAAHEP)—agency supporting the process of medical assisting certification through program endorsement; accredits over 2100 entry-level programs in 23 health science professions.

community college—educational institution that provides 2-year undergraduate education

competency—skill in a defined area

practicum—educational learning opportunity outside the classroom that gives students hands-on experience; final phase of an accredited medical assisting program

proprietary school—a private business enterprise that sells vocational/occupational courses (e.g., medical assisting) to the general public for training or employment purposes

recertification—process of certificate renewal

registered medical assistant (RMA)—credential awarded a medical assistant who has passed the RMA certification examination

scope of practice—range of skills and duties a health care professional is expected to have and operate within

technical educational program—program designed to give students skills without higher education; also called vocational program

vocational program—program designed to give students skills without higher education; also called technical educational program

Abbreviations

AAPC—American Academy of Professional Coders

ABHES—Accrediting Bureau of Health Education Schools

AHDI—Association for Healthcare Documentation Integrity

AHIMA—American Health Information Management Association

AMT—American Medical Technologists

CAAHEP—Commission on Accreditation of Allied Health Education Programs

CCS—certified coding specialist

CEU—continuing education unit

CLC—certified laboratory consultant

CMA—certified medical assistant

CMAS—certified medical administrative specialist

CMAA—certified medical administrative assistant

CMT—certified medical transcriptionist

COLT—certified office laboratory technician

CPC—certified professional coder

CPR—cardiopulmonary resuscitation

HIPAA—Health Insurance Portability and Accountability Act

LPN—licensed practical nurse

MLT—medical laboratory technician

MT—medical technologist

NAHP—National Association of Health Professionals

NCCT—National Center for Competency Testing

NCMA—National Certified Medical Assistant

NHA—National Healthcareer Association

NP—nurse practitioner

PA—physician assistant

RMA—registered medical assistant

RPT—registered phlebotomy technician

Introduction

With dramatic changes in health care over the past decade, including shorter hospital stays and managed care, physicians must rely on allied health personnel like medical assistants to help care for patients. With technology advancing and patient safety increasingly a focal point, many physicians today insist on hiring medical assistants who have been formally trained in accredited medical assisting programs. Part of this training includes complete knowledge of the medical assistant's role in patient care.

As health care facilities move toward implementation of electronic health records as mandated by the government, those facilities must prove that the medical records contain vital information. The inclusion of this information is referred to as meeting the *meaningful use* rule. Only credentialed medical assistants meet the meaningful use rule. This means that a medical assistant must be certified or any provider orders entered by the MA into the patient's medical record will not count toward giving the physician credit for meeting the rule.

Educational Requirements of the Medical Assistant

Vocational programs, **technical educational programs**, and **community colleges** all offer medical assisting education. Programs take from six months to two years to complete. Many two-year programs award **associate degrees** as well as medical assisting certificates and diplomas. Other medical assisting programs are located in **proprietary schools**. A proprietary school is a private business enterprise that sells vocational/occupational courses (e.g., medical assisting) to the general public for training or employment purposes. The courses are typically fast-paced. Though many of the proprietary schools are accredited, they are not associated with earning college credits for the completion of courses. Students will receive a certificate of completion for the program.

Medical Assisting Accreditation

Medical assisting programs are typically **accredited** by one of two associations: (1) **Commission of Accreditation of Allied Health Education Programs (CAAHEP)** or (2) **Accrediting Bureau of Health Education Schools (ABHES)**. The AAMA curriculum review board approves the work of both agencies. Some states require medical assistants to become certified, licensed, or registered. Those states dictate which of the accrediting bodies are acceptable for the medical assistant to go through for education.

The Commission on Accreditation of Allied Health Education Programs (CAAHEP) was formed in 1994. Prior to that, the organization was called the Committee on Allied Health Education and Accreditation (CAHEA) The CAHEA was part of the American Medical Association (AMA). CAAHEP accredits over 2,100 entry-level programs in 23 health science professions.

The Accrediting Bureau of Health Education Schools (ABHES) has been recognized by the U.S. Secretary of Educa-

tion since 1968. ABHES accredits private and postsecondary institutions offering allied health education programs in medical assisting, medical laboratory technician, and surgical technology programs.

Accredited medical assisting programs must teach in all areas of the AAMA Occupational Analysis, which lists medical assisting competencies for graduation, including **administrative**, **clinical**, and general skills (**Figure 2-1 ■**). To help keep the analysis grid current, the AAMA periodically surveys medical assistants nationwide to identify current job duties.

Critical Thinking Question 2-1

Referring to the case study at the beginning of the chapter, what evidence supports the argument that medical assistants should have a standardized base of knowledge?

Critical Thinking Question 2-2

Refer back to the case study at the beginning of the chapter. How might Carrie explain to Karla why medical assistants who have completed accredited programs have more health care knowledge than those lacking formal training?

The Medical Assisting Education Review Board (MAERB) completes program reviews for CAAHEP, providing recommendation for accreditation of medical assisting programs. MAERB provides ongoing reviews of medical assisting programs as well as providing medical assisting instructors with the opportunity to attend workshops on promoting standardization of program reviews.

Taking a Certified or Registered Medical Assistant Exam

Medical assisting certification or registration is voluntary, but the AAMA strongly encourages it as a means of guaranteeing **competency**. Many physicians require medical assistants to have certification or registration as a condition of employment, in part because in many states, many malpractice insurance carriers offer discounts to physicians who employ only certified or registered medical assistants. Certification or registration means medical assistants have been trained to a standard required by the AAMA, which implies they have education that renders them able to behave legally and ethically and helps avoid patient injuries as well as breaches of patient confidentiality (**Figure 2-2 ■**). **Figure 2-3 ■** outlines the Medical Assistant's Creed. To sit for the Certified Medical Assistant exam, students must be graduates of a CAAHEP or ABHES accredited school.

General, Clinical, and Administrative Skills* of the CMA (AAMA)

General Skills

◆ Communication
- Serve as patient advocate professional and health coach in a team approach in health care
- Recognize and respect cultural diversity
- Adapt communications to individual's understanding
- Employ professional telephone and interpersonal techniques
- Recognize and respond effectively to verbal, nonverbal, and written communications
- Utilize and apply medical terminology appropriately
- Receive, organize, prioritize, store, and maintain transmittable information utilizing electronic technology
- Serve as "communication liaison" between the physician and patient

◆ Legal Concepts
- Recognize professional credentialing criteria
- Identify and respond to issues of confidentiality
- Perform within legal (including federal and state statutes, regulations, opinions, and rulings) and ethical boundaries
- Document patient communication and clinical treatments accurately and appropriately
- Maintain medical records
- Follow employer's established policies dealing with the health care contract
- Comply with established risk management and safety procedures

◆ Instruction
- Identify basics of office emergency preparedness
- Function as a health care advocate to meet individual's needs
- Educate individuals in office policies and procedures
- Educate the patient within the scope of practice and as directed by supervising physician in health maintenance, disease prevention, and compliance with patient's treatment plan
- Identify community resources for health maintenance and disease prevention to meet individual patient needs
- Maintain current list of community resources, including those for emergency preparedness and other patient care needs
- Collaborate with local community resources for emergency preparedness
- Educate patients in their responsibilities relating to third-party reimbursements

◆ Operational Functions
- Perform inventory of supplies and equipment
- Perform routine maintenance of administrative and clinical equipment
- Apply computer and other electronic equipment techniques to support office operations
- Perform methods of quality control

Clinical Skills

◆ Fundamental Principles
- Identify the roles and responsibilities of the medical assistant in the clinical setting
- Identify the roles and responsibilities of other team members in the medical office
- Apply principles of aseptic technique and infection control
- Practice Standard Precautions, including handwashing and disposal of biohazardous materials
- Perform sterilization techniques
- Comply with quality assurance practices

◆ Diagnostic Procedures
- Collect and process specimens
- Perform CLIA-waived tests
- Perform electrocardiography and respiratory testing
- Perform phlebotomy, including venipuncture and capillary puncture
- Utilize knowledge of principles of radiology

◆ Patient Care
- Perform initial-response screening following protocols approved by supervising physician
- Obtain, evaluate, and record patient history employing critical thinking skills
- Obtain vital signs
- Prepare and maintain examination and treatment areas
- Prepare patient for examinations, procedures and treatments
- Assist with examinations, procedures, and treatments
- Maintain examination/treatment rooms, including inventory of supplies and equipment
- Prepare and administer oral and parenteral (excluding IV) medications and immunizations (as directed by supervising physician and as permitted by state law)
- Utilize knowledge of principles of IV therapy
- Maintain medication and immunization records
- Screen and follow up test results
- Recognize and respond to emergencies

Administrative Skills

◆ Administrative Procedures
- Schedule, coordinate, and monitor appointments
- Schedule inpatient/outpatient admissions and procedures
- Apply third-party and managed care policies, procedures, and guidelines
- Establish, organize, and maintain patient medical record
- File medical records appropriately

◆ Practice Finances
- Perform procedural and diagnostic coding for reimbursement
- Perform billing and collection procedures
- Perform administrative functions, including bookkeeping and financial procedures
- Prepare submittable ("clean") insurance forms

*All skills require decision making based on critical thinking concepts.

Figure 2-1 ■ General, clinical, and administrative skills of the CMA (AAMA).
Source: *Printed with permission of the American Association of Medical Assistants.*

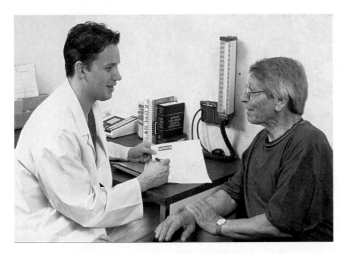

Figure 2-2 ■ Certification or registration means medical assistants have education that renders them able to behave legally and ethically.
Source: Pearson Education/PH College. Photographer: Michal Heron.

I believe in the principles and purposes of the profession of medical assisting.

I endeavor to be more effective.

I aspire to render greater service.

I protect the confidence entrusted to me.

I am dedicated to the care and well-being of all patients.

I am loyal to my physician-employer.

I am true to the ethics of my profession.

I am strengthened by compassion, courage, and faith.

Figure 2-3 ■ Medical Assistant's Creed.
Source: Printed with permission of American Association of Medical Assistants.

Critical Thinking Question 2-3

Referring back to the case study at the beginning of the chapter, how might Carrie explain to Karla how certification or registration discounts on physicians' medical malpractice insurance policies impact job opportunities for medical assistants?

Becoming a Certified Medical Assistant (CMA; AAMA)

The CMA (AAMA) Certification Examination is offered via computer-based testing. Candidates are able to select locations and flexible testing times at conveniently located computer-based testing centers throughout the United States.

Current exam fees and requirements can be found on the CAAHEP and ABHES websites (refer to the Resource Guide at the end of this chapter). Exam fees are nonrefundable.

After taking the computer-based exam, students receive preliminary immediate pass/fail results. The CMA (AAMA) Certification/Recertification Examination is available year-round. Applications to sit for the exam are due at least 90 days in advance of the first of the month the applicant intends to sit for the exam. The exam is offered online. The AAMA exam consists of 200 questions. The exam is administered in four 40-minute segments. Applicants have an optional 20-minute total for breaks between the segments and have 160 minutes to answer all exam questions.

The AAMA informs the applicant of application status within 75 days after the application postmark deadline. Applicants also can inquire about enrollment status via e-mail (mailto: info@aama-ntl.org). It is important to include the following information in the e-mail:

- Your name
- Your graduation date
- Your accreditation code
- OR
- Your school name, school city, and school state.

In addition to applying for the exam, applicants must pay a fee and provide appropriate documentation. AAMA members and CAAHEP program graduates both enjoy significant enrollment fee discounts. Documentation requirements depend on the applicant's enrollment category. Applicants fall into one of the two following categories:

- Graduating students or recent graduates of a CAAHEP or an ABHES accredited medical assisting program
- Nonrecent graduates of a CAAHEP or an ABHES accredited medical assisting program

Since 1998, applicants for the Certification Examination for Medical Assistants have been required to complete accredited medical assisting programs that include classes in clinical and administrative competencies (Table 2-1) and end with a

---

TABLE 2-1 Sample Accredited Medical Assisting Classes		
Medical terminology	Medical law and ethics	Clinical surgical skills
Phlebotomy skills	Introduction to pharmacology	Clinical ambulatory skills
Intercultural communications	Administrative and office management skills	Medical billing and coding
Medical practice finances	Computer applications in the medical office	Anatomy and physiology
Medication administration	Disease and pathology	Cardiopulmonary resuscitation (**CPR**) and first aid skills
Clinical laboratory skills	Patient relations	Practicum

**TABLE 2-2 CMA (AAMA) Certification/
Recertification Examination Content Outline**

General	Administrative	Clinical
Medical terminology	Data entry	Principles of infection control
Anatomy and physiology	Equipment	Treatment area
Psychology	Computer concepts	Patient preparation and assisting the physician
Professionalism	Records management	Patient history interview
Communication	Screening and processing mail	Collecting and processing specimens; diagnostic testing
Medicolegal guidelines and requirements	Scheduling and monitoring appointments	Preparing and administering medications
	Resource information and community services	Emergencies
	Maintaining the office environment	First aid
	Office policies and procedures	Nutrition
	Practice finances	

Source: Printed with permission of the American Association of Medical Assistants.

required **practicum**. The practicum is an educational learning opportunity outside the classroom that provides students with hands-on learning experience.

Practicums involve working as a medical assistant under a provider's supervision. The AAMA requires a minimum of 60 hours, but many medical assisting programs require practicums of more than 240 hours. Although practicums are unpaid, students earn credits toward their medical assisting certificates.

Students who complete accredited programs and pass the Certification Examination for Medical Assistants earn the title of **certified medical assistant (CMA)** and may include the initials CMA (AAMA) after their name **Figure 2-4 ■**). Those who fail the exam may reapply for a retake. This requires the same 90-day application wait process as taking the exam the first time. Because the CMA (AAMA) exam is taken electronically, medical assistants are alerted to their pass or fail status at the end of the exam. Table 2-2 lists the CMA (AAMA) examination content outline.

Critical Thinking Question 2-4

Referring back to the case study at the beginning of the chapter, how could Carrie explain to Karla how a practicum supports the educational goals of an accredited medical assisting program?

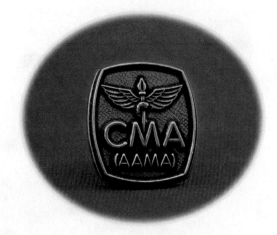

Figure 2-4 ■ CMA (AAMA) pin.
Source: Printed with permission of the American Association of Medical Assistants (AAMA).

HIPAA Compliance

All accredited medical assisting programs include training on Health Insurance Portability and Accountability Act (**HIPAA**) regulations. HIPAA is a federal law that is mandated for all health care professionals for safeguarding patient information. An understanding of HIPAA and how it applies to the work the medical assistant performs is vital to the success of every medical assistant.

CMA (AAMA) Recertification To maintain CMA (AAMA) status, medical assistants must complete **recertification** every 5 years. They can retake the Certification Examination for Medical Assistants or acquire 60 continuing education units (**CEUs**) in administrative, clinical, or general categories by attending informational seminars or lectures. Of those 60 continuing education credits, 30 must be approved by the AAMA. Recertification via CEU is discounted for AAMA members.

Becoming a Registered Medical Assistant (RMA)

Another medical assisting credential, this one received through the **American Medical Technologists (AMT)** agency, is **registered medical assistant (RMA)** (AMT). Since 1972, medical assistants have been able to earn RMA (AMT) status by taking a voluntary certification exam that today is given on paper or electronically. Examinations are available year round. Table 2-3 outlines the exam's contents.

To sit for the RMA (AMT) certification exam, a medical assistant must meet one of the following requirements:

1. Graduation from a:
   - Medical assistant program accredited by the ABHES or CAAHEP

   or

TABLE 2-3 RMA Certification Examination Content Outline		
General Medical Assisting Knowledge *(86 items)*	**Administrative Medical Assisting** *(51 items)*	**Clinical Medical Assisting** *(73 items)*
Anatomy and physiology	Insurance	Asepsis
Medical terminology	Financial book-keeping	Sterilization
Medical law	Medical receptionist/ Secretarial/ Clerical	Instruments
Medical ethics		Vital signs and mensuration
Human relations		Physical exami-nations
Patient education		Clinical pharma-cology
		Minor surgery
		Therapeutic modalities
		Laboratory procedures
		Electrocardiog-raphy (ECG)
		First aid and emergency response

Source: Reprinted by permission of American Medical Technologists (AMT).

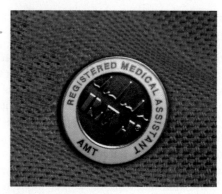

Figure 2-5 ■ RMA (AMT) pin.
Source: Reprinted by permission of American Medical Technologists (AMT.)

- Medical assistant program with institutional accreditation by a regional or national accrediting commission that is approved by the U.S. Department of Education and that includes at least 720 hours of training in medical assisting skills and a clinical practicum of at least 160 hours.
  - Applicants must have graduated from their accredited program within the past four years. Applicants who graduated more than four years prior to applying must provide proof of recent medical assisting experience.

or

- Formal medical services training program of the U.S. Armed Forces
  - Applicants must have graduated from their accredited program within the past four years. Applicants who graduated more than four years prior to applying must provide proof of recent medical assisting experience.

2. At least five years of medical assisting employment experience, no more than two of which may have been as an instructor in a medical assistant program.

3. Applicant may be currently working as an instructor in an accredited medical assisting program, have completed a course on instruction related to medical assisting, and have a minimum of five years of experience teaching both clinical and administrative classes.

4. Applicant may have taken and passed another certification program's medical assisting examination, provided that program has been approved by the AMT Board of Directors. No examination is required.

In addition to one of the preceding requirements, applicants must also be:

- Of good moral character
- At least 18 years old
- A graduate of an accredited high school or acceptable equivalent

In paper format, the RMA (AMT) exam is available at least four times a year, depending on exam location. AMT has announced that it will stop taking registrations for paper testing as of 10/1/2015; there will be no more testing by paper after 1/1/2016. The electronic version is available every day of the year, except Sundays and holidays, at over 200 locations in the United States and Canada. In the electronic version, scores appear on the screen moments after students complete the exam. With the paper version, notification can be expected within four weeks.

The RMA (AMT) exam questions consist of 41% in general medical assisting knowledge, 24% in administrative medical assisting, and 35% in clinical medical assisting. Applicants who pass the exam earn the RMA (AMT) distinction (**Figure 2-5** ■). Those who fail can retake the exam 90 days after their initial attempts. The AMT requires members to pay annual dues to remain registered.

Becoming a Certified Medical Administrative Specialist

The American Medical Technologists (AMT) offer certification as a Medical Administrative Specialist. Applications for this certification may be downloaded from the AMT Web site at: www.americanmedtech.org. Once the application is filled out, it can be mailed to American Medical Technologists (see the Resource Guide at the end of this chapter for the mailing address), or it may be submitted online on the AMT Web site. Approximately four to six weeks after submitting the application, candidates will receive written confirmation that approval to take the test has been granted. Exams may be taken either on paper, or in computerized format. Results for paper examinations take six to eight weeks to arrive; computerized examination scores are given on completion of the exam. The fee for taking this certification exam can be found by vising the Web site. The criteria for eligibility to take the Certified Medical Professional examination are:

1. Applicant must be of good moral character.
2. Applicant must meet one of the following criteria:
   - Route 1 (Education): Applicant shall be a graduate of, or scheduled to graduate from, an accredited medical office administrative program.
   - Route 2 (RMA Certification): Applicant shall be certified as a Registered Medical Assistant (RMA), or equivalent, and possess a minimum of two years of recent full-time experience working as a medical office administrative specialist.
   - Route 3 (Work Experience): Applicant shall have been employed as a medical office administrative specialist for a minimum of five of the past seven years. Proof of high school graduation (or equivalent) is required.
3. Applicant shall take and pass the appropriate AMT certification examination.

   Table 2-4 outlines the **CMAS** examination content.

Becoming a National Certified Medical Assistant (NCMA)

The National Center for Competency Testing (**NCCT**) offers a National Certified Medical Assistant (**NCMA**) designation to assistants who qualify and pass an examination. Table 2-5 includes the NCCT Medical Assistant Certification exam content categories.

To qualify for the National Certified Medical Assistant examination, applicants must meet two requirements:

1. High school graduate, or equivalent
2. Meet one of the following requirements:
   - Route 1: Graduation from an NCCT-approved MA program within the last 10 years.
   - Route 2: Two years of qualifying full-time employment (4,160 hours) or equivalent part-time employment as an MA within the last 10 years.

For current examination fee amounts, applicants should visit the NCCT Web site (www.ncctinc.com).

Becoming Certified with the National Association of Health Professionals

The National Association of Health Professionals (**NAHP**) offers certification for medical assistants. A medical assistant seeking certification with NAHP must be a graduate of an accredited medical assisting program that has been approved by NAHP. The applicant must have graduated within 10 years of applying for this certification exam. If an applicant has not graduated from an accredited medical assisting program, they may qualify for this exam if they have had formal medical training in the U.S. Armed Forces of no less than two years. A third option for applicants to take this exam is to have been employed as a medical assistant for a period of no less than two years. For this last option, applicants must provide a letter or letters on employer's letterhead indicating their recommendation and documenting the time of employment. The employment mentioned in the recommendation letters cannot have ended more than 10 years from the date of the application.

The NAHP exam consists of 100 exam questions, and applicants must pass the test with a score of 70% or higher. The test may be taken three times on one application within a year. If the test is not passed in three tries, a new application must be submitted. The NAHP also certifies phlebotomy technicians, coding specialists, ECG technicians, administrative health assistants, pharmacy technicians, dental assistants, patient care technicians, and surgical technicians.

Becoming a Certified Medical Administrative Assistant (CMAA)

The National Healthcareer Association (**NHA**) offers certification as a Certified Medical Administrative Assistant (**CMAA**). Applicants seeking medical administrative assistant certification must have successfully completed a medical administrative assistant training program within the last year or have recently worked in the field for a minimum of one year. At the time of publication of this text, the NHA was in the process of revising its test plan. For the most up-to-date information regarding the NHA test plan, number of test questions, and time allotted to take the exam, please visit their website at www.nhanow.com.

Critical Thinking Question 2-5

Refer back to the case study at the beginning of this chapter. After considering the various certification options available to Carrie, what factors might she consider when determining which certification is best for her?

Gaining Multiple Medical Assisting Statuses

Medical assistants who are certified by more than one of the certification bodies may use all of the credentials. All certified or registered medical assistants are encouraged to join their local, state, and federal professional organizations. Although these organizations require fees to join, they help medical

TABLE 2-4 AMT (CMAS) Competencies and Examination Specifications

Medical Assisting Foundations (13% of examination)	Basic Clinical Medical Office Assisting (8% of examination)	Medical Office Clerical Assisting (10% of examination)	Medical Records Management (14% of examination)	Health Care Insurance Processing, Coding, and Billing (17% of examination)	Medical Office Financial Management (17% of examination)	Medical Office Information Processing (7% of examination)	Medical Office Management (15% of examination)
Medical terminology	Basic health	Appointment management and scheduling	Systems	Insurance processing	Fundamental financial management	Fundamentals of computing	Office communications*
Anatomy and physiology	History interview	Reception	Procedures	Coding	Patient accounts	Medical office computer applications	Business organization management*
Legal and ethical considerations	Basic charting	Communication	Confidentiality	Insurance billing and finances	Banking		Human resources*
Professionalism	Vital signs and measurements				Payroll		Safety
	Asepsis in the medical office						Supplies and equipment
	examination preparation						Physical office plant
	Medical office emergencies						Risk management and quality assurance
	Pharmacology						*Note: Asterisked areas addressed by the medical office management job function may or may not be performed by the certified medical administrative specialist at entry-level practice. Nevertheless, the competent specialist should have sound knowledge of these management functions at certification level.

Source: Reprinted by permission of American Medical Technologists (AMT).

TABLE 2-5 NCCT (NCMA) Certification Exam Content Categories

Content Categories
Anatomy and physiology
Medical office management
Medical procedures
Medical terminology
Pharmacology

Source: © 2013 National Center for Competency Testing. Reprinted by permission of NCCT.

assistants maintain the skills needed in today's competitive job market through such benefits as:

- Educational presentations that offer CEUs
- Access to information on upcoming legislation related to the profession
- Subscriptions to professional journals
- Group insurance plans
- Professional malpractice insurance policies
- Networking opportunities

The Medical Assistant's Scope of Practice

Some states dictate the **scope of practice** for medical assisting in that state. To practice according to local laws, medical assistants must know, and stay on top of, the legal parameters in their state.

Currently, medical assistants must work under the direction and supervision of physicians, nurse practitioners (**NP**s), or physician assistants (**PA**s). Medical assistants are not licensed to make independent medical assessment of patients or to offer advice. In some states, medical assistants can perform procedures such as urinalysis, strep tests, blood pressure checks, weight checks, EKGs, venipuncture, and injections of certain medications. A growing number of states are currently looking into licensing medical assistants, which would require that a defined scope of practice for this profession be developed.

In coming years, the scope of practice in medical assisting is expected to grow. With the increase in the number of patients entering the health care system, both due to an aging population in the United States and inclusion of more covered individuals under the Affordable Care Act, the need for an expanded scope of practice for medical assistants is expected. In Washington State, as an example, the scope of practice for medical assistants (called Health Care Assistants in that state) was expanded in 2012 to include the administration of eye, ear, and skin medications, under the orders of a physician. Although medical assisting is not currently a licensed profession, that might change.

Patient Education

It is important for patients to understand the knowledge, skills, and scope of practice of all health care professionals, including the medical assistant. When patients incorrectly identify the medical assistant as a nurse, they should be politely corrected so they understand the medical assistant's role. For example, the medical assistant might say, "I am Dr. Smith's medical assistant. I have different skills from a nurse, and we perform different duties in the physician's office."

Certification Requirements for Other Allied Health Professionals

Health care is a very diverse community of professionals who work together as a team to care for patients. Allied health professionals have industry-specific associations; some have certification or registration exams. Postname initials indicate a professional's certification or registration status.

The American Medical Technologists (AMT)

In addition to the RMA (AMT) and CMAS (AMT) certifications discussed previously, the AMT offers certification or registration as medical technologist (**MT**), medical laboratory technician (**MLT**), certified office laboratory technician (**COLT**), certified laboratory consultant (**CLC**), and registered phlebotomy technician (**RPT**).

AAPC

AAPC (formerly known as the American Academy of Professional Coders) is an organization for professionals focusing on medical billing and coding. The AAPC offers a voluntary credentialing program with examinations that confer certified professional coder (**CPC**) status, as well as several other credentials in the area of coding, billing, and practice management.

The American Health Information Management Association (AHIMA)

The American Health Information Management Association (**AHIMA**) is a national organization of professionals who work in medical records, coding, and health information management. This group was founded in 1928 to improve the quality of medical records. Currently, it is working to educate its membership on the changes required as health care records move toward becoming electronic. AHIMA offers a voluntary credentialing program with examinations that confer certified

PROCEDURE 2-1 Adapt to Change

Theory and Rationale

Because physicians, supervisors, or office managers will often ask medical assistants to start a new task, it is crucial for medical assistants to adapt efficiently and effectively to changing priorities.

Materials

- Notepad
- Pen

Competency

1. Listen closely as a new task is requested.
2. Ask questions to clarify the request, if needed.
3. Take notes about the task, if needed.
4. Begin working on the new task while maintaining a positive and professional attitude.

---

coding specialist (**CCS**) status, as well as several other credentials in coding and health information management.

The Association for Healthcare Documentation Integrity (AHDI)

In 1978, The Association for Healthcare Documentation Integrity (**AHDI**) was established as part of an effort to achieve recognition for the medical transcription profession. AHDI sets standards of education and practice for the medical transcription profession and offers a voluntary certification exam to individuals who wish to become Certified Medical Transcriptionists (CMTs). The **CMT** credential is awarded on successfully passing the AHDI certification examination for medical transcriptionists.

REVIEW

Chapter Summary

- Types of certifications and registrations in the field dictate the educational requirements of medical assisting.
- Medical assisting certification or registration can help the medical assistant stay abreast of industry developments and maintain the skills needed to remain competitive in the workplace.
- Like certification and registration, professional organizations offer a number of benefits aimed at keeping the medical assistant optimally efficient and effective.
- The scope of medical assisting practice is expected to continue to grow and change.
- Medical assisting is just one allied health profession that has created organizations to keep its members aligned and active.

Chapter Review

Multiple Choice

1. The certification examination is offered through the AAMA:
   a. 1 time each year
   b. 2 times each year
   c. 3 times each year
   d. 4 times each year
   e. throughout the year

2. To recertify as a CMA (AAMA), the medical assistant must:
   a. obtain 60 hours of CEUs within 5 years
   b. retake the Certification Examination for Medical Assistants
   c. obtain permission from their employers
   d. a or b
   e. a and b

3. _____ is an organization for professionals focusing on medical billing and coding.
   a. AAPC
   b. CMA
   c. RMA
   d. HIPAA
   e. AAMA

4. Which of the following is true about medical assistants and the meaningful use rule?
   a. The medical assistant must be over the age of 35.
   b. The medical assistant must be attending nursing school.
   c. The medical assistant must have been working in the field no less than five years.
   d. The medical assistant must be certified or registered as a medical assistant, having passed a national medical assistant's exam.
   e. The medical assistant must be certified in health care records management.

5. Medical assistants must work under the direction of:
   a. physicians
   b. nurse practitioners
   c. physician assistants
   d. a, b, and c
   e. a and b

6. The AMT offers certification or registration to which of the following groups of professionals?
   a. CMAs
   b. CMASs
   c. CPCs
   d. RNs
   e. LPNs

7. Which of the following offers medical assisting education?
   a. Vocational programs
   b. Technical educational programs
   c. Community colleges
   d. Proprietary schools
   e. All of the above

True/False

T F 1. Accredited medical assisting programs must include practicums.

T F 2. Malpractice insurance carriers may offer discounts to physicians who hire only certified or registered medical assistants.

T F 3. The scope of medical assisting practice varies from state to state.

T F 4. One requirement of the AMT RMA examination is to be at least 21 years of age.

T F 5. Certification or registration signals that the medical assistant has been trained to a certain standard.

T F 6. AHIMA focuses mainly on the area of medical records, billing, and coding.

T F 7. The term mandatory credentialing generally refers to a profession where licensing is required.

Short Answer

1. Name the types of education facilities that may offer accredited medical assisting programs.
2. What are the benefits of professional medical assisting organizations?
3. With regard to meaningful use, what is the benefit for medical assistants to be certified?
4. Name the agencies that accredit medical assisting programs.
5. Why is the scope of medical assisting practice soon expected to grow?
6. Why is it important to correct patients who misidentify medical assistants?

Research

1. Where does your local medical assisting association meet?
2. How would you go about becoming a member of your local medical assisting group?
3. What is the scope of practice of a medical assistant in your state?

Practicum Application Experience

A patient at the practicum site asks the medical assistant to differentiate between a nurse and a medical assistant. How should the medical assistant respond?

Resource Guide

AAPC
2480 South 3850 West, Suite B
Salt Lake City, UT 84120
Phone: (800) 626-2633
Fax: (801) 236-2258
e-mail: info@aapc.com, www.aapc.com

Accrediting Bureau of Health Education Schools (ABHES)
777 Leesburg Pike, Suite 314
N. Church Falls, VA 22043
Phone: (703) 917-9503
Fax: (703) 917-4109
www.abhes.org

American Association of Medical Assistants
20 N. Wacker Dr., Ste. 1575
Chicago, IL 60606
Phone: (312) 899-1500
Fax: (312) 899-1259
www.aama-ntl.org

Association for Healthcare Documentation
4230 Kiernan Avenue, Suite 130
Modesto, CA 95356
Phone: (800) 982-2182
Fax: (209) 527-9633
e-mail: www.ahdionline.org

American Health Information Management Association
233 N. Michigan Avenue, 21st Floor
Chicago, IL 60601-5800
Phone: (312) 233-1100
Fax: (312) 233-1090
e-mail: info@ahima.org, www.ahima.org

American Medical Technologists
10700 West Higgins Road, Suite 150
Rosemont, IL 60018
Phone: (800) 275-1268
Fax: (847) 823-0458
www.amt1.com

Commission on Accreditation of Allied Health Education Programs (CAAHEP)
1361 Park Street
Clearwater, FL 33756
Phone: (727) 210-2350
Fax: (727) 210-2354
www.caahep.org

National Center for Competency Testing
7007 College Boulevard, Suite 385
Overland Park, KS 66211
Phone: (800) 875-4404
Fax: (913) 498-1243
www.ncctinc.com

National Healthcareer Association
11161 Overlook Road
Leawood, KS 66211
Phone: (800) 499-9092
Fax: (913) 661-6291
www.nhanow.com

3

Roles and Responsibilities of the Health Care Team

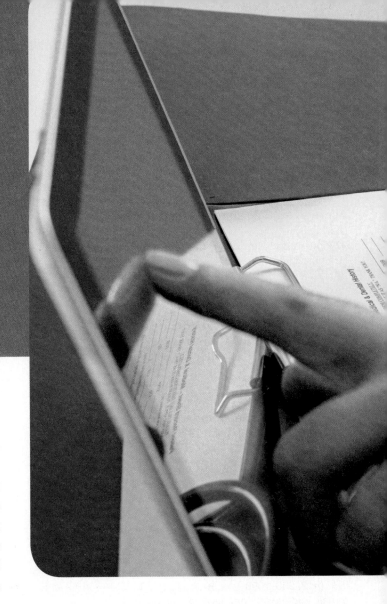

Case Study

Read the following case study and answer the critical thinking questions presented throughout the chapter.

William Johanson is a medical assistant working with Dr. Chan. William frequently arrives to work late for his shift. Because William also works a late-night part-time job, he doesn't always have time in the morning to shower before coming in for his medical assisting job. This causes William to sometimes have poor hygiene, something that patients have occasionally complained about. During his lunch hour, William is often overheard in the lunchroom gossiping with other coworkers about patients he took care of that day. William also has several visible tattoos and facial piercings.

Objectives

After completing this chapter, you should be able to:

3.1 Define and spell the key terminology in this chapter.

3.2 List career opportunities for the medical assistant.

3.3 List the qualities of a professional medical assistant.

3.4 Describe the proper attire of a medical assistant.

3.5 List techniques for improving time-management skills.

3.6 Define the responsibilities of other members of the health care team and their education requirements.

3.7 Define various medical practice specializations.

Key Terminology

administrative skills—clerical-type responsibilities (e.g., typing, filing)

advocate—to defend the rights of others; one who defends or acts on behalf of another

ambulatory care centers—health care clinics where patients are seen for short visits

attitude—state of mind; way of carrying one's self

body language—nonverbal means of communication (e.g., gestures, expressions)

clinical skills—abilities gained through hands-on patient care

confidentiality—state of privacy or secrecy

courtesy—polite behavior

credibility—the quality of being worthy of trust; believable

dependability—capable of being relied on

empathy—ability to identify with and understand another person's feelings

flexibility—willingness to change when needed or requested

initiative—energy or aptitude displayed in starting a task without prompting

loyalty—devotion to another

multidisciplinary—combining many fields of study

rapport—trust and affection between parties

respect—to hold in high esteem

Abbreviations

ACPE—Accreditation Council for Pharmacy Education

ADN—associate degree in nursing

AMA—American Medical Association

ASCP—American Society of Clinical Pathologists

BSN—bachelor of science degree in nursing

CAM—complementary alternative medicine

DO—doctor of osteopathy

DEA—Drug Enforcement Agency

DME—durable medical equipment

FDA—Federal Drug Administration

HIPAA—Health Insurance Portability and Accountability Act

HUC— health unit coordinator

LPN—licensed practical nurse

LVN—licensed vocational nurse

MD—medical doctor

MLT—medical laboratory technologist

MPJE—Multistate Pharmacy Jurisprudence Exam

NAPLEX—North American Pharmacist Licensure Exam

NP—nurse practitioner

OTC—over the counter

PA—physician assistant

PT—physical therapist

PTA—physical therapist assistant

RN—registered nurse

Certification Exam Coverage

AAMA (CMA) Exam Coverage:

- Professionalism
  - Supporting professional organization
  - Accepting responsibility for own actions
- Working as a team member to achieve goals
  - Member responsibility
  - Promoting competent patient care
- Time management
  - Establishing priorities
  - Managing routine duties

AMT (CMAS) Exam Coverage:

- Professionalism
  - Employ human relations skills appropriate to the health care setting
  - Display behaviors of a professional medical administrative specialist
  - Participate in appropriate continuing education

AMT (RMA) Exam Coverage:

- Patient relations
  - Identify and employ professional conduct in all aspects of patient care
- Patient relations
  - Recognize the importance of professional development through continuing education

NCCT (NCMA) Exam Coverage:

- Medical Office Management
  - Patient instruction
  - Organizational skills

AAMA (CMA) certification exam topics are reprinted with permission of the American Association of Medical Assistants.

AMT (CMAS) certification exam topics are reprinted with permission of American Medical Technologists.

AMT (RMA) certification exam topics are reprinted with permission of American Medical Technologists.

NCCT (NCMA) certification exam topics © 2013 National Center for Competency Testing. Reprinted with permission of NCCT.

Introduction

Medical assistants, along with physicians, pharmacists, nurses, and other staff, work as part of a health care team that cares for patients. Some patients receive care from multiple specialists, while others see only single primary care physicians. Medical assistants must practice the art of listening to patients and relay information effectively between patients and all other members of the health care team. Medical assistants should be skilled in the areas of all necessary administrative and clinical competencies and must always practice only within their scope of practice.

Working in Health Care Today

Health care is constantly changing and growing. As the population ages and the demand for health care continues to rise, more and more patients will seek medical care. As this increase in the need for health care rises, medical assistants will become more in demand. According to the U.S. Department of Labor Web site (2014), "Employment [for medical assistants] is expected to grow by 29 percent from 2012–2022, much faster than the average for all occupations. Demand will stem from physicians hiring more medical assistants to do routine administrative and clinical duties so that physicians can see more patients." The number of medical assisting jobs in the United States as of 2012 was 571,690, with an additional 162,900 jobs expected by the year 2022.

The Medical Assistant's Career Opportunities

Medical assistants today can work in a variety of health care specialties or in more administrative capacities, depending on the needs of the medical practice. According to the U.S. Department of Labor, most medical assistants today work in **ambulatory care centers** under the direction of physicians; some work in public and private hospitals, including inpatient and outpatient facilities; and some work in the offices of other health practitioners, such as chiropractors, optometrists, and podiatrists. The remaining medical assistants work in public and private educational services, state and local government agencies, employment services, medical and diagnostic laboratories, and nursing care facilities.

Medical assistants earn varying amounts depending on their experience, skill levels, and locations. In the United States in 2012, the median annual earnings of medical assistants was $30,780. Table 3-1 lists quick facts on medical assistants and the job outlook for this profession. This data is updated by the U.S. Department of Labor and can be found on their Web site: http://www.dol.gov/.

TABLE 3-1 Quick Facts: Medical Assistants	
2012 median pay	$14.80 per hour $30,780 per year
Entry level education	High school diploma or equivalent
On-the-job training	Moderate term on-the-job training
Number of jobs, 2012	571,690
Job outlook, 2012–2022	29% growth (much faster than average)
Employment change, 2012–2022	162,900 new jobs

Source: US Department of Labor: www.dol.gov

Choosing Medical Assisting as a Career

Medical assisting is a career with multiple responsibilities, and it requires a set of unique qualities, including, but not limited to, loyalty, empathy, dependability, and flexibility. The following sections discuss medical assisting responsibilities and the desirable medical assisting attributes sought out by potential employers.

Medical Assisting Responsibilities

As mentioned earlier, the medical assistant helps the physician on the health care team provide patient care. To help keep patients safe, the medical assistant must be proficient in their **clinical skills**, which include taking vital signs, collecting specimens, and may include administering medications and immunizations. Specific clinical duties for the medical assistant depend on the scope of practice in the state where the medical assistant is employed. The following is a list of some, but not all, duties the clinical medical assistant may be responsible for in the medical office:

- Disinfection procedures
- Preparing, administering, and documenting various types of medication via various routes
- Obtaining vital signs (temperature, pulse, respirations, blood pressure), and obtaining weight and height measurements
- Preparing the patient for physical examination and assisting the physician
- Preparing the patient for surgical procedures
- Obtaining and preparing specimens for microbiological examination
- Hematology procedures
- Medical imaging procedures (e.g., performing the general procedure for an X-ray examination)
- Pulmonology and pulmonary testing (spirometry, measuring oxygen saturation, peak flow testing, etc.)

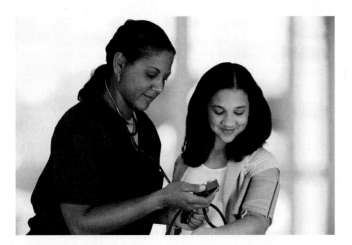

Figure 3-1 ■ Medical assistants must develop a rapport with patients.
Source: Fotolia © Rob.

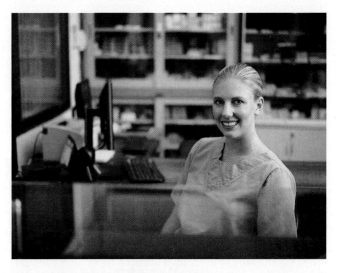

Figure 3-2 ■ This medical assistant's responsibilities are weighted in the administrative arena.
Source: Fotolia © Diego Cervo.

- Assisting with the examination and treatment of various body system disorders
- Responding to emergency situations

While patient care is part of medical assisting, the medical assistant's main responsibility is to be the patient's **advocate.** Because medical assistants will likely spend more time with patients than the physicians, medical assistants must develop a **rapport** with patients. Patients must be able to trust medical assistants, because those patients are more likely to share their personal information with medical assistants they trust (**Figure 3-1** ■).

In addition to clinical skills, medical assistants are responsible for performing **administrative skills.** The types of administrative duties medical assistants perform depend on the type, size, and needs of the practice, as well as the medical assistants' preferences. The following is a list of some, but not all, duties the administrative medical assistant may be responsible for in the medical office:

- Front desk reception (opening and closing the office, greeting and registering patients, collecting payments at the front desk, closing the office)
- Telephone procedures (answering the telephone in a professional manner, taking telephone messages, calling a pharmacy with prescription orders)
- Understanding medical law and ethics and how they apply to the preparation of patient paperwork (informed consent forms, authorization for the release of medical records, etc.)
- Patient education and identifying community resources
- Patient scheduling using various systems
- Medical records management
- Composing and managing written and electronic correspondence
- Using computers effectively in the medical office

- Equipment, maintenance, and supply inventory
- Creating and maintaining office policies and procedures
- Insurance billing and authorization
- Diagnostic and procedural coding
- Payroll, accounts payable, and banking procedures
- Billing, collections, and credit procedures
- Managing the medical office
- Responding to emergency situations

Medical assistants may choose to apply for positions that have responsibilities weighted in the clerical or clinical arenas. In small clinics, medical assistants often perform both administrative and clinical functions. In large offices, job duties are often more specialized. Medical assistants in these offices may work in the clinical or administrative areas exclusively (**Figure 3-2** ■).

Positive Medical Assisting Qualities

To be highly valued in today's competitive job market, medical assistants should have good clinical and administrative skills. The most sought-after medical assistants can perform varied duties in the medical office, applying their skills where those skills are needed most. To ensure they gain the proper skills, medical assistants should complete accredited programs. They should have a good understanding of medical terminology, and they should be well versed in the scope of their professional duties.

In addition to the proper background and training, good medical assistants have sound interpersonal skills. For a list of some desired qualities, see Table 3-2. Because many patients will stop seeing physicians when they feel uncomfortable with

TABLE 3-2 Desirable Medical Assisting Qualities	
Quality	**Explanation**
Loyalty	• Being faithful to one's employer, performing to the best of one's abilities, and arriving to work on time and ready to perform the job. Loyalty is staying with an employer through good days and bad.
Respect	• Treating coworkers and patients with honor. Staff should demonstrate respect for physicians by using the title "Doctor" in front of patients, and doctors should show respect for their staff in return. Any corrective comments or disciplinary action should occur in private.
Dependability	• Completing tasks on time and to the best of one's abilities. Dependability is arriving to work on time and staying to the end of the assigned shift. Late arrivals and frequent cancellations disrupt the whole office. Emergencies do happen, but dependable employees can generally be counted on to arrive and work when scheduled.
Courtesy	• Extending polite words and compassion to patients and coworkers. Professional words and actions demonstrate courtesy.
Initiative	• Taking action without being asked. A person with initiative knows what needs to be done and does it.
Flexibility	• Willingness to exceed the job description whenever needed by changing one's schedule, if needed, or replacing someone who cannot work. Flexibility is the willingness to work late when the physician is running late and patients are still in the office. This is the ultimate sign of teamwork.
Credibility	• Trustworthiness. Credibility is the feeling employers have toward employees when those employees have demonstrated that they are open and honest in their communications and actions. Credibility is the ability to convey knowledge and wisdom.
Confidentiality	• Ability to keep patient information private, to avoid sharing that information with inappropriate parties, like coworkers or neighbors.
Attitude	• Overall approach. Positive attitudes foster positive work environments, while poor attitudes cultivate poor ones.

the office staff, patients should always feel welcome and cared for in the medical office. For example, good medical assistants remember patients' names. It helps make patients feel important and builds patient rapport.

◦ In Practice

A new patient in town, Isaiah Rodriguez, arrives at the office needing a physician. According to Isaiah, his last physician had an unpleasant receptionist. Isaiah tells the medical assistant, "If I didn't like my doctor so much, I would have found another one." He adds that the person who answered his call for this appointment seemed like she was in a hurry. How should the medical assistant handle this situation? What can the medical assistant say to Isaiah? Should the medical assistant bring the situation to the doctor's attention? Why or why not?

Effective medical assistants communicate well with patients as well as with other members of the health care team. Medical assistants should have **empathy** for others, and they should be comfortable in their role as patient advocates. Empathy is the concept of identifying with what the patient is feeling or experiencing. Sympathy, on the other hand, is sharing the feelings of another, typically feelings of sorrow or sadness. In a country as diverse as the United States, medical assistants should know the prevailing cultural customs in their areas and keep their personal beliefs separate from patient care. Medical assistants should also maintain patient confidentiality, disclosing personal patient information only when providing information to other providers, to governmental agencies, for mandatory reporting, or when directed to do so by a patient or a court order.

Living and working in the same community can pose special challenges for health care staff who work with private patient information. Medical assistants know confidential patient information and are obligated by the Health Insurance Portability and Accountability Act (**HIPAA**), as well as ethical considerations, to keep that information private. In small communities, patients may ask about other patients outside the office. Medical assistants should never breach patient privacy, whatever the setting.

The medical assisting profession changes as health care advances. In order to keep up with these changes, medical assistants should join their local professional associations and attend meetings with these groups. Often, these local association meetings provide medical assistants with continuing education opportunities. These continuing education meetings may offer medical assistants credits toward applying for recertification as a medical assistant. Requirements regarding the number of continuing education hours and credits required for medical assistants vary from one state to another.

HIPAA Compliance

The Health Insurance Portability and Accountability Act (HIPAA) requires that medical assistants carefully guard patient confidentiality. Medical assistants should never release patient information without a patient's written authorization or a court order except to coordinate treatment, protect the public, make required reports to governmental agencies, with the patient's written authorization, or with a court order.

▸▸▸ Pulse Points

Patient Confidentiality

The responsibility of protecting patient confidentiality extends beyond the work day. Never discuss patients by name outside the office, even when with coworkers. Always imagine that the patients, or people who know them, can hear the conversation. Imagine how breaching patient confidentiality would affect you and the physician.

Like ethical behavior, a professional image is a critical part of medical assisting. Medical assistants are often a patient's first contact with the office, and their behavior and appearance directly reflect the office and the physicians. Demonstrating professionalism means avoiding eating, drinking, and chewing gum while working or in patient view and maintaining a professional attitude. Part of maintaining a professional attitude includes remaining calm and polite and preventing patients from sensing any stress or irritation. Good medical assistants keep their personal feelings to themselves, never indicating disagreement with patients' health care or lifestyle choices. **Body language**, like facial expressions, may indicate disapproval. Table 3-3 provides examples of body language in different cultures.

Critical Thinking Question 3-1

Thinking back to the case study at the beginning of the chapter, imagine that a patient overhears William talking about a patient from earlier in the day. What might that patient think about William's professionalism? Do you imagine the patient would feel comfortable sharing private details with William? Why or why not?

Good medical assistants give the same level of professional care to all patients, even those who are rude and unpleasant. Good assistants also use proper grammar when communicating with patients, and that means avoiding slang terms or phrases. Patients who speak English as a second language might be unfamiliar with slang terms and misinterpret their meanings.

TABLE 3-3 Body Language in Different Cultures

Culture	Examples
Asian-Pacific	• An open mouth, as when yawning, is considered rude. • Smiling can mean happiness, anger, confusion, or sadness. • Pointing with fingers is considered rude.
Chinese	• Being physically intimidating, such as moving into a person's personal space without first gaining permission, especially with an older person, is considered very rude. • Pointing is appropriate with an open hand, never with just one finger.
Japanese	• Bowing is a traditional greeting. • Staring is considered rude. • Standing with the hands in pockets is considered rude. • The "OK" symbol (the thumb and forefinger joined in a circle) may be interpreted as the signal for money.
Korean	• Prolonged direct eye contact is considered rude. • Entering a room without knocking is considered rude. • Spitting and burping in public is acceptable.
Filipino	• Hugging upon first meeting is acceptable. • Greetings include raised eyebrows. • Staring is considered rude.
Arabic	• Failing to face a person while speaking is considered rude. • Men stand when women enter a room. • Men may shake hands with women only when the women offer their hands. • Only the right hand is used for eating.
Hispanic	• Pointing with the index finger has a sexual meaning. • Standing close together is appropriate.

Good personal hygiene, like professional behavior, is part of a professional image. Medical assistants should practice good personal hygiene for their body and their clothing. For example, American Medical Association (**AMA**) studies have shown that artificial nails may harbor bacteria, which is difficult to remove with hand washing. As a result, artificial nails should not be worn on the job. Medical assistants should also avoid wearing excessive or obtrusive jewelry, because hands will be washed and gloves donned several times a day. Body piercings, except for posts in the ear lobes, should not be visible, and tattoos and other body art should be covered during office hours. Hair should be clean and pulled back, and scented lotions and perfumes should be minimized out of respect for patients with allergies. These are policies that are dictated by the employers, so medical assistants will need to be aware of how their employer wishes them to comply with dress codes.

Uniforms, including shoes, should be clean and in good repair. The medical assistant's nametag should be in plain view and clearly identify the name and role of the medical assistant. Policies for dress, jewelry, hairstyles, piercings, and tattoos will vary from office to office, so medical assistants should review these policies when they are hired (**Figure 3-3** ■). Certain cultural manners of dress are appropriate for the medical assistant, including head coverings for both men and women whose faith mandates this.

Critical Thinking Question 3-2

Referring to the case study at the beginning of the chapter, what is it about William's appearance that may make him seem less professional than patients would like to see in their medical assistant?

Critical Thinking Question 3-3

Refer back to the case study at the beginning of the chapter. Given William's unprofessional appearance due to poor hygiene, do you think patients might think he is less than capable of taking care of patient needs? How would you react if you had such a medical assistant taking care of you during your own physician visit?

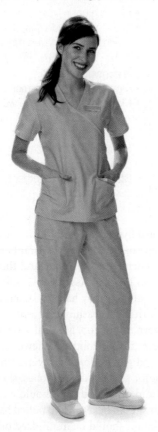

Figure 3-3 ■ The medical assistant must maintain a professional image.
Source: Fotolia © Eric Simard.

The Medical Assistant's Role Outside of the Office

In some ways, health care workers are held to a higher standard than those in many other fields. The medical assistant's professional image is expected to extend beyond the medical office, and the rules of patient confidentiality apply in all environments. When medical assistants work in the communities where they live, they are likely to see patients outside the clinical

▶▶▶ Pulse Points

Maintaining a Professional Image

- **Leave personal problems at home.** As much as possible, avoid bringing personal problems to work. When personal problems become overwhelming, consider taking a day or two off to address them.

- **Avoid office gossip.** Refuse to gossip and spread rumors, because doing so is unproductive and can be harmful. Even when true, office information should be kept confidential. Consider how you would feel if you were the subject.

- **Conduct no personal business during work hours.** Personal business takes time from the employer. Respect your employer's time, and conduct personal business, like telephone calls or texting, during breaks or before or after work. Remember that patients might overhear your conversations, so always act professionally and courteously. When you must make a personal call during business hours, do so from a private room or outside the building.

- **Stay out of office politics.** Avoid office politics, because they are particularly destructive. Do not take credit for coworkers' accomplishments or blame others for your mistakes.

- **Do not procrastinate.** Practice prioritization rather than procrastination. Rank activities so you can complete them in an acceptable time frame. When a project seems too big to handle, try breaking it into smaller pieces, or seek help.

- **Be mindful of what is posted on social media sites.** Though employers might be legally restricted from using information found on employees' social media sites as cause for disciplinary action, any information that breaches HIPAA legislation may be cause for termination. Medical assistants should be aware that anything posted on a social media site might be seen by employers, or even patients. The information placed on a social media site is irretrievable once it is posted.

setting. Medical assistants must remember that they represent the medical office at all times, not just during business hours. This professional standard extends to areas such as social media that have become commonplace only in the last few years. When the medical assistant posts something unprofessional on a social media site, such as Facebook or Twitter, that information might be seen by employers or even patients in the facility where the medical assistant is employed.

Critical Thinking Question 3-4

Refer back to the case study at the beginning of the chapter. How might William's gossiping about patients be a problem with regard to HIPAA regulations? What might his supervisor tell him about HIPAA law to help him understand how to protect patient privacy?

Effective Time Management

In a busy health care setting, demands on the medical assistant's time can seem overwhelming. Depending on the office, one medical assistant might support several physicians. Especially in these situations, it is important for medical assistants to track their job duties and to know who to consult when their priorities conflict. In most cases, the medical assistant will have only one supervisor; the supervisor is the person who should be consulted if the medical assistant is given conflicting orders from different physicians.

Good organization is key to medical-office time management. A time-management outline, which prioritizes projects, is one way for medical assistants to manage their time effectively (**Figure 3-4** ■). Writing down tasks is a good habit to develop. It is easier to divide big projects into smaller tasks or to organize tasks into a workable schedule. List items according to their due dates, and then categorize those items depending on how long they will take to complete. To stay on top of tasks, at the end of each day make a "to-do" list for the following day (**Figure 3-5** ■). Crossing items off the list as they are completed gives a sense of accomplishment and helps to ensure all tasks are completed.

Many medical assistants are expected to perform tasks other than patient care. These tasks, such as stocking supplies in exam rooms or calling in prescriptions to pharmacies, will need to be fit in between the times patients are seen in the office. Good time management includes fitting those tasks into the day, perhaps while the physician is with the patient, rather than rushing to get through the tasks at the end of the day. The medical assistant who feels he or she has too many tasks to reasonably complete during the day should consult the supervisor for guidance on how tasks should be prioritized.

If these techniques fail to help the medical assistant manage time effectively, try keeping a journal of each activity

---

TIME MANAGEMENT OUTLINE

8-9 a.m. Meet with lead RN and MA

9-945 a.m. Return telephone calls from previous work day

945-1030 a.m. Update schedules for staffing for next work day

1030-1130 a.m. Meet with suppliers

1130-12 p.m. Meet with MDs

12-1 p.m. Lunch

1-2 p.m. Make rounds through the departments to check in with staff members

2-3 p.m. Make telephone calls to patients regarding patient satisfaction details

3-4 p.m. Meet with lead RN and MA

4-5 p.m. Go over schedule for next work day, determine needs that may arise

Figure 3-4 ■ Effective time management may be easier with the use of a time-management outline.

and the time it takes. The following steps are involved in creating and using such a time-management journal:

1. At the beginning of the work day, place a notepad and pen in your clinic jacket.
2. Each time you perform a task, list the task and the exact time it took from beginning to end.

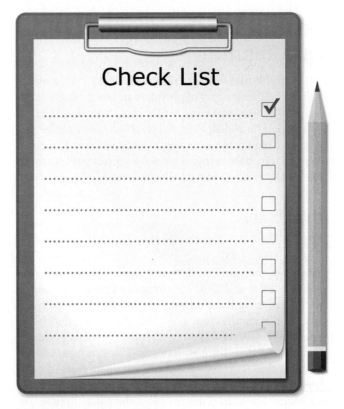

Figure 3-5 ■ Using a checklist is a good way to stay organized.
Source: Fotolia. © Aleksandr Bryliaev.

3. Note any conflicts, such as overlapping requests from supervisors.

4. At the end of the day, analyze the data. Determine if any tasks were unneeded or could be combined. For example, you might be making multiple trips to the file room for patient's charts instead of pulling all charts at the beginning of each shift. You might need data from more than one day to obtain an accurate picture of an average work day.

5. When you find no tasks to omit or combine, schedule a meeting with your supervisor to try to achieve a more efficient workflow.

It is important for medical assistants to collaborate with their supervisors on time-management initiatives. Office managers and physicians should strive to keep their employees happy and efficient, and medical assistants who raise concerns about their use of time show that they are responsible members of the health care team.

Critical Thinking Question 3-5

Referring to the case study at the beginning of the chapter, how might William's frequent tardiness be a problem for his coworkers? If you were William's coworker, what might you do if you were the one who had to pick up William's job responsibilities each time he arrives late for his shift?

Members of the Health Care Team

Today's health care team is **multidisciplinary**, which means that many different types of providers and medical specialists help provide a patient's care. Medical assistants should have a good working knowledge of the types of care these professionals provide so they can accurately relay information to patients when doctors make referrals, as well as direct patients to the appropriate members of the health care team.

Physicians

The term *physician* refers to a medical doctor (**MD**) or doctor of osteopathy (**DO**). Many people use these terms interchangeably, but generally the term refers to one who practices medicine. MDs and DOs are similar in many ways, and in most states, these two professionals are seen as virtually the same. For example, both complete the same educational requirements (see the following section); both obtain graduate medical education (through residencies, internships, and fellowships) that takes between three and eight years to complete; both can practice in any specialty; and they must both pass examinations in order to obtain their state license. The main difference between an MD and a DO is that a DO receives additional training in the musculoskeletal system.

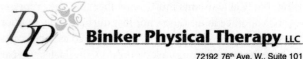

Binker Physical Therapy LLC

Molly K. Malone PT
Espen Ford OT

72192 76th Ave. W., Suite 101
Wynnwood, WA 98088

Phone: 425-555-9991
Fax: 425-555-9995

Date _____

Patient's Name _____

Diagnosis _____

_____

ICD-9 Codes _____

Requested Treatment _____

☐ Evaluate & Treat

☐ Specific Treatment _____

_____

_____

Frequency: _____ times per week for _____ weeks.

Precautions _____

_____

_____

Physician Re-check Date _____

Physician's signature below constitutes letter of medical necessity.

_____
Physician's Signature

Figure 3-6 ■ Sample referral form for sending a patient out for physical therapy.

The DO treats the "whole" person, focusing not only on specific illnesses or symptoms, but rather treating the body as an integrated whole. The additional training on the musculoskeletal system provides the osteopathic physician with a more in-depth understanding of how illness can affect different parts of the body. There are more physicians with the MD degree, mainly because there are far more medical schools than osteopathy schools.

Physicians typically head the health care team, directing other medical-office staff. Physicians diagnose and treat patients, as well as refer patients to other members of the health care team. **Figure 3-6** ■ is an example of a referral form that would be used to send a patient to a physician outside the practice.

The Physician's Education Requirements

Medical training for physicians varies around the world, but all physicians must pass a licensure examination to practice medicine in the United States, as well as apply for a license in whichever states they wish to practice.

In the United States, physicians must first obtain at least a four-year undergraduate or bachelor's degree, which usually consists of varied premedical courses. After that, they must then attend four years of medical school, followed by a residency program. Residency programs usually concentrate on the fields the physicians wish to practice in, such as dermatology or emergency medicine. Residency programs vary from two to six years.

Pharmacists

Pharmacists play an important role in patient care. They distribute the drugs prescribed by health care providers and educate patients about the medications they are taking. Some pharmacists work for pharmacies, while others own them. Many large health care facilities, including hospitals, have pharmacies on their premises, which can be convenient for patients. Some pharmacists work for drug manufacturers researching new medications. **Figure 3-7** ■ shows an example of a sample prescription that would be filled by a pharmacist.

Pharmacists who work in community or retail pharmacies often counsel patients and answer questions about medications, both prescriptions and over-the-counter (**OTC**) medications, including possible side effects or drug interactions. Pharmacists may also advise patients about the use of durable medical equipment (**DME**), diet, exercise, or stress management. Patients

who are allergic to certain substances might also need accommodations. Pharmacists understand that they need to be aware of any cultural accommodations a patient might require with regard to taking medications. Pharmacists also need to be connected to an online system for identifying medications that patients bring in from outside the United States. This is important, as some medications may conflict with those prescribed by the patient's physician here in the United States.

The Pharmacist's Education Requirements

A license to practice pharmacy is required in all 50 of the United States, the District of Columbia, and all U.S. territories. To obtain a license to practice, pharmacists must graduate from a college of pharmacy that is accredited by the Accreditation Council for Pharmacy Education (**ACPE**) and pass an examination. All states require pharmacists to pass the North American Pharmacist Licensure Exam (**NAPLEX**), which tests pharmacy skills and knowledge. The District of Columbia and 43 of the United States also require pharmacists to pass the Multistate Pharmacy Jurisprudence Exam (**MPJE**), which tests knowledge of pharmacy law.

As of 2013, 129 colleges of pharmacy were accredited in the United States. Pharmacy programs grant the degree of Doctor of Pharmacy (Pharm D), which requires at least six years of college, including extensive courses in all aspects of drug therapy.

Pharmacy Technicians

Pharmacy technicians typically work under the direction and supervision of a licensed pharmacist. This position requires dispensing prescription drugs and other medical devices to patients and often instructing patients on their use. Pharmacy technicians may also perform certain administrative duties, such as reviewing prescription refill requests, contacting physician offices regarding prescriptions, and checking with insurance companies to determine patient coverage for needed medications. Pharmacy technicians typically work in pharmacies and in hospitals.

Education Requirements for Pharmacy Technicians

Becoming a pharmacy technician usually requires earning a high school diploma or the equivalent. Pharmacy technicians typically learn through on-the-job training, or they may complete a postsecondary education program. Though no mandated regulatory agency regulates pharmacy technicians, each state dictates the training requirements this professional needs to perform his or her work.

Physician Assistants

Physician assistants (**PAs**) are clinicians who are licensed to practice medicine under the supervision of a physician or a

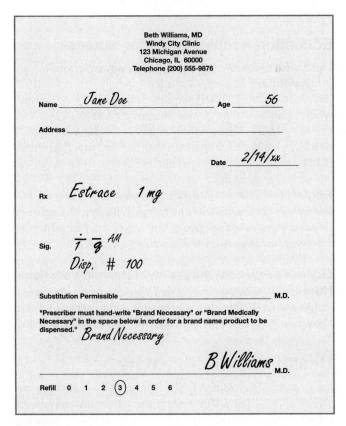

Figure 3-7 ■ Sample prescription.

surgeon. PAs can treat patients, including taking medical histories, performing examinations, interpreting laboratory tests and X-rays, and making diagnoses. PAs will often perform such tasks as suturing, splinting, and casting. In 48 states, PAs can also prescribe medications.

The Physician Assistant's Education Requirements

As of 2013, there were 141 accredited PA programs in the United States. All states require PAs to complete an accredited, formal education program and pass a national exam to obtain a license. PA programs are generally two or more years long, and admission requirements vary. Many programs require at least two years of college and some health care experience before admission.

Nurse Practitioners

Nurse practitioners (**NPs**) provide services similar to those of the PA. The main differences between these two professions are that the NP is also a trained nurse, and NPs require more training than PAs. Most NPs have advanced nursing degrees and many are able to open their own clinical practices, depending on the laws in their states. NPs are also allowed to prescribe medications and have Drug Enforcement Administration (**DEA**) registration numbers in most states. NPs can serve as patients' primary care providers and can see patients of all ages.

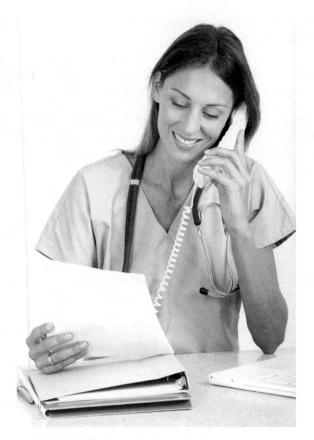

Figure 3-8 ■ A nurse performing telephone triage.
Source: Shutterstock © kurhan.

The Nurse Practitioner's Education Requirements

To be licensed as NPs, applicants must first complete the education and training needed to be a registered nurse (**RN**). In most states, NPs are also required to have a master's degree in nursing. Once applicants have secured their RN degree, they must complete an advanced nursing education program. Many of these programs specialize in a field like family practice, adult health, acute care, or women's health. NPs must be licensed by the states where they practice.

Nurses

Nurses are employed in varied health care settings. Nurses may work in hospitals, with insurance companies, or in home health care settings. In most medical practices today, depending on their degree, nurses perform triage roles or help physicians with complex cases (**Figure 3-8** ■). Medical assistants assist the physician in other cases. Each state outlines the scope of practice for nurses. Typically, nurses are able to perform more invasive procedures and administer more classifications of medications than medical assistants are allowed within scope of practice. As with all medical professions, the nursing scope of practice is dictated by the state within which the nurse practices.

Education Requirements for Nurses

Unlike the education requirements of many other health care professions, nursing education has many levels. A bachelor degree in nursing (**BSN**) requires four years of education, whereas an associate degree in nursing (**ADN**) takes two years. Typically, nurses with more advanced degrees (e.g., RN or BSN) have higher-level duties than licensed practical nurses (**LPNs**) or licensed vocational nurses (**LVNs**).

Registered Nurses   Registered nurses (**RNs**) usually follow one of these education pathways: a bachelor's degree in nursing, an associate's degree in nursing, or a diploma from an approved nursing program. RNs must be licensed.

Licensed Practical Nurses and Licensed Vocational Nurses   To become an LPN or LVN, one must complete a state-approved educational program, which typically takes about one year to complete. LPNs and LVNs must be licensed.

Health Unit Coordinators

Many medical offices and facilities hire health unit coordinators (**HUCs**). These staff members are commonly tasked with duties such as transcribing physicians' orders, scheduling diagnostic studies and appointments for followup care, ordering and maintaining office supplies, and maintaining patient medical records and consent forms.

Education Requirements for Health Unit Coordinators

Health unit coordinators may be trained on the job, with no prior medical training, or they may go through certificate programs to learn the tasks in a formal environment. Many medical offices hire medical assistants in the role of the health unit coordinator.

Medical Laboratory Technologists

Medical laboratory technologists (MLTs) are staff members who collect samples and perform tests to analyze bodily fluids, tissues, and other substances. Although many medical laboratory technologists work in hospital settings, they are also employed in ambulatory care settings where a laboratory is present. These laboratories are typically those that perform mid- to high-level tests with equipment that requires training to use.

Education Requirements for Medical Laboratory Technologists

Medical laboratory technologists typically have a 4-year college degree, and some states require these technologists to be licensed. The American Society of Clinical Pathologists (**ASCP**) is the agency that provides certification for medical laboratory technicians.

Registered Dietitians and Nutritionists

Registered dietitians are the members of the health care team that provide dietary and nutrition advice to patients. They are experts in food and nutrition, and they advise individuals on what they should eat to lead a healthy lifestyle or to achieve health-related goals. Dietitians and nutritionists work in varied settings, including nursing homes, hospitals, clinics, and facilities that care for patients that may have special dietary needs, such as diabetics.

Education Requirements for Registered Dieticians and Nutritionists

Registered dieticians typically complete a bachelor's degree and pass a national examination administered by the Commission on Dietetic Registration. Most have also participated in supervised training through an internship or as part of their coursework.

Phlebotomists

Phlebotomists draw blood for tests, transfusions, research, or blood donations. Phlebotomists are employed in ambulatory care settings as well as in hospitals and skilled nursing facilities.

Some phlebotomists work for agencies that provide home care, requiring the phlebotomist to go to patients' homes to draw blood samples.

Education Requirements for Phlebotomists

To be certified as a phlebotomist, applicants must attend a phlebotomy technician program and then sit for a national examination. A phlebotomist's training is more extensive than the phlebotomy training that medical assistants receive in their programs.

Physical Therapists

Physical therapists (**PTs**) are licensed professionals that work with injured or ill patients to help restore function, improve mobility, relieve pain, and prevent injuries. PTs are often an important part of rehabilitation and treatment of patients with chronic conditions or injuries. These professionals typically work in private offices and clinics, hospitals, and nursing homes.

Education Requirements for Physical Therapists

Physical therapists must complete an accredited physical therapy degree, a degree that is typically a Doctor of Physical Therapy. Physical therapists must also be licensed in the state in which they practice.

Physical Therapy Assistants and Physical Therapy Aides

Physical therapy assistants (**PTAs**) and physical therapy aides work under the direction and supervision of physical therapists. These individuals help patients who are recovering from injuries and illnesses regain movement and manage pain. Most physical therapy assistants and aides work in physical therapists' offices or in hospitals.

Education Requirements for Physical Therapy Assistants and Physical Therapy Aides

Physical therapy assistants must complete a two-year degree program that is accredited by the Commission on Accreditation in Physical Therapy Education. PTAs must pass a national exam to be licensed or certified to work with patients. Each state outlines the specific requirements and scope of practice for PTAs. Physical therapist aides generally have a high school diploma and receive on-the-job training.

Medical Practice Specializations

Medical and surgical specialties today are varied. Table 3-4 lists several common medical specialties and the services they provide. Table 3-5 outlines several common surgical specialties.

TABLE 3-4 Common Medical Specialties	
Specialty Type	**Service(s) Provided**
Allergist	Diagnoses and treats allergic conditions
Cardiologist	Diagnoses and treats heart and cardiovascular system conditions
Dermatologist	Diagnoses and treats skin disorders
Emergency physician	Treats patients with emergent needs, such as in emergency rooms
Endocrinologist	Diagnoses and treats hormone-related disorders
Family practitioner	Acts as a primary care physician for patients of all ages, treating varied illnesses and performing routine screenings (e.g., physical examinations)
Gastroenterologist	Diagnoses and treats disorders related to the stomach and intestines
General practitioner	Same as the family practice physician (see two above), except may not accept child patients
Gerontologist	Diagnoses and treats conditions of the elderly population
Gynecologist	Diagnoses and treats conditions related to the female reproductive system
Hematologist	Diagnoses and treats conditions associated with blood disorders
Infertility practitioner	Diagnoses and treats disorders related to infertility problems and helps achieve pregnancy via medical means
Intensive care physician	Treats patients in the hospital intensive care unit
Internist	Focuses on the prevention and treatment of adult diseases
Neonatologist	Diagnoses and treats newborns
Nephrologist	Diagnoses and treats conditions associated with the kidneys
Obstetrician	Treats pregnant women through the postpartum period
Oncologist	Diagnoses and treats patients with cancerous conditions
Ophthalmologist	Diagnoses and treats eye conditions
Orthopedist	Diagnoses and treats conditions associated with the musculoskeletal system
Otolaryngologist	Diagnoses and treats conditions associated with the ears, nose, and throat
Pediatrician	Treats children
Podiatrist	Diagnoses and treats feet conditions
Proctologist	Diagnoses and treats conditions associated with the colon, rectum, and anus
Psychiatrist	Diagnoses and treats mental disorders
Pulmonologist	Diagnoses and treats conditions associated with the respiratory system
Radiologist	Interprets radiographs (X-rays) and other imaging studies (e.g., ultrasounds or mammograms)
Rheumatologist	Diagnoses and treats conditions associated with arthritis or other joint disorders
Urologist	Diagnoses and treats conditions associated with the urinary system

Complementary and Alternative Medicine Providers

Complementary and alternative medicine (**CAM**) is another term for holistic or natural medicine. CAM providers treat patients with such alternative practices as chiropractic treatments (**Figure 3-9 ■**), acupuncture, naturopathy, massage,

biofeedback, hypnosis, and dietary supplements. For examples of these treatments, see Table 3-6.

In the United States, CAM is a $10 billion per year industry. Most of those revenues come directly from patients, not their insurance carriers, because traditional health insurance does not cover many CAM therapies. Medical assistants must alert patients that CAM therapies might not be reimbursed.

TABLE 3-5 Common Surgical Specialties

Surgical Specialty Type	Description
Cardiothoracic	Treats chest diseases and heart and lung conditions
Cosmetic	Repairs or reconstructs body parts as necessary either due to accidents or disease, or as elective surgery
General	Treats varied surgical cases
Maxillofacial	Repairs face and mouth disorders
Neurological	Repairs disorders of the neurologic system
Orthopedic	Repairs conditions of the musculoskeletal system
Vascular	Repairs conditions of the blood vessels

TABLE 3-6 Complementary and Alternative Medicine Examples

Treatment Type	Treatment Objective
Acupressure	Use hand pressure on various body areas to restore balance.
Acupuncture	Insert needles into various body areas to restore balance.
Biofeedback	Teach patients to control their involuntary body responses to treat pain and disease.
Chiropractic	Manipulate the spine and extremities to rectify misalignments, relieve pain, and treat disease.
Dietary supplements	Administer such substances as vitamins, herbs, or minerals, usually by mouth, to promote health and treat certain diseases.
Hypnosis	Induce a trance-like state to access the subconscious mind.
Magnetic therapy	Apply magnets to various body areas to correct the body's energy fields.
Massage	Use touch to relieve pain and encourage muscle relaxation.
Naturopathy	Use nutrition and exercise to promote healing and well-being.
Yoga	Use breathing exercises and poses to encourage relaxation and flexibility.

With any treatment, it is always good to verify a patient's coverage with the insurance carrier.

Because alternative therapies might not be covered by traditional insurance, the CAM industry, especially the dietary supplements industry, is highly competitive for the consumer's dollar. A 2007 survey by the American Medical Association

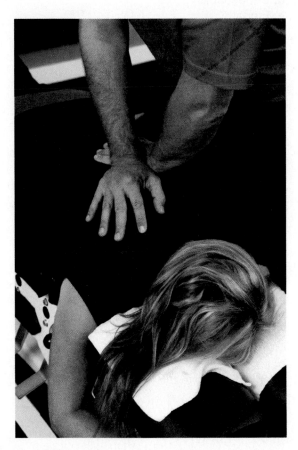

Figure 3-9 ▇ A chiropractor adjusting his patient.
Source: Fotolia © Rainer Plendl.

(AMA) found that 37% of adults in the United States said they use some form of CAM. The most commonly used CAM therapies include vitamins and herbal supplements.

CAM Approaches

Many traditional health care providers recommend or use some CAM techniques with their patients. Most patients who use CAM do so because they want more natural, drug-free types of treatment. Some patients may wish to pursue some form of CAM while undergoing traditional medical treatment. For example, a patient receiving chemotherapy for cancer might use massage for relaxation and comfort.

Even when an office does not endorse or practice CAM, patients will often ask for advice on treatments or supplements they have heard about from friends, family, neighbors, or advertisements. As a result, all members of the health care team, including the medical assistant, should have a working knowledge of each of the common CAM therapies.

Patients should always be advised to investigate thoroughly any alternative therapy and discuss that therapy with their physician before starting it. Patients have the right to seek CAM either with or instead of traditional medicine, so health care workers should respect that right even when it conflicts with their personal beliefs.

REVIEW

Chapter Summary

- Medical assistants perform varied tasks, both clinical and administrative, and keep the medical office running smoothly. The scope of medical assisting is expected to expand and to continue offering varied challenges and responsibilities.

- Effective medical assistants today have sound clinical and administrative skills, good interpersonal skills, and a professional image that extends outside the office.

- Organization and the proper tools are key to efficient time management in the medical office.

- Many medical assistants work in ambulatory care settings, insurance companies, and other care settings, but the growing nature of the industry will continue to offer medical assistants new and varied career opportunities with other members of the health care profession.

- Because the medical assistant is just one member of the health care team, he or she should know the roles and responsibilities of other staff and learn to interface with those staff properly.

- Contemporary medical and surgical specialties offer patients a wide variety of services and treatments.

- Complementary alternative medicine (CAM) is a growing alternative to traditional medical techniques.

Chapter Review

Multiple Choice

1. _____ is being faithful to the employer, performing to the best of one's abilities, and arriving to work on time.
   a. Loyalty
   b. Respect
   c. Courtesy
   d. Initiative
   e. Empathy

2. _____ is treating others in a manner that honors them.
   a. Loyalty
   b. Respect
   c. Courtesy
   d. Dependability
   e. Empathy

3. _____ is completing tasks on time and to the best of one's abilities, arriving to work on time, and staying to the end of the shift.
   a. Loyalty
   b. Respect
   c. Courtesy
   d. Dependability
   e. Empathy

4. _____ is extending polite words and compassion to others and keeping words and actions professional.
   a. Respect
   b. Courtesy
   c. Initiative
   d. Dependability
   e. Empathy

5. _____ is completing tasks without waiting to be asked.
   a. Respect
   b. Courtesy
   c. Initiative
   d. Dependability
   e. Empathy

6. Which of the following professional degrees has many associated levels of education?
   a. Physician
   b. Nurse
   c. Physician assistant
   d. Pharmacist
   e. Medical assistant

7. The American Medical Association (AMA) has shown that _____ may harbor bacteria that are not removed with normal washing.
   a. artificial nails
   b. tattoos
   c. nylon stockings
   d. jewelry
   e. all of the above

True/False

T F 1. According to the U.S. Department of Labor Bureau of Labor Statistics, medical assisting is projected to be the fastest growing occupation from 2010–2020.

T F 2. Massage uses touch to relieve pain and encourage muscle relaxation.

T F 3. Acupuncture is the practice of inducing a trance-like state.

T F 4. Natural medicine is sometimes called holistic medicine.

T F 5. CAM services are nearly always covered in full by health insurance.

T F 6. Chiropractic is only for the treatment of back pain.

T F 7. Nurses are allowed to perform minor invasive procedures in some states, depending on that state's scope of practice.

T F 8. Medical assistants are not obligated to maintain professional images when outside the office.

Short Answer

1. What is the pharmacist's role on the patient's health care team?
2. Explain how a PA differs from an NP.
3. Why would a patient seek CAM services?
4. Explain why medical assistants should not wear scented perfumes, lotions, or colognes while working.
5. Explain why it is important for medical assistants to know their coworkers' job duties.

Research

1. Think back to your last visit as a patient with a health care provider. Did the staff you encountered act in a professional manner? Describe the visit and what you felt was professional, or unprofessional, about the actions.
2. Speak with some of your friends about how they would describe professionalism in the health care setting. What is the same or different about their ideas?
3. Using the Internet as a resource, look up definitions for professionalism. What do you find?

Practicum Application Experience

Markus is helping his patient, Sun Chien, complete her paperwork on her first office visit when she mentions that she is seeing a chiropractor. When Markus asks Sun to describe the symptoms for which Sun seeks chiropractic care, she tells him she does not believe the doctor will care about her seeing a chiropractor. How should Markus respond to Sun?

Resource Guide

American Association of Medical Assistants
20 N. Wacker Dr., Suite 1575
Chicago, IL 60606
Phone: (312) 899-1500
Fax: (312) 899-1259
www.aama-ntl.org

Harris, P. R., and Moran, R. T. (1977). *Managing cultural differences.* Houston: Gulf Publishing Co.

Mayo Clinic—Stress and Time Management Techniques
www.mayoclinic.com
Search for "time management."

National Center for Complementary and Alternative Medicine
9000 Rockville Pike
Bethesda, MD 20892
http://nccam.nih.gov/

U.S. Department of Labor Bureau of Labor Statistics
Postal Square Building
2 Massachusetts Ave., NE
Washington, DC 20212-0001
Phone: (202) 691-5200
Fax: (202) 691-6325
www.bls.gov/

4

Medicine and the Law

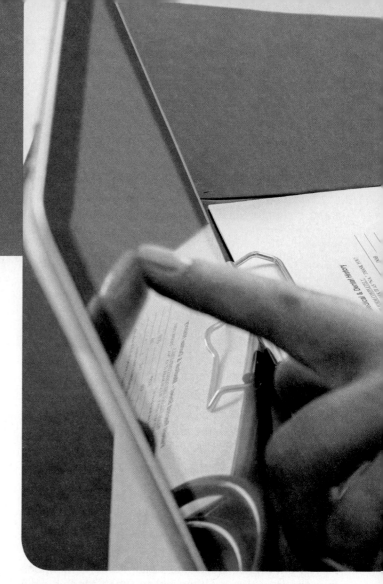

Case Study

Read the following case study and answer the critical thinking questions presented throughout the chapter.

Victoria Mason is a registered medical assistant in Dr. Kozlowski's office. Victoria takes a telephone call from a man named Bart. He tells Victoria that one of his employees is a patient of Dr. Kozlowski's and asks her to tell him when his employee was last in the office and what treatment she received.

Objectives

After completing this chapter, you should be able to:

4.1 Define and spell the key terminology in this chapter.

4.2 Explain the sources of law.

4.3 Classify varied laws as they apply to health care.

4.4 Understand and classify types of consent.

4.5 Define the types of malpractice, and describe the types of malpractice insurance policies available.

4.6 Describe how medical malpractice is proven.

4.7 Describe how to prevent and defend against medical malpractice claims.

4.8 Describe the concept of tort reform and how it applies to malpractice cases.

4.9 Outline the physician's public duties and describe causes for disciplinary action.

4.10 Compare the duties of the physician and the patient in the physician–patient relationship.

4.11 Define the types of contracts in health care.

4.12 Define the Good Samaritan Act.

4.13 List ways in which administrative medical assistants can help maintain patient confidentiality through proper medical records handling.

4.14 Describe the Health Insurance Portability and Accountability Act (HIPAA) and how it affects health care clinics and providers

4.15 List and describe various types of advance directives.

4.16 Discuss employment laws and their impact on health care.

4.17 Outline important information contained in the patients' bill of rights.

4.18 Identify the monitoring agencies that address ambulatory health care.

4.19 Define the Controlled Substances Act and discuss the rules of compliance.

Competency Skills Performance

1. Prepare an informed consent for treatment form.
2. Obtain authorization for the release of patient medical records.
3. Respond to a request for copies of a patient's medical record.

Key Terminology

administrative law—legislation passed by administrative governmental agencies

advance directives—directions for medical staff to follow in the event the patient cannot speak for herself

appeal—request for review of a denied service or claim, in an attempt to see the insurance company's denial reversed or overturned

assault—threat of causing physical harm to another without their consent

assumption of risk—defense to medical malpractice in which the provider must prove the patient was fully informed of a procedure's risks

battery—act of harming another person without the person's consent

civil law—legislation that governs actions between two or more citizens

commercial law—legislation that governs business transactions

common law—legislation derived from the Old English legal system that is based on precedence

comparative negligence—defense to medical malpractice in which the physician proves the patient was partly responsible for the patient's injury

constitutional law—law outlined in the U.S. Constitution

contract law—legislation that relates agreements between two parties

contributory negligence—defense to medical malpractice in which the physician proves an injury would not have occurred if not for the patient's actions

criminal law—legislation that relates to crimes

damages—money a patient is awarded for damages or injuries the patient sustained

defamation of character— intentional false or negative statements about a person that causes damages

discovery rule—legislation that states the statute of limitations begins when an injury was discovered or should have been discovered

duress—act of coercing someone into an act

expert witness—person deemed by the court to be an authority on a particular subject matter

expressed consent—agreement, either verbally or in writing, from the patient before a procedure is performed

expressed contract—a contract that identifies all the elements are specifically stated

Family Medical Leave Act (FMLA)—law pertaining to employees' ability to take unpaid leave for medical conditions, birth or adoption of a child, or to care for a family member

felony—a crime considered to be of a serious nature; characterized as any offense punishable by imprisonment for more than one year, or by death

Four Ds of Negligence—elements patients must prove in malpractice (i.e., duty, dereliction of duty, direct cause, and damages)

fraud—deceitful act done to conceal the truth

Good Samaritan Act— a law that may protect a person from negligence for voluntarily performing life-saving care

Health Insurance Portability and Accountability Act (HIPAA)—legislation that addresses patient privacy

implied consent—agreement through actions only

implied contract—agreement to a contract through actions only

informed consent—process in which a physician reviews with a patient the risks associated with a procedure, the risks of nontreatment, and accepted treatment alternatives

intentional tort—act of purposefully harming another

international law—legislation that relates to the actions that occur between two or more countries

invasion of privacy—the intentional prying or intruding into another person's confidential information or matters

malpractice—a breach of duty

malfeasance—state of performing an incorrect treatment resulting in injury to the patient

malpractice insurance policy—insurance to cover actions that have hurt a patient

misdemeanor—crime of a less serious nature; characterized as any offense punishable by no more than one year in prison

misfeasance—state of performing a procedure incorrectly resulting in injury to the patient

negligence— not acting responsibly resulting in patient harm

nonfeasance—the act of delaying or failing to perform a treatment

Patient Care Partnership—A list from the American Hospital Association (AHA) of patients' expectations, rights, and responsibilities while under care in the hospital setting

portability—state of being able to move an insurance policy from one employer to another

precedent—legal decision that sets the standard for subsequent, like cases

protected health information (PHI)—any information about health status, provision of health care, or payment for health care that can be linked to a specific individual

regulatory law—legislation that relates to government regulations

res ipsa loquitur—the Latin phrase for, "the thing speaks for itself"

res judicata—Latin phrase for "the thing has been decided"

respondeat superior—Latin phrase for "let the master answer"

settled—state in which an offer of money is extended and accepted to drop a lawsuit

Key Terminology (continued)

standard of care—the established requirements that dictate how and when care is to be provided

statute of limitations—period after an injury happens within which a patient may file a malpractice lawsuit

subpoena—a formal written document that legally requires a person or persons, via court order, to appear in court

subpoena duces tecum—a formal written document that requires a person or persons to produce records or documents in court, via court order

tort law—legislation that relates to one party injuring another

undue influence—to persuade someone to do something they do not want to do

unintentional tort—to harm another person accidentally

Abbreviations

AAMA—American Association of Medical Assistants
ADA—Americans with Disabilities Act
AHA—American Hospital Association

AHIMA—American Health Information Management Association
AIDS—acquired immune deficiency syndrome
CDC—Centers for Disease Control and Prevention
CLIA—Clinical Laboratory Improvement Amendments Act
CMS—Centers for Medical and Medicaid Services
CPR—cardiopulmonary resuscitation
DEA—Drug Enforcement Agency
DNR—do not resuscitate
EIN—employer identification number
FDA—Food and Drug Administration
FMLA—Family Medical Leave Act
HIPAA—Health Insurance Portability and Accountability Act
HIV—human immunodeficiency virus
IRS—Internal Revenue Service
MSA—medical savings account
OSHA—Occupational Safety and Health Act
PHI—protected health information
STI—sexually transmitted infection
TJC—The Joint Commission

Certification Exam Coverage

AAMA (CMA) Exam Coverage:

- Patient interviewing techniques
  - Legal restrictions

- Medicolegal guidelines and restrictions
  - Medical practice acts
  - Revocation/suspension of license
    1) Criminal/unprofessional conduct
    2) Professional/personal incapacity

- Legislation
  - Advance directives
  - Occupational Safety and Health Act (OSHA)
  - Food and Drug Administration (FDA)
  - Clinical Laboratory Improvement Act (CLIA '88)
  - Americans with Disabilities Act (ADA)
  - Health Insurance Portability and Accountability Act (HIPAA)

- Documentation/reporting
  - Sources of information
  - Drug Enforcement Administration (DEA)
  - Internal revenue service (e.g., personnel forms)
  - Employment laws
  - Personal injury occurrences

- Physician–patient relationship
  - Contract
    1) Legal obligations
    2) Consequences for noncompliance
  - Responsibility and rights
    1) Patient
    2) Physician
    3) Medical assistant
  - Professional liability
    1) Current standard of care
    2) Current legal standards
    3) Informed consent
  - Arbitration agreements
  - Affirmative defenses
    1) Statute of limitations
    2) Comparative/contributory negligence
    3) Assumption of risk
  - Termination of medical care
    1) Establishing policy
    2) Elements for withdrawal
    3) Patient notification and documentation
  - Medicolegal terms and doctrines

AAMA (CMA) certification exam topics are reprinted with permission of the American Association of Medical Assistants.

- Maintaining confidentiality
  - Agent of physician
    1) Patient rights
    2) Releasing patient information
  - Intentional tort
    1) Invasion of privacy
    2) Slander and libel

AMT (CMAS) Exam Coverage:

- Legal and ethical considerations
  - Apply principles of medical law and ethics to the health care setting
  - Recognize legal responsibilities of, and know scope of practice for the medical administrative specialist
  - Know basic laws pertaining to medical practice
  - Know and observe basic disclosure laws (patient privacy, minors, confidentiality)

AMT (RMA) Exam Coverage:

- Medical law
  - Types of consent used in medical practice
  - Disclosure laws and regulations (including HIPAA security and privacy acts, state and federal laws)
  - Laws, regulations, and acts pertaining to the practice of medicine

- Scope of practice acts regarding medical assisting
- Patient bill of rights legislation
- Licensure, certification, and registration
  - Identify credentialing requirements of medical professionals
  - Understand the application of the Clinical Laboratory Improvement Amendments of 1988 (CLIA '88)
- Terminology
  - Define terminology associated with medical law
- Legal responsibilities
  - Understand protection and limits of the Good Samaritan Act
  - Understand scope of practice when providing first aid
  - Understand mandatory reporting guidelines and procedures

NCCT (NCMA) Exam Coverage:

- Medical office management/general office procedures
  - Legal and professional concepts
  - Patient instruction
  - Cultural awareness

Introduction

Medical assistants face many situations that involve medical law. Laws tend to allow little room for opinion. Each state has unique laws governing health care and the medical assisting profession. It is crucial for medical assistants to know the laws of their states and to uphold those laws at all times. That adherence to the laws pertaining to the practice of medicine can help the medical assistant build a solid career.

The Sources of Law

The common law that exists in the United States originated from England. The common law was a body of law based on custom and the concept of precedence. Precedence is an act or an instance that may be used as an example, or standard, in subsequent similar cases. The concept of common law is still used today, but in limited form. For example, when the U.S. Supreme Court decided Roe v. Wade, that decision requires all courts in the United States to abide by that ruling.

Statutes are laws created by federal, state, or local legislators. Statutes are upheld by law enforcement, and cases may end up in local, state, or federal court systems. Medicare, Medicaid, and the Food and Drug Administration (**FDA**) are a few examples of federal agencies that create health care-related statutes.

Administrative Law

Administrative law is passed by administrative governmental agencies such as the Internal Revenue Service (**IRS**). Administrative law addresses issues of taxation, public transportation, manufacturing, the environment, and public broadcasting.

Comparing Criminal and Civil Law

The United States' judicial system has two main types of law: (1) criminal and (2) civil.

Criminal Law

Criminal law, also called penal law, focuses on issues between the government and citizens, such as **constitutional law** (law outlined in the U.S. Constitution), administrative law, and **international law** (legislation that relates to the actions that occur between two or more countries). Criminal law focuses on the public's safety and welfare, addressing people who commit crimes or other criminal offenses. **Civil law** is legislation that governs the actions between two more citizens.

Classified by severity as either felonies or misdemeanors, criminal laws vary from one state to another. In addition to state criminal laws, there are federal criminal laws. While all states have laws against such serious crimes as rape or murder, the laws for less serious crimes like theft or drug use may vary from one jurisdiction to another.

Felonies

Felonies are considered serious crimes, whereas misdemeanors are considered less serious offenses. States have varying definitions for each. Table 4-1 lists general felony categories. Some states, like New Jersey, classify felonies in four degrees. Other states place felonies in "classes," like Class A or Class 1. In cases like these, Class 1 is the most serious while Class 6 is the least.

Misdemeanors

Like felony classifications, **misdemeanor** classifications vary from state to state. Misdemeanors include such crimes as petty theft, prostitution, simple **assault**, and disorderly conduct. Because they are considered lesser crimes than felonies, misdemeanors are generally punished with lesser sentences. Felony convictions hold the possibility of more than one year in prison whereas misdemeanor convictions hold the possibility of no more than one year in prison.

Civil Law

Most cases involving the medical profession are primarily concerned with civil law because those cases are typically issues relating to **contract law** (legislation that relates agreements between two parties), **commercial law** (legislation that governs business transactions), and **tort law** (legislation that relates to one party injuring another). Contract and commercial laws address the rights and obligations one has to another, such as the doctor–patient relationship. Tort law deals with the injuries one has suffered at the hands of another, such as in cases of medical malpractice.

Tort Law

Torts are one of two types: unintentional or intentional. An **unintentional tort** occurs when a mistake is made. The vast majority of medical malpractice cases fall into this category, because unintentional torts usually involve negligence. **Negligence** is defined as not acting responsibly resulting in patient harm. In contrast, an **intentional tort** occurs when someone purposefully does something that injures someone else. Table 4-2 defines intentional torts and gives health care examples.

TABLE 4-1 Felony Categories

Felony Degree	Action of Person Being Charged
First	Committed the crime with forethought
Second	Assisted in the crime
Third	Assisted in the crime before or after the crime occurred
Fourth	Assisted the person who committed the crime

TABLE 4-2 Intentional Torts

Assault	Threat of causing physical harm to another without their consent. *Example:* Telling a patient their temperature will be taken whether they want it to be or not after they refuse to allow it.
Battery	Act of harming another person without the person's consent. *Example:* Taking a patient's temperature against the patient's will.
Defamation of character	Intentional false or negative statements about a person that causes damages. *Example:* Telling patients they should not see the cardiologist across the street because that cardiologist has a drinking problem.
Duress	Act of coercing someone into an act. *Example:* Telling patients they must have a tetanus vaccine or they will develop a life-threatening infection. The patients feel they have no choice but to comply, even though they do not want the vaccine.
Fraud	Deceitful act made to conceal the truth. *Example:* Falsifying a patient's medical record to conceal a medical mistake.
Invasion of privacy	The intentional prying or intruding into another person's confidential information or matters. *Example:* Releasing a patient's medical records without the patient's consent or a court order.
Undue influence	Intentionally persuading people to do things they do not want to do. *Example:* Convincing single mothers that they should give their children up for adoption when they clearly do not want to.

Critical Thinking Question 4-1

How does the case study outlined at the beginning of this chapter illustrate one of the torts in Table 4-2? Please specify the tort.

Understanding and Classifying Consent

Before patients are accepted for care in a medical office, they must give their consent to be examined and/or treated by the physician or health care provider and sign a consent form. Before asking the patient or parent/guardian to consent for any examination or treatment, it is the responsibility of the provider to explain the suggested care. Part of this explanation must be to outline the benefits and risks, if any, as well as any accepted alternative to the treatment. Once that information has been explained to the patient and the patient has been given the opportunity to ask any questions, the patient should be asked to sign a consent form. This is the process of obtaining informed consent from the patient. The following information must be included on a consent form:

- Name of the procedure to be performed
- Name of the physician or health care provider who will perform the procedure
- Name of the person administering the anesthesia (if applicable)
- Any potential risks to the patient from the procedure
- Any risks to the patient if the procedure is *not* elected
- Any accepted alternative treatments and their risks
- Any exclusions the patient has requested
- A statement indicating that all the patient's questions have been answered
- The patient's and witnesses' signatures and the date signed

Only certain parties are legally able to sign consent forms. Patients who can sign a consent form include

- Any mentally competent adult over age 18
- The parent or legal guardian of a child, mentally incompetent adult, or temporarily incapacitated adult
- Emancipated minors, defined as under age 18 but:
  - Are married or self-supporting and responsible for their debts
  - Have received a court order declaring them emancipated
- A minor who is:
  - In the armed services
  - Being seen for treatment for sexually transmitted infections
  - Pregnant

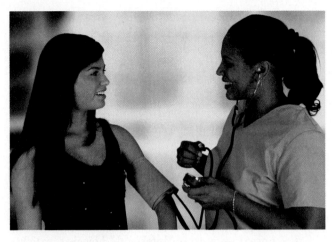

Figure 4-1 ■ This patient has given implied consent to have her blood pressure taken.
Source: Shutterstock © Rob Marmion.

- Being seen for information regarding birth control or abortion
- Being seen for treatment regarding drug or alcohol abuse

Consent forms must be written in the languages patients speak. Most facilities that treat patients from other cultures have consent forms in multiple languages

Health care has two types of consent: (1) implied and (2) expressed. **Implied consent** is given when patients indicate through action only that they agree to submit. When patients are told they need to give blood samples and they roll up their sleeves while saying nothing, they are giving implied consent (**Figure 4-1** ■).

▶▶▶ Pulse Points

Consent for Children and Mentally Incompetent Adults

Children or people who are mentally incompetent or temporarily incapacitated cannot legally give consent, just as they cannot legally enter into contracts. The parents or guardians of these patients must give consent for these patients.

▶▶▶ Pulse Points

Signing Consent Forms

Patients must never be coerced or threatened into signing consent forms. Consent must be gained voluntarily and only after the patient has been fully informed of the procedure. Patients who fail to completely understand procedures, have any unanswered questions, or cannot read consent forms should never sign those forms.

Expressed consent occurs when patients agree either verbally or in writing to consent to a procedure. In health care, any invasive procedure should be done only after a patient has signed a consent form. This helps prove the patient knew the risks involved and agreed to them before the service.

Whether consent is implied or expressed, it must always be informed, meaning patients must be told the benefits and risks of any procedure, the risks of not having the procedure, and any accepted alternative treatments to the procedure (**Figure 4-2** ■). Patients must also be clearly informed of any pain associated with the procedure or recovery and if they will require any assistance after the procedure. The physician is responsible for obtaining informed consent. For the consent to be truly "informed," however, patients must have the opportunity to ask the physician any and all questions. This task should never be delegated to the medical assistant. It is, however, appropriate for the medical assistant to witness the patient's signature on the consent form.

▶▶▶ Pulse Points

The Value of Signed Consent Forms

Lack of a valid, signed informed consent form has been cause for malpractice claims to be filed against health care providers. Without a signed consent form prior to a procedure, for example, the patient may sue the provider for performing that procedure without proper consent.

▶▶▶ Pulse Points

When Patients Refuse Treatment

Physicians have the right to refuse to perform elective surgery on patients who refuse to receive blood if needed. An example would be a surgeon who recommends his patient have a surgery where blood loss may happen, and the patient has stated that she will not consent to the transfusion of blood.

PEARSON GENERAL HOSPITAL

COMPLETE ORIGINAL IN INK FOR HOSPITAL CHART
PATIENT MUST BE AWAKE, ALERT AND ORIENTED WHEN SIGNING

DATE: _____ TIME: _____ ☐ AM ☐ PM

I AUTHORIZE THE PERFORMANCE UPON_____
OF THE FOLLOWING OPERATION (state nature and extent):_____
_____
_____

TO BE PERFORMED UNDER THE DIRECTION OF DR. _____

1. I HAVE BEEN ADVISED THAT THERE IS A FAVORABLE LIKELIHOOD OF SUCCESS, BUT I UNDERSTAND THAT A COMPLETELY SUCCESSFUL OUTCOME MAY NOT BE ACHIEVABLE, AND THERE ARE NO GUARANTEES REGARDING THE OUTCOME. I ALSO UNDERSTAND THAT CERTAIN ADVERSE EVENTS COULD OCCUR AS A RESULT OF THE PERFORMANCE OF THE PROCEDURE OR TREATMENT, INCLUDING PAIN, INFECTION, LACERATION OR PUNCTURE OF INTERNAL ORGANS, BLEEDING, NERVE DAMAGE OR EVEN IN RARE CASES, DEATH. I UNDERSTAND THAT HOSPITALIZATION OR OTHER INSTITUTIONAL CARE, HOME CARE OR CARE BY HEALTH PROFESSIONALS MAY BE NEEDED FOLLOWING THE PROCEDURE OR TREATMENT, RELATED TO FULL RECOVERY, RECUPERATION OR CONVALESCENCE. I UNDERSTAND THE ALTERNATIVES TO THIS PROCEDURE, INCLUDING MY RIGHT TO REFUSE TO CONSENT TO IT, AND I NEVERTHELESS HAVE DECIDED TO CONSENT TO PERFORMANCE OF THE PROCEDURE OR TREATMENT.

2. I CONSENT TO THE PERFORMANCE OF OPERATIONS AND PROCEDURES IN ADDITION TO OR DIFFERENT FROM THOSE NOW CONTEMPLATED, WHETHER OR NOT ARISING FROM PRESENTLY UNFORESEEN CONDITIONS WHICH THE ABOVE NAMED DOCTOR OR HIS/HER ASSOCIATES OR ASSISTANTS MAY CONSIDER NECESSARY OR ADVISABLE IN THE COURSE OF THE OPERATION.

3. I CONSENT TO THE DISPOSAL BY HOSPITAL AUTHORITIES OF ANY TISSUES OR PARTS WHICH MAY BE REMOVED.

4. THE NATURE AND PURPOSE OF THE OPERATION/PROCEDURE, POSSIBLE ALTERNATIVE METHODS OF TREATMENT, THE RISK AND BENEFITS INVOLVED, AND THE COURSE OF RECUPERATION HAVE BEEN FULLY EXPLAINED TO ME. NO GUARANTEE OR ASSURANCE HAS BEEN GIVEN BY ANYONE AS TO THE RESULTS THAT MAY BE OBTAINED.

5. I UNDERSTAND AND AGREE WITH THE ABOVE INFORMATION. I HAVE NO QUESTIONS WHICH HAVE NOT BEEN ANSWERED TO MY FULL SATISFACTION. I UNDERSTAND THAT I HAVE THE RIGHT TO ASK FOR FURTHER INFORMATION BEFORE SIGNING THIS CONSENT.

I have crossed out any paragraph above which does not apply or to which I do not give consent.

PATIENT SIGNATURE: _____   WITNESS SIGNATURE: _____
(OR PARENT OR GUARDIAN IF PATIENT IS UNDER 18 YEARS OF AGE)   (OF PATIENT, PARENT OR GUARDIAN SIGNATURE)

RELATIONSHIP: _____   WITNESS SIGNATURE: _____
    ☐ **TELEPHONE CONSENT** (2ND WITNESS NEEDED FOR TELEPHONE CONSENT)

Figure 4-2 ■ Sample informed consent form.

PROCEDURE 4-1 Prepare an Informed Consent for Treatment Form

Theory and Rationale

While the task of explaining the procedures, risks, and alternatives falls to the physician, the medical assistant is often the person who discusses the paperwork with the patient and obtains the patient's signature.

Materials

- Informed consent for treatment form
- Blue or black ink pen
- Copy machine

Competency

1. As the physician goes over the details of the upcoming procedure with the patient, fill in the informed consent form. The form must include:
   - The name of the procedure or treatment to be performed
   - The expected benefits of the procedure
   - Any possible risks of the procedure
   - Any accepted alternatives to the procedure and the risks or benefits associated with each
   - The fact that the patient may choose to forego the procedure and the possible risks or benefits associated with that choice
2. Be certain the form lists the patient's name, birth date, and the place the procedure is to be performed (in office, hospital, etc.).
3. Show the consent form to the physician for him or her to verify that all information is correct.
4. After the physician has left the room, go over the form with the patient. If the patient has further questions about the procedure, have the patient wait in the treatment room while you ask the physician to return to answer the questions. If the patient has no further questions about the procedure, have the patient sign the consent form.
5. Sign the consent form as a witness to the patient's signature.
6. Go over any specifics with the patient about the procedure day, such as any restrictions to eating or drinking on the day of the surgery, or where the patient should park her car.
7. Make a copy of the consent form for the patient. Place the original form in the patient's file.

Patients may refuse treatment for any reason, including religious and personal beliefs. For example, a patient with end-stage cancer may refuse chemotherapy because the side effects may decrease the quality of life. A Jehovah's Witness may refuse blood products on religious grounds. When patients refuse treatment, they or their parents or guardians should sign a refusal-of-consent form. This form must indicate that the patient was given information on the risks and benefits of having the procedure or not. If the patient refuses to sign a refusal-of-consent form, the physician may refuse to treat the patient, or can make a notation in the patient's chart of the refusal to sign.

Many cases have been brought to the court system regarding refusal of treatment. Each time, courts have found that mentally competent adults are within their legal rights to refuse medical care, even if that care is life-sustaining.

Medical Malpractice

Doctors are sued for varied reasons. Some are sued for making serious errors, such as giving the wrong medications, performing the wrong surgeries, or failing to properly diagnose or treat patients. Other doctors, though few, commit Medicare or insurance fraud, or falsify patient records to conceal errors.

Malpractice is a breach of duty. There are three different ways that a person can breach their duty:

- **Malfeasance** is the state of performing an incorrect treatment resulting in injury to the patient, such as operating on the wrong patient.
- **Misfeasance** is the state of performing a procedure incorrectly resulting in injury to the patient, such as performing a minor surgery on a patient and accidentally severing a nerve, leaving the patient with loss of sensation.
- **Nonfeasance** is the act of delaying or failing to perform a treatment such as a physician missing the presence of a tumor on a patient's x-ray and therefore not suggesting further treatment of the tumor. In the event the patient has a bad outcome directly due to the missed diagnosis, the patient may bring a case of nonfeasance malpractice against the physician.

The Doctrine of *Respondeat Superior*

Staff in the medical office can cause the office to be sued. If the medical assistant makes an error, for example, the lawsuit will usually be filed against the doctor who employs the medical assistant. This is called the doctrine of **respondeat superior**, which is Latin for, "Let the master answer." Under this doctrine,

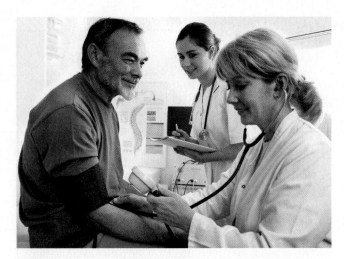

Figure 4-3 ■ The physician and medical assistant work closely together to maintain safe care for their patients.
Source: Shutterstock © Alexander Raths.

physicians are responsible for the actions of their health care employees (**Figure 4-3** ■).

In many malpractice lawsuits, the patient is unaware of the exact person(s) responsible for the alleged injury. In these cases, the patient will often list the hospital or medical facility under the doctrine of *respondeat superior*, claiming that the employer is responsible for the acts of the employees, even if the exact employee is not named.

Medical assistants can still be named in malpractice lawsuits, however, so each should seriously consider carrying a **malpractice insurance policy**. Because medical assistants have a low risk of injuring patients, insurance rates are generally low. Policies are available through local or state medical-assisting associations.

Critical Thinking Question 4-2

Thinking back to the case study at the beginning of this chapter, if the medical assistant were to release any information about the patient to the patient's employer, how might the concept of *respondeat superior* come into play?

Malpractice Insurance Policies

Malpractice insurance policies are known as occurrence policies. An occurrence policy covers policyholders regardless of when claims are filed, provided the policies were in effect at the time of the alleged malpractice events. If Dr. Rasheem is covered by Unified Insurance under an occurrence-made policy on June 1, 2015, when an alleged malpractice event occurs, and then switches to a different company before the claim filing date of December 10, 2015, she would still be covered for the claim under her Unified Insurance policy.

▸▸▸ Pulse Points

Individual Malpractice Insurance Policies for Medical Assistants

Medical assistants may choose to purchase their own individual malpractice insurance policy. This type of policy would cover the medical assistant's personal assets should a patient name the medical assistant in a malpractice lawsuit. Because medical assistants are covered under the provider's malpractice policy under the doctrine of respondeat superior, many medical assistants choose not to purchase their own coverage. Purchasing such a policy might be done for the reason of providing peace of mind to the medical assistant in knowing he or she is covered in the event the provider's insurance policy is somehow found to be invalid. Individual malpractice insurance policies for medical assistants are fairly inexpensive. For a quick online quote on malpractice insurance premiums, visit www.hpso.com.

Proving Medical Malpractice

The vast majority of medical malpractice lawsuits fail to reach court. Most malpractice lawsuits are either **settled**, meaning the two sides agree on a financial award to the injured patient, or they are dismissed due to lack of proof. To prove medical malpractice, the patient must prove all of the following **Four Ds of Negligence**:

- **Duty**—Physicians have a duty to care for patients once they have taken those patients on. The patients must prove the physician breached this duty.
- **Dereliction of duty**—Physicians must meet **standard of care** (established requirements that dictate how and when care is to be provided) guidelines for a health care provider with the same training, under the same circumstances. The patients must prove the physician failed to perform to this standard.
- **Direct cause**—Patients must prove that the physicians' actions, or lack of action, directly caused the patients' injuries.
- **Damages**—Patients must prove they sustained **damages** due to the negligence. These damages must be physical injury or financial loss directly caused by the injury sustained.

Medical Malpractice Awards

Public Citizen, a non-partisan public research group that focuses on many areas of health care, reported in 2010 that personal injury attorneys accept about 1 out of every 20 cases they review, but most cases are found in the physician's favor. Only 1 in 10 cases accepted by an attorney result in an award or a settlement for the patient. When injured patients win cases, judges or juries may make one of the three following types of awards:

- **Nominal**—These are small awards or payments that are made when the negligence is proven but the damages are minimal.

- **Compensatory**—This is money that is awarded to the patient or the patient's family to compensate for the cost of medical care, the disability, mental suffering, any loss of income, and the loss of future income due to the injury.

- **Punitive**—Awards like these are made when judges or juries feel the health care providers should be punished for their actions. Courts may feel the providers were reckless or purposefully ignored signals that should have alerted them to the injuries. Punitive damages are typically high dollar amounts. Several states do not allow for punitive damages. In those states that do not allow punitive damages, a punitive award in damages may still be made against a medical equipment manufacturer. In these cases, the patient must prove that the medical equipment manufacturer knew of a malfunction or defect with the equipment that is found to cause the patient's injury.

Preventing Medical Malpractice Claims

Patients file malpractice lawsuits for many reasons; lack of understanding is chief among them. Scientific advances in health care have allowed doctors to perform procedures that were considered too risky until recently. As procedures have become more complicated, patient risk has increased, and this has increased the likelihood of both poor outcomes and malpractice lawsuits, especially when the physician has failed to thoroughly explain the risks to patients. Physicians can help avoid lawsuits by completely explaining the risks of the procedures and obtaining the patients' **informed consent**. Informed consent should be written in detail and signed by both the patient and the health care provider (**Figure 4-4** ■). Medical assistants can help avoid lawsuits by making sure to answer

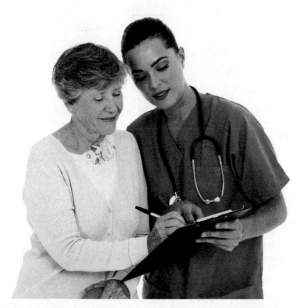

Figure 4-4 ■ The medical assistant will frequently witness a patient's signature on a consent form.

Source: Fotolia © michaeljung.

questions the patient may have and knowing when to alert the provider to patient concerns.

Another means of lawsuit reduction has been gaining popularity over the past decade, and that is if health care providers apologize to patients, those patients will be less likely to file malpractice claims. Many believe that patients sue because they are angry and only pursue legal recourse because they failed to receive acknowledgments of the errors, and apologies. In research activities at the University of Michigan, health care providers were instructed to apologize to their patients when errors occurred. After one year, malpractice defense costs decreased from $3 million to $1 million. Today, 36 states have some form of law that allows health care providers to apologize to patients after injuries without those apologies being used as proof of negligence in lawsuits.

Defending Against Medical Malpractice Claims

Once a medical malpractice suit has been filed, the best defense is the medical record. Especially in the area of medical malpractice, an accurate and complete medical record is of paramount importance. This record is the authoritative description of all care that was provided to a patient. It has all consent forms signed by the patient, as well as descriptions of the questions the patient asked and the answers the physician gave about needed care or treatment. The medical assistant, like all members of the health care team, must be sure to accurately document all patient care issues and concerns in the patients' medical records.

The Statute of Limitations

Each state has a **statute of limitations** that sets the time frame within which an injured patient can file a malpractice lawsuit. Normally, this time frame begins from the date of the injury. According to something called the **discovery rule**, some states allow the time frame to begin when the injury was discovered or should have been discovered. This rule helps in cases in which the patient fails to discover the injury for several years after the injury has occurred. Other states allow the statute to begin when a minor child reaches the age of majority, allowing injured children to bring suits on their own behalf once they reach adulthood. Table 4-3 outlines the statute of limitations for each state.

▶▶▶ Pulse Points

Patient Safety

Every member of the health care team is responsible for patient safety. Any team member who witnesses something that seems wrong is compelled to speak with the physician about it out of the patient's hearing range. Team members who remain silent may be considered partly responsible for a patient's injuries.

TABLE 4-3 Statute of Limitations for Medical Malpractice in Each State

State	Statute of Limitations for Medical Malpractice
Alabama	2 years from the date of injury or 6 months from the date the injury was discovered to a maximum of 4 years from the date of injury.
Alaska	2 years from the date of injury. 2 year discovery rule.
Arizona	2 years from the date of injury. 2 year discovery rule.
Arkansas	2 years from the date of injury. 1 year discovery rule, if after statute of limitations has run.
California	3 years from the date of injury or 1 year from the date the injury was discovered or should have been discovered. In the event a foreign object is found inside the plaintiff, the statute begins at the date the object was discovered or should have been discovered and runs for 3 years.
Colorado	2 years from the date of injury 3 year discovery rule. If malpractice knowingly concealed or foreign object, then 2 years from discovery with no 3 year limitation
Connecticut	2 years from the date of injury to a maximum of 3 years from the date of injury regardless of discovery.
Delaware	2 years from the date of injury or within 4 years if the injury was unknown and could not reasonably have been discovered.
Florida	2 years from the date of injury or date the injury was discovered or should have been discovered to a maximum of 4 years from the date of injury.
Georgia	2 years from the date of injury or up to 5 years from the date of discovery.
Hawaii	2 years from the date of injury or reasonable date of discovery. In the event an object is left inside a patient, a claim may be filed up to 1 year from the date of discovery. All claims must be filed within 6 years of the injury.
Idaho	2 years from the date of injury.
Illinois	2 years from the date of injury or up to 4 years if the injury could not reasonably have been discovered within 2 years.
Indiana	2 years from the date of injury.
Iowa	2 years from the date of injury or discovery of the injury. All claims must be filed within 6 years of the injury.
Kansas	2 years from the date of injury or up to 4 years if the injury could not reasonably have been discovered within 2 years.
Kentucky	1 year from the date of injury or up to 5 years if the injury could not reasonably have been discovered within 1 year.
Louisiana	1 year from the date of injury or up to 3 years from the date of discovery.
Maine	3 years from the date of injury.
Maryland	5 years from the date of injury or 3 years from the date the injury was discovered, whichever is greater.
Massachusetts	3 years from the date of injury or 3 years from the date of discovery. All claims must be filed within 7 years of the date of injury.
Michigan	2 years from the date of injury or 6 months from the date of discovery. All claims must be filed within 6 years of the date of injury.
Minnesota	4 years from the date of injury.
Mississippi	2 years from the date of injury or 2 years from the date of discovery. All claims must be filed within 7 years of the date of injury.
Missouri	2 years from the date of injury or date of discovery up to 10 years from the date of injury.
Montana	3 years from the date of injury or discovery up to 5 years from the date of injury.
Nebraska	2 years from the date of the injury or 1 year from the date the injury was discovered. All claims must be filed within 10 years of the date of injury.

TABLE 4-3 Statute of Limitations for Medical Malpractice in Each State (*Continued*)

State	Statute of Limitations for Medical Malpractice
Nevada	4 years from the date of injury or 2 years from the date the injury was discovered.
New Hampshire	3 years from the date of the injury or 3 years from the date of the discovery.
New Jersey	2 years from the date of the injury or 2 years from the date the injury was discovered or should have been discovered.
New Mexico	3 years from the date of injury.
New York	30 months from the date of injury. In the event a foreign object is left inside a patient, the claim must be filed within 1 year of the discovery.
North Carolina	3 years from the date of injury or 2 years from the date the injury was discovered or should have been discovered.
North Dakota	2 years from the date of injury or the date the injury was discovered or should have been discovered. All claims must be filed within 6 years of the injury.
Ohio	1 year from the date of injury or 1 year from the date of discovery. All claims must be filed within 4 years of the date of injury.
Oklahoma	3 years from the date of injury.
Oregon	2 years from the date of injury or the date the injury was discovered or should have been discovered. All claims must be filed within 5 years of the injury.
Pennsylvania	2 years from the date of injury.
Rhode Island	3 years from the date of injury or 3 years from the date of discovery.
South Carolina	3 years from the date of injury or the date the injury was discovered or should have been discovered. In the event a foreign object is left inside a patient, the claim must be filed within 2 years of the discovery. All claims must be filed within 6 years of the date of injury.
South Dakota	2 years from the date of injury.
Tennessee	1 year from the date of injury.
Texas	2 years from the date of injury.
Utah	2 years from the date of injury or the date the injury was discovered or should have been discovered. In the event a foreign object is left inside a patient, the claim must be filed within 1 year of the discovery. All claims must be filed within 4 years of the date of injury.
Vermont	3 years from the date of injury or 2 years from the date injury was discovered or should have been discovered. All claims must be filed within 7 years of the injury.
Virginia	2 years from the date of injury or the date the injury was discovered or should have been discovered. In the event a foreign object is left inside a patient, the claim must be filed within 1 year of the discovery. All claims must be filed within 10 years of the date of injury.
Washington, D.C.	3 years from the date of injury.
Washington State	3 years from the date of injury or 1 year from the date the injury was discovered or should have been discovered. All claims must be filed within 8 years of the injury.
West Virginia	2 years from the date of injury or the date the injury was discovered or should have been discovered.
Wisconsin	3 years from the date of injury or 1 year from the date the injury was discovered or should have been discovered. All claims must be filed within 5 years of the injury.
Wyoming	2 years from the date of injury or the date the injury was discovered or should have been discovered.

Using Assumption of Risk as a Defense

Assumption of risk is a defense to medical malpractice that physicians can use to prove the physician made the patients aware of the risks of the recommended procedures and decided to proceed regardless of those risks. Under this defense, patients cannot sue the physicians when one of those risks occurs. This defense relies, however, on a detailed consent form signed by the patient.

Contributory and Comparative Negligence

The **contributory negligence** defense is one in which a physician might have been at fault for a patient's injuries but can prove that the patient aggravated his injuries or in some way worsened them. For example, assume a physician sends a patient home with a sling instead of a cast and tells the patient to limit the motion of the arm to avoid aggravating the injury. If the patient then lifts groceries, worsening the fracture, that patient could be proven to have contributed to negligence.

Most states give patients no awards in contributory negligence cases. When awards are allowed, the court will normally assign a percentage of the award based on how responsible the patient was for the injury. For example, if the court finds the physician is 50 percent responsible for an injury and the patient is also 50 percent responsible, the physician will be ordered to pay 50 percent of the damages. These types of cases are typically called **comparative negligence**.

Res Judicata and Res Ipsa Loquitur

Res judicata is Latin for the phrase, "The thing has been decided." If patients lose their malpractice lawsuits, they cannot bring other suits against the physician for the same injuries. Once a case has been decided in a physician's favor, the case must be dropped.

The doctrine of **res ipsa locuitur**, the Latin phrase for, "The thing speaks for itself" pertains to a case where the negligence is obvious. In all other malpractice cases, the patient must prove the physician's negligence. Cases of res ipsa loquitur are ones in which the malpractice is obvious. A wrong limb may have been amputated or an instrument left inside a patient.

The Standard of Care

The standard of care is a crucial tool for deciding most medical malpractice cases. To determine if a health care provider has performed within the standard of care, one or both sides in the lawsuit will call on **expert witnesses**. An expert witness is a person deemed by the court to be an authority on a particular subject matter. While expert witnesses must be licensed or certified, they need not be licensed or certified in the state where they are testifying.

Alternative to Litigation

In many states, parties in a malpractice suit are required to participate in mediation before they can go to trial. The process of mediation involves a mediator hired by the attorneys involved in the case. The mediator hears both sides of the case and attempts to bring the parties to a successful solution. If one or both sides do not agree with the mediator, and an agreement cannot be reached, the parties may go to trial.

In some states, malpractice cases may go to arbitration. This situation is one where both parties agree to abide by the decision of the arbitrator, whose decision is legally binding.

Tort Reform

Some sources claim that the number of malpractice cases has risen over the past few years, causing an increase in medical malpractice insurance premiums, but those sources have been called into question by some public safety groups. The medical malpractice insurance industry is cyclical, exhibiting the ups and downs of any other insurance industry. In fact, the number of malpractice cases that have awarded money to patients has decreased over the past decade and, once inflation is factored in, the amount of money awarded to patients has remained flat. Medical malpractice insurance carriers make most of their profits by investing premiums in the stock market. As the stock market ebbs and flows, so do the profits of insurance carriers.

Capping the Money Awarded to Injured Patients

Thirty-two states have capped the awards that can be given to injured patients. These caps typically range from $250,000 to $1 million and fail to factor in the number of physicians' prior malpractice cases, or if patients were injured due to physicians' reckless behavior. Twelve states have laws in place stating that capping awards in malpractice cases would be unconstitutional.

Studies have shown that capping the money awarded to injured patients has not lowered medical malpractice premiums. Instead, premiums have continued to rise, even in states with caps. For example, a recent report in *The New York Times* found that caps on awards have reduced the payout of malpractice awards for the decade between 1991 and 2002 by 16 percent. Meanwhile, in the same time period, malpractice policy premiums went up 48 percent. Many studies have found that patients who suffer the most severe injuries are typically compensated far less than patients with similar injuries in states without caps.

There is a social cost of capping awards to injured patients, as well, and it is high. With too little money to cover their medical costs and expenses after an injury, patients often rely on their states' public health care systems (Medicaid), which means the taxpayers in those states pay for the injuries instead of the providers who are responsible for them.

Repeat Offender Providers

Studies in many states have shown that the vast majority of patient injuries arise from the same small handful of health care providers. Public Citizen, a nonprofit consumer rights group, performed a study in 2005 comparing the malpractice payouts in the United States to the number of doctors making payments. Their findings concluded that 5.5% of U.S. physicians were responsible for 57.3% of all medical malpractice payouts

The Physician's Public Duties and Consequences

Physicians have certain responsibilities surrounding the reporting of certain events. Physicians who deliver babies must report birth certificates, for example. Physicians who are the last to care for patients who have died are typically responsible for completing death certificates. All states list reporting requirements in the event of certain infectious or communicable diseases. Such lists can be obtained from state or local health departments and should be updated yearly.

Reporting Vaccine Injuries

According to the 1986 National Childhood Vaccine Injury Act, vaccine injuries must be reported by physicians' offices to alert other physicians to possibly contaminated batches of vaccine. To report a vaccine injury, the medical assistant should obtain the patient's name and age, as well as the name and lot number of the vaccine. The Department of Health and Human Services provides a form on their website that must be filled out regarding the vaccine injury. The report must be documented in the patient's file.

Other Reportable Conditions

Most states compose a list of conditions and diseases that must be reported to local, county, or state agencies. This list is typically kept by the state's department of health and may change as new diseases are discovered. The list of reportable conditions will contain a mandatory reporting period. The medical office staff must report the conditions within that time period to be within the rules of the law. In cases of conditions that could spread quickly, such as an airborne illness, the condition might need to be reported within 1 to 3 days. In cases of conditions that are slower to spread, such as sexually transmitted infections, the reporting requirement might be up to 5 days. **Figure 4-5** ■ shows the New York State Department of Health Communicable Disease Reporting Requirements.

Reporting Cases of Abuse

Any incapacitated person, elderly person, or child who shows signs of suspected abuse or neglect must be protected. To that end, physicians are required to report all cases of suspected abuse to the proper authorities. After accidents, abuse is thought to be the second leading cause of death in children under age 5. Each state outlines its own definitions for the various degrees of child abuse. Spousal abuse, known as domestic violence, is defined in each state's law. In most states, domestic violence is not something the health care provider must report, unless the victim would like to file a complaint against the abuser. Like other crimes, first degree abuse is the most serious offense.

When patients of any age sustain violent injuries, including injuries from gunshots or knives or criminal acts (like assault), attempted suicide, or rape, those injuries must be reported. The law protects health care workers from being sued for reporting suspected abuse. Failure to report suspected abuse may expose the health care worker to criminal charges.

Elder abuse is defined as abuse of an elderly person in one of the following areas:

- Physical abuse—physically harming the elderly person
- Emotional abuse—humiliating and verbal abuse of the elderly person
- Financial abuse—abusing the finances of the elderly person
- Sexual abuse—forcing sexual activity from the elderly person
- Neglect—depriving the elderly person of food, heat, clothing or medications

Revoking Medical Licenses

Each state has its own medical practice act. These acts list the duties and responsibilities of the physician and outline the actions that might be cause for disciplinary action, including suspension or revocation of the physician's license. In general, the more serious the action, the more serious the disciplinary action. For example, physicians who are convicted of felonies or proven to have abused patients can face license revocation.

The Physician-Patient Relationship

Both physicians and patients have responsibilities in their relationships. A partnership between the physician and patient is necessary to the delivery of high quality and effective health care, and in the treatment and prevention of disease.

The Role of the Patient

Patients are free to choose their physicians. They can also choose whether they want to begin care or limit their care. Patients have the right to understand their treatment components, as well as side effects or benefits. All this information must be detailed for the patient before the procedure.

The Role of the Physician

Physicians have the right to refuse treatment to new patients, or even existing ones, unless those patients have life-threatening, emergent conditions. With proper notification, physicians can

Communicable Disease Reporting Requirements

Reporting of suspected or confirmed communicable diseases is mandated under the New York State Sanitary Code (10NYCRR 2.10,2.14). The primary responsibility for reporting rests with the physician; moreover, laboratories (PHL 2102), school nurses (10NYCRR 2.12), day care center directors, nursing homes/hospitals (10NYCRR 405.3d) and state institutions (10NYCRR 2.10a) or other locations providing health services (10NYCRR 2.12) are also required to report the diseases listed below.

Anaplasmosis
Amebiasis
(Animal bites for which rabies prophylaxis is given[1]
(Anthrax[2]
(Arboviral infection[3]
Babesiosis
(Botulism[2]
(Brucellosis[2]
Campylobacteriosis
Chancroid
Chlamydia trachomatis infection
(Cholera
Cryptosporidiosis
Cyclosporiasis
(Diphtheria
E.coli O157:H7 infection[4]
Ehrlichiosis
(Encephalitis

(Foodborne Illness
Giardiasis
(Glanders[2]
Gonococcal infection
Haemophilus influenzae[5] (invasive disease)
(Hantavirus disease
Hemolytic uremic syndrome
Hepatitis A
(Hepatitis A in a food handler
Hepatitis B (specify acute or chronic)
Hepatitis C (specify acute or chronic)
Pregnant hepatitis B carrier
Herpes infection, infants aged 60 days or younger
Hospital associated infections (as defined in section 2.2 10NYCRR)

Influenza, laboratory-confirmed
Legionellosis
Listeriosis
Lyme disease
Lymphogranuloma venereum
Malaria
(Measles
(Melioidosis[2]
Meningitis
   Aseptic or viral
   (Haemophilus
   (Meningococcal
   Other (specify type)
(Meningococcemia
(Monkeypox
Mumps
Pertussis
(Plague[2]
(Poliomyelitis

Psittacosis
(Q Fever[2]
(Rabies[1]
Rocky Mountain spotted fever
(Rubella (including congenital rubella syndrome)
Salmonellosis
(Severe Acute Respiratory Syndrome (SARS)
Shigatoxin-producing E.coli[4] (STEC)
Shigellosis[4]
(Smallpox[2]
Staphylococcus aureus[6] (due to strains showing reduced susceptibility or resistance to vancomycin)
(Staphylococcal enterotoxin B poisoning[2]

Streptococcal infection (invasive disease)[5]
   Group A beta-hemolytic strep
   Group B strep
   Streptococcus pneumoniae
(Syphilis, specify stage[7]
Tetanus
Toxic shock syndrome
Transmissable spongiform encephalopathies[8] (TSE)
Trichinosis
(Tuberculosis current disease (specify site)
(Tularemia[2]
(Typhoid
(Vaccinia disease[9]
Vibriosis[6]
(Viral hemorrhagic fever[2]
Yersiniosis

WHO SHOULD REPORT?

Physicians, nurses, laboratory directors, infection control practitioners, health care facilities, state institutions, schools.

WHERE SHOULD REPORT BE MADE?

Report to local health department where patient resides.

Contact Person _____

Name _____

Address _____

_____

Phone _____ Fax _____

WHEN SHOULD REPORT BE MADE?

Within 24 hours of diagnosis:
- Phone diseases in bold type,
- Mail case report, DOH-389, for all other diseases.
- In New York City use form PD-16.

SPECIAL NOTES

- Diseases listed in **bold type** (warrant prompt action and should be reported **immediately** to local health departments by phone followed by submission of the confidential case report form (DOH-389). In NYC use case report form PD-16.
- In addition to the diseases listed above, any unusual disease (defined as a newly apparent or emerging disease or syndrome that could possibly be caused by a transmissible infectious agent or microbial toxin) is reportable.
- Outbreaks: while individual cases of some diseases (e.g., streptococcal sore throat, head lice, impetigo, scabies and pneumonia) are not reportable, a cluster or outbreak of cases of any communicable disease is a reportable event.
- **Cases of HIV infection, HIV-related illness and AIDS are reportable on form DOH-4189 which may be obtained by contacting:**

        Division of Epidemiology, Evaluation and Research
        P.O. Box 2073, ESP Station
        Albany, NY 12220-2073
        (518) 474-4284
   In NYC: New York City Department of Health and Mental Hygiene
        For HIV/AIDS reporting, call:
        (212) 442-3388

1. Local health department must be notified prior to initiating rabies prophylaxis.
2. Diseases that are possible indicators of bioterrorism.
3. Including, but not limited to, infections caused by eastern equine encephalitis virus, western equine encephalitis virus, West Nile virus, St. Louis encephalitis virus, La Crosse virus, Powassan virus, Jamestown Canyon virus, dengue and yellow fever.
4. Positive shigatoxin test results should be reported as presumptive evidence of disease.
5. Only report cases with positive cultures from blood, CSF, joint, peritoneal or pleural fluid. Do not report cases with positive cultures from skin, saliva, sputum or throat.
6. Proposed addition to list.
7. Any non-treponemal test ≥1:16 or any positive prenatal or delivery test regardless of titer or any primary or secondary stage disease, should be reported by phone; all others may be reported by mail.
8. Including Creutzfeldt-Jakob disease. Cases should be reported directly to the New York State Department of Health Alzheimer's Disease and Other Dementias Registry at (518) 473-7817 upon suspicion of disease. In NYC, cases should also be reported to the NYCDOHMH.
9. Persons with vaccinia infection due to contact transmission and persons with the following complications from vaccination; eczema vaccinatum, erythema multiforme major or Stevens-Johnson syndrome, fetal vaccinia, generalized vaccinia, inadvertent inoculation, ocular vaccinia, post-vaccinial encephalitis or encephalomyelitis, progressive vaccinia, pyogenic infection of the infection site, and any other serious adverse events.

ADDITIONAL INFORMATION

For more information on disease reporting, call your local health department or the
   New York State Department of Health
   Bureau of Communicable Disease Control at
   (518) 473-4439
   or (866) 881-2809 after hours.
In New York City, 1 (866) NYC-DOH1.
To obtain reporting forms (DOH-389), call (518) 474-0548.

PLEASE POST THIS CONSPICUOUSLY

Figure 4-5 ■ New York State Department of Health Communicable Disease Reporting Requirements.

Source: http://www.health.ny.gov/forms/instructions/doh-389_instructions.pdf

change their policies or their availabilities. When physicians are away from their practice for a period, like vacation, they must arrange for other physicians to cover their practice in the event of emergency. To simply close an office, with no emergency referral, can be seen as abandonment of the patient and may result in a malpractice lawsuit.

Contracts in Health Care

A contract is an agreement between two or more parties that the law will recognize. All contracts must have the three following components:

1. An offer (the initiation of the contract)
2. Acceptance of the offer (both parties agree to the terms of the contract)
3. Some form of consideration (the exchange of fees for service)

Contracts can be verbal or written. In health care, a contract can be initiated when a patient calls the office to schedule an appointment. The offer is accepted when the administrative medical assistant schedules the appointment. The patient is obligated to pay a fee for the service of seeing the physician, and the physician is obligated to treat the patient.

Physicians and patients operate using two types of contracts: (1) implied and (2) expressed.

Implied Contracts

Much like in implied consent discussed earlier, in an **implied contract**, nothing is written or spoken. Instead, patients imply through their actions alone that they agree to the contracts. For example, simply by arriving for care at the medical office, patients imply that they will abide by the patient's portion of the doctor–patient contract and will pay for the services (**Figure 4-6 ■**).

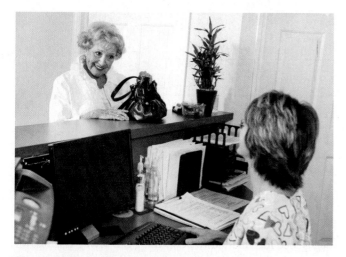

Figure 4-6 ■ By arriving for care in the medical office, the patient implies that she will abide by the patient's portion of the doctor–patient contract, as well as pay for services rendered.
Source: Shutterstock © Lisa F. Young.

Expressed Contracts

Unlike implied contracts, **expressed contracts** have elements that are spoken or written; they identify all of the elements are specifically stated. Expressed contracts occur when patients either verbally or in writing state that they will be responsible for their portion of contracts. For example, patients who sign payment agreements stating they will make payments of $100 per month for the next 6 months enter into an expressed contract. **Figure 4-7 ■** shows a sample expressed contract.

▸▸▸ Pulse Points

Verbal Contracts

Not all contracts need to be written to be valid. A verbal contract can be just as binding as a signed one. The challenge that parties face with a verbal contract lies in proving the contract exists.

Terminating Contracts

The doctor–patient contract is typically resolved once the patient has completed the prescribed course of treatment outlined by the physician. While the patient may choose to end the doctor–patient relationship at any time, the physician must follow legal protocol to end the relationship.

Patients may choose to end the relationship with their physician for various reasons, and they might or might not share those reasons with their provider. When patients do state reasons for ending their medical relationship, those reasons must be charted in the patients' charts. Physicians should send the patients letters acknowledging the termination and offer to refer the patients to other health care providers, if desired.

For their part, physicians may choose to terminate the doctor–patient relationship due to patients' noncompliance with treatment programs. They may also end patient relationships for personal reasons. Whatever the reason, physicians must follow legal protocol to avoid accusations of patient abandonment. A physician may be accused of abandoning his patient if the patient has a chronic illness that needs ongoing care and is unable to schedule care with the physician. This protocol includes sending a letter to a patient indicating the intent to terminate the relationship. This letter must include:

- A statement clearly indicating the intent to terminate the relationship and the date the termination is to be effective
- The reason for the termination of the relationship
- A statement that the patient's medical records will be available for transfer to another physician
- An offer to refer the patient to another physician
- A statement strongly encouraging the patient to seek care with another physician as needed

September 4, 20xx

I, _Walter Backous_, agree to make payments of $100 per month to Morton Family Practice. My payment will be made by the _15th_ of each month and will begin on the _15th of September, 20xx_.

Walter Backous	_9/11/20xx_
Parent or Guardian's Signature	Date

John Smith	_9/11/20xx_
Witness's Signature	Date

Figure 4-7 ■ Sample expressed contract agreement.

A termination-of-care letter (**Figure 4-8** ■) must give the patient at least 30 days before the termination is effective. During that time, the present physician must continue to see the patient if the patient desires. Termination letters should be sent via certified mail with a signed return receipt requested. Copies of termination letters and signed receipts must be placed in patients' medical records.

The Good Samaritan Act

The **Good Samaritan Act** is a law that may protect a person from negligence for voluntarily performing life-saving care. If, for example, health care workers rendered cardiopulmonary resuscitation (**CPR**) at their local grocery store and the patient died or survived with poor outcomes, those health care workers would be protected if the health care worker performed the treatment according to their training. All states have Good Samaritan Acts.

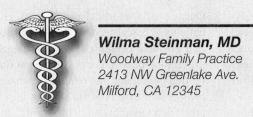

Wilma Steinman, MD
Woodway Family Practice
2413 NW Greenlake Ave.
Milford, CA 12345

August 25, 20xx

Gloria Sanchez
891 NW Wallingford Ave.
Milford, CA 12345

Dear Ms. Sanchez:

Because you have missed your last four follow-up appointments to monitor your condition, I will no longer be able to provide you medical services. I believe your condition requires attention and strongly encourage you to seek care with a physician. When you have chosen a new physician, please advise this office by requesting, in writing, the transfer of your medical records.

If you wish, I would be happy to give you a referral. I will be available to treat you for no longer than 30 days from the receipt of this letter.

Sincerely,

Wilma Steinman, M.D.

Wilma Steinman, M.D.

Figure 4-8 ■ Sample termination of care letter.

Maintaining Patient Confidentiality Through Proper Records Handling

Because medical assistants are patient advocates, they must keep patients' best interests, notably patient confidentiality, at the forefront of their work. Medical assistants must never reveal patient information without a patient's signed HIPAA authorization form or a court order. As a result, when patients' family members call the office, medical assistants can tell them nothing about the patients. Similarly, medical assistants are forbidden from releasing information to insurance companies, even bills for services, without patients' consent.

Critical Thinking Question 4-3

Referring back to the case study at the beginning of this chapter, assume that Victoria revealed information about Dr. Kozlowski's patient to the patient's employer. What is the potential impact on Victoria?

Releasing Medical Records

Requests for patients' medical records are common. Patients might need to see specialists, obtain second opinions, or seek care at different facilities. Any request for copies of patients' medical records must be accompanied by the patients' signed authorization. The medical assistant must be certain the authorization is directed to the correct facility and that it contains a date for when the signature was made. In addition to verifying the authorization, the medical assistant must also be completely clear about the nature of the request and must follow HIPAA guidelines regarding the release of any medical information. Patients may authorize the release of their entire records, or they may authorize the release of information for one date of service only. Some physicians require their staff to alert them of any requests for records. In these offices, the medical assistant pulls the patient's file, attaches the request for copies, and gives the file to the physician for review. Often, release forms for copies of medical records will have a separate box to check if information on HIV or AIDS testing or treatment is requested.

Before sending any copies of medical records, however, the medical assistant must review the file to ensure that it is complete and that it contains only information about that patient. Some facilities provide counseling services that include patients and their family members. For these records, the medical assistant must obliterate any nonpatient specific information from the copied record before sending.

In rare cases, medical offices may release original patient records. These requests are most often received via subpoena for court cases in which the judge or attorneys wish to see original material. When original medical records are required, the medical assistant should make a complete copy of every item in the chart, and keep the copies in the office, recorded in a log, as proof of the contents at the time of release.

Occasionally patients will ask to rescind the authorization to release information previously given. When this occurs, the patient will need to sign a separate form that states their previously given authorization is now rescinded. Many legal documents used for obtaining medical records have a disclosure included that states the amount of time the authorization is to be valid. For example, a form may say, "This authorization is valid for 90 days from the date of the signature." In the event one of these forms is used, the patient will not need to sign a separate form in order to rescind the authorization, unless the patient wishes to withdraw their authorization before the 90-day time period.

Critical Thinking Question 4-4

Looking back at the case study at the beginning of this chapter, what do you think the medical assistant should do if the employer tells the assistant that the patient has given the employer permission to call regarding the patient's health care?

Subpoenas of Medical Records

Occasionally, medical offices may receive a subpoena for patients' medical records. The term **subpoena** is a Latin term that means a person or persons is legally required, via court order, to appear in court. **Subpoena duces tecum** is a formal written document that requires a person or persons to produce records or documents, via court order, in court. Subpoenas can arise from lawsuits due to injury, such as from a car accident. A judge must sign a subpoena, which authorizes the physician to release the information without the patient's signature. Medical facilities are not required to notify the patient of the subpoena, but many will as a courtesy. HIPAA requires medical facilities to keep records of all patient-record disclosures, however, and to make those records available to patients upon request.

Disclosing Minors' Medical Information

In most states, children under 18 may receive certain types of medical treatment without their parents' consent. Such treatments are limited to those for family planning (i.e., birth control or abortion), sexually transmitted infections (**STIs**), mental health, human immunodeficiency virus (HIV), acquired immune deficiency syndrome (AIDS), or alcohol or drug rehabilitation. Because laws for releasing minors' information vary from state to state, medical assistants must be very clear about the laws in the states where they practice.

Minors may receive copies of only those documents their parents cannot see. For example, minors could request and receive copies of their STI treatments, but they could not receive copies of the vaccines they received, except in cases where the minor is emancipated. Parents, in contrast, could receive copies of their children's vaccination record, not their STI treatments.

Guarding Super-Protected Medical Information

A few areas of medical information are considered "super-protected." While the definition varies from state to state, super-protected information is usually any material pertaining to family planning; STIs; mental illness; HIV or AIDS treatment, diagnosis, or testing; and alcohol or drug rehabilitation. Super-protected information normally requires a separate authorization before it can be released to a third party. In other words, if the medical assistant were to receive a request for copies of a patient's file, she would be unable to release super-protected information without a specific request from the patient.

Faxing Medical Records

Medical records should be faxed only when no other method of data transfer is available, because the risk of unintended recipients is too high. The American Health Information Management Association (**AHIMA**) recommends fax use for confidential patient information only when sending copies via postal service or messenger does not suffice. Medical offices should use a HIPAA-compliant fax cover sheet such as the one in **Figure 4-9** ■ any time they fax patient information. Patients may request portions of their medical record be emailed to

Anne Wager, MD

Quan Lee, MD
8282 Arlington Way
Arlington, WA 12345
360-555-4545

Facsimile transmittal

To: _____   Fax number: _____

From: _____   Date: _____

Re: _____   No. of pages, including cover sheet: _____

___ Urgent   ___ For Review   ___ Please Comment   ___ Please Reply

Comments:

CONFIDENTIAL INFORMATION
The information in this facsimile message and any accompanying documents is confidential. This information is intended for use only by the
individual or entity named above. If you are not the intended recipient of
this information, you are hereby notified that any disclosure, copying, or
distribution of this information is strictly prohibited. Please notify the
sender immediately by telephone. Thank you.

Figure 4-9 ■ Sample HIPAA compliant fax cover sheet.

other providers or to the patient. Medical assistants will want to be sure these patients have signed a proper consent form that lists the exact information that is to be sent.

Disclosing Medical Records Improperly

Disclosing confidential patient information without proper authorization (**Figure 4-10** ■) or subpoena is cause for a lawsuit. Patients who feel they have been harmed by improper disclosure may sue a medical office for defamation of character, invasion of privacy (HIPAA violation), or breach of confidentiality. When

information is disclosed improperly, the office is responsible for reporting the event to the HIPAA authorities.

Critical Thinking Question 4-5

In the case study at the beginning of the chapter, imagine the patient's employer obtained a subpoena for her
medical information. How would the medical assistant
determine which information to release? What is the
proper procedure?

Johnston Medical Center
123 Center Avenue
Johnston, MD 12345
(234) 555-1456

Date: _____

I hereby authorize: _____ to release photocopies of the below-defined medical records.

Medical records to be released:

_____

_____

_____

_____

Patient name: _____

Date of birth: _____

Release medical records to: _____

I do_____ do not_____ place limitations on history of illness or diagnostic and therapeutic information, including any treatment for alcohol, drug abuse, psychiatric disorders, or HIV infection.

Date: _____Signature: _____

Witness:_____

Figure 4-10 ■ Sample release of records form.

PROCEDURE 4-2 Obtain Authorization for the Release of Patient Medical Records

Theory and Rationale

The release of patient medical records requires strict attention to detail and relevant laws. The Health Insurance Portability and Accountability Act (HIPAA) requires health care providers to obtain patients' consent to release those patients' health information. The ability to properly obtain authorization for the release of patient medical records is vital to the medical assistant.

Materials

- Release-of-records authorization form
- Blue or black ink pen
- Copy machine
- Patient medical record

Competency

1. When the patient states all or a portion of his record are to be released to a third party, ask the patient to sign and date a release-of-records form.

2. Verify the address where the patient would like the copies of the record sent.

3. Verify the records the patient would like released. If the patient requests specific release dates, ask her to write those dates on the release-of-records form.

4. Verify if the patient would like super-protected information (**HIV/AIDS**, mental health, drug or alcohol rehabilitation information, sexually transmitted infection information, or information about family planning) to be sent, and ask the patient to check the appropriate box on the authorization form to allow the release of that information.

5. Identify which information in the medical record must be copied.

6. Copy the appropriate documents from the medical record.

7. Send the copies to the requested location.

8. Make a notation of the release of information in the patient's medical record.

PROCEDURE 4-3 # Respond to a Request for Copies of a Patient's Medical Record

Theory and Rationale

Releasing personal patient information without the patient's consent or a court order violates HIPAA. In fact, improperly copying documents in a patient's medical record could subject the physician to a lawsuit. Therefore, knowing how to properly respond to a request for copies of the patient's medical record is imperative for the medical assistant. In some facilities, the physician may be involved in choosing the documents that are to be released. Most facilities, however, leave this procedure up to the assistant who has been properly trained on how to follow HIPAA procedures in the release of information from patient files.

Materials

- Release-of-records authorization form
- Blue or black ink pen
- Copy machine
- Patient's medical record

Competency

1. Verify that the release-of-records form has been signed and dated by the patient or the patient's legal representative.

2. Carefully review the release form for any specific date or information requests.
3. Check if the patient has authorized release of super-protected information (HIV/AIDS, mental health, drug or alcohol rehabilitation information, sexually transmitted infection information, or information about family planning).
4. Verify that you have the correct patient file.
5. Locate the documents to be copied.
6. Review the documents to be copied to verify that they carry the correct patient name and contain the information requested in the authorization to release information and only that information.
7. Copy the appropriate documents.
8. Send the copies to the requesting agency.
9. File the release-of-records request in the patient's medical record with a notation of the documents that were copied and sent.

The Health Insurance Portability and Accountability Act (HIPAA)

The **Health Insurance Portability and Accountability Act (HIPAA)** of 1996 was enacted to reform health care mainly by:

1. Improving **portability** and continuity in group and individual insurance
2. Combating waste, fraud, and abuse in health insurance and health care delivery
3. Promoting the use of medical savings accounts (**MSAs**)
4. Improving access to long-term care services and coverage
5. Simplifying health insurance administration
6. Providing a means of paying for reforms and related initiatives

HIPAA is divided into the seven following titles:

Title I	Health Care Access, Portability, and Renewability
Title II	Preventing Health Care Fraud and Abuse; Administrative Simplification; Medical Liability Reform
Title III	Tax-Related Health Provisions
Title IV	Application and Enforcement of Group Health Plan Requirements
Title V	Revenue Offsets
Title XI	General Provisions, Peer Review, Administrative Simplification
Title XXVII	Assuring Portability, Availability, and Renewability of Health Insurance Coverage

HIPAA titles are nonsequential because some portions of the original legislation failed to pass.

Title II of HIPAA

Title II of HIPAA, which relates to health care providers, has three main goals, which are to:

- Prevent fraud and abuse in health care delivery and payment
- Improve Medicare and other programs through an efficient and effective standard
- Establish standards and requirements for all electronic transmission of certain health information

Title II dictated that, by July 2002, all health care providers begin using employer identification numbers (**EINs**) whenever they transmitted patient data electronically. The second portion of Title II imposed a privacy rule that addressed the:

- Rights individuals should have for their private health information

- Procedures that should be established for patients to exercise their rights to private health information
- Uses and disclosures of private patient health information that should be authorized or required

This rule requires all providers of health care or health care products to notify patients in writing how the patients' private health information would be handled and under what circumstances it would be released. The deadline for compliance was April 2003.

The third portion of Title II addresses the issue of electronically transmitting private health information. HIPAA mandates security measures to standardize electronic claim formats and eliminate outdated forms. The Security Ruling in Title II outlines the security measures that must be in place for health care providers to submit patient health information electronically.

HIPAA and Computer Privacy

HIPAA requires password protection for all computers used in health care. All employees who access the computers must have their own passwords and log off when leaving their desks. In addition, computers must face away from patient areas of the clinic.

To be HIPAA-compliant, the medical office must keep its computer systems secure. Knowing the proper procedure for keeping private patient information from being inappropriately viewed is an important function of the administrative medical assistant.

Before stepping away from an office computer for a moment or for the evening, be certain the computer is logged out so no one can obtain private patient information without logging in with a password.

1. Look around the desk area to be certain nothing in sight has private information viewable.
2. Cover or remove any files or papers that may contain patient information and may be viewable to patients.
3. When returning to the workstation, log back into the computer system using a personal password.
4. Ensure that your password is changed periodically and that it is not written anywhere near the computer station.

The HIPAA Security Rule establishes national standards to protect individuals' electronic personal health information that is created, received, used, or maintained by a covered entity. The security rule requires appropriate administrative, physical and technical safeguards to ensure the confidentiality, integrity, and security of electronic protected health information.

The HIPAA Privacy Officer

While every member of the medical office should be well versed in HIPAA, every office must designate one person as the HIPAA privacy officer. The privacy officer is responsible for overseeing all aspects of the office's compliance with federal and state laws related to privacy, security, and confidentiality,

and helping patients who may question or file complaints about suspected violations.

The HIPAA privacy officer may be the person responsible for developing privacy policies and procedures in the medical office. These policies are known as the HIPAA Compliance Plan and will include policies for how protected health information may be disclosed and documented. Medical office staff who are not sure about a disclosure question should consult with the privacy officer for clarification, before releasing information.

Critical Thinking Question 4-6

Refer back to the case study at the beginning of the chapter. Assume that the patient was fired after the medical office gave her employer her private health information without her permission. How should the patient go about filing a complaint with HIPAA authorities?

HIPAA Records Violations

Patients who believe medical offices have inappropriately disclosed medical information may contact HIPAA authorities directly. Every medical office must have the complaint forms on file and help patients filing the proper paperwork. Normally, HIPAA authorities will only issue fines or written warnings when violations were intentional or offices have logged a number of violations. Patients who believe their health care privacy, or the health care privacy of another individual, has been violated may report that violation directly to the Office of Civil Rights in writing. This may also be done electronically, via email (OCRComplaint@hhs.gov), fax, or online through the complaint portal (https://ocrportal.hhs.gov/ocr/index.html).

HIPAA Compliance

Patients can give anyone verbal access to their medical information by notifying the medical office in writing. Permission for verbal access is restricted solely to giving verbal information about a patient's medical care; providing copies, either on paper or electronically, is not permitted with verbal access permission. Such information becomes part of the patients' permanent medical records. For example, if Julius Reiman gives written permission for his wife, Ruth, to have knowledge of his care, the physician can talk to Ruth about Julius's care or condition.

The HIPAA Business Associate Agreement

HIPAA legislation stipulates that only those persons in the office who must have access to private patient information should have access. The office cleaners might work for the physician, but they do not need access to any private patient information.

Employees of medical offices are covered under HIPAA and are required to keep confidential information from leaving the office. Anyone who is not an employee of the medical office but who might come into contact with private patient information must sign a HIPAA Business Associate Agreement. Such people include

- Copy-machine repairperson
- Computer software support technician
- Medical assistant performing a practicum in the clinic
- Medical assistant performing a shadow project
- Consultants
- Professional staff (e.g., accountants or lawyers)
- Cleaning staff
- Transcriptionists

▶▶▶ Pulse Points

What Is an Employee?

Employees are people who work for wages and have payroll taxes taken out of their checks. People who perform work for the office but have no payroll taxes taken from their checks are not employees. These people must sign a HIPAA Business Associate Agreement if they might come into contact with patient private health information.

Protected Health Information (PHI)

Any information in the patient's chart that can be identified as belonging to the patient is considered **protected health information (PHI)**. HIPAA law specifically addresses PHI in stating that this information must be kept confidential, unless released at the patient's request or via court order.

Penalties for HIPAA Violations

The fines for HIPAA violations range from $100 to $25,000. Criminal penalties can also apply if it is determined that an individual knowingly obtained or disclosed personal health information without the proper authority. The most severe penalties under HIPAA legislation apply to anyone who commits an offense with the intent to sell, transfer, or use another person's health information. Table 4-4 outlines the penalties for HIPAA violations.

Advance Directives

Today, many patients use **advance directives** to outline their wishes should they be unable to speak for themselves. Advance directives consist of living wills, orders outlining patients' desire to not be resuscitated, and durable power of attorney for health care. Any "Do Not Resuscitate" (**DNR**) order must be written and signed by the patient's doctor. A do-not-resuscitate order outlines the patient's wishes regarding life-saving measures, should the patient be unable to speak for himself. A copy

---

TABLE 4-4 Penalties for HIPAA Violations

General penalty for the failure to comply with requirements and standards:

- $100 to $50,000 if the violation occurred due to ignorance of the law; $1,000 to $50,000 for violations considered reasonable cause; $10,000 to $50,000 for violations considered due to willful neglect, where the violator corrected the actions; $50,000 for violations due to willful neglect, where the violator did not correct the actions.

Wrongful disclosure of protected health information:

- A person who knowingly and in violation of HIPAA regulations:
  - Uses or causes to be used a unique health identifier
  - Obtains private health information relating to an individual
  - Discloses individually identifiable health information to another person

Shall be punished by:

  - A fine of not more than $50,000, imprisoned for not more than 1 year, or both
  - If the offense is committed under false pretenses, be fined not more than $100,000, imprisoned for not more than 5 years, or both
  - If the offense is done with the intent to sell, transfer, or use private health information for commercial purposes or to cause harm, be fined not more than $250,000, imprisoned not more than 10 years, or both

---

should rest in the patient's file. Concealing or altering an advance directive is a misdemeanor. Creating an advanced directive falsely is a felony.

Living wills, which are legal in every state, state patients' desires should those patients become incapacitated (**Figure 4-11 ■**). Instructions address patients' desire for life-support procedures.

Patients might sometimes give power of attorney to other people. The power of attorney names people who can speak or act for the patients in the event the patients cannot speak for themselves. Power-of-attorney documents normally address patients' desires for life support, but authorized parties may do such things as sign contracts or access bank accounts (**Figure 4-12 ■**).

Patients may write a list of medical directives. These are instructions for medical personnel to follow regarding care of the patient, should the patient be unable to speak for himself. Unlike the do not resuscitate order, medical directives will contain instructions regarding other types of medical care that will or will not be provided and, not just life-saving care.

Patients may sign a health care proxy. This is a legal document that assigns legal authority to another individual to speak for, and make medical decisions for the patient, should the patient be unable to speak for himself. This type of document may be signed by a patient who is undergoing surgery, or who expects to become incapacitated and unable to speak for himself for a period of time.

LIVING WILL OF _____

I, _____, a resident of the City of _____,

_____ County, State of _____, being of sound and disposing

mind, memory and understanding, do hereby willfully and voluntarily make, publish, and declare this to be my LIVING WILL, making known my desire that my life shall not be artificially prolonged under the circumstances set forth below, and do hereby declare:

1. This instrument is directed to my family, my physician(s), my attorney, my clergyman, any medical facility in whose care I happen to be, and to any individual who may become responsible for my health, welfare, or affairs.

2. Death is as much a reality as birth, growth, maturity, and old age. It is the one certainty of life. Let this statement stand as an expression of my wishes now that I am still of sound mind, for the time when I may no longer take part in decisions for my own future.

3. If at any time I should have a terminal condition and my attending physician has determined that there can be no recovery from such condition and my death is imminent, where the application of life-prolonging procedures and "heroic measures" would serve only to artificially prolong the dying process, I direct that such procedures be withheld or withdrawn, and that I be permitted to die naturally. I do not fear death itself as much as the indignities of deterioration, dependence, and hopeless pain. I therefore ask that medication be mercifully administered to me and that any medical procedures be performed on me which are deemed necessary to provide me with comfort or care or to alleviate pain.

4. In the absence of my ability to give directions regarding the use of such life-prolonging procedures, it is my intention that this declaration shall be honored by my family and physician as the final expression of my legal right to refuse medical or surgical treatment and accept the consequences for such refusal.

5. In the event that I am diagnosed as comatose, incompetent, or otherwise mentally or physically incapable of communication, I appoint _____ to make binding decisions concerning my medical treatment.

6. If I have been diagnosed as pregnant and my physician knows that diagnosis, this declaration shall have no force or effect during the course of my pregnancy.

7. I understand the full import of this declaration and I am emotionally and mentally competent to make this declaration. I hope you, who care for me, will feel morally bound to follow its mandate. I recognize that this appears to place a heavy responsibility on you, but it is with the intention of relieving you of such responsibility and of placing it on myself, in accordance with my strong convictions, that this statement is made.

IN WITNESS WHEREOF, I have hereunto subscribed my name and affixed my seal at _____,

_____, this _____ day of _____, 20 _____, in the presence of the subscribing witnesses whom I have requested to become attesting witnesses hereto. _____

Declarant

The declarant is known to me and I believe him/her to be of sound mind.

_____

_____Witness Address

_____

_____Witness Address

Subscribed and acknowledged, before me by _____, and subscribed and sworn to before the witnesses, on the _____ day of _____, 20_____.

_____

(SEAL)

NOTARY PUBLIC State of _____ My Commission

Expires:_____

Copies of this instrument have been given to:

Receipt and acknowledged & date:

Figure 4-11 ■ Sample living will.

DURABLE POWER OF ATTORNEY FOR HEALTH CARE

I, _____, (Printed or typed full name) am of sound mind, and I voluntarily make this designation. I designate _____, (insert name of patient advocate) my _____, (Spouse, child, friend . . .) living at _____ (Address of patient advocate) as my patient advocate to make care, custody and medical treatment decisions for me in the event I become unable to participate in medical treatment decisions. If my first choice cannot serve, I designate _____ (Name of successor) living at _____ _____ (Address of successor) to serve as patient advocate.

The determination of when I am unable to participate in medical treatment decisions shall be made by my attending physician and another physician or licensed psychologist.

In making decisions for me, my patient advocate shall follow my wishes of which he or she is aware, whether expressed orally, in a living will, or in this designation.

My patient advocate has authority to consent to or refuse treatment on my behalf, to arrange medical services for me, including admission to a hospital or nursing care facility, and to pay for such services with my funds. My patient advocate shall have access to any of my medical records to which I have a right.

My specific wishes concerning health care are the following: (if none, write "none")

_____
_____
_____
_____
_____
_____

I may change my mind at any time by communicating in any manner that this designation does not reflect my wishes.

It is my intent that my family, the medical facility, and any doctors, nurses and other medical personnel involved in my care shall have no civil or criminal liability for honoring my wishes as expressed in this designation or for implementing the decisions of my patient advocate.

Photostatic copies of this document, after it is signed and witnessed, shall have the same legal force as the original document.

I sign this document after careful consideration. I understand its meaning and I accept its consequences.

Signed: _____ Date: _____

Address: _____

NOTICE REGARDING WITNESSES

You must have two adult witnesses who will not receive your assets when you die (whether you die with or without a will), and who are not your spouse, child, grandchild, brother or sister, an employee of a company through which you have life or health insurance, or an employee at the health care facility where you are a patient.

STATEMENT OF WITNESSES

We sign below as witnesses. This declaration was signed in our presence.

The declarant appears to be of sound mind, and to be making this designation voluntarily, without duress, fraud or undue influence.

Signed by witness: _____
(Print or type full name)
Address: _____
Signed by witness: _____
(Print or type full name)
Address: _____

Figure 4-12 ■ Sample durable power of attorney for health care.

Employment Law and Health Care

Title VII of the Civil Rights Act of 1964 was passed to protect employees from discrimination in the workplace. Under this act, employers cannot refuse to hire, refuse to equally compensate, or fire an employee based on race, color, sex, religion, or national origin.

During an interview, candidates cannot be asked questions that would reveal their age, marital status, religion, height, weight, or arrest record unless the information somehow relates to the job for which they are interviewing. For example, candidates who must reach objects on a shelf during the day can be polled about height to ensure they have the proper reach. Arrests are a forbidden topic, because mistakes can be made in the criminal justice system. Employers can, however, ask about convictions, as well as drug use. Drug screening before employment is also legal.

Sexual Harassment

Title VII of the Civil Rights Act protects employees against sexual harassment. Sexual harassment is defined as any unwelcome sexual advance or request for sexual favors in the workplace. This can include verbal or physical conduct of a sexual nature if it is used as a condition of employment, is a basis for promotion, or creates a hostile workplace. In plain terms, sexual harassment occurs when one employee feels uncomfortable with another employee on a sexual level.

To keep from being sued for allowing a hostile work environment, employers must act on any employee complaints. Employees who are being sexually harassed but fail to complain to the employer cannot sue the employer for allowing a hostile work environment. The employer must be given a chance to remedy the situation. In the event the physician employer is harassing the employee, that employee may either report the harassment to management, or to the department of health in the state where the harassment is occurring.

The Americans with Disabilities Act and Health Care Employment

The Americans with Disabilities Act (**ADA**) prohibits employers from refusing to hire people with disabilities unless those disabilities prevent the people from performing the essential duties of a job. Employers would be justified in turning down wheelchair candidates for ditch-digging jobs, for example. A written, complete job description that includes any physical duties that are required helps candidates know if they can meet the requirements (**Figure 4-13** ■).

The ADA applies only to employers with 15 or more employees, and a disability is defined as any condition that causes a person's major life activities to be limited. The act covers those who are HIV positive or have AIDS, cancer, a history of mental illness, and alcoholism.

The ADA's Requirements

The ADA requires employers to provide their employees basic accommodations for disabilities, such as extra-wide parking spaces close to the door, accessible bathrooms, break rooms, and work-area accommodations. If an employer has 15 or more employees and one of those employees suddenly becomes disabled, the employer must provide accommodations so the employee can continue to work. However, the employer has two years to provide the accommodations, and the accommodations must be reasonable for the employer, meaning they are not of excessive cost.

Family Medical Leave Act (FMLA)

The **Family Medical Leave Act (FMLA)** was enacted in 1993. This federal law entitles eligible employees to take unpaid leave for specific family and medical reasons, while continuing coverage under the employer-provided health insurance plan. In order to be eligible, employees must have worked for their employer for at least one year, and have worked at least 1250 hours in the previous 12 months immediately preceding the leave. Employers with 50 or more employees are required to provide FMLA coverage for their employees who are eligible. Employers must hold the employee's job during the leave, or have a similar job available to the employee upon return from the leave.

Under the FMLA, employees may take up to 12 work weeks off in a 12-month period of time for one of the following reasons:

● Birth or adoption of a son or daughter
● To care for a spouse, son, daughter, or parent with a serious health condition
● For a serious health condition that makes the employee unable to perform the essential functions of his/her job
● For a qualifying event arising out of the military service of a spouse, son, daughter, or parent on covered active duty

Many states have additional laws in place to allow employees to take time off to care for a sick family member, or other qualifying event. Washington State, for example, passed the Washington State Family Care Act in 1988. This law allows employees to take time off to care for a sick family member when the FMLA does not apply. Most commonly, this law is useful for employees who have not yet reached one year of employment and are therefore ineligible for the FMLA. States that have these additional leave laws may place certain

Job Title: Certified Medical Assistant
Department: Pediatrics
Reports To: Clinical Manager

SUMMARY:

Under general supervision, is responsible for the physical care of patients through tasks of routine difficulty; responsible for maintaining the clinical area of the clinic.

ESSENTIAL DUTIES AND RESPONSIBILITIES:

Includes the following. Other duties may be assigned. Assists physicians with surgical procedures. Takes and records patients' blood pressure, temperature, pulse, respiration and weight. Makes routine entries into patients' charts. Shares responsibilities for use of equipment and supplies. Administers specified medication, by injection, orally or topically, and notes time and amount on patients' charts. Sterilizes equipment and supplies. Makes suggestions to improve work methods, trains new employees; makes routine entries into logs, records supplies and materials used. Completes requisitions for supplies and forwards to supervisor for approval.

QUALIFICATIONS:

To perform this job successfully, an individual must be able to perform each essential duty satisfactorily. The requirements listed below are representative of the knowledge, skill, and/or ability required. Reasonable accommodations may be made to enable individuals with disabilities to perform the essential functions.

EDUCATION:

Successful completion of an accredited medical assisting program.

LANGUAGE SKILLS:

Ability to read and comprehend simple instructions, short correspondence, and memos. Ability to write simple correspondence. Ability to effectively present information in one-on-one and small group situations to patients and other employees of the organization.

MATHEMATICAL SKILLS:

Ability to add and subtract two digit numbers and to multiply and divide with 10's and 100's. Ability to perform these operations using units of American money and weight measurement, volume and distance.

REASONING ABILITY:

Ability to apply common sense understanding to carry out instructions furnished in written, oral, or diagram form.

CERTIFICATES, LICENSES, REGISTRATIONS:

Must have certification of completion of CMA (AAMA) or RMA (AMT) certification examination.

PHYSICAL DEMANDS:

The physical demands described here are representative of those that must be met by an employee to successfully perform the essential functions of this job. Reasonable accommodations may be made to enable individuals with disabilities to perform the essential functions. While performing the duties of this job, the employee is regularly required to stand; walk; use hands to finger, handle, or feel; reach with hands and arms; and talk or hear. The employee is occasionally required to sit; climb or balance; and stoop, kneel, crouch, or crawl. The employee must regularly lift and/or move up to 50 pounds. Specific vision abilities required by this job include close vision, distance vision, color vision, peripheral vision, depth perception, and ability to adjust focus.

The employee must have the ability to work overtime hours.

WORK ENVIRONMENT:

The work environment characteristics described here are representative of those an employee encounters while performing the essential functions of this job. Reasonable accommodations may be made to enable individuals with disabilities to perform the essential functions. While performing the duties of this job, the employee is occasionally exposed to outside weather conditions. The noise level in the work environment is usually moderate.

Figure 4-13 ■ Sample detailed job description.

restrictions on when employees are able to access leave through the state laws. For example, the Washington Family Care Act requires employees to use their vacation and sick leave time for the leave, and cannot take the time unpaid as they can with the FMLA.

The Patients' Bill of Rights

The American Hospital Association (**AHA**) first adopted a Patients' Bill of Rights in 1972 and modified it in 1992. The AHA revamped this document in 2003, renaming the new version The Patient Care Partnership. This agreement is provided to all patients upon entering the inpatient hospital setting. The Patient Care Partnership outlines patients' expectations, rights, and responsibilities while in the hospital setting and explains the quality of care the patient can expect to receive, recognizing that a clean and safe environment should be provided to all patients.

Patients should expect to be involved in their care while in the hospital and should be involved in discussing their condition with the medical providers. These discussions should include the patient's treatment plan. Patients are directed to provide their health care team with all information relating to their treatment, including past illnesses and allergic reactions. The **Patient Care Partnership** assures patients that they can expect protection of their privacy while in the hospital setting, that they will be properly prepared for discharge when the time comes, and that they will be provided with help in filing insurance claims, if needed. The Patient Care Partnership can be viewed on the American Hospital Association Web site: http://www.aha.org/.

In March 1997, President Bill Clinton appointed a committee to study the quality of health care in the United States. As part of its work, the committee issued a list of Consumer Bill of Rights and Responsibilities, which contained the Patients' Bill of Rights in **Figure 4-14** ■

I. Information Disclosure You have the right to receive accurate and easily understood information about your health plan, health care professionals, and health care facilities. If you speak another language, have a physical or mental disability, or just do not understand something, assistance will be provided so you can make informed health care decisions.

II. Choice of Providers and Plans You have the right to a choice of health care providers that is sufficient to provide you with access to appropriate high-quality health care.

III. Access to Emergency Services If you have severe pain, an injury, or a sudden illness that convinces you that your health is in serious jeopardy, you have the right to receive screening and stabilization emergency services whenever and wherever needed, without prior authorization or financial penalty.

IV. Participation in Treatment Decisions You have the right to know all your treatment options and to participate in decisions about your care. Parents, guardians, family members, or other individuals that you designate can represent you if you cannot make your own decisions.

V. Respect and Nondiscrimination You have a right to considerate, respectful, and nondiscriminatory care from your doctors, health plan representatives, and other health care providers.

VI. Confidentiality of Health Information You have the right to talk in confidence with health care providers and to have your health care information protected. You also have the right to review and copy your own medical record and request that your physician amend your record if it is not accurate, relevant, or complete.

VII. Complaints and Appeals You have the right to a fair, fast, and objective review of any complaint you have against your health plan, doctors, hospitals, or other health care personnel. This includes complaints about waiting times, operating hours, the conduct of health care personnel, and the adequacy of health care facilities.

Figure 4-14 ■ Patients' Bill of Rights.

Many states have enacted their own patients' bills of rights. Contents vary, but most include patients' rights for obtaining care, completing the **appeal** process, and handling abuses by insurance carriers.

OSHA and Ambulatory Care

Under the Occupational Safety and Health Act (**OSHA**), employers are required to provide a safe working environment for their employees. OSHA controls and monitors employers for compliance, and employees can make complaints directly to OSHA if they feel their workplace is unsafe.

With regard to health care, OSHA has rules that protect workers from exposure to blood-borne pathogens. OSHA requires that health care workers use standard precautions when they are likely to come into direct contact with patients and that they use protective equipment to protect from blood and bodily fluids. **Figure 4-15** ■ lists the standard precautions recommended by the Centers for Disease Control and Prevention (**CDC**).

Under OSHA rules, all health care facilities must keep a list of all employees who might be exposed to blood-borne pathogens. All facilities must have a written exposure-control plan that outlines the steps to follow in the event of an accidental needle stick or other blood-borne exposure (**Figure 4-16** ■). In many states, OSHA also dictates that any employee who has the potential to become exposed to bodily fluids in the workplace must be given the opportunity to receive the Hepatitis B vaccine series free of charge.

The Clinical Laboratory Improvement Amendments Act (CLIA) and Ambulatory Care

The Centers for Medicare and Medicaid Services (**CMS**) regulates all laboratory testing performed on humans in the United States, with the exception of testing done for medical research. CMS achieves this regulation via the Clinical Laboratory Improvement Amendments Act (**CLIA**) of 1988. These rules apply to any lab, including ambulatory care settings, that is performing any work with specimens. The rules are in place to ensure safe, accurate laboratory testing. CLIA regulations are based on the complexity of the test method. The more complicated the test, the more stringent the requirements. Every facility that performs laboratory testing must establish a quality assurance program that includes quality control, personnel policies, patient test management, and proficiency testing. Facilities are inspected every two years to ensure compliance with federal CLIA regulations.

The Joint Commission (TJC) and Ambulatory Care

The Joint Commission (**TJC**) is a private organization that sets standards for health care administration and patient safety. Hospitals that receive federal funding, such as Medicare and Medicaid, are required to be Joint Commission certified, while private hospitals and doctors' offices are not. Many facilities, including clinics that are not required to be Joint Commission certified still seek this accreditation because it is a sign of excellence in patient safety.

The Controlled Substances Act

The Controlled Substances Act of 1970 regulates the manufacture, distribution, and dispensing of narcotics and nonnarcotic drugs that are considered to have a high potential for abuse. This act is enforced by the Drug Enforcement Agency (**DEA**) and was designed to limit the illegal use of controlled substances in addition to preventing substance abuse by health care professionals. This law requires that any health care provider who dispenses, administers, or prescribes narcotics or any other controlled substances must be registered with the DEA. Violation of this act is a criminal offense punishable by fines and/or imprisonment.

Compliance with the Controlled Substances Act is mandatory and includes the following:

- Health care providers who keep a supply of controlled substances in the office for dispensing or administration must use a triplicate order form from the DEA.
- A record of every controlled substance transaction must be kept and maintained for two to three years and must be available for inspection by the DEA at any time.
- All controlled substances must be kept in a locked cabinet out of the patient's view, and only those staff members who need access should have it.
- Any theft of controlled substances must be reported to the local police and the nearest DEA office.
- Prescription pads must be kept in a safe place to avoid theft.
- Any health care provider who ceases practice must return all unused order forms to the DEA.
- Only a limited supply of prescription pads may be kept in the office. Rather than ordering enough pads to last a year, order just enough for a month or two so missing pads will be more easily and quickly noticed.
- No prescription pads should be kept in the examination rooms or any other location where they are unattended and could be stolen.
- Prescription pads in the office should be inventoried regularly so theft will be quickly noticed.
- Local law enforcement and the DEA must be notified when a prescription pad is stolen.

Hand Washing

[x] Wash hands after touching blood, body fluids, secretions, excretions, and contaminated items, whether or not gloves are worn.

[x] Wash hands immediately after gloves are removed, between patient contacts, and when otherwise indicated to avoid transfer of microorganisms to other patients or environments. It may be necessary to wash hands between tasks and procedures on the same patient to prevent cross-contamination of different body sites.

[x] Use a plain soap for routine hand washing.

[x] Use an antimicrobial agent for specific circumstances, as defined by the infection-control program.

Gloves

[x] Wear gloves when touching blood, body fluids, secretions, excretions, and contaminated items.

[x] Put on clean gloves just before touching mucous membranes and nonintact skin.

[x] Change gloves between tasks and procedures on the same patient after contact with material that may contain a high concentration of microorganisms.

[x] Remove gloves promptly after use, before touching noncontaminated items and environmental surfaces, and before treating another patient.

Mask, Eye Protection, Face Shield

[x] Wear a mask and eye protection or a face shield to protect mucous membranes of the eyes, nose, and mouth during procedures and patient-care activities that are likely to generate splashes or sprays of blood, body fluids, secretions, and excretions.

Gown

[x] Wear a gown to protect skin and to prevent soiling of clothing during procedures and patient care activities that are likely to generate splashes or sprays of blood, body fluids, secretions, or excretions.

[x] Remove a soiled gown as promptly as possible.

Patient-Care Equipment

[x] Handle used patient care equipment soiled with blood, body fluids, secretions, and excretions in a manner that prevents skin and mucous membrane exposures, contamination of clothing, and transfer of microorganisms to other patients and environments.

[x] Ensure that reusable equipment is not used for the care of another patient until it has been cleaned and reprocessed appropriately.

[x] Ensure that single-use items are discarded properly.

Environmental Control

[x] Ensure that the facility has adequate procedures for the routine care, cleaning, and disinfection of environmental surfaces, beds, bedrails, bedside equipment, and other frequently touched surfaces.

Linen

[x] Handle, transport, and process used linen soiled with blood, body fluids, secretions, and excretions in a manner that prevents skin and mucous membrane exposures and contamination of clothing.

Occupational Health and Bloodborne Pathogens

[x] Take care to prevent injuries when using needles, scalpels, and other sharp instruments or devices; when handling sharp instruments after procedures; when cleaning used instruments; and when disposing of used needles.

[x] Never recap used needles, or otherwise manipulate them using both hands or use any other technique that involves directly the point of a needle toward any part of the body.

[x] Do not remove used needles from disposable syringes by hand, and do not bend, break, or otherwise manipulate used needles by hand.

[x] Place used disposable syringes and needles, scalpel blades, and other sharp items in appropriate puncture-resistant containers.

[x] Use mouthpieces, resuscitation bags, or other ventilation devices as alternatives to mouth-to-mouth resuscitation methods in areas where the need for resuscitation is predictable.

Patient Placement

[x] Place a patient who contaminates the environment or who does not or cannot be expected to assist in maintaining appropriate hygiene or environmental control in a private room.

Figure 4-15 ■ CDC Recommended Standard Precautions.

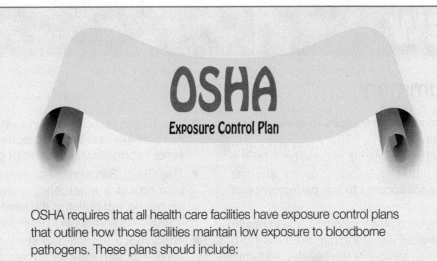

OSHA
Exposure Control Plan

OSHA requires that all health care facilities have exposure control plans that outline how those facilities maintain low exposure to bloodborne pathogens. These plans should include:

☒ Exposure determinations. What does the facility define as an "exposure?"

☒ The schedule and method of implementation for each of the bloodborne pathogens regulations, including:

  • Methods of compliance

  • Hepatitis B vaccination and postexposure evaluation and followup

  • Communication of hazards to employees

  • Recordkeeping

☒ Provisions for the initial reporting of exposure incidents

☒ Hepatitis B vaccination series for unvaccinated employees

☒ Effective procedures for:

  • Evaluating the circumstances surrounding exposure incidents

  • Gathering sharps injury information

  • Periodically determining the frequency of use and the types and brands of sharps involved in exposure incidents

  • Identifying and selecting appropriate and currently available engineering control devices

  • Actively involving employees in the review and update of the exposure control plan for the procedures they perform

Figure 4-16 ■ OSHA exposure control plan.

REVIEW

Chapter Summary

- U.S. laws arise from varying sources to achieve varying legal purposes.
- Obtaining consent from patients is done both for the release of that patient's information to another source, as well as for consent to the performance of a procedure.
- Malpractice is a serious, wide-ranging issue in health care that the medical assistant can address both individually and as a member of the health care team.
- Tort reform is a concept that has been addressed in many states in the United States. Most legislation in this area is aimed at reducing the amount of money an injured victim may recover after a malpractice incident.
- Physicians have a number of public duties to perform to ensure patient safety and confidentiality are upheld.
- Both physicians and patients have duties they should uphold in the physician–patient relationship. Many of these are dictated by law, especially the physician's responsibilities.
- Contracts in health care encompass the consent for care and payment for services rendered.
- Medical assistants play a crucial role in patient confidentiality procedures.

- The Health Insurance Portability and Accountability Act (HIPAA) is a law that outlines how patient personal information is to be kept confidential.
- The Good Samaritan Act mandates that a person who provides emergency assistance while outside his normal job duties in the health care setting cannot be sued for additional injuries sustained by the victim.
- The various federal and state organizations driving current health care practices demand compliance from all members of the medical staff.
- Health care professionals must be vigilant about all relevant legislation, including the patients' bill of rights.
- Various advance directives exist to provide legal means for an individual to express her health care wishes in the event she cannot speak for herself.
- The patients' bill of rights is a list of rights patients have upon entering a particular health care facility.
- Various monitoring agencies such as The Joint Commission and OSHA provide rules and regulations that protect the safety of patients and employees in the health care setting.
- The Controlled Substances Act defines the ways in which controlled substances are to be monitored, recorded, and prescribed.

Chapter Review

Multiple Choice

1. *Res judicata* is Latin for:
   a. The physician is responsible
   b. The thing speaks for itself
   c. Let the master answer
   d. The thing has been decided
   e. There is a master–servant relationship in place

2. Which of the following is the threat of causing harm to another without their consent?
   a. Assault
   b. Battery
   c. Duress
   d. Invasion of privacy
   e. Coercion

3. Which of the following refers to the release of private information about another person without the person's consent?
   a. Assault
   b. Battery
   c. Duress
   d. Invasion of privacy
   e. Coercion

4. Which of the following refers to the actual physical touching of another person without the person's consent (includes physical abuse)?
   a. Assault
   b. Battery
   c. Duress
   d. Invasion of privacy
   e. Coercion

5. Which of the following is the act of coercing someone into an act?
   a. Assault
   b. Battery
   c. Duress
   d. Invasion of privacy
   e. Violation

True/False

T F 1. In most states, children under age 18 may receive medical attention for a sexually transmitted infection without parental consent.

T F 2. Patients win most medical malpractice cases.

T F 3. Patients may refuse treatment for any reason.

T F 4. Hospitals that receive federal funding, such as Medicare and Medicaid, are required to be Joint Commission certified.

T F 5. The statute of limitations for medical malpractice cases is the same in every state.

T F 6. Classes of felony crimes are the same in every state.

T F 7. The physician must report any vaccine injuries.

Short Answer

1. In addition to the examples provided in the text, what other type of persons would the medical office need to have an HIPAA Business Associate Agreement for?
2. What is the Good Samaritan Act?
3. What are the Four Ds of Negligence?
4. Differentiate "implied consent" from "expressed consent."
5. Explain what is meant by "informed consent."
6. Describe the steps the physician must take to legally terminate the physician–patient relationship.
7. Explain the function of the HIPAA Privacy Officer in the medical office.

Research

1. Are there caps on the medical malpractice awards allowed in your state? If so, what are they?
2. Search the Internet for a medical malpractice case. What were the specifics of the case?

Practicum Application Experience

Joe Rutigliano is a patient of Dr. Mallory's. As Joe is leaving the office after his appointment, he overhears Dr. Mallory and her medical assistant discussing his treatment plan in the hallway. He believes other patients also overhear their conversation, and he is upset. What should the medical assistant do?

Resource Guide

American Association of Medical Assistants
20 N. Wacker Dr., Suite 1575
Chicago, IL 60606
Phone: (312) 899-1500
Fax: (312) 899-1259
http://www.aama-ntl.org/

Health Care Providers Service Organization
159 E. County Line Road
Hatboro, PA 19040-1218
Phone: (800) 982-9491
Fax: (800) 739-8818
www.hpso.com

Public Citizen
1600 20th St. NW
Washington, DC. 20009
Phone: (202) 588-1000
www.citizen.org

Sorry Works
P.O. Box 531
Glen Carbon, IL 62034
Phone: (618) 559-8168
http://www.sorryworks.net

5

Medicine and Ethics

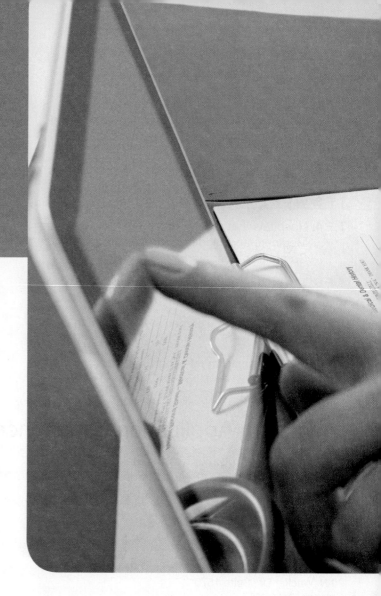

Case Study

Read the following case study and answer the critical thinking questions presented throughout the chapter.

Montel Warman is a patient in a busy family practice office. Montel has been diagnosed with a rare form of cancer. The physician asks Montel if he would be willing to participate in a clinical trial for a new medication. The physician tells Montel that the new medication has the possibility of aggressively attacking his cancer cells and placing the disease into remission. The new medication also has been shown to have serious side effects, including the advancement of the cancer, in laboratory settings. The physician gives Montel all of the information on the clinical trial and asks him if he would like to participate.

Objectives

After completing this chapter, you should be able to:

5.1 Define and spell the key terminology in this chapter.

5.2 Discuss the history of ethics in medicine.

5.3 Describe ethical considerations of the medical assistant, and the importance of performing within the scope of practice.

5.4 Explain how the medical assistant can use the Blanchard and Peale Ethical Model to assist in ethical decision making.

5.5 List ethical issues in the management of patient care, as outlined by the American Medical Association.

5.6 Define bioethics, and list examples of bioethical issues the medical assistant should be aware of in the workplace.

5.7 Describe the ethical issues surrounding clinical research in health care.

5.8 Discuss the ethical nature of employer-mandated medical care.

Key Terminology

abuse—the neglect, or physical, emotional, or financial misconduct of another.

artificial insemination—fertilization of sperm and egg through a nonsexual process

bioethics—issues surrounding life-and-death situations in health care (e.g., cloning, artificial insemination, abortion)

cloning—the process of producing an identical copy of something biological via DNA replication

medical ethics—the concepts that govern the actions of health care professionals

morals—codes or guidelines used to determine behavior or a course of action

values—internal points of reference used to differentiate between what is good and what is bad

Abbreviations

AAMA—American Association of Medical Assistants

AI—artificial insemination

CMA—certified medical assistant

Certification Exam Coverage

AAMA (CMA) Exam Coverage:

● Working as a team member to achieve goals
  • Promoting competent patient care

● Legislation
  • Anatomical gifts
  • Reportable incidents
    1) Public health statuses (e.g., communicable diseases, vital statistics, substance abuse/chemical dependency, abuse against persons)
    2) Wounds of violence

● Performing within ethical boundaries
  • Ethical standards
    1) AAMA Code of Ethics
    2) AMA Code of Ethics
  • Patient rights
  • Current issues in bioethics

AMT (CMAS) Exam Coverage:

● Legal and ethical considerations
  • Apply principles of medical law and ethics to the health care setting
  • Know the principles of medical ethics established by the AMA
  • Recognize unethical practices and identify ethical responses for situations in the medical office

AMT (RMA) Exam Coverage:

● Medical ethics
  • Identify and employ proper ethics in practice as a medical assistant
  • Identify the principles of ethics established by the American Medical Association
● Recognize unethical practices and identify the proper response

Introduction

Medical ethics deal with issues of right and wrong, and often take more thought than legal issues because people have different views about what is right. **Medical ethics** are the concepts that govern the behavior of health care professionals. Throughout their career, every medical assistant should have a clear understanding of what society and the medical assisting profession expect with regard to ethics.

AAMA (CMA) certification exam topics are reprinted with permission of the American Association of Medical Assistants.

AMT (CMAS) certification exam topics are reprinted with permission of American Medical Technologists.

AMT (RMA) certification exam topics are reprinted with permission of American Medical Technologists.

History of Ethics in Medicine

Ethics in medicine has evolved over time and continues to evolve today. As people's **values** and **morals**—their sense of right and wrong—change over time, so do concepts of what is considered ethical. Even within the same group, individuals may feel differently about the ethics in a particular situation. For this reason, societies and professional organizations have come up with ethical guidelines for their citizenry.

Hippocratic Oath

Introduced during the life of Hippocrates, a classical Greek physician who lived between 460 and 377 B.C.E. the Hippocratic Oath was the first basic guide for medical ethics. What began as a short phrase, "Do no harm," has since become a 181-word vow that is recited at modern medical school graduation ceremonies by new graduates.

Ancient Ethical Creeds

One hundred years after the time of Hippocrates, the societies of China and India began to establish their own ethical creeds. These cultures documented their guidelines for those practicing medicine in that era, concentrating on humility, concern, and compassion for the patients they treated. Medical care in ancient times was generally practiced by clerics, and religious themes influenced the practice of medicine, as well as the ethics of that practice.

The Nuremberg Code

Upon discovery of the atrocities performed on the prisoners kept in camps during World War II, legal courts were convened to prosecute those responsible for the killing of prisoners. These trials were called the Nuremberg Trials, named after the city where they were held. During the Nuremberg Trials, judges in 1947 developed a guideline for future conduct of researchers when performing any kind of medical experimentation that involves humans. Ten points regarding permissible experimentation on human beings, known as the Nuremberg Code, were contained within the verdict released at the end of the Nuremberg Trials (**Figure 5-1** ■). This code addressed the proper and ethical control of human experimentation, and was the first medical ethics code to introduce the concept of informed consent. This code considers the way any human experimentation is formulated and concentrates on the value or damage that is brought upon those participating in the experiment. The Nuremberg Code has served as the foundation for all medical research since its publication in 1947.

Declaration of Helsinki

Almost twenty years after the publication of the Nuremberg Code, the World Medical Association published the Declaration of Helsinki in 1964. Like the Nuremberg Code, the Declaration

1. The voluntary consent of the human subject is absolutely essential.
2. The experiment should be such as to yield fruitful results for the good of society, unprocurable by other methods or means of study, and not random and unnecessary in nature.
3. The experiment should be so designed and based on the results of animal experimentation and a knowledge of the natural history of the disease or other problem under study that the anticipated results will justify the performance of the experiment.
4. The experiment should be so conducted as to avoid all unnecessary physical and mental suffering and injury.
5. No experiment should be conducted where there is an a priori reason to believe that death or disabling injury will occur; except, perhaps, in those experiments where the experimental physicians also serve as subjects.
6. The degree of risk to be taken should never exceed that determined by the humanitarian importance of the problem to be solved by the experiment.
7. Proper preparations should be made and adequate facilities provided to protect the experimental subject against even remote possibilities of injury, disability, or death.
8. The experiment should be conducted only by scientifically qualified persons. The highest degree of skill and care should be required through all stages of the experiment of those who conduct or engage in the experiment.
9. During the course of the experiment the human subject should be at liberty to bring the experiment to an end if he has reached the physical or mental state where continuation of the experiment seems to him to be impossible.
10. During the course of the experiment the scientist in charge must be prepared to terminate the experiment at any stage, if he has probable cause to believe, in the exercise of the good faith, superior skill and careful judgment required of him that a continuation of the experiment is likely to result in injury, disability, or death to the experimental subject.

Figure 5-1 ■ The ten points of the Nuremberg Code.
Source: U.S. Department of Health and Human Services.

of Helsinki concentrates on human subjects of research studies. Some of the concepts covered in this ethical guideline for the medical profession include well-informed subjects, a focus on the safety and well-being of those involved, and protection for those subjects who might not be able to speak for themselves.

The Declaration of Helsinki has been revised by the World Medical Association six times, with the most recent revision published in 2008.

Professional Codes of Ethics

Every professional association has its own code of ethics that details the actions that are considered ethical by that profession, and medical assisting is no exception. The American Association of Medical Assistants (**AAMA**) has a code of ethics that addresses five areas the medical assistant must strive for, including:

1. Rendering services with respect for human dignity

2. Respecting patient confidentiality, except when the law requires information

3. Upholding the honor and high principles set forth by the AAMA

4. Continually improving knowledge and skills for the benefit of patients and the health care team

5. Participating in community services that promote the good health and welfare of the general public

Since 1999, the AAMA has had a policy of sanctioning medical assistants who violate its disciplinary standards. Under this policy, called the AAMA's Disciplinary Standards and Procedures for CMAs, sanctions range from being denied eligibility to sit for the certification examination to permanent revocation of the certified medical assistant (**CMA**) credential.

Critical Thinking Question 5-1

Referring back to the case study at the beginning of the chapter, if the medical assistant at the family practice were asked to find information about the ethics involved in clinical research, would he be able to find that information by going to his national or state professional association for medical assistants?

Ethical Considerations

All medical assistants can expect to face legal and ethical situations that might require them to act to protect the patient yet remain within the bounds of law and the scope of practice. Sometimes, physicians might ask medical assistants to perform duties outside the scope of practice. Because this is illegal, the medical assistant should be comfortable declining to accept the task. To do so could cause patient injury and a lawsuit against both the medical assistant and the physician (**Figure 5-2** ■).

Similarly, some medical assistants will witness the physician or other members of the health care team perform procedures outside of the scope of practice for the medical assistant. In some practices, physicians may train medical assistants to perform some of these tasks. Because there are variations, medical assistants must be fully versed in their state's scope of practice. Some procedures, like the application of a cast, might seem easy to perform after being shown by the physician, but if it is outside the scope of medical-assisting practice, it might be illegal to perform even with the physician's supervision. Even if the physician and medical assistant believe no injury will come to the patient, practicing outside the scope of practice is both illegal and unethical.

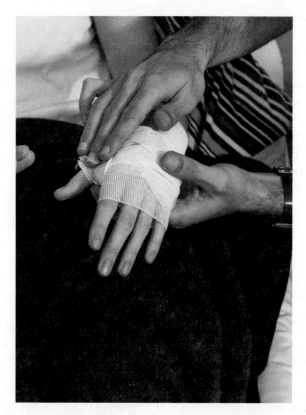

Figure 5-2 ■ The medical assistant should perform only those tasks that are within his or her scope of practice.
Source: Shutterstock © MAErtek.

Patients are sometimes the source of an unethical request to the medical assistant or other health care professional. Patients who have been in an accident or who are abusing a substance may ask the medical assistant to refrain from adding that information into their medical record. Some patients may pretend to have symptoms they are not actually experiencing to receive medications.

There are occasions when the medical assistant is tempted to do something unethical. Medical assistants who take supplies or medications from the office are not acting in an ethical manner, for example. Medical assistants who falsify their time sheets, call out sick when they are not ill, or provide inaccurate information to patients, physicians, or insurance companies are also acting in an unethical, and often unsafe, manner.

Treating Patients without Bias

Medical assistants will be faced with a variety of issues and situations in which they might feel uncomfortable on a personal level. Those personal feelings might be perceived as having a bias against the patient or co-worker who is involved in or living a different lifestyle from the medical assistant. Patients and coworkers should never sense that the assistant disapproves of the activity or lifestyle difference. Examples of these differences include but are not limited to prescription of medical marijuana for a medical condition, or homosexuality or transgenderism.

Ethical Model

An unethical physician might ask the medical assistant to break the law. Medical assistants are legally bound by law and scope of practice to treat patients lawfully and ethically and to document correctly in patients' charts. If medical assistants wonder whether actions cross ethical or legal boundaries, they should consider the following questions based on the Blanchard and Peale Ethical Model:

1. Is the action legal?
2. Is the action ethical?
3. How will the action make me feel?
4. How would I feel if the action, and my involvement, was published in the local newspaper? If I had to explain my actions to my child/spouse/parent?

If the medical assistant is uncomfortable with any of the answers to these four questions, the action likely crosses an ethical or legal boundary and the medical assistant should decline to participate. Any local Association of Medical Assistants chapter is a good place to call when in doubt about an action. Bad actions can hinder future employment. Prospective employers must believe new staff are ethical and will practice within their legal scopes of practice. Medical assistants who are associated with a medical practice or a physician who is practicing unethically or illegally will unfortunately gain that same reputation (**Figure 5-3** ■).

Critical Thinking Question 5-2

If the physician in the case study at the beginning of the chapter were to answer questions about suggesting Montel's participation in the clinical trial based on the Blanchard and Peale Ethical Model, how do you think he would answer each of the questions in her situation?

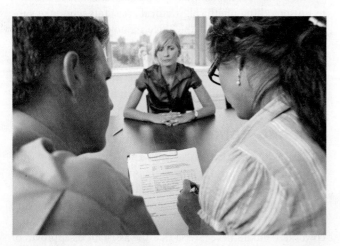

Figure 5-3 ■ The medical assistant might find it difficult to gain future employment if a negative work history becomes known.
Source: Shutterstock © StockLite.

In Practice

Jan has been working as an administrative medical assistant for Dr. Borse for seven years. Dr. Borse frequently asks Jan to add charges to a patient account for services he did not perform.

Jan is paid well and feels she is harming no patients by complying with the doctor's requests. Dr. Borse says he only submits the false claims to make up for the money he loses by treating Medicare and Medicaid patients. One day, Dr. Borse is arrested for insurance fraud; he eventually serves two years in prison and loses his license to practice medicine. Jan is originally arrested too, as a participant in the crime. Because she testifies against her employer, she is not charged with a crime. In the months after this event, Jan has a very hard time getting a new job. Dr. Borse's story has been in all the local papers, and employers do not want to work with unethical staff.

How could Jan have changed the course of events? What advice would have helped Jan while she was working with Dr. Borse?

Raising Ethical Issues in Health Care

The American Medical Association (AMA) has outlined several areas surrounding ethics in the management of patient care, some of which include:

- With regard to organ transplantation, physicians must not consider age in the decision of who gets the organ. Priority must be given to the patient who has the strongest chance of obtaining long term benefit; a person's individual worth to society must not be considered.

- With regard to clinical research, physicians must fully inform any patient involved in research and must give that patients the highest of level of respect and care. The goal of any research program must be to obtain some type of scientific data.

- With regard to obstetrics, physicians must perform abortions within the boundaries of state and federal laws. If physicians do not wish to perform abortions, they must

Critical Thinking Question 5-3

Referring back to the case study at the beginning of the chapter, if the physician suspects that Montel may be reluctant to participate in the study if he is informed of the possible serious side effects, what would ethical guidelines from the American Medical Association prompt the physician to do?

refer patients to physicians who will perform the procedure. If a patient undergoes genetic testing, the physician must give the results to both parents.

Other ethical standpoints by the AMA include areas surrounding finances in the health care setting. These include:

- Patient care should not be dictated by the patient's ability to pay. In other words, a physician should not order expensive tests for a patient who can pay and skip tests for one who cannot.

- Physicians can charge for missed appointments only when they notify the patients of the policy ahead of time.

- Patients must be able to receive copies of their medical record, regardless of any amounts owed the office. The physician cannot hold the medical record hostage for payment of the bill.

- Physicians can charge interest on medical bills in accordance with state law if they notify patients of the policy ahead of time.

- Fees for service must be reasonable and fair and must be based on Current Procedural Terminology (**CPT**) code guidelines regarding the nature of the care involved.

Bioethics

As medical technology advances, the issue of **bioethics** will continue to expand current thought—as well as some individuals' comfort zones. Bioethics addresses areas that affect human life. Within bioethics, what is right for one person might not be right for another. The goal is to make decisions on a case-by-case basis, taking into consideration the individuals who are involved.

Abortion

Though abortion is legal in all 50 states, each state is allowed to make laws regarding how the procedure is accessed. In some states, if a woman is under the age of 18, she might be required to obtain permission from one or both parents before obtaining an abortion. It is estimated that one out of three women in the United States will have had an abortion by the time she is 45 years old. Though this procedure is more common than many people might think, abortion is a bioethical issue to be considered when working in health care (**Figure 5-4** ■).

Abortions can be done by one of two methods. The first is a medication abortion (the patient takes an oral medication to terminate the pregnancy) and the second is a surgical procedure. Even though a medical assistant might not be working in a clinic that provides any type of abortion procedure, he might need to schedule or refer a patient for those services at the physician's request. Assistants who have a moral objection to abortion should notify their employers of their inability to assist in the process of scheduling or preparing referrals. This refusal should never be done in front of or in hearing range of the patient, however.

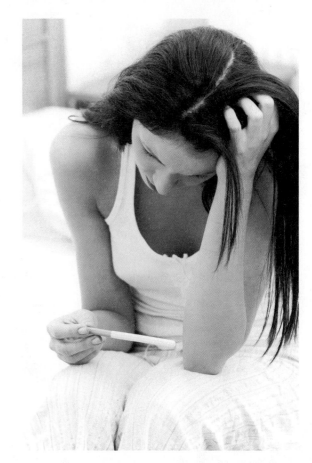

Figure 5-4 ■ A patient who is faced with an unwanted pregnancy may choose to undergo an abortion.
Source: Shutterstock © Piotr Marcinski.

Abortion is a bioethical issue because of the belief some people hold that termination of a pregnancy is killing the unborn or potential child. There are various beliefs as to when life begins; those who believe life begins at conception would likely disapprove of abortion under any circumstances. Those who believe life begins at a later stage in embryonic or fetal development might find abortion is ethical only up to that point in development.

Abuse

Abuse can take one of many different forms. Physical abuse is the actual infliction of pain or injury, such as slapping, bruising, or restraining, on another. Sexual abuse is any nonconsensual sexual contact of any kind with an adult. Sexual contact with a disabled person or a child is considered abuse as the victim is not capable of consenting to the act. Neglect is the failure of a caregiver, parent, or guardian to provide food, shelter, health care, or protection to the person being cared for. Exploitation is the illegal taking, misuse, or concealment of funds or property of a vulnerable adult or child. Emotional abuse is the infliction of mental pain on another through verbal or nonverbal acts. Abandonment is the desertion of a vulnerable adult or child by the person who has the responsibility to care for the victim.

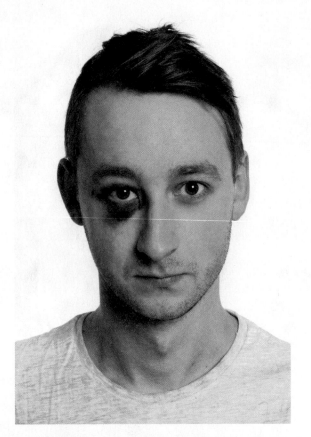

Figure 5-5 ■ Domestic violence victims might be male or female.
Source: Shutterstock © Berents.

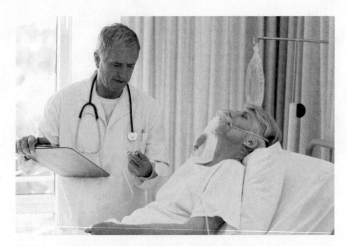

Figure 5-6 ■ When resources are limited, there may be times when patients are unable to receive the care they need.
Source: Shutterstock © wavebreakmedia.

Any form of abuse of a child, or vulnerable adult, must be reported to the local law enforcement agency. Failure to make this report can cause the physician to face legal charges, should the victim incur further harm. When the medical assistant suspects a patient might have been abused, the assistant should inform the physician of the findings and the reason for suspicion and allow the physician to make the determination as to whether the suspicion is valid and a report should be made.

Spousal abuse is also known as domestic violence. Domestic violence can take many forms, including emotional, sexual and physical abuse, and threats of abuse. Men are sometimes abused by partners, but domestic violence is most often directed toward women. Domestic violence can happen in heterosexual or same-sex relationships (**Figure 5-5** ■).

The medical assistant will need to work with the physician to document any abuse, though the patient may refuse to file legal charges against the abuser. In these cases, the physician should only report the abuse if the abuser is thought to be an imminent danger to others or if the abuser used a weapon, such as a knife or a gun.

Allocation of Health Resources

With many health care resources in short supply, health care providers and organizations are sometimes faced with the ethical dilemma of deciding who gets the resource and who goes without. Scarce health care resources might be in the form of supplies, such as medications or immunizations and vaccinations. When this shortage occurs, organizations—or, in the case of vaccinations, a governmental agency—will step in to decide who should receive that resource. Other scarce resources can be in the form of equipment, such as respirators (**Figure 5-6** ■). In the event of an influenza pandemic, if there were more patients needing respirators than a hospital has, the hospital administration would need to decide how those resources were best used.

In health care today, many of the available resources are spent on patients who are at the end of their lives or who are critically ill. The Centers for Medicare and Medicaid states that 30 percent of all funding for Medicare patients is spent in the final year of patients' lives. This care is sometimes seen as futile, as the patient might be declining quickly, and yet health care providers, patients, and family members may be unable or unwilling to realize when it is time to stop certain treatments.

Allocation of resources is a bioethical issue because it forces those in charge of the resources to determine who is most deserving of the resources. This creates a system in which one life is determined to be more valuable than another, and the resource is allocated to that life that is considered more worth saving.

Artificial Insemination

Artificial insemination (**AI**) is the process of introducing sperm into the female reproductive tract by some means other than sexual intercourse. AI is a fairly easy and effective treatment for certain types of infertility. The process of AI includes the insertion of a thin tube through which sperm is injected into the female reproductive tract, and it is seen as unethical by some who feel that it is bypassing the natural process. AI does not typically involve increased risk of multiple embryos being fertilized, as with some forms of infertility treatments.

Infertility Treatments

Generally, as a woman passes the age of 35, her chances of getting pregnant begin to decrease. While the number of patients who seek treatment for infertility has risen over the past 20 years, this is not because the condition of infertility has risen. The rise in treatment is due to the number of women over the last 20 years who put off starting a family until later in life. Many of these women put their careers at the forefront of their lives until their mid- to late thirties, before they look to have children.

There are a variety of options for treatment of infertility. Medical insurance often does not cover the costs of infertility treatment as it is seen as an elective procedure. The first step for a couple having trouble conceiving is to seek the advice of a physician who specializes in infertility treatment. This specialist will often run a series of diagnostic tests on both partners to determine the cause of the infertility. In the event the woman is having trouble ovulating, treatment may include medications that cause her body to ovulate. Another option for infertility may be for the physician to harvest eggs from the woman and fertilize those eggs with sperm from the partner (or donor, in some cases). This process is called in vitro fertilization (**Figure 5-7** ■). The fertilized eggs are then inserted into the woman's uterus with the goal of having one or two of the fertilized eggs implant and result in a pregnancy.

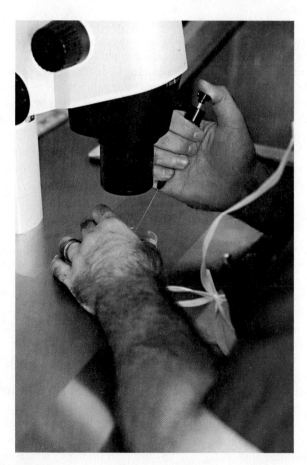

Figure 5-7 ■ In vitro fertilization takes place in a laboratory.
Source: Shutterstock © Michael Zysman.

Medications to force ovulation and in vitro fertilization can both result in pregnancy with multiple embryos. Pregnancies with multiple embryos are often considered high-risk, and the outcome for the infants can be poor, depending upon the number of fetuses. In some cases, fertilization of a ripe egg occurs within the uterus of the woman via introduction of sperm via medical methods. This is called in vivo fertilization.

Both in vitro and in vivo fertilization are seen as bioethical issues because they bypass the natural process. With the higher risk of multiple pregnancies, many believe in vitro fertilization creates the possibility that one or more of the fertilized embryos will not survive to birth or might be aborted. With the process of in vitro fertilization, many eggs can become fertilized, while only a small number are implanted into the uterus. Those fertilized eggs that are not implanted are seen by those who believe life begins at conception as the loss of a potential life. In addition, the infants in a multiple pregnancy have a higher chance of being born with disabilities.

Stem Cell Research

Stem cells are cells that can develop into many different cell types in the body during early life. They are distinguished from other cell types in that they are capable of renewing themselves through cell division and, under certain conditions, they can be induced to become cells with special functions. Scientists work mainly with two kinds of stem cells—those taken from embryonic tissue and those taken from adult tissue. The science behind embryonic stem cell research was discovered in the early 1980s. In 2006, scientists discovered certain conditions under which adult cells can be manipulated into becoming a cell similar to a stem cell (**Figure 5-8** ■).

Stem cell research is considered a bioethical issue because embryos must be destroyed in order to perform embryonic stem cell research. Because some people believe that life begins at conception, the destruction of an embryo for any reason is seen as killing a potential person.

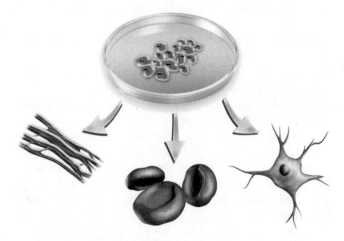

Figure 5-8 ■ Stem cells can be manipulated into becoming muscle, blood, or nerve cells.
Source: Shutterstock © Andrea Danti.

Surrogacy

Surrogate pregnancy is when one woman carries a child for another. There are two types of surrogacy. Traditional surrogacy occurs when a surrogate mother is artificially inseminated and carries the baby to term. With traditional surrogacy, the child is genetically related to the surrogate mother as well as the donor father. Gestational surrogacy occurs when an egg is removed from a donor mother and fertilized with the sperm from a donor father. The fertilized egg is then transferred into a surrogate, who carries the child to term. With gestational surrogacy, the child is not genetically related to the surrogate mother. Couples may use surrogacy in situations where the woman is unable to carry a child to term, or when a couple consists of two men and a surrogate mother is needed to carry their desired child.

Couples using a surrogate mother will want to work with an attorney who is experienced in handling surrogate cases. There have been cases in which the surrogate mother changes her mind about giving up the baby at the end of the pregnancy, and the legality of parental rights is then called into question.

Surrogacy is seen as a bioethical issue as it bypasses the natural way of becoming pregnant. There may be some stigma for the surrogate mother who carries the child to birth, and some confusion as to who the child's parents are.

Cloning

The term **cloning** refers to the process of producing an identical copy of something biological via DNA replication. The copied biological material is referred to as the clone. Scientists have successfully cloned a range of biological materials, such as genes, cells, and tissues. In order to clone an animal, scientists remove a cell from the animal they wish to clone. The removed cell is then used to transfer the DNA of the donor animal into an egg cell that has had its own DNA removed. The egg is then allowed to develop and is implanted into the womb of an adult female animal. When the animal gives birth, the young animal is a clone, with identical genetic makeup as the donor animal.

Cloning can happen naturally in the example of identical twins. The process of creating identical twins can also take place in a laboratory with scientists separating a fertilized egg into two cells, allowing those cells to continue to divide, then implanting the two eggs into a surrogate mother, where they finish the development process.

Reproductive cloning is an imperfect process. The cloning process is inefficient, and cloned animal embryos have not been found to live long. A variety of defects have been noted in clones, such as defective internal organs, premature aging, and problems with the immune system. Improvements have been made to this process in the past decade, and it is expected that one day in the near future cloned biological material may remain stable.

There are several medical reasons to perform cloning. In medical research today, animals are bred to carry certain disease-causing mutations, which are then studied in the laboratory setting. Cloning this type of animal could reduce the amount of time it takes to create new test subjects. Some medical researchers are looking into the ability to create stem cells via cloning. Other scientific research focuses on cloning stem cells from a particular individual, with the goal of growing new needed organs.

Cloning has been seen as a way to revive endangered or even extinct species. To do this, scientists would need a source of DNA from the endangered or extinct species and some closely related species to provide an egg donor and surrogate mother.

At present, a biotechnology company in the United States will clone a pet. This process is costly and produces only a genetic copy of the deceased pet. Just as in human twins, genetic identity does not translate to identical personalities or traits. Cloning a deceased pet may result in an animal that is genetically identical to the lost pet, but the clone may be vastly different in personality traits.

Research into cloning has involved the idea of creating agricultural animals that are efficient producers of high-quality milk or meat. Because it is not possible to determine the quality of beef cattle meat until the animal is slaughtered, cloning the dead animal is seen as a way to produce quality beef with little risk of ending up with a poor quality animal.

Because the process of cloning requires the destruction of a donor egg cell, which could have become another, individual life form, cloning is seen by some as unethical. Many scientists and lawmakers view human cloning as unethical. The idea of cloning to create a more intelligent human, or to create humans that could be harvested for organs needed by others, is seen by some as the unethical slope that cloning will follow. Some religious groups find the concept of human cloning to be objectionable; these groups believe that life should not be created by man, only by God. Currently, laws in the United States ban the cloning of humans.

Genetic Counseling

Genetic counseling is often offered to couples with a family history of birth defects and who wish to have a child. When visiting a genetic counselor, these couples undergo a family health history review as well as a discussion of how their ethnic makeup might make them more prone to genetic defects. Women above the age of 35 are typically at higher risk for bearing children with some birth defects, such as Down syndrome. Genetic counselors serve the function of helping couples make an informed decision about the likelihood of a particular genetic defect appearing in their offspring (**Figure 5-9** ■).

Genetic counseling can be considered a bioethical issue as it is commonly performed so that parents can make decisions regarding going forward with having a child. Some people may see this as discounting the value of a child with certain disabilities.

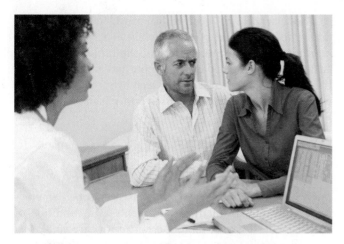

Figure 5-9 ■ Couples concerned about possible genetic defects may choose to consult a genetic counselor.
Source: Shutterstock © Monkey Business Images.

Physician-Assisted Suicide

Physician-assisted suicide is the process by which a physician provides to patients the education and the means to end their own lives. This process does not include the physician administering any treatment or procedure. Physician-assisted suicide is a passive form of assisting the patient in ending his own life; it is the patient who takes the action, using the information and means provided by the physician. Many physicians feel it is unethical to assist a patient in ending his own life. These physicians often feel that their job is to heal patients, not to help them to die. Other physicians feel that patients who are at the end of their lives due to a terminal illness are best helped by providing them with education and the means to end their lives, at the time and place of the patients' choosing.

In states that allow physician-assisted suicide, mechanisms are in place to guide physicians in helping patients who seek this service. Patients must have a terminal illness, with a short period of time within which they are expected to die. These patients are required to undergo psychological examinations to verify they are not making the choice to end their lives due to depression or other mental illness. Once a patient meets the prerequisites, physicians who choose to provide this service will educate the patient on how to end her life with medications and will provide a prescription to the patient for those medications. In states that allow physician-assisted suicide, physicians are allowed to choose for themselves whether they will provide this service to patients. Some health care organizations, particularly those that are faith-based, do not allow the physicians they employ to provide physician-assisted suicide services or to advise patients seeking care in their facility.

Organ Donation

Several human organs can be transplanted, including the cornea, liver, kidney, heart, lung, and skin, but every year approximately 6,000 Americans die waiting for organ transplants. To address the donation of human organs, the National Conference of Commissioners for Uniform State Laws passed the Uniform Anatomical Gift Act. Most states allow people to indicate their wish to become organ donors by making a notation on their driver's license. All states abide by the following rules:

- Donors must be mentally competent and over age 18 to donate their own bodies. Parents or legal guardians may consent for a child or dependent adult to become an organ donor. The next of kin may provide consent as well.
- A physician who is also on the transplant team must not determine the death of the donor.

No financial compensation may be made for organ donation. Like the allocation of resources in short supply, organ donation is a bioethical issue: health care providers and committees have to determine which patient is the best candidate for the organ. With so many Americans dying while they wait for an organ, it might be considered unethical to allow one person to die while another gets the available organ.

The sale of one's own organs is also seen as a bioethical issue. Allowing individuals to sell their own organs for financial gain could be seen as preying on the poor in society. The assumption is that only those experiencing financial difficulty would sell their own organs, creating a system in which the wealthy could afford to purchase the organ they need, while the poor who need organs would go without. This ethical concern is a large part of the reason why it is illegal to sell organs in the United States.

Treating Patients with HIV/AIDS

In the early 1980s, when HIV and AIDS were first discovered and diagnosed in patients, people with AIDS were not likely to live long. Today numerous antiretroviral drugs exist that treat HIV infection. Though these treatments do not cure people with HIV or AIDS, they suppress the virus, sometimes to the point where the virus can no longer be detected. With the virus suppressed, people infected with HIV and AIDS are now able to live longer lives. It is important to note that, even with the virus suppressed, those infected with HIV and AIDS are able to transmit the virus to others. The American Medical Association advises physicians to treat patients with HIV or AIDS, unless those patients are outside the physician's range of expertise. The refusal to treat any patient with any type of disease or illness is seen as unethical. Those who work in health care have an ethical—and often legal—obligation to provide care to patients who are in need.

Clinical Research

Clinical research typically consists of researchers studying the effects of a medicine or treatment on a particular disease or condition. These studies are called clinical trials and are designed to test whether a particular strategy or treatment is both safe and beneficial to patients needing the care. Clinical trials start in a laboratory, where scientists develop and research treatments and drugs. These laboratory settings often include animals on whom scientists test their treatments and theories. Because animals respond different to treatments than humans may, the next step in a clinical trial would be for the researchers to move from animals to humans.

Clinical trials are strictly planned and monitored to ensure that no individual is taken advantage of or unnecessarily injured in the research process. There are three possible outcomes to a clinical trial: (1) the strategy improves patient outcomes, (2) the strategy offers no benefit, or (3) the strategy causes harm rather than good. Clinical trial research may be performed in a variety of different settings and designs. Most clinical trials include a group of individuals that receive the treatment or medicine and another group that does not. The group not receiving the treatment will receive a placebo, which is a treatment that appears to be the same as the real medicine, but is instead made of an inert harmless substance. Participants in the groups do not know whether they are receiving the treatment or the placebo. In some situations, the scientists performing the research know which individuals are receiving the medicine or treatment and which are receiving the placebo. In other situations, the scientists do not know which participants are in which group; this second type of trial is known as a double-blind clinical research trial. In some situations, scientists choose the participants of each group, and in other examples, the participants are chosen at random.

Because there has been ethical consideration about certain types of clinical research trials, every trial today is monitored to ensure the safety of the individuals and to ensure that all participants are protected and informed of the process. Clinical research is seen by some as an ethical issue because harm may be caused rather than benefit.

Employer-Mandated Medical Care

Many health care employers today insist that their employees receive certain medical treatments as a condition of employment. It is very common for health care employers to require medical staff to be immunized against a variety of diseases, including mandating the receipt of an annual influenza vaccine. This practice of mandating immunizations has been challenged in some health care organizations. Employees with a documented medical reason for not receiving the immunization(s) are typically excused from having the vaccine. Some organizations allow employees to claim a religious exemption to receiving the vaccine; others do not allow this exception. There have been cases of health care unions opposing the mandate of vaccine receipt. In 2004, Virginia Mason Medical Center in Seattle made flu shots mandatory for all staff and volunteers. The Washington State Nurses' Association opposed this requirement. In 2006, the U.S. District Court ruled in favor of the Nurses' Association.

REVIEW

Chapter Summary

- The concepts surrounding medical ethics have been around since the time of Hippocrates.
- Medical ethics govern the behavior of health care professionals. Each professional association has its own code of ethics that details the actions that are considered ethical by that profession.
- Medical ethics pertain to health care professionals acting only within their legal scope of practice.
- There are ethical-decision-making models that medical assistants can use in making ethical decisions in the health care field.
- The American Medical Association outlines several ethical issues that pertain to physician care.

- Medical bioethics includes topics such as abortion, genetic counseling, cloning, physician-assisted suicide, and organ donation.
- Clinical research is performed to determine the benefits of certain types of care or medications on a particular population.
- Many health care employers today mandate that their employees receive certain types of medical care as a condition of employment. Most often, this care consists of vaccinations against a variety of illnesses and diseases.

Chapter Review

Multiple Choice

1. Abuse can take the form of:
   a. slapping
   b. bruising
   c. pinching
   d. restraining
   e. all of the above

2. Which of the following is true about infertility treatment?
   a. It is covered by most major insurance carriers.
   b. It always results in multiple-fetus pregnancies.
   c. Treatment for infertility is the same for all patients.
   d. It is expensive and paid for out-of-pocket by the patient.
   e. Patients have to try becoming pregnant naturally for two years before they are eligible for infertility treatment.

3. The Declaration of Helsinki was published in:
   a. 1944
   b. 1954
   c. 1964
   d. 1974
   e. 1984

4. The Nuremberg Code was written at the end of which war?
   a. World War I
   b. World War II
   c. The Korean War
   d. The Vietnam War
   e. The Civil War

5. Which of the following is part of the AMA Code of Ethics?
   a. Physicians may not charge patients interest on health care bills.
   b. Physicians must notify patients of any charge associated with copying medical records.
   c. Physicians may refuse to treat a patient for any reason.
   d. Physicians may charge whatever they wish for the services they provide.
   e. Physician may dismiss patients who are unable to pay their bill.

True/False

T F 1. Surrogacy is always done using the egg of the surrogate mother.

T F 2. Physician-assisted suicide is legal in all 50 states.

T F 3. Reproductive cloning results in a replica that will typically outlive the original animal.

T F 4. Any form of abuse of a child or vulnerable adult must be reported to the local law enforcement agency.

T F 5. Even if the physician and medical assistant believe no injury will come to the patient, practicing outside scope of practice is both illegal and unethical.

Short Answer

1. What are the four steps in an ethical model, and how do they apply in an everyday situation, such as talking about a patient with coworkers outside the medical office?
2. What is the process of in vitro fertilization, and how it is used to treat infertility?
3. Explain why the Nuremberg Code was written.
4. Why is care at the end of a patient's life so expensive?
5. How is physician-assisted suicide handled in a faith-based medical institution?

Research

1. Search the Internet for a medical ethics case. What were the specifics of the case?
2. Research the concept of cloning. What are the various arguments for and against this procedure?
3. Talk with your own physician about physician-assisted suicide. What are his or her thoughts on providing this service to patients?

Practicum Application Experience

Chelsea Palabrica is a patient of Dr. Vallen's. When Dr. Vallen told Chelsea that she is pregnant, Chelsea requested a referral for a pregnancy termination. Dr. Vallen takes Chelsea to the medical assistant's desk and requests the medical assistant call to schedule Chelsea for the procedure. The medical assistant objects to abortion and does not wish to proceed with the task that is asked of her. What can the medical assistant do?

Resource Guide

American Association of Medical Assistants
20 N. Wacker Dr., Suite 1575
Chicago, IL 60606
Phone: (312) 899-1500
Fax: (312) 899-1259
http://www.aama-ntl.org/

Bioethics.com
http://bioethicsnews.com

Donate Life America
http://donatelife.net/understanding-donation/
organ-donation/

National Society of Genetic Counselors
383 Colorow Drive
Salt Lake City, UT 84108
Phone: (801) 585-3470
http://www.nsgc.org/

Learn.Genetics
The University of Utah Genetic Science Learning Center
http://learn.genetics.utah.edu/content/tech/cloning/

Physician-assisted suicide: legal and ethical considerations
http://www.ncbi.nlm.nih.gov/pubmed/17549931

Stem Cell Research & Therapy
http://stemcellres.com/

6

Interpersonal Communication Skills

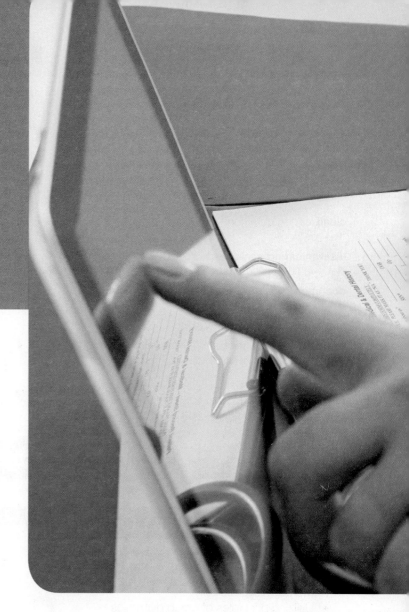

Case Study

Read the following case study and answer the critical thinking questions presented throughout the chapter.

Katerina Bolshoy is a Russian patient who speaks broken English. The registered medical assistant, who does not speak Katerina's language, must schedule several appointments for Katerina, as well as explain insurance coverage to her. The RMA is concerned with how she will communicate this important information to the patient.

Objectives

After completing this chapter, you should be able to:

6.1 Define and spell the key terminology in this chapter.

6.2 List and describe the elements of the communication process.

6.3 Describe both verbal and nonverbal communication and how each can be used most effectively.

6.4 Discuss the importance of active listening when communicating with patients.

6.5 Describe interviewing techniques the medical assistant can use with patients.

6.6 Identify factors that hinder communication.

6.7 List and describe techniques for communicating with distressed or difficult patients and patients with special needs.

6.8 Describe various patient defense mechanisms.

6.9 Maintain professional patient communication.

6.10 Explain how to communicate effectively with members of the health care team and other facilities.

6.11 Discuss developmental stages of the life cycle and their impact on communication.

6.12 Describe the steps involved in patient education.

6.13 Outline a plan for educating patients on a variety of topics.

Key Terminology

active listening—giving full attention during an exchange of information

assess—to make a judgment about something

body language—the process of communicating nonverbally through movements and gestures (e.g., facial expressions)

close-ended question—question that can be answered with "yes" or "no"

discriminating—acting against a person's interest due to a perceived difference in race, gender, economic, or other status

documenting—process of capturing information in the patient's chart

empathy—identification with another person's feelings

evaluation—to judge or interpret the value of something (e.g., a patient's progress)

examples—illustrations of concepts or ideas

feedback—information that is reflected back to an individual in an interpersonal exchange (e.g., during patient–provider communication)

implementation—process of taking action; putting a plan in place

open-ended question—question that requires more than a "yes" or "no" answer

personal space—area around a person deemed the "comfort zone"

planning—process of researching the actions or steps needed to implement a plan or project

professional distance—maintaining a professional relationship with patients and coworkers to remain objective and avoid the appearance of impropriety

reflecting—the practice of repeating patient information so that the patient knows he or she has been understood

stereotyping—to falsely believe that all individuals with particular characteristics (e.g., race, gender, economic status) are the same; judging individuals based on your own opinions

sympathy—feelings of pity for someone else's trouble or misfortune

therapeutic communication—face-to-face process of interacting with the patient that focuses on the patient's physical and emotional well-being

Certification Exam Coverage

AAMA (CMA) Exam Coverage:

- Working as a team member to achieve goals
  - Member responsibility
  - Utilizing principles of group dynamics
- Adapting communication according to an individual's needs
  - Blind
  - Deaf
  - Elderly
  - Children
  - Seriously ill
  - Mentally impaired
  - Illiterate
  - Non-English speaking
  - Anxious
  - Angry/distraught
  - Culturally different
- Recognizing and responding to verbal and nonverbal communication
  - Body language
  - Listening skills
  - Eye contact

- Barriers to communication
- Identifying needs of others
- Professional communication and behavior
  - Professional situations
    1) Tact
    2) Diplomacy
    3) Courtesy
    4) Responsibility/Integrity
  - Therapeutic relationships
    1) Impartial behavior
    2) Empathy/sympathy
    3) Understanding emotional behavior
- Patient interviewing techniques
  - Types of questions
    1) Exploratory
    2) Open-ended
    3) Direct
  - Evaluating effectiveness
    1) Observation
    2) Active listening
    3) Feedback
  - Legal restrictions

AAMA (CMA) certification exam topics are reprinted with permission of the American Association of Medical Assistants.

- Patient interviewing techniques
- Resource information and community services
  - Patient advocate
    1) Services available
    2) Appropriate referrals
    3) Follow-up

AMT (CMAS) Exam Coverage:

- Professionalism
  - Employ human relations skills appropriate to the health care setting
  - Display behaviors of a professional medical administrative specialist
- Communication
  - Employ effective written and oral communication

AMT (RMA) Exam Coverage:

- Human relations
  - Patient relations
    1) Identify age-group specific responses and support
    2) Identify and employ professional conduct in all aspects of patient care

    3) Understand and properly apply communication methods
    4) Identify and respect cultural and ethnic differences
    5) Respect and care for patients without regard for age, gender, sexual orientation, or socioeconomic level
  - Interpersonal relations
    1) Employer/administration
    2) Coworkers
    3) Vendors
    4) Business associates
    5) Observe and respect cultural diversity in the workplace
  - Patient education
    1) Identify and apply proper written and verbal communication to instruct patient
  - Oral and written communication
    1) Employ active listening skills

NCCT (NCMA) Exam Coverage:

- General office procedures
  - Oral and written communication skills
  - Patient instruction
  - Cultural awareness

Introduction

Communication is the process of sharing ideas between two or more people. It is the transfer of information and can take different forms, such as sending messages verbally and nonverbally. Communication skills are vital for anyone working in health care, including the medical assistant. The medical assistant must have a firm understanding of the communication process in order to share information accurately with patients, physicians, and coworkers and respond appropriately.

The Communication Process

The communication process includes a source, message, channel, receiver, and feedback. The *source*, or sender, is the individual sending the message. The message includes the content (written or spoken) that is being delivered. An example of a verbal message is one that is sent over the telephone; another example is one that is spoken directly from one person to another. An example of a nonverbal message is one that is sent

using a computer, such as an e-mail message. The *channel* is the way in which the message is sent and can include the senses (i.e., hearing, sight, taste, smell, or touch). The *receiver* is the individual who receives the message. Another important part of the communication process is that of **feedback**. After the receiver has received the message, feedback is necessary to ensure comprehension; it is used to determine if further clarification is necessary, or if the message received is correct (Figure 6-1). All components of the communication process are important; if any part of the communication process breaks down, the correct message will not be received (**Figure 6-1 ■**).

Competency Skills Performance

1. Use effective listening skills in patient interviews.
2. Communicate with a hearing-impaired patient.
3. Communicate with a sight-impaired patient.
4. Communicate with a patient via interpreter.
5. Prepare a patient's specialist referral.
6. Identify community resources.
7. Use the Internet to find patient education materials.

AMT (CMAS) certification exam topics are reprinted with permission of American Medical Technologists.

AMT (RMA) certification exam topics are reprinted with permission of American Medical Technologists.

NCCT (NCMA) certification exam topics © 2013 National Center for Competency Testing. Reprinted with permission of NCCT.

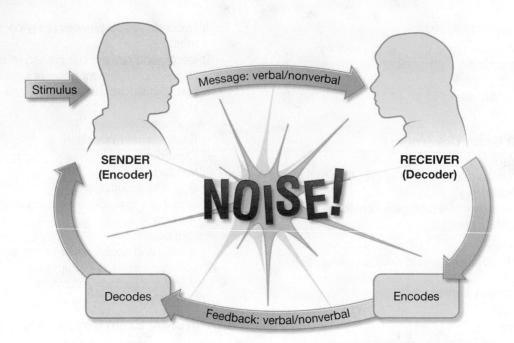

Figure 6-1 ■ The communication process includes a sender and receiver.

Verbal Communication

Verbal communication uses spoken words to transfer messages. Professional medical assistants adopt polite tones of voice, avoid slang, use proper grammar, have a positive attitude, and present information pleasantly. When communicating with patients, patients' families, physicians, and coworkers, medical assistants should follow these "five Cs" of better communication:

- **Content**—Address all areas of interest and fully answer all questions.
- **Conciseness**—Get to the point; say what needs to be said in as few words as possible.
- **Clarity**—Choose words that accurately and precisely convey meaning.
- **Coherence**—Create a logical, easy-to-follow train of thought.
- **Check**—Ask for feedback or clarification to ensure comprehension.

These guidelines should be employed by medical assistants for all means of communication, both verbal and nonverbal (discussed in the next section).

Communication must be geared to patients' ability to understand, which often means using basic terms rather than medical terminology. This applies even when patients are also health care professionals. Such patients might work in different fields and lack knowledge about the procedures they are undergoing.

Some patients may be embarrassed to admit a lack of understanding, and that can be dangerous. Patients who fail to understand could fail to follow medical directions. Feedback, which involves questioning patients to ensure comprehension, is the best way to avoid this situation. Medical assistants must ensure that patients understand what is being said. When communication barriers like language or disabilities limit patient comprehension, medical assistants must arrange for interpreters or family members to help facilitate the patient exchange.

Part of medical assisting is communicating carefully to ensure patients never feel demeaned. Sometimes, communication can be unintentionally offensive. Tone of voice, which is a person's characteristic style of speaking or quality of voice, is important to consider when communicating with patients. Voice tone can impact a patient's perception of the message you are sending. Facial expression and projection are also critical (**Figure 6-2** ■). Medical assistants who project the image that something is important inspire patients to do the same.

Critical Thinking Question 6-1

Referring to the case study at the beginning of the chapter, how can the registered medical assistant enhance communication with nonnative English speakers like Katerina?

Nonverbal Communication

Some communication is verbal, while other communication is nonverbal. Nonverbal communication includes writing, using body language, and therapeutic touch to relay a message.

Written Communication

Written communication is one form of nonverbal communication that is crucial to both medical documentation and

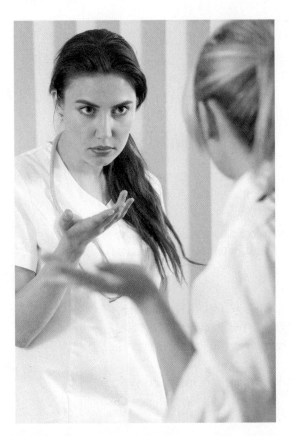

Figure 6-2 ■ Facial expression, voice tone, and projection impact the receiver's perception of the message being sent.
Source: Fotolia © Photo_Ma.

patient education. Medical assistants should use patients' charts both to capture patient information and to document that patients have understood the information given to them.

In health care, patients typically receive written instructions after they are given verbal instructions, to ensure patient comprehension. **Figure 6-3** ■ provides a sample of written instructions given to the parent of a child who was seen in the medical office for eczema.

▶▶▶Pulse Points

English as a Second Language

Remember that patients might not use English as their primary language. As a result, they might fail to understand phrases or slang common in English.

Critical Thinking Question 6-2

Referring to the case study at the beginning of the chapter, what is the value of written communication for patients like Katerina, who speak English as a second language? What characteristics would make that written communication most effective?

Reading and Using Body Language

Research has shown that nonverbal communication sends primary messages more often than spoken words, and **body language** is an important part of nonverbal communication. Facial expressions, gestures, and eye movements can say more than words. For example, a shrug of the shoulders can be interpreted as a lack of interest.

Body language can help clarify verbal communication. A patient might, for example, claim to feel no pain but grimace when touched. The real message, then, is that the patient needs attention. Medical assistants should use nonverbal communication to ensure patient exchanges are effective and accurate. When patients say one thing but do another, medical assistants should ask appropriate questions to ensure that patients provide accurate information.

Patients will read medical assistants' body language as well, so it is important for medical assistants to use neutral stances, even when patients are difficult. Medical assistants should always be professional and nonjudgmental, whatever the patient communication. Patients need to trust their medical assistants and should feel comfortable sharing personal information (**Figure 6-4** ■).

Therapeutic Touch

Nonverbal communication includes the use of touch. Touch can be very helpful to some patients. For example, touching a patient's arm during a time of sadness can relay a sense of kindness that most patients will appreciate. Some cultures do not welcome therapeutic touch. The medical assistant will need to be aware of a patient's cultural preferences before initiating any kind of touch with the patient. A patient in a good deal of emotional pain may appreciate a hand on the arm or shoulder (**Figure 6-5** ■).

Some patients prefer no touch. All people have a comfort zone called **personal space**. In general, personal space varies by culture. People from some cultures desire closeness, while others do not. Medical assistants can determine patients' personal spaces by observing how those patients react to differing levels of interaction. If, for example, the medical assistant reaches out to touch the patient's arm and the patient pulls away, the patient is likely uncomfortable and the medical assistant should withdraw the hand.

Therapeutic Communication

Communicating with the patient in a therapeutic way is to use body language, as well as words, to encourage the patient to share thoughts and feelings and to open up to the medical assistant about his condition. There are several techniques involved in **therapeutic communication**, the first of which is allowing for silence. By remaining silent, the medical assistant encourages the patient to talk and share what is on his mind. Providing acceptance in response to what the patient is saying also encourages the patient to continue to share. This can be

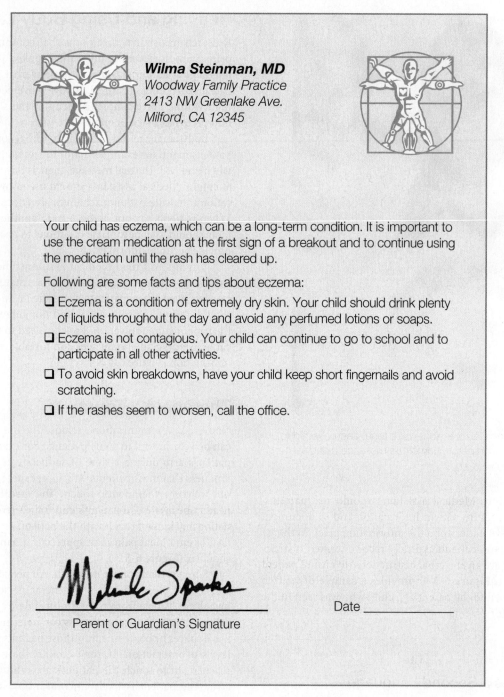

Wilma Steinman, MD
Woodway Family Practice
2413 NW Greenlake Ave.
Milford, CA 12345

Your child has eczema, which can be a long-term condition. It is important to use the cream medication at the first sign of a breakout and to continue using the medication until the rash has cleared up.

Following are some facts and tips about eczema:

❑ Eczema is a condition of extremely dry skin. Your child should drink plenty of liquids throughout the day and avoid any perfumed lotions or soaps.

❑ Eczema is not contagious. Your child can continue to go to school and to participate in all other activities.

❑ To avoid skin breakdowns, have your child keep short fingernails and avoid scratching.

❑ If the rashes seem to worsen, call the office.

_____
Parent or Guardian's Signature

Date _____

Figure 6-3 ■ Sample written instructions.

done with body language, such as nodding of the head, or words such as, "I follow what you're saying."

Offering recognition to the patient for changes observed is another form of therapeutic communication. This is done by noticing the patient's manner of dress, achievement of an accomplishment, or other noticeable change. Offering leading statements is a method of therapeutic communication that allows the patient encouragement to continue speaking. Using a phrase such as, "Please go on" lets the patient know the assistant wishes to hear more.

The medical assistant will use therapeutic communication with the patient during various parts of his or her office visit, for example, at check-in, when discussing the patient's insurance plan, when scheduling appointments, and when explaining procedures.

Active Listening

Medical assistants should always focus on patients' body language and spoken words. **Active listening** is the process of giving full

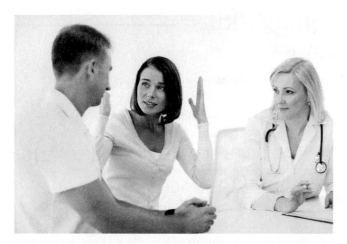

Figure 6-4 ■ This patient's body language reflects her anger. The medical assistant must remain calm and show the patient with his body language that he is listening and he cares.
Source: Fotolia © Syda Productions.

attention during an exchange and minimizing interruptions. In the medical office, interruptions like telephone calls tell patients that they are less important than the callers.

Active listening is more listening than talking. This means the medical assistant should listen without interruption while the patient speaks, and then give the patient feedback so they feel understood. This is especially important when the patient is angry or upset. When medical assistants try to hurry conversations or fail to show **empathy** for patients, situations can worsen. Empathy, which is understanding patients' feelings, differs from **sympathy**, which is pity.

Because patients oftentimes spend more time with the medical assistant than with the doctor, they often feel more comfortable sharing information with the medical assistant. Studies have shown that patients grow less likely to share information as a person's authority rises. Therefore, the medical assistant should share any patient concerns with the physician, chart all medically relevant information, and notify the doctor when appropriate.

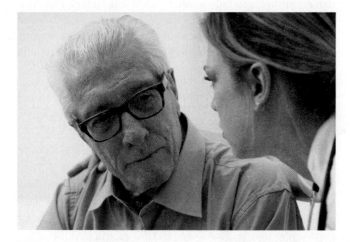

Figure 6-5 ■ A medical assistant comforts a patient in distress.
Source: Fotolia © Rido.

Pulse Points

Empathetic Listening

Part of empathetic listening is making direct eye contact with the patient, nodding, and keeping an interested facial expression.

Appraising Communication Abilities

When examining an individual's communication abilities, it is important to note both verbal and written communication skills. Exceptional communication skills are indicative of a person who is considered the go-to person when others need help with communication projects. This person is able to write and speak without grammatical errors, communicate in a concise manner, give excellent presentations, and is comfortable in front of a large group.

Interviewing the Patient

Administrative medical assistants are often asked to obtain information from patients in the office. Medical assistants should always remain professional and organized and begin any patient conversation with introductions. With a working pen or within the electronic medical record to document information in patient charts, the assistant should then conduct the interview in a private room. When the interview concludes, the medical assistant should let the patient know who will be entering the room next and when. When the medical assistant expects the physician or other provider to be delayed, the patient should be informed.

Interviewing Techniques

Medical assistants may use different communication styles when interviewing patients. Some are more appropriate than others depending on the patient and the situation. **Open-ended questions** are appropriate when more than a "yes" or "no" response is needed. An example is, "Mrs. Dow, would you please describe your symptoms?" **Close-ended questions**, in contrast, can be answered with "yes" or "no." An example of this type of question is, "Mrs. Dow, have you had anything to eat or drink since midnight last night?"

Reflecting is another interviewing technique. This is the practice of repeating the patient's statement so the patient knows she has been understood. This technique allows the medical assistant to clarify parts of conversations. For example, a medical assistant might say, "Mrs. Dow, you said that for two weeks you have been having pain in your right shoulder and arm, and that the pain has been running down to your right hand. Is that right?"

Asking for **examples** is a technique that can help the medical assistant better understand the patient. In this case, a medical assistant may say, "With '1' being no pain, and '10' being extreme pain, can you tell me how you would rate the pain level you are having, Mrs. Dow?"

PROCEDURE 6-1 Use Effective Listening Skills in Patient Interviews

Theory and Rationale

Effective listening skills are vital for the medical assistant. By listening carefully to the patient and documenting appropriately, the medical assistant performs a valued function for the physician. Watching for the patient's nonverbal communication and paraphrasing the patient's statements verifies comprehension.

Materials

- Patient history form
- Pen or electronic medical record

Competency

1. Smile, and introduce yourself to the patient.
2. Identify the patient by verifying the patient's birth date.

3. Verify that you have the correct paper or electronic patient chart.
4. Maintain a professional persona.
5. Maintain eye contact with the patient.
6. Ask the patient open-ended questions.
7. Do not interrupt the patient.
8. Paraphrase the patient's statements to verify comprehension.
9. Watch for the patient's nonverbal communication.
10. Summarize the patient's statements, and conclude the interview.
11. Document appropriate information in the patient's medical record.

Allowing for periods of silence in conversations gives patients time to collect their thoughts or to think of answers. When patients fail to answer questions right away, the medical assistant should give them time before asking more questions.

Another communication tool to use when speaking with patients is the indirect question. An indirect question is considered polite, especially when speaking with strangers. A sample direct question is, "Where is your son?" An indirect question is, "I was wondering if you know where your son is?" The following is a list of common phrases that are used for asking indirection questions:

- *Do you know...?*
- *I was wondering...*
- *Can you tell me...?*
- *Do you happen to know...*
- *Have you any idea...?*

Medical assistants may also use exploratory interviewing techniques with the patient. This includes asking questions that require the patient to provide an answer that includes their personal perception of the topic. An example of this type of question would be, "Tell me how you think this happened."

Critical Thinking Question 6-3

Referring to the case study at the beginning of the chapter, how would the reflecting conversation technique help ensure that medical assistants understand the concerns of patients like Katerina? What sort of questions would support this technique?

Factors That Hinder Communication

Various factors can impede communication. Culture is one, because messages can be perceived differently. Medical assistants will encounter patients who think differently than they do, but assistants must treat all patients with dignity and respect. Some patients are not comfortable with direct communication. The medical assistant may encounter some patients who prefer less direct communication, and would rather conduct some form of small-talk before getting directly to the point.

In some cultures, agreement is seen as an act of politeness. Patients may say that they agree with the suggestions of the medical assistant or physician, even though the patient does not actually agree and has no intention of following the advice. **Stereotyping** is prejudging patients based solely on gender, ethnic background, or other identifying factors. **Discriminating** is taking some sort of action against a person based solely on a stereotype. Whatever the medical assistant's personal feelings about a patient, he or she must always remain professional.

▶▶▶Pulse Points

Body Language and Culture

Different cultures have different body-language norms. Some cultures consider direct eye contact a sign of disrespect, for example. As patient advocates, medical assistants must know the norms of their patients' cultures and observe those norms as signs of respect for patients' needs. See Table 6-1 for examples of cultural norms and body language.

TABLE 6-1 Cultural Norms and Body Language	
Eye Contact	• U.S. and Canada—seen as conveying attention and interest in the speaker. • Middle Eastern—between members of the same gender, seen as a symbol of trust. Between members of opposite genders, seen as inappropriate. Many Middle Eastern cultures believe a woman should look down when talking with a man. • Asian, African, Latin—extended eye contact is seen as rude or disrespectful.
Shaking Hands	• Northern European—quick, firm handshake • Southern European, Central and South American—long, warm grasp, often using both hands to shake the hand of the other person • Turkey—firm handshake is seen as aggressive and rude • African—limp handshake is the norm • Islamic—men never shake the hands of women outside the family
Formal Greetings	• U.S. and Western cultures—handshake and introduction by name • Japanese—bow to the other person • Italian—kissing the other person's cheeks
Personal Space and Touching	• U.S.—approximately arm's length from one another, touching typically welcomed only in informal groups • Chinese—close enough to touch one another while speaking • Strict Judaism—males only touch their wives • Latinos—touching is common

Communicating in Special Circumstances

Patients who are young, hearing impaired, sight impaired, mentally unable to understand, or sedated present special communication challenges. In all cases, medical assistants must always include the patients and their interpreters or guardians in conversations. Patients should always feel part of the process.

Communicating with Hearing-Impaired Patients

Communicating with hearing-impaired patients presents some special challenges. Many hearing-impaired people can read lips. When this is the case, medical assistants must speak slowly, facing the patient in a well-lighted room. The medical assistant can touch the patient's arm to get his attention, and then begin the conversation.

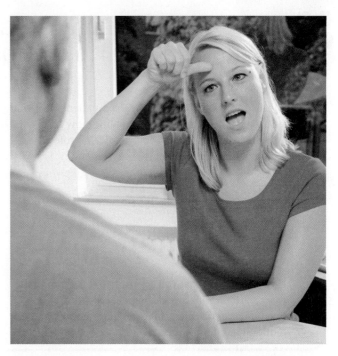

Figure 6-6 ■ Hearing impaired patients will often bring an interpreter.
Source: Fotolia © Dan Race.

When hearing-impaired patients have an interpreter, the conversation is still with the patient, not the interpreter (**Figure 6-6** ■). Medical assistants should face their patients and speak with them directly. The medical assistant should speak to the patient, even though the interpreter is acting as a go-between. In other words, the medical assistant should speak to the patient as if the interpreter is not in the room.

Communicating with Sight-Impaired Patients

Patients with sight impairments present communication challenges and raise special considerations about medical facilities. Medical assistants must escort patients who cannot see well to treatment rooms or the restroom, being careful to alert the patients to any steps, ramps, or slopes. Once in the treatment room, the medical assistant should place the patient's hand on the chair or table where the patient should sit. The medical assistant should then familiarize the patient with the room's layout and important features, such as the sink and door.

Sight-impaired patients often bring service animals to the medical office (**Figure 6-7** ■). These animals must stay with the patients throughout the visit, including when the patients use the restroom or visit the lab or radiology facilities. To ensure patient safety and honor the Americans with Disabilities Act (ADA), patients with service animals like guide dogs must be allowed to keep the animals with them at all times. These animals are working, however, so medical assistants should not pet or play with these animals unless invited to do so by the patient. Federal law mandates that the medical office allow the animal to accompany the patient at all times, without restrictions. While the medical assistant is permitted by law to

PROCEDURE 6-2 Communicate with a Hearing-Impaired Patient

Theory and Rationale

Communicating with hearing-impaired patients is a skill needed in any medical facility. Knowing how to get the patient's attention and how to communicate professionally and accurately is an important skill to master.

Materials

- Patient's paper or electronic file
- Blue or black ink pen or electronic medical record

Competency

1. Alert the patient that you are ready to take him to the examination room by entering the reception area, touching the patient's arm to get his attention, and motioning to follow.

2. If the patient has an interpreter, also have the interpreter enter the examination room.

3. When speaking, look directly at the patient and speak slowly.

4. When the patient can read lips, verify understanding through patient questioning. When comprehension is lacking, write instructions for the patient.

5. When asking a patient to change into a gown, ask the patient to flip a switch or crack the door open when ready. People with hearing impairments cannot hear a knock that announces the physician's arrival.

6. At the end of the patient's visit, chart all communications, including verification of the patient's understanding in the patient's medical record.

ask the patient if the animal is a service animal, and inquire as to the service the animal provides, proof of the animal's training may not be asked for from the patient. In the event the owner of the animal is not in control of the animal, the medical office staff may ask that the animal be removed from the building. Examples of an instance where the animal is not under control would be if the animal is not house-trained, or if the animal poses a threat to another person in the building.

Communicating with Patients with Speech Impairments

Patients with speech impairments might be difficult for the medical assistant to understand. When communication is

difficult, the medical assistant should ask the patient to repeat herself. If the medical assistant still cannot understand the patient, the medical assistant should ask the patient to write down what she is saying. At no time should the medical assistant act frustrated or hurried. Part of patient advocacy is being certain to correctly relate patient information to the physician.

Communicating with Patients via Interpreters

Patients who cannot communicate due to language barriers should be accompanied to the medical office by interpreters (**Figure 6-8** ■). The office may arrange interpreters, or the patient may bring a friend or family member to serve the role. The most important issues are that patients can understand the information being communicated to them and that health care professionals clearly understand what the patients are communicating. In communities with a high proportion of patients who speak languages other than English, the medical office will likely seek medical professionals who speak the community's prevalent language, in which case interpreters might be unnecessary. The names and contact information of interpreters who accompany patients should be clearly noted in the patients' files so the interpreters can be contacted for comment or clarification.

There may be times when the medical assistant will need to communicate with the patient via an interpreter over the telephone, rather than in person. This can be a challenge, as face-to-face conversation typically provides a better way to communicate with the patient. In some instances, the patient might be in the exam room with the patient, and the interpreter's services are enlisted on the telephone. Medical assistants will need to use licensed interpreters for any type of interpretation services. These licensed professionals are bonded and understand the importance of keeping patient information confidential.

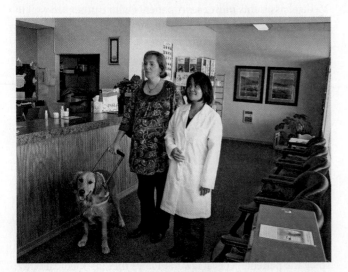

Figure 6-7 ■ A patient with her guide dog.

Source: Pearson Education/PH College. Photographer: Dylan Malone.

PROCEDURE 6-3 Communicate with a Sight-Impaired Patient

Theory and Rationale

Communicating with sight-impaired patients is a skill needed in any medical facility. The administrative medical assistant may be called on to gather information from sight-impaired patients to facilitate paperwork completion in the office.

Materials

- Patient's paper or electronic file
- Blue or black ink pen or electronic medical record

Competency

1. Alert the patient that you are ready to visit the examination room by entering the reception area, touching the patient's arm, and offering your arm for the patient to hold.

2. Ensure that the patient's service animal accompanies him to the examination room.

3. Alert the patient to any steps, doorways, ramps, or slopes along the way.

4. Take the patient to a private area, outside of other patients' views or hearing ranges.

5. Place the patient's hand on the chair or table where you would like him to sit.

6. Arrange for the service animal to sit directly next to the patient.

7. Ask the patient the questions on the history form, and write down the answers. Ensure the patient's responses are clearly understood.

8. At the end of the patient's visit, chart all communications, including how the patient's understanding was verified in the patient's medical record.

9. Sign and date the patient history form and note that the history form was completed for the patient due to sight impairment.

Communicating with Mentally Ill Patients

Most patients who are mentally incompetent visit the medical office with their legal guardians. The medical assistant should speak with such patients first and then their guardians. Some patients have a mental illness and are mentally incompetent to speak for themselves. In these situations, the medical assistant must be certain the patient understands any instructions. Some effective techniques are to repeat patients' statements, ask patients to repeat what they have been told, or demonstrate the skills the patients have been shown.

Communicating with Angry or Distressed Patients

To avoid angering or distressing patients, the medical assistant should try to avoid the emotions' triggers. For example, the medical assistant can help avoid anger over a bill by reviewing the bill with the patient. The medical assistant should always explain things up front and give the patient written information on any relevant office policies.

When patients become angry or distressed, the medical assistant must always remain calm and professional (**Figure 6-9** ■). Typically, the best response to an angry patient is, "I'm sorry you're upset. Let's see if we can work this out." Most patients calm when the medical assistant responds calmly and demonstrates a sincere desire to help. The medical assistant often needs to resolve conflict with the patient. This is best done by remaining calm and asking the patient what it is the medical assistant can do to assist with the problem. When patients continue to escalate their anger, the medical assistant must recognize when it is time to call for a supervisor, or, in cases where the patient becomes aggressive, to call security. The medical assistant should involve the supervisor in any conversation where the patient remains unhappy or upset, despite the efforts of the medical assistant. Any time the patient becomes threatening, whether physically or via threats to sue the physician or clinic, the medical assistant will need to involve the supervisor or physician.

Figure 6-8 ■ Interpreters should accompany those patients who cannot communicate due to language barriers.

Source: Pearson Education/PH College. Photographer: Dylan Malone.

PROCEDURE 6-4 Communicate with a Patient Via Interpreter

Theory and Rationale

Communicating with a patient via an interpreter is something the administrative medical assistant may need to do both over the telephone when scheduling an appointment, and when the patient arrives in the office for a visit. It is imperative that patients understand the information being communicated to them and that health care professionals understand what patients are communicating.

Materials

- Patient's paper or electronic file
- Pen or electronic medical record

Competency

1. When the patient arrives in the office with an interpreter, obtain the name of the interpreter and verify the spelling.
2. Obtain the interpreter's contact information for the patient's medical record. If the interpreter has a business card, attach it to or enter it into the patient's file.
3. Communicate with the patient directly; do not speak directly to the interpreter.
4. When any of the interpreter's comments are unclear, ask for clarification.
5. Document all essential parts of the interview in the patient's chart.

Communicating with Young Patients

When communicating with young patients, it is important that the medical assistant use words and questions the patients will understand. When the patients cannot articulate their feelings, the medical assistant can have them draw pictures. When talking to a young patient, the medical assistant should sit down in order to be at eye level with the patient. Before beginning any procedure on a young patient, even a simple one, the medical assistant should explain the procedure and show the equipment that will be used (**Figure 6-10** ■).

Young patients might sometimes be subjected to undesirable procedures. Vaccinations and blood draws, for example, can be uncomfortable and may require the patient to remain still for a few moments. For these types of procedures, parents can be helpful in or out of the room. Medical assistants should use their best judgment about parent presence and reassure the patient as much as possible. When the procedure concludes, the medical assistant should always praise the patient for being brave or "grown up." To help the patients view the medical office in a positive light, the office may reward young patients with a small prize, like a sticker.

▶▶▶Pulse Points

Working with Young Patients

Treat young patients with respect. Do not lie to them. Misinformation about pain, for example, can create a long-standing distrust of health care professionals. Be honest, and demonstrate on stuffed animals or dolls first so the patients can understand the plan and prepare.

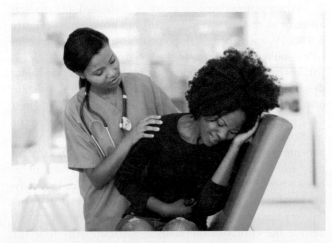

Figure 6-9 ■ The medical assistant must remain calm when communicating with an emotional patient.
Source: Fotolia © michaeljung.

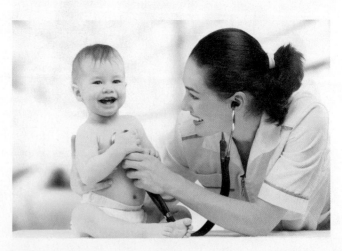

Figure 6-10 ■ The medical assistant should use simple words and phrases with very young children.
Source: Fotolia © Konstantin Yugenov.

Communicating with Grieving Patients

Communicating with grieving patients can be uniquely challenging. First, medical assistants must remember that the patients might be grieving for unique reasons: the loss of a loved one, a job, or a relationship. It is important for the medical assistant to remember that the level of grief a person experiences is directly related to the importance of the person or thing lost. Patients may also grieve the diagnoses of chronic or terminal illnesses. Second, medical assistants must remember that people feel grief in individual ways. Therefore, medical assistants should never belittle someone for feeling grief. Every person is entitled to grieve and for whatever reason. People feel what they feel. Medical assistants are not entitled to judge why.

Dr. Elisabeth Kübler-Ross was a pioneer in the field of working with dying or grieving patients. She advocated hospice care and wrote several books about the dying process. Kübler-Ross developed a list of the five stages of grief, noting that not every person experiences the stages in the same way or for the same period (Table 6-2).

It is important to remember that there is no "right" way to grieve. Medical assistants should listen to grieving patients and allow those patients time to express themselves. As appropriate, medical assistants should touch patients reassuringly on the arm or shoulder. Because there is no right thing to say, medical assistants should focus on offering support and empathy.

TABLE 6-3 National Resources

Organization	Focus Area(s)
American Cancer Society www.cancer.org	Patients, families, friends and survivors of cancer
American Diabetes Association www.diabetes.org	Diabetes and related nutrition and recipes, prevention, and research
American Lung Association www.lungusa.org	Hayfever, asthma, lung cancer, and other respiratory illnesses
National Domestic Violence Hotline www.ndvh.org	Domestic violence, including a toll-free number to call 24 hours per day, 365 days per year
International Child Abuse Network www.yesican.org	Twenty-four-hour chat groups on child abuse, incest, and parenting; Web site is in English and Spanish
American Heart Association www.americanheart.org	Heart attack/stroke warning signs, high blood pressure, and healthy lifestyles; Web site is in English and Spanish
Centers for Disease Control and Prevention HIV/AIDS www.cdc.gov/hiv/	Information on HIV/AIDS transmission, current research, and Internet links to testing centers or support groups

Medical assistants can also offer information as needed. With physicians' permission, medical assistants can refer patients to a number of community and national resources that are available through hospice or other support groups (Table 6-3).

Different types of losses cause different types of grief. For the patient who has lost a loved one to a long-term illness, the grief process likely began when that illness was diagnosed. For the patient who has lost a loved one to a sudden illness or accidental injury, the grief can be extreme. For the patient who has lost a loved one due to a death that holds some form of stigma, such as suicide, or death due to a drug overdose, the patient will likely be feeling the trauma of both the loss and the stigma attached. No matter the type of loss, any grieving patients should be treated with compassion and understanding and given extra time for their visit, if possible.

Defense Mechanisms

Defense mechanisms are people's characteristic, usually unconscious, ways of protecting themselves in stressful situations. Just as everyone has physical defenses that combat disease, everyone also has mental and emotional defenses to deal with stress and *anxiety*. These mechanisms may be engaged consciously or unconsciously, usually in combination with others. Table 6-4 lists some common defense mechanisms the MA might encounter in patients. The MA should also examine his or her own defense mechanisms as they arise in interactions with patients and coworkers.

TABLE 6-2 Kübler-Ross's Five Stages of Grief

Stage	Description
Denial	• Patients have difficulty accepting the loss that has happened or is happening to them. This stage often lasts until the patient comes to accept the diagnosis given or the death that has occurred.
Anger	• Patients experience anger, often with the person who has died. Patients might also turn their anger toward the health care provider who has given them the news of the terminal diagnosis. Patients might also focus their anger on the deity of their religion.
Bargaining	• Patients make irrational offers or promises in an attempt to reverse the diagnosis or death. This may manifest in situations where patients say, "I will do volunteer work in my community for the rest of my life if I can have John back."
Depression	• Patient might become clinically depressed over the loss or diagnosis. In this stage, the patient might need to seek professional help, such as counseling or medications prescribed by their health care provider.
Acceptance	• The patient accepts the terminal diagnosis or death and begins to accept the new reality.

TABLE 6-4 Common Defense Mechanisms	
Compensation	• Trying to overcome some inability or inferiority. It helps to maintain one's self-respect and raise self-esteem.
Conversion	• Changing an emotional problem into a physical symptom or other method of release that eases tension and anxiety related to conflict.
Denial	• Avoiding or escaping the unpleasant or distasteful realities of living by ignoring or refusing to admit their existence.
Displacement	• Transferring into another situation an emotion that was felt in a past situation where its expression would have been socially unacceptable.
Identification	• Unconsciously imitating the mannerisms, behavior, and feelings of another person.
Overcompensation	• Repressing unconscious attitudes and wishes and replacing them with conscious attitudes and behavior that are the opposite of the unconscious ones. Often referred to as *reaction formation*.
Projection	• Blaming someone else for one's own failures or for specific events.
Rationalization	• Explaining, excusing, or defending ideas, actions, and feelings. It helps to "save face" in embarrassing and anxiety-producing situations.
Regression	• Escaping frustration and conflict anxiety by returning to methods used at an earlier stage of life.
Repression	• Unconsciously storing unpleasant, unacceptable thoughts, desires, and impulses in the mind. The repressed information does not enter conscious awareness and may not be remembered unless there is an emotional trigger. Repression is sometimes termed *selective forgetting*.
Substitution	• Accepting something in place of a desired object or need when the original cannot be obtained. The substitution helps to achieve at least some fulfillment.
Suppression	• Storing away or forgetting unpleasant, emotionally painful experiences. This is a conscious forcing of unpleasant, anxiety-producing experiences into the unconscious mind.

Source: Frazier, M., & Morgan, C. Clinical Medical Assisting: Foundations and Practice, *First Edition. © 2008. Reprinted by permission of Pearson Education, Inc. Upper Saddle River, NJ.*

Defense mechanisms protect a person's self-esteem but do not effectively deal with conflict. It is important to recognize the coping style of the patient, the patient's family, staff, and physicians. For example, denial is one of the most common defense mechanisms. A patient with a serious condition may refuse to believe what is happening. This refusal to accept reality is a factor in the patient's treatment and education.

An understanding of the psychological principles discussed in this chapter will improve your therapeutic communication skills and your interactions with patients.

▸▸▸Pulse Points
The Influence of Culture and Age

The following are examples of different approaches to the same situation—a patient has just been diagnosed with insulin-dependent diabetes.

• You are teaching a 7-year-old boy how to give himself insulin injections. It is natural for the child to be worried. He may not listen well or remember instructions. One way to handle the situation is to find out more about the child's home situation, then instruct one or both parents in giving the insulin injection along with the child. The child will feel more secure when his parents are involved. It also satisfies the child's emotional needs, paving the way for easier learning. A parent or responsible caretaker should be present in the room during the teaching experience.

• A woman with a hearing impairment who is on Medicare and Social Security thinks she is going to die because she has no money for insulin and syringes. Explain that you will help her contact the appropriate agencies to help pay for the medications. Stress that she should contact you if she needs any other help. By relieving her concerns about money, you now have a patient ready to learn.

• A Hispanic man learns he will have to take insulin for the rest of his life. He tells you, "I might as well die!" After talking with the man, you learn he is afraid he will no longer be able to work. Assure him that working should not be a problem. Tell him that learning how to take care of himself will help him continue taking care of his family.

Maintaining Professional Patient Communication

The most effective medical assistants form positive relationships with their patients through mutual respect and professionalism. Medical assistants must be role models and earn their patients' trust and admiration. In short, medical assistants are professionals and must always act as such. A medical assistant's bad days and personal stress should always be hidden from patients, and any personal problems or coworker difficulties should be concealed. Voice and body language should mask any negative feelings. When the medical assistant cannot keep her patient interactions free of personal stress, she should consider asking her employer to find a temporary replacement.

Medical assistants must speak respectfully and appropriately to patients, as well as to anyone within the patients' range of hearing. In addition, medical assistants should always use proper forms of address when speaking with patients. Elderly patients, for example, might prefer to be called either "Mrs. Thompson" or "Margaret."

To ensure patient respect, medical assistants should not assume they can shorten anyone's name; it is rude to shorten a person's name without permission. It is acceptable with permission, however. Take a patient named Richard, for example. The medical assistant should ask the patient if he would like to be called Richard. If he indicates he prefers to be called Rick, then the medical assistant should make a note in his chart so that all members of the health care team can address him properly.

The medical assistant should never use pet names for patients, like "Honey" or "Sweetie." It could offend some patients. The medical assistant should also avoid referring to patients by their conditions, such as "Back pain is in Room 2." In the same vein, the medical assistant should maintain patient confidentiality by only calling out full patient names outside the hearing of other patients.

HIPAA Compliance

To be Health Insurance Portability and Accountability Act (HIPAA)-compliant, the medical assistant should not call patients by their full names in the reception area. Instead, the assistant should use first or last name only. When two patients have the same first name, the last name is appropriate. For example, instead of "Jim," the medical assistant should call out "Mr. Costas."

Keeping a Professional Distance

It is important, both for the patient and the medical assistant, to keep a **professional distance**, but doing so can be difficult. Most health care professionals chose the field because they care about people and find it hard to remain detached when patients are hurting, dying, or in need. Medical assistants could become very stressed if they became attached to every patient, and some patients might take advantage of medical assistants who are willing to go above and beyond the call of duty. Medical assistants need not abandon their concern for patients. They simply must keep a professional distance to maintain a professional image.

In addition to maintaining a professional distance, medical assistants must be very careful to avoid revealing personal details about themselves or the physician. It is acceptable for medical assistants to reveal an engagement when a patient notices an engagement ring, but the assistants should not tell the patient where they live or discuss personal relationships. Such details have no place in the patient–health care professional relationship.

▶▶▶Pulse Points

Finding Community Resources for Patients

Do not offer to drive patients to the store or to pay for prescriptions. Medical assistants serve patients best by finding them the appropriate community resources and making referrals with the doctor's permission.

Communicating with Coworkers

The medical assistant must maintain professional communication with coworkers and the doctors at all times while in the office. The medical assistant should minimize any nonwork conversations, remembering that patients might overhear them.

Just as in any work setting, the medical assistant may dislike some coworkers. Personal feelings aside, all members of the health care team should treat each other professionally and respectfully. Should medical assistants ever need to speak to a supervisor about coworkers, they should do so in a private setting. They should be professional, stating only facts, not opinions.

When communicating with the doctor in front of patients, the medical assistant must always address the doctor as "Dr." Even when the doctor is relaxed and informal, patients must have a level of respect for the doctor as an authority, and that image starts with the behavior of the other members of the health care team. Similarly, patients should never suspect that medical assistants are irritated with the physician.

All members of the health care team should be careful to use correct medical terminology and no slang when speaking with physicians and coworkers. The medical assistant should speak slowly, confidently, and always honestly. Jokes and nonwork conversation have no place in the medical office when patients are present.

In Practice

Mark Minton, CMA (AAMA) is completing paperwork in the reception area. Two of his coworkers, who are standing behind him at the front desk, begin a conversation about last night's episode of their favorite television show. Their conversation is loud enough to be heard in the reception area. What should Mark do?

PROCEDURE 6-5 Prepare a Patient's Specialist Referral

Theory and Rationale

Administrative medical assistants are often required to schedule patients to see specialists. This procedure must always be done in a private place and preferably with the patient present. Knowing the steps in this procedure and how to communicate the necessary information to the patient, is part of being the patient's advocate in the medical office.

Materials

- Telephone
- Blue or black ink pen or electronic medical record
- Patient's paper or electronic file
- Referral form to a specialist

Competency

1. Verify the patient file is correct.
2. Verify the referral form for the specialist is correct.
3. Verify the doctor's instructions (e.g., What does the doctor want the patient to be seen for? How soon does the patient need to be seen?).

4. Choose a private location, out of the hearing range of other patients.
5. If the pending referral is not an emergency and the patient is in the clinic, ask the patient for a convenient time or day to see the specialist.
6. Call the specialist's office, and ask to speak to the person who handles the schedule.
7. Provide personal identification and the name of the referring doctor or clinic.
8. State the reason for the call.
9. Give patient information as requested by the specialist's office.
10. Set an appointment date and time. If the patient is in the clinic, verify the date and time.
11. Document the appointment's date and time on the referral form. If the patient is in the clinic, give the patient the referral form. Choose to mail the referral form when there is time before the appointment.
12. Document the call's results in the patient's chart.

Communicating with Other Facilities

Patient confidentiality is the most important factor when communicating with other facilities. When medical assistants schedule patients in another facility, they should give those facilities only the information needed to schedule the patients. This usually includes patient name and contact information, reason for referral, referring physician, and patient's insurance carrier. Any other information about the patient should come from the patient.

When making appointments for patients with other facilities, medical assistants must be out of hearing range of all other patients in the office. The assistants should have a telephone location for these types of calls, one that is not in the clinic hallway or at the front desk. Calling from the treatment room where the patient is waiting or from a private area is best.

Developmental Stages of the Life Cycle and Their Impact on Communication

Human development is a lifelong process. The individual faces certain tasks during each stage, builds on previous growth when entering each new stage, and gradually progresses to a higher level of development. The physical and emotional stages of the life cycle are often presented in psychology courses; understanding these stages helps in communication with all patients, regardless of age.

The stages of development are a complex subject that is presented more in depth during psychology courses. Depending on what theorist you subscribe to, you may believe that individuals will pass through life stages one at a time in chronological order without ever returning to the previous stage, they may skip stages and successfully navigate others in a random order, or they may pass unilaterally through stages and remain in one or more at any given time. It is important to understand that there is no "appropriate" method of development with people, because they will develop at an individual pace according to their own needs and environment.

An individual's ability to communicate and to interpret messages is greatly affected by his or her developmental stage. Jean Piaget, a Swiss philosopher and developmental theorist known for his theory of cognitive development as well as for his work studying children, conceived of physical and emotional stages of the life cycle (Table 6-5). It is important to communicate with each person at his or her developmental level. As an example, an older female patient of 70-plus years might be beginning to prepare for the loss of her mate or for her own death. She might not hear or understand instructions about medications, activity, or treatment because she is preoccupied with other concerns. A common mistake made by people who work with the elderly is to speak in baby-like, patronizing tones. The usual response is annoyance or feeling insulted, and the elderly person might simply stop listening.

In terms of personality and relationships, American psychoanalyst Erik Erikson (1902–1994) believed that the development of trust, or lack of trust, in the first year of life is the

TABLE 6-5 Approximate Physical and Emotional Stages of the Life Cycle, According to Jean Piaget

6 weeks	The baby begins to smile and develop facial expressions.
10 weeks	The baby begins to roll from prone to a supine position.
4 to 6 months	The baby raises its head and shoulders while lying in supine position.
6 to 8 months	The baby sits without support. Eye color may change.
8 to 12 months	The baby learns to crawl, stand, take steps, feed him- or herself, and develop autonomy.
1 year	The baby understands commands and simple conversation.
18 months	The toddler walks alone, feeds self, stacks objects, and is becoming more independent.
20 to 24 months	The toddler begins to learn bowel and bladder control and explores the environment.
3 to 4 years	The child talks in complete sentences.
4 to 5 years	The child dresses and undresses him- or herself.
5 to 6 years	The child's eye and body coordination improves. The child can skip and draw figures.
6 to 8 years	The child enters school, and physical skills improve.
8 to 13 years	The adolescent's rate of physical growth increases and adult sexual characteristics develop.
13 to 18 years	The teenager undergoes puberty and strives for independence.
18 to 20 years	The young adult becomes more independent, may continue his or her education, and/or may marry and have children.
20 to 30 years	The adult attempts to build a firm, safe foundation for the future. There may be a continuation of the educational process, marriage, and children.
30 to 40 years	The adult experiences more freedom, continuing to work and raise children.
40 to 50 years	The adult evaluates the first part of his or her life and continues working. The children may begin leaving the nest.
50 to 60 years	The adult experiences a sense of comfort, acceptance of life. Children continue leaving the home. The individual experiences freedom and success.
60 to 70 years	The adult looks forward to or begins retirement. Losing the mate and living alone become real possibilities. Fewer home commitments mean greater sense of freedom to explore, travel, start a new hobby. Their rich fullfillment of life offers a great education they can pass on to younger generations.
70 plus years	The adult faces the facts of aging, may lose the mate and friends to illness and death, and begins to prepare for his or her own death. Fewer financial burdens bring the ability to fulfill wants and desires of traveling, gifts, vacations. More time can be spent enjoying family, friends and hobbies.

The last stage of life, old age, is often divided into three stages: early old age (55-65), old age (65-85), and very old age (85 and older). Adults in early old age become more aware of their own mortality, and significant lifestyle changes may occur. Some begin to acknowledge health problems, physical limitations, and a likely decline in earning power or working capacity in the years ahead.

Among the 65- to 85-year-old group, many have retired, are forced to live on lower incomes, and are experiencing progressively worse health problems. Living arrangements may change because of their financial situations or because they can no longer care for themselves. Some have lost partners, family members, and friends through death.

Most adults over age 85 have gone through all the experiences mentioned above. Many are in long-term care facilities, many have severe memory problems, and many have no income. Others are in excellent health, are able to care for themselves travel and live life to the fullest.

The aging process affects different people in different ways. It is important not to stereotype the elderly—each person is unique in terms of genetic makeup, health status, financial status, and life experience.

Source: Frazier, Margie; Malone, Christine; and Morgan, Connie. Medical Assisting: Foundations and Practice, First Edition. © 2010. Reprinted by permission of Pearson Education, Inc. Upper Saddle River, NJ.

foundation for the development of an individual's coping skills (Table 6-6). In each of the developmental stages described by Erikson, the positive resolution of any crisis is based on positive coping characteristics: trust, independence, initiative, competence, and integrity. Negative coping characteristics that contribute to negative resolution include mistrust, insecurity, and dependency, among others. An awareness of Erikson's life stages will help you better understand what patients experience as they grow and age, and will provide a foundation for more effective therapeutic communication with patients.*

Educating the Patient

Any patient education the medical assistant does in the office must be done under the direction of the physician. Part of patient education includes helping patients accept their condition and providing positive reinforcement. To educate patients properly,

*Source: Frazier, Margaret Schell; Malone, Christine; and Morgan, Connie. Comprehensive Medical Assisting: Foundations and Practices. © 2010, pages 82–84. Reprinted by permission of Pearson Education, Inc. Upper Saddle River, NJ

TABLE 6-6 Erik Erikson's Life Stages and Developmental Tasks	
1. Infancy	Develop trust.
2. Early childhood	Develop independence and self-direction.
3. Play age	Develop initiative.
4. School age	Develop competence.
5. Adolescence	Develop self-identity.
6. Early adulthood	Develop intimacy and love.
7. Middle adulthood	Develop concern for others and continue productivity.
8. Old age	Develop integrity.

Source: Frazier, Margie and Morgan, Connie. Clinical Medical Assisting: Foundations and Practice, *First Edition. © 2008. Reprinted by permission of Pearson Education, Inc. Upper Saddle River, NJ.*

the medical assistant must first **assess** the best way to teach them. For this step, the medical assistant will want to know how much pain patients are experiencing or if they are distressed. Patients cannot fully comprehend information when distracted by pain or anxiety.

After assessment, the medical assistant must gather the patient's information. Normally, this is found in the patient's medical record, but the medical assistant might need to gather information from the doctor, the patient's family members, or other health care facilities.

Planning the patient's education includes taking the information gathered during the assessment and determining how to proceed in educating the patient. This step may include gathering pamphlets or printed information on the patient's condition or gathering equipment that will be used to demonstrate a new skill to the patient.

The **implementing** step is the actual teaching phase. During this step, it might help for the medical assistant to demonstrate what she wants the patient to learn and then have the patient demonstrate the skill. For example, the medical assistant might show the patient how to use a pair of crutches and then ask the patient to demonstrate using the crutches (**Figure 6-11** ■).

The next step in patient education is **documenting** what has been taught to the patient, the tools used in the teaching process, how well the patient demonstrated the skill, and any concerns the medical assistant might have, such as for a patient who states an unwillingness to follow the doctor's instructions.

The **evaluation** step of patient education involves checking to see how well a patient is using the information given to her. Some evaluation might need to be done over the phone if the doctor asks the patient to call in to let the medical assistant know how she is doing. If the medical assistant discovers the patient is failing to comply with the doctor's instructions, either because she is unable or unwilling, the medical assistant will need to determine if there is a misunderstanding. If the patient is refusing to follow through, the refusal must be charted and the doctor notified right away. Patients have the

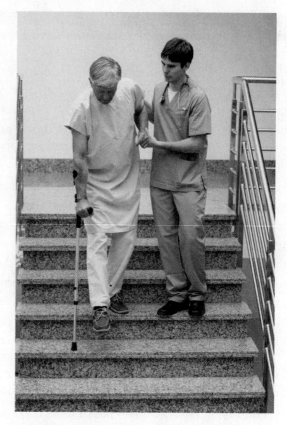

Figure 6-11 ■ A medical assistant aiding a man who is learning to use crutches.
Source: Fotolia © WavebreakmediaMicro.

right to refuse treatment, but if they do so, their choices must be clearly documented.

Working through Miscommunication

Miscommunication can be disastrous, so medical assistants must be careful to be completely clear and watch for signs that patients might not understand instructions fully. Medical assistants should be watching the patient's body language for signs he might not completely understand what is being discussed. The patient who furrows his brow, or looks confused, is one who might not fully comprehend the conversation. Communicating with the patient cannot be hurried, so assistants will need to ensure they are comfortable with the patient's levels of understanding before moving on.

Taking Time for Patient Education

Depending on the disease or illness, patient education can take several visits. Serious illnesses can be difficult to comprehend, and patients may need multiple visits to comprehend all the relevant information. When patients are willing to bring family members, those family members can be very helpful in patient-education initiatives. Written instructions or information are also helpful, because they serve as reference materials outside the medical office.

Teaching to Different Learning Styles and Personality Differences

The medical assistant needs to determine the patient's learning style prior to any education process. While some people learn best with visual cues, some are more auditory learners, and others might need to touch and hold an item to fully learn its use. Some patients prefer to learn things quickly, or to have someone show them something, then go home and learn on their own. Other patients need to be walked through a learning process several times before they are able to practice on their own. The medical assistant will need to determine which method is most appropriate for each patient, and to tailor the learning to that learning, or personality, style.

▸▸▸Pulse Points

Proper Charting of Patient Instruction

The party who signs the patient's medical chart is assumed to have performed the tasks described. For example if, after entering information on patient instruction, the medical assistant signs the chart, the assistant indicates that he or she did the teaching. When that is not the case, notes must reflect this fact.

Maslow's Hierarchy of Needs

Patients must be ready to learn for education to occur. They must be motivated and see a need to learn what the medical assistant is trying to teach. Abraham Maslow was an American psychiatrist who came up with a theory that said people will be motivated by their needs and that lower level needs must be met before higher ones. For example, it is impossible to teach people about proper nutrition when they cannot access food.

Maslow arranged human needs on a pyramid with basic needs at the bottom and higher needs at the top (**Figure 6-12** ■). The following is a brief description of these needs:

- **Physical:** These include the most basic needs that are vital to mere survival, such as water, food, air, and sleep.

- **Security and safety:** These include the need for steady employment or other source of income, access to health care, and shelter from the environment.
- **Love/Social:** These include the need for belonging, affection, romantic attachments, and friendships.
- **Self-esteem/Status:** These include the need for things that reflect on the self-esteem, such as recognition, feelings of personal worth, and accomplishment.
- **Self-actualization/Self-fulfillment:** This level includes an individual's ability to look at and work on personal growth and the fulfillment of his or her potential.

The medical assistant's job is to determine where patients are on this pyramid before teaching those patients new skills.

Establishing a Proper Learning Environment

The teaching environment must be conducive to learning. It must be quiet and free from interruptions, and it should be well lighted. Hallways, the reception area, and any locations in view of other patients are inappropriate places for teaching. Patients must feel relaxed, comfortable, and able to ask questions (**Figure 6-13** ■).

Assume the medical assistant is teaching a patient how to use a piece of equipment. The equipment should be in the office, and the medical assistant should be very familiar with the equipment's use and repair. The medical assistant should always provide written instructions on how to use any machinery.

Medical assistants must have solid knowledge of the skills they are trying to teach. When assistants are uncomfortable or less knowledgeable, they should request help before teaching patients. If a patient asks a question and the medical assistant does not know the answer, he should let the patient know he will find the answer and get back to the patient.

Using Teaching Resources

Teaching resources may be available for purchase, or the medical office can create its own. The medical assistant may use such teaching tools as CDs, food labels, videos, or pamphlets

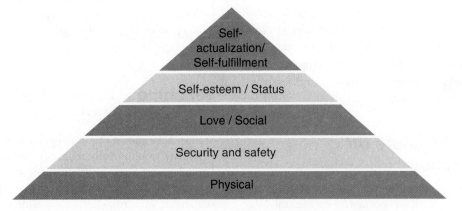

Figure 6-12 ■ Maslow's hierarchy of needs.

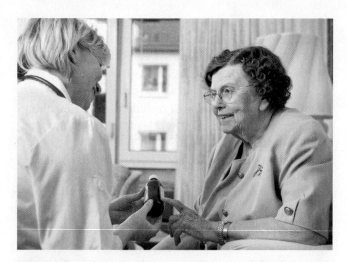

Figure 6-13 ■ Patients must feel relaxed and comfortable, and able to ask questions.
Source: Fotolia © Alexander Raths.

in helping to demonstrate a new skill to a patient. Because people learn through seeing, hearing, and touching, and different patients may have different learning styles, the medical assistant might need to incorporate more than one teaching approach to educate the patient.

Understanding the Patient's Skills and Abilities

Before teaching a patient new skills, the medical assistant must be aware of any of the patient's physical impairments. For example, the assistant must know if the patient cannot open a bottle of pills due to severe arthritis, especially when educating the patient about medication use throughout the day. In cases like this, the medical assistant may need to improvise and devise other ways to help the patient accomplish the doctor's directives.

▶▶▶Pulse Points

Preventing Childhood Injuries

Preventable injuries are the leading cause of childhood death in the United States. Medical assistants working in family practices or pediatric offices should have educational materials on how to keep children safe and distribute the materials to new parents. Simple tips for preventing choking, drowning accidents, and fire hazards can help prevent tragedies.

The Impact of Culture on Patient Education

A patient's culture may prevent the medical assistant from teaching that patient certain skills. It is important for the medical assistant to know this and to come up with alternatives that are acceptable to both the physician and the patient. For example, if a medical assistant is teaching a patient about proper nutrition, and the patient's culture is one that does not consume meat, the medical assistant must consult the physician regarding alternatives.

In some cultures, the patient might not be the person in charge of making health care decisions for himself. It may be the oldest male member of the family, or the oldest female. In these situations, the assistant will need to include both the patient and the person who makes the decisions in the conversation.

Though various cultures have different mechanisms for communicating about health care, it is important for the assistant to refrain from stereotyping patients based on their culture. Two patients from the same culture may have very different means of communicating in health care. In order to keep from offending the patient, the assistant should follow the patient's lead in communication.

The Impact of Finances on Patient Education

Financial difficulties can prevent patients from achieving desired educational goals. For example, patients might be unable to pay for appropriate shoes to begin a walking or exercise program.

In cases such as this, the patient might not be able to comply with the physician's directions for care, and might end up with a less than favorable outcome. The medical assistant must address any such restrictions before undertaking education. This must be done in a way that is not offensive to the patient. An appropriate method for determining if the patient is able to comply with instructions is for the assistant to ask, "Is there any reason why you would be unable to follow these directions?" If the patient mentions a financial constraint, the assistant may be able to direct the patient to resources in the community that provide financial assistance for items such as medicines or equipment. In the event the patient is unable to pay for the care or to find alternate methods for obtaining the care, the assistant will need to alert the physician who can then suggest an alternative method of treatment that the patient is able to access.

● In Practice

Dr. Lopez has asked the medical assistant to schedule Sara Hardy for three followup visits, but Sara is not covered by insurance and states that she can afford just one visit. How should the medical assistant proceed?

Teaching Patients about Preventive Medicine

Studies have shown that if people practiced preventive medicine, they would greatly reduce the cost of health care in the United States. Preventive medicine includes such things as mammograms or prostate exams, yearly physical exams, and scheduled immunizations for children. Medical assistants should promote health screenings to patients. They should keep

Name of
medication:_____

Dosage:_____

You will be taking this medication _____ times each day.

This medication is being prescribed for the following
health condition:_____

Possible side effects of this medication include:
_____

If you experience any of the following signs or symptoms,
please call the office right away:_____
_____

Figure 6-14 ■ Sample medication-teaching tool.

educational literature available and ask patients about their last physical examinations to encourage screening appointments.

Preventing Medication Errors

Medication errors are far too common and are mostly preventable. Medical assistants can help prevent such errors by properly teaching patients about their medications. Patients do not always read the information the pharmacist gives them, and they sometimes fail to take time to consult with the pharmacist. **Figure 6-14** ■ is a sample medication-teaching tool that can be implemented in any medical office. In order to be sure the provider is aware of all the medications a patient is taking, the medical assistant should ask the patient to bring in a list of their current medications, or even to bring in all of their current medication bottles.

The medical assistant must be sure to think or ask about a patient's lifestyle before teaching her about the medications she needs to take. Does the patient work nights? If a prescription says to take a medication three times per day, does that mean the patient must rise in the middle of the night? The assistant should ensure that the patient is clear on how to administer medications and know the proper administration routes.

▸▸▸Pulse Points

Preventing Injuries in the Elderly

Falls are common with the elderly, and most are preventable. Medical practices that treat elderly patients should distribute pamphlets detailing how to prevent falls. Such pamphlets should include details like removing throw rugs and ensuring steps are lined with slip-resistant material.

Providing Dieting or Weight-Loss Information

Because patients will ask for information on dieting or weight loss, medical assistants should have information on hand to teach basic nutrition. This information should include copies of the new food guide (ChooseMyPlate) and information on reading food labels (**Figures 6-15** ■ and **6-16** ■). The Choose-MyPlate food guide outlines the types of foods and food groups that are necessary for a balanced diet. Many people are

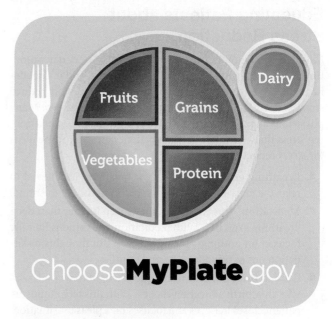

Figure 6-15 ■ ChooseMyPlate.
Source: choosemyplate.gov

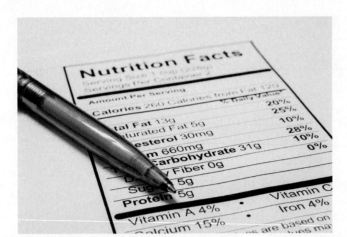

Figure 6-16 ■ Food label listing nutritional information.
Source: Fotolia © paulojgon.

unaware of the proper foods to eat to maintain a healthy lifestyle, and giving this information to the patient is one way to help him make healthy changes in his diet. However, the physician must authorize any information given to patients.

Delivering Information on Exercise

Teaching patients about exercise is a common task. Medical assistants should have pamphlets on the benefits of exercise. Patients must be taught the importance of easing into exercise programs, how to stretch and warm up properly, and how to keep from injuring themselves. Any patients over age 35 or with an underlying health conditions should seek the advice of her physician before beginning any new exercise program.

Educating Patients about Stress Reduction

Most people are under various levels of stress every day. Sometimes that stress gets to be too much to handle, and it impedes health. Having information on how to handle and reduce stress is one tool to help patients maintain good health. Many physicians suggest their patients find a mechanism for reducing stress that works best for that patient's lifestyle. Some ideas for stress reduction are:

- **Breathing exercises.** Deep, slow breathing is believed to relax the muscles, oxygenate the blood, and calm the mind.
- **Meditation.** This technique goes a step further than deep breathing exercises. With meditation, the mind is literally focused on nothing—taking the stressful thoughts or situation out of mind for a period of time.
- **Guided imagery.** This technique is taught to women who take childbirth education classes. With this technique, the patient closes her eyes and focuses on a pleasant situation.
- **Visualization.** Taking guided imagery one step further, visualization is the technique of thinking of a task that needs to be done and thinking of doing it well. During a

stressful situation, this technique might be used to visualize a resolution that is less stressful.

- **Exercise.** Many people find that exercise has the benefit of reducing stress.
- **Sex.** Though in stressful situations many people tend to have less sex, physicians recommend sex as a stress reliever.
- **Music.** Listening to relaxing music is a well-known mechanism for reducing stress levels.
- **Yoga.** This type of exercise incorporates breathing techniques and imagery, which can greatly reduce a person's stress level.

Teaching Patients about Smoking and Substance Abuse Cessation

Patients who smoke or abuse other substances will sometimes ask for help in stopping. Physicians may advise patients to stop smoking for health reasons. Therefore, medical assistants should have on hand information that has been approved by the physician to let patients know what resources are available, both locally and nationally or on the Internet. The American Cancer Society (ACS) Web site (www.cancer.org) contains valuable resources for people who wish to quit smoking. The ACS points out that tobacco addiction is both psychological and physical. For this reason, most people who wish to quit smoking may need to try some combination of medicine, some method to change personal habits, and some level of emotional support. On the ACS Web site, patients or health care professionals can find links to information on:

- Using nicotine replacement therapy
- Various nicotine substitutes
- Choosing the right method to quit smoking
- Telephone support to help stop smoking
- Support groups
- Success rates

The National Institute on Drug Abuse (NIDA) maintains a Web site (www.nida.nih.gov), which provides a wealth of information on drug abuse and addiction. There the patient or health care professional will find information and resources for combating abuse of:

- Alcohol
- Club drugs
- Cocaine
- Heroin
- Inhalants
- LSD
- Marijuana
- Ecstasy
- Methamphetamine
- PCP
- Prescription medications
- Tobacco
- Anabolic steroids

Educating Patients on Dietary Supplements

Many patients seek information or guidance regarding dietary supplements when they come in for care. In 1994, Congress passed the Dietary Supplement and Education Act, which defines dietary supplements as products that are

- Intended to supplement a diet
- Made of one or more dietary ingredient (e.g., vitamins, minerals, or herbs)
- Intended for oral administration
- Labeled as dietary supplements

All medications must meet FDA approval. Products found to be ineffective or unsafe will likely be removed from the market, but they do not require approval to appear on the market.

In addition, there is no standard within dietary supplements of the same type. Products may contain vastly different ingredients, even when they are marketed as the same items.

▶▶▶Pulse Points

Dietary Supplements

Many patients take dietary supplements in addition to prescribed medications. Because physicians might not prescribe those supplements, patients might fail to mention the supplements when listing their medications. Because some supplements can conflict with medications, be sure to ask patients about any supplements they might be taking when helping those patients complete their medical history forms.

TABLE 6-7 Common Dietary Supplements

Supplement	Recommended Daily Amount	Intended Benefits	Possible Adverse Reactions
Vitamin A	5000 IU	Protects cells from free radicals that can cause disease	Birth defects, bone abnormalities, liver disease
Vitamin B$_6$	2 mg	Treats asthma and heart disease	Balance problems, decreased sense of touch
Vitamin B$_{12}$	6 micrograms	Aids in metabolism, formation of red blood cells, and maintenance of the central nervous system	Skin rash
Vitamin C	60 mg	Increases the body's reactions to free radicals	Gastrointestinal distress
Vitamin D	400 IU	Treats tuberculosis, rheumatoid arthritis, and skin disorders	Bone demineralization, tendonitis
Vitamin E	30 IU	Increases the body's reactions to free radicals	Increased blood coagulation, stroke
Vitamin K	80 micrograms	Aids in blood clotting	Temporary redness of the face and neck
Biotin	300 micrograms	Treats brittle fingernails and thinning hair	None noted
Calcium	1000 mg	Prevents osteoarthritis and strengthens teeth and bones	Constipation, bloating, gas, and flatulence
Chromium	120 micrograms	Helps regulate glucose levels	At high levels, anemia and liver dysfunction
Copper	2 mg	Treats arthritis and serves as an antioxidant and anticancer agent	Nausea, vomiting, and diarrhea
Folate	400 micrograms	Reduces risk of neural tube defects in the fetus	Sleep changes
Iodine	150 micrograms	Treats thyroid disorders	Acne, skin rash
Iron	18 mg	Treats anemia	Nausea, vomiting, bloating
Magnesium	400 mg	Treats various heart disorders	Diarrhea
Manganese	2 mg	Treats osteoarthritis and premenstrual syndrome	Increased liver dysfunction
Niacin	20 mg	Decreases cholesterol	Stomach pain, vomiting, nausea, diarrhea
Potassium chloride	3400 mg	Treats hypertension	Nausea, vomiting, diarrhea
Selenium	70 micrograms	Decreases cancer risk	Tissue damage of the hair, nails, nervous system, and teeth
Thiamin	1.5 mg	Helps protect against metabolic changes in alcoholics	None noted
Zinc	15 mg	Prevents and lessens the severity of the common cold	Nausea and vomiting

Given that dietary supplements need not meet standard requirements, the FDA requires that all manufacturers of dietary supplements refrain from stating that their products treat or cure disease. The agency also requires that disclaimers accompany any benefits on product labels. A sample disclaimer might read, "This statement has not been evaluated by the Food and Drug Administration. This product is not intended to diagnose, treat, cure, or prevent disease."

Because vitamins and minerals are needed in the diet to achieve optimal health, the FDA has established recommended daily amounts for them. Many people take vitamin and mineral supplements, even when eating well-balanced diets. Medical assistants should therefore have a good working knowledge of dietary supplements and should regularly ask patients which supplements they are taking. Medical assistants should know the uses of supplements and any possible adverse reactions. Table 6-7 lists common dietary supplements with their recommended daily amounts, benefits, and possible adverse reactions. Many physicians recommend dietary supplements to their patients for various health care concerns.

Because some patients may have beliefs regarding dietary supplements that are culturally based, physicians and medical assistants will need to be aware if the patient requires any additional information or accommodations. Some patients do not realize that dietary supplements may help or hinder their medical care and may not realize that they should mention any dietary supplements to the medical team.

Using the Internet for Education

The Internet has patient education materials, but the medical assistant should use only reputable Web sites to gather information on conditions, medications, or illnesses (Table 6-8).

TABLE 6-8 Reputable Web Sites for Patient Education

Web Site	Information
American Lung Association	Smoking cessation, asthma, hay fever, lung cancer (www.lungusa.org)
American Diabetes Associations	Nutrition and recipes, weight loss and exercise, diabetes prevention (www.diabetes.org)
Hospice	Guides for caregivers of and patients with terminal illnesses, talking to children about death, pain control, advance directives, finding a local hospice, healing after a loss (www.americanhospice.org)
American Heart Association	High blood pressure, controlling cholesterol levels, diet, and nutrition (www.americanheart.org)
Alzheimer's Association	Living with Alzheimer's, guides for caregivers (www.alz.org)
American Parkinson Disease Association	Local support groups (www.apdaparkinson.org)
ALS Association	Local support groups, guides for caregivers (www.alsa.org)
Web MD	Information for patients on medications and health care conditions (www.webmd.com)
eMedicine	Health information for consumers on first aid for medical emergencies, accidents and injuries, symptoms and treatment of disease and health conditions (http://www.emedicinehealth.com)

 PROCEDURE 6-6 Identify Community Resources

Theory and Rationale

Medical assistants will frequently be asked to give patients referrals to community resources at the physician's request. Having this information in an easy and quick-to-locate format is one way to provide patients with excellent care.

Materials

- A computer with Internet access
- Written pamphlets and brochures
- Telephone directories

Competency

1. Locate the name, address, telephone number, and Web site address for each of the following need categories in your community:
   a. Homeless services
   b. HIV/AIDS resources
   c. Disability services
   d. Domestic violence aid
   e. Public assistance
   f. Housing authority/services
   g. Ombudsman services
   h. Foster care for children
   i. Foster care for adults
   j. Seniors services
   k. Legal aid
   l. Rape victim aid
   m. Crime victim aid
   n. Culturally specific services (Native American, Military, etc.)
   o. Medical assistant services (Medicaid, etc.)
2. Identify at least 1 to 3 resources for each need category.
3. Create a written document to give to patients.

PROCEDURE 6-7 Use the Internet to Find Patient Education Materials

Theory and Rationale

The Internet is a fast way to locate educational resources and information. Often, the information can be printed and distributed to patients or incorporated into an educational piece created by the medical office.

Materials

- Computer and printer
- Paper or electronic patient chart
- Blue or black ink pen or electronic medical record

Competency

1. Using the computer, locate reputable Web sites for desired materials.

2. Print copies of materials.
3. Show materials to the physician for approval.
4. Give/mail the materials to the patient.
5. Explain the materials to the patient as needed.
6. Place a copy or scan the materials in the patient's file.
7. Document how the materials were given to the patient and any verbal education provided with the materials.

Reputable Web sites are typically those that are associated with a university or college, the government, reputable news sources, and nonprofit organizations. Web sites that are maintained as "personal sites"—sites that are created and maintained by one person containing that person's beliefs—are not typically considered a reputable source for patient education materials. The physician should approve any material before the assistant gives it to patients.

REVIEW

Chapter Summary

- Communication is the process of sharing ideas between two or more people; it is sending and receiving messages verbally and nonverbally.
- Good communication skills are vital to anyone who works in health care, but especially for the medical assistant, who must demonstrate superior verbal and nonverbal communication.
- The medical assistant must have a firm understanding of the communication process in order to share information accurately with patients, physicians, and coworkers and respond appropriately.
- Listening is a crucial component of communication in health care.
- The medical assistant must identify barriers to communication and work to overcome them using the appropriate tools and techniques.

- Patient populations, including those with special needs and/or disabilities, dictate the ways in which the medical assistant should interact with them.
- A number of community resources are available when it comes time for patient referrals.
- Just as they do with patients, medical assistants must communicate properly, professionally, and respectfully with the other members of the health care team and other facilities.
- Patient education is a vital part of the medical assistant's job duties.
- Patient education consists of supplying information about the patient's condition and treatment options and on supplying the patient with resources where they might seek further information.

Chapter Review

Multiple Choice

1. What is the proper way to address an elderly patient?
   a. Mrs. _____
   b. By first name
   c. "Honey" or "Sweetie"
   d. By the description of the patient's condition or complaint
   e. b and c

2. The opinion that all people living in homeless shelters are likely to have lice is an example of:
   a. Stereotyping
   b. Discriminating
   c. Facilitating
   d. Harassing
   e. a and b

3. Which of the following is *not* an example of keeping a professional distance?
   a. Giving a patient transportation options to the clinic
   b. Offering to pay a patient's copayment
   c. Telling the patient about a new personal relationship
   d. Calling the patient to remind her to take her medications
   e. Driving the patient to the pharmacy to pick up his medications

4. When calling another facility to schedule a patient, the most important factor to remember is:
   a. To end the call quickly
   b. To get the earliest appointment
   c. To maintain patient confidentiality
   d. To give all information about the patient's care for all conditions to the other facility
   e. To give the person on the other end of the call the best customer service possible

True/False

T F 1. Body language is far less important than verbal communication.

T F 2. Empathy and sympathy are really the same thing.

T F 3. When working with a hearing-impaired patient, the medical assistant should speak directly to the interpreter.

T F 4. When working with child patients, it is best to communicate directly with the parent during the visit rather than the child.

T F 5. Addressing the physician as "Dr." in front of patients gives patients the impression that the doctor is an authority figure who should be respected.

T F 6. Part of developing a good patient relationship includes sharing personal problems with the patients.

T F 7. Sometimes the information the medical assistant must go over with the patient may take more than one visit.

T F 8. Patients will often share more information with the medical assistant than they will with the physician.

T F 9. It is best to use proper medical terminology to demonstrate competence when speaking with patients.

T F 10. A clinic's office policy dictates whether to allow service animals to accompany their owners to treatment rooms.

Short Answer

1. What is a good communication technique to use with angry patients?
2. What are the five stages of grief?
3. Why would writing down patient instructions help the patient?
4. What is the difference between an open-ended question and a close-ended question? Provide an example of each.
5. When might it be appropriate to use therapeutic touch with a patient?
6. Describe the method you would use to communicate effectively with a hearing-impaired patient.

Research

1. Search the Internet for books to read about communication skills. Which ones sound as if they might be helpful to the medical assistant?
2. What are the local resources for hearing-impaired people in your area?
3. What are the local resources for sight-impaired people in your area?

Practicum Application Experience

Dr. Roberts wants Beth Parcher, a sight-impaired patient, to be scheduled for a series of physical therapy appointments and has asked the medical assistant to schedule the appointments. How will the medical assistant ensure Beth completely understands what Dr. Roberts wants her to do? How will the assistant ensure Beth is clear about the appointments scheduled for her?

Resource Guide

American Lung Association
61 Broadway, 6th Floor
New York, NY 10006
Phone: (800) LUNGUSA
www.lungusa.org

American Diabetes Association
National Call Center
1701 North Beauregard Street
Alexandria, VA 22311
Phone: 1-800-DIABETES
www.diabetes.org

American Hospice Foundation
2120 L Street NW, Suite 200
Washington, DC 20037
Phone: (800) 347-1413
www.americanhospice.org

American Heart Association National Center
7272 Greenville Avenue
Dallas, TX 75231
Phone: (800) AHA-USA-1
www.americanheart.org

Alzheimer's Association
225 N. Michigan Ave, Floor 17
Chicago, IL 60601
Phone: (312) 335-5886
www.alz.org

American Parkinson Disease Association Inc.
135 Parkinson Avenue
Staten Island, NY 10305
Phone: (800) 223-2732
www.apdaparkinson.org

The ALS Association
27001 Agoura Road, Suite 150
Calabasas Hills, CA 91301
Phone: (818) 880-9007
www.alsa.org

Online Communication Skills Test
http://discoveryhealth.queendom.com/

Seven Challenges: A guide to cooperative communication skills
http://www.newconversations.net/

7

Written Communication

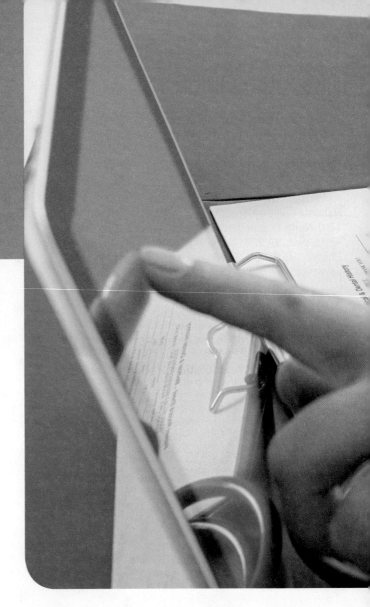

Case Study

Read the following case study and answer the critical thinking questions presented throughout the chapter.

Dr. Calvin Jones brings the certified medical assistant a business card from the medical equipment salesperson he just had lunch with and asks the assistant to type a letter to the salesperson. In the letter, the physician would like to thank the salesperson for showing him a new electrocardiogram (**ECG**) machine and indicates that while he is uninterested in purchasing the machine now, the salesperson should call after the first of the year to assess the physician's willingness to purchase one at that time.

Objectives

After completing this chapter, you should be able to:

7.1 Define and spell the key terminology in this chapter.

7.2 Write letters to patients and other health care professionals using correct grammar, spelling, and punctuation.

7.3 List and describe components of the business letter.

7.4 Detail the process of proofreading a business letter.

7.5 Discuss the use of the photocopier in the medical office.

7.6 List accepted health care abbreviations.

7.7 Describe appropriate memo use in the medical office.

7.8 Mail written communication and classify mail, including its size and postage requirements.

7.9 Develop a policy for incoming and outgoing e-mail to patients.

7.10 Manage incoming mail and correspondence.

Competency Skills Performance

1. Compose a business letter.
2. Send a letter to a patient about a missed appointment.
3. Proofread written documents.
4. Prepare a document for photocopying.
5. Fold documents for window envelopes.
6. Open and sort mail.
7. Annotate written correspondence.

Key Terminology

annotation—process of reading a document and highlighting pertinent information

body—main portion of a business letter

closing—ending portion of a business letter

electronic mail—message sent electronically from one person to another; also called e-mail

font—style of type

letterhead—professional-quality stationery with a business's contact information (e.g., name, address, telephone and fax numbers)

logo—image that represents a business entity or brand

memo—interoffice note

postage meter—electronic scale used for weighing packages and printing postage labels

proofreading—process of reading and reviewing a document for errors

proofreader's marks—notations used when reading and reviewing a document for errors

reference initials—in a professional letter, the all-capital initials of the author followed by the all-lowercase initials of the person who typed the letter (e.g., AJF/ cmm)

salutation—greeting

spell check—software that verifies word spellings

subject line—in a professional letter, the subject of the letter

thesaurus—resource for locating alternate words with similar meanings

Abbreviations

ECG—electrocardiogram

JCAHO—Joint Commission on the Accreditation of Healthcare Organizations (now TJC)

MLOCR—multiline optical character reader

OCR—optical character recognition

PDR—Physician's Desk Reference

TJC—The Joint Commission (formerly **JCAHO** – Joint Commission on the Accreditation of Healthcare Organizations)

UPS—United Parcel Service

USPS—United States Postal Service

Certification Exam Coverage

AAMA (CMA) Exam Coverage:

- Fundamental writing skills
  - Sentence structure
  - Grammar
  - Punctuation
- Formats
  - Letters
  - Memos
  - Reports
  - Envelopes
  - Chart notes
- Proofreading
  - Proofreader's marks
  - Making corrections from rough draft

- Screening and processing mail
  - U.S. Postal Service
    1) Classifications
    2) Types of mail services
  - Processing machine/meter
  - Processing incoming mail
    1) Labels
    2) Optical character recognition (OCR) guidelines

AMT (CMAS) Exam Coverage:

- Communication
  - Employ effective written and oral communication

AMT (RMA) Exam Coverage:

- Transcription and dictation
  - Transcribe notes from dictation system
  - Transcribe letter or notes from direct dictation

AAMA (CMA) certification exam topics are reprinted with permission of the American Association of Medical Assistants.

AMT (CMAS) certification exam topics are reprinted with permission of American Medical Technologists.

AMT (RMA) certification exam topics are reprinted with permission of American Medical Technologists.

Certification Exam Coverage (continued)

- Patient education
  - Patient instruction—identify and apply proper written and verbal communication to instruct patients
- Oral and written communication
  - Compose correspondence employing acceptable business format

- Employ effective written communication skills adhering to ethics and laws of confidentiality

NCCT (NCMA) Exam Coverage:
- General office procedures
  - Oral and written communication skills
  - Patient instruction

Introduction

The ability to compose written documents is crucial for the administrative medical assistant. Physicians regularly ask medical assistants to type letters to patients and other health care providers. Often, physicians will provide just basic facts and ask their medical assistants to compose letters with more detail. To perform these tasks well, the medical assistant must understand medical terminology as well as proper grammar, sentence structure, and punctuation.

Writing to Patients and Other Health Care Professionals

Any written correspondence from the medical office reflects the physician and the office. Typographical, grammatical, and punctuation errors are not only confusing, they reflect poorly on the medical office and may endanger the patient. Therefore, letters to patients and other health care professionals should be accurate, professional, and to the point. Each paragraph should address one topic and have no more than three to six sentences (**Figure 7-1** ■).

To compose and correct documents properly, every medical office should have a comprehensive medical dictionary, a **thesaurus** for acceptable alternative words, a desk dictionary, current coding books for procedure and diagnostic coding, and a *Physician's Desk Reference (PDR)*. Many of these items are available in electronic format, which is often easier to reference than using an actual book.

The Role of Spell-Checking

To help ensure written correspondence is error free, most computer software programs have built-in **spell check** capa-

bilities, but medical assistants should not rely on such programs alone. Some words might pass spell checking because they are spelled correctly, but they might be used incorrectly. For example, the words "two," "to," and "too" all pass computerized spell checking, but each has a distinct meaning that is sometimes confused with the others. An understanding of meaning is therefore important. Also, many spelling-verification programs lack the ability to check medical terms. As a result, medical assistants should keep medical dictionaries on hand for supplementary reference. While spell-check programs can be valuable tools, the medical assistant should take the time to read all documents for errors before giving those documents to physicians for final review and signing.

Critical Thinking Question 7-1

Referring to the case study at the beginning of this chapter, how can the medical assistant help ensure the typed letter contains no errors?

Proper Spelling, Grammar, and Punctuation Use

Many words in the English language, especially medical words, are commonly misspelled. Table 7-1 presents some examples. When medical assistants are unsure of correct spellings of medical terms, they should consult a comprehensive medical dictionary. Commonly used medical dictionaries include *Taber's Cyclopedic Medical Dictionary* and *Mosby's Medical Dictionary*.

Like accurate spelling, proper grammar is essential to a medical office's written correspondence. Poor grammar is unprofessional and reflects poorly on the physician and the

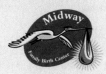

Jack Tsong, MD
Midway Family Birth Center
55 Long Island Way
Seattle, WA 12345

July 25, 20xx

Suzanne Haufe
4728 California Ave E
Seattle, WA 12345

Dear Suzanne:

On behalf of my entire staff, I would like to welcome you to Midway Family Birth Center. Our goal is to provide our patients the highest quality service. If you ever feel we fall short, please bring it to my attention. I would consider it a personal favor.

It is an honor that you have placed your care in our hands. We look forward to working with you to meet your health goals.

Sincerely,

Jack Tsong, MD

Jack Tsong, MD
JKT/cmm

Figure 7-1 ■ Sample patient letter.

TABLE 7-1 Commonly Misspelled Words		
acceptable	accidentally	accommodate
acquire	a lot	apparent
believe	calendar	category
cemetery	changeable	collectible
column	conscience	conscientious
conscious	discipline	embarrass
foreign	gauge	guarantee
harass	height	immediate
inoculate	judgment	leisure
liaison	maintenance	maneuver
miniature	minuscule	noticeable
occurrence	personnel	possession
privilege	publicly	questionnaire
receive	recommend	referred
relevant	schedule	threshold

office. Part of the medical assistant's role is to correct any grammar issues in physicians' drafts but retain the original intent of the content. Table 7-2 identifies common grammatical errors.

Proper punctuation is another vital focus area in written documentation. Table 7-3 outlines the rules of use for common punctuation marks.

Critical Thinking Question 7-2

Referring to the case study at the beginning of this chapter, what are the possible ramifications for Dr. Jones if the medical assistant does not use accurate grammar, spelling, and punctuation?

TABLE 7-2 Common Grammatical Errors

Error	Example
Noun/verb mismatch	"The office feels this is a bad idea." (The office cannot feel, but people can.)
Adjective used as a adverb	"I did good on that exam." (The word *well* should replace *good.*)
Sentence that ends with a preposition	"This is something we need to work on." (A proper rewrite is, "This is something on which we need to work.")
Run-on sentence	"This lab is a dangerous place, patients should not be back here." (A semicolon should replace the comma.)
Misuse of words that sound alike but differ in spellings and meanings	"Their here, just two quiet." (The sentence should read, "They're here, just too quiet.")
Fragmented sentence	Working very hard to understand the patient. (There is no subject-verb relationship. The sentence should read, "The medical assistant works very hard to understand what the patient is saying.")
Subject and predicate mismatch	Except for irregular plurals for nouns and verbs, either the subject (noun) or the predicate (verb) has to have an "s" on it. For example: The cat plays. The cats play. Singular nouns require an "s" on the verb; plural nouns require no "s" on the verb. For example: The man walks. The men walk.

Sentence Structure

In order to compose a proper sentence, certain components must be present. Every sentence must have a subject and a predicate in order to be a proper sentence. The subject is whom or what the sentence is about. The predicate is the word that says something about the subject. As an example, consider the sentence: "The patient arrived at 2:00 P.M." The subject is the word that the verb describes. In the example sentence, the verb "arrived" is describing the subject "patient." The predicate is what the subject did. In the example sentence, the predicate is "arrived at 2:00 P.M."

Numbers in Correspondence

In general, medical assistants should use words for quantities from one to ten in office correspondence but numbers for quantities over ten, like 24 or 876. When writing any unit of measurement, however, such as a medication dosage or weight or height,

TABLE 7-3 Rules of Use for Common Punctuation Marks

Mark	Use(s)
Period (.)	Indicates the end of a sentence and separates the parts of an abbreviation.
Comma (,)	Separates words, phrases, or two independent clauses and sets off elements that interrupt or add information in a sentence.
Semicolon (;)	Sets apart independent clauses and items in a list that contain commas.
Colon (:)	Follows a salutation in a business letter, precedes a list, separates independent clauses, helps express time.
Apostrophe (')	Indicates a missing letter from a contracted word and the possessive case of nouns.
Diagonal (/)	Separates the numbers in dates (e.g., 6/1/12) and fractions (e.g., 1/2) and sometimes indicates abbreviations (e.g., w/o).
Parentheses ( )	Sets off part of a sentence that is not part of the main thought.
Quotation marks (" ")	Indicates a direct quote.
Ellipsis (…)	Shows that a thought trails off or represents missing material (e.g., "I was going to, but …").

always use numbers. For example, the medical assistant should type, "The patient is taking 5 milligrams of the medication every hour." Numbers also always apply for the time of day, such as "1:00 P.M." Numbers that begin a sentence should be spelled out.

Rules for Medical-Term Plurals

The rules for creating plurals of medical terms can create confusion. Table 7-4 serves as a guide to the proper approaches.

TABLE 7-4 Pluralization Rules for Medical Terms

Singular Form	Plural	Example
a	ae	bulla to bullae
ax	aces	thorax to thoraces
ex or ix	ices	appendix to appendices
on	a	ganglion to ganglia
um	a	ilium to illia
us	i	mellitus to melliti
y	ies	idiosyncrasy to idiosyncrasies
nx	ges	phalanx to phalanges

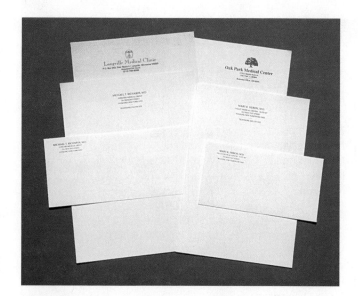

Figure 7-2 ■ Sample physician letterhead stationery and envelopes.

Source: Pearson Education/PH College. Photographer: Michal Heron.

Components of the Business Letter

All business letters, including those from medical offices, have the same basic components. First, each letter should appear on **letterhead**. Most medical offices have professionally printed letterhead that carries the offices' names and addresses, telephone and fax numbers, e-mail addresses, and physicians' names (**Figure 7-2** ■). Letterhead may also contain a **logo,** some form of artwork that indicates the type of practice or other item of significance. For example, a pediatric office might have a logo that depicts children, while a chiropractic office might have a logo that includes a spine.

After letterhead, every piece of correspondence that is composed in the medical office must contain a nonabbreviated date, such as May 26, 2014, three lines down from the letterhead content at the top. Normally, a letter carries the date that the physician wrote or dictated it, not the date the medical assistant types it.

Three to six lines after the date comes the next component of the business letter: the inside address. The inside address appears against the left margin and includes the recipient's name, title, company name, and address (**Figure 7-3** ■). Table 7-5 lists the two-letter abbreviation for each state.

The **salutation** component of the business letter serves as the greeting. It typically appears two lines down from the inside address and carries the same name as the inside address. The salutations of a formal letter should include the recipient's proper names and courtesy title, such as "Dear Dr. Hagen." A more informal letter may not include a salutation. Table 7-6 provides guidelines for courtesy titles. For more informal correspondence, such as between two physicians who know each other well, a salutation may use first name only, as in "Dear Shawn." When unsure of name spellings, medical assistants should ask for verification.

Critical Thinking Question 7-3

Referring to the case study at the beginning of the chapter, which courtesy title is appropriate for a letter to the sales representative, and why?

The **subject line** is that part of the business letter that describes the letter's purpose. The subject line should appear two lines down from the salutation and should begin with the abbreviation "RE:" which stands for "regarding." A subject line might read, "RE: Sally Luder," for example. The subject line is the patient's name when the letter is about the patient (**Figure 7-4** ■).

The **body** is the main part of the business letter. It should start two lines down from the subject line, and each of its paragraphs should address only one issue (see Figure 7-4).

The **closing** part of the letter typically appears two lines down from the ending portion of the body. The most common closing in a business letter is "Sincerely," but closing choice is at the physician's discretion. Four or five lines should be left between the closing and the physician's typed name to accommodate the physician's handwritten signature (see Figure 7-4).

Reference initials typically appear four to five lines down from the closing. Reference initials include the all-capital

Shawn D. Hagen, DC
19713 Scriber Lake Road
Lynnwood, WA 98036

Figure 7-3 ■ Sample inside address.

TABLE 7-5 Two-Letter State Abbreviations

State	Abbreviation	State	Abbreviation
Alabama	AK	North Carolina	NC
Alaska	AL	North Dakota	ND
Arkansas	AR	Nebraska	NE
Arizona	AZ	New Hampshire	NH
California	CA	New Jersey	NJ
Colorado	CO	New Mexico	NM
Connecticut	CT	Nevada	NV
Delaware	DE	New York	NY
Florida	FL	Ohio	OH
Georgia	GA	Oklahoma	OK
Hawaii	HI	Oregon	OR
Iowa	IA	Pennsylvania	PA
Idaho	ID	Rhode Island	RI
Illinois	IL	South Carolina	SC
Indiana	IN	South Dakota	SD
Kansas	KS	Tennessee	TN
Kentucky	KY	Texas	TX
Louisiana	LA	Utah	UT
Massachusetts	MA	Virginia	VA
Maryland	MD	Vermont	VT
Maine	ME	Washington	WA
Michigan	MI	Wisconsin	WI
Minnesota	MN	West Virginia	WV
Missouri	MO	Wyoming	WY
Mississippi	MS		
Montana	MT		

TABLE 7-6 Guidelines for Courtesy Titles

- "Mr." is the appropriate title for males.
- Professional titles such as "MD" or "DO" replace the courtesy title. For example, "John Aye, MD," should replace "Dr. John Aye."
- "Ms." is used when a woman's marital status is unknown, the woman is divorced, or when the woman prefers.
- "Mrs." is used for a married woman.
- "Miss" is used for a young girl or an unmarried woman who prefers it. When in doubt, use "Ms." rather than "Miss."
- Two people at the same address should appear separately (e.g., "Mr. Joseph Paterniti and Ms. Beth Dorio").

initials of the physician who dictated or wrote the letter, followed by the all-lowercase initials of the medical assistant who typed the letter (**Figure 7-5 ■**).

An enclosure notification should be included two lines below the reference initials to notify the recipient of any other information that might be enclosed with the letter. The notification can be rendered as "Enclosures" or "ENC.," followed by the number (in parentheses) of items that are enclosed. For example, a letter with two enclosures would have an enclosure notification that reads "Enclosures (2)" or "ENC. (2)." When there are no enclosures, this notation is omitted.

When a copy of the letter is to be sent to another party, the notation "c:" followed by the other party's name should appear two lines down from the enclosure indication. For example, when Sally Luder is to receive a copy of the letter, the copy notation would read, "c: Sally Luder."

Margins and line-spacing are often left to the preference of the letter writer, the provider, or the office manager. The goal is to make the letter look as professional as possible. If there is little text, the margins may be larger and the line spacing may be two lines so that the text appears centered on the paper.

Sometimes, business letters exceed one page. When they do, all subsequent pages must begin with the date of the letter, followed by the subject line. Pages after the first page require no letterhead, but they should appear on paper that matches the color and quality of the letterhead. Subsequent pages should be numbered.

Margins in the Professional Business Letter

When using a word processing software, the margins will typically default to being 1″ at the top and 1″ at the bottom, and 1 1/2″ on both the right and left sides of the documents. Though this is the default for margins, this spacing can and should be altered in certain situations. For letters that are short, such as only one or two paragraphs, margins may be increased in order to center the text. Centering the text creates a more appealing visual for the document.

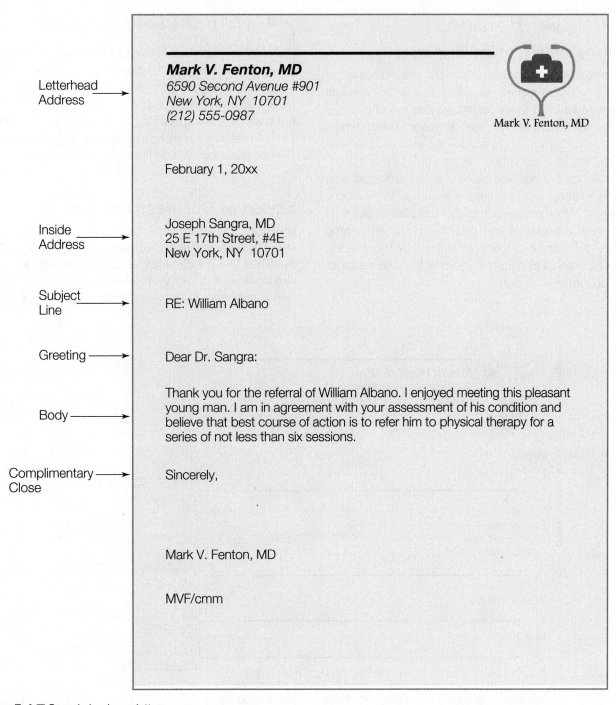

Letterhead Address

Mark V. Fenton, MD
6590 Second Avenue #901
New York, NY 10701
(212) 555-0987

Mark V. Fenton, MD

February 1, 20xx

Inside Address

Joseph Sangra, MD
25 E 17th Street, #4E
New York, NY 10701

Subject Line

RE: William Albano

Greeting

Dear Dr. Sangra:

Body

Thank you for the referral of William Albano. I enjoyed meeting this pleasant young man. I am in agreement with your assessment of his condition and believe that best course of action is to refer him to physical therapy for a series of not less than six sessions.

Complimentary Close

Sincerely,

Mark V. Fenton, MD

MVF/cmm

Figure 7-4 ■ Sample business letter.

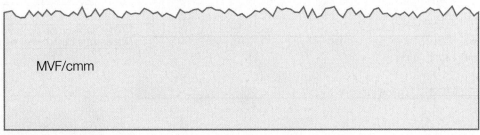

MVF/cmm

Figure 7-5 ■ Sample reference initials.

▸▸ Pulse Points

Signing Letters for the Physician

Occasionally, the physician will be out of the office when letters must be mailed, so she may ask her medical assistant to send those letters without the physician's signature. The review process, however, should remain the same. The physician should still read or otherwise review the letters and give her approval before the letters are sent. Approved letters can be stamped with notes such as, "Read but not signed due to time constraints." When offices lack preprinted stamps like this, the medical assistant can print the physician's name where the signature belongs and follow the printing with a personal signature to indicate that the assistant signed for the physician.

● In Practice

Dr. Mohammad asks Joanne Brennan, his new administrative medical assistant, to type a letter to a patient while he dictates. During dictation, Dr. Mohammad uses words unfamiliar to Joanne, so she guesses at how to spell some of the words, thinking that the patient probably won't notice.

What might happen if Joanne continues to guess at word spellings? Why is this issue important?

Styles of Business Letters

Medical offices use varied letter styles, including block (**Figure 7-6A ■**), modified block (**Figure 7-6B ■**), and modified block with indentations (**Figure 7-6C ■**). Block and modified block are the most common styles, but the physician's preference dictates letter style.

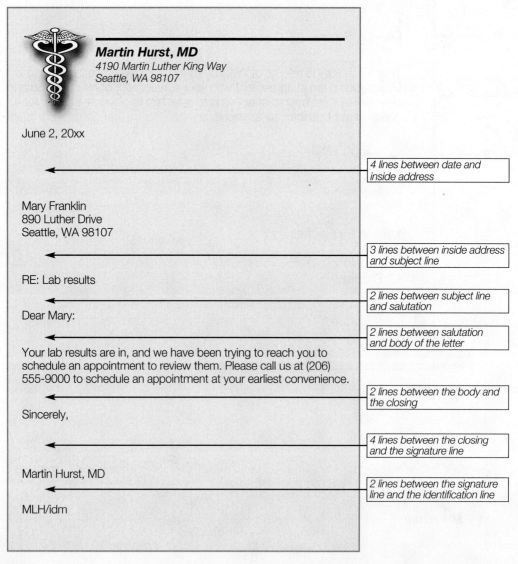

Martin Hurst, MD
4190 Martin Luther King Way
Seattle, WA 98107

June 2, 20xx

4 lines between date and inside address

Mary Franklin
890 Luther Drive
Seattle, WA 98107

3 lines between inside address and subject line

RE: Lab results

2 lines between subject line and salutation

Dear Mary:

2 lines between salutation and body of the letter

Your lab results are in, and we have been trying to reach you to schedule an appointment to review them. Please call us at (206) 555-9000 to schedule an appointment at your earliest convenience.

2 lines between the body and the closing

Sincerely,

4 lines between the closing and the signature line

Martin Hurst, MD

2 lines between the signature line and the identification line

MLH/idm

A

Figure 7-6 ■ Styles of business letters. A. Block style.

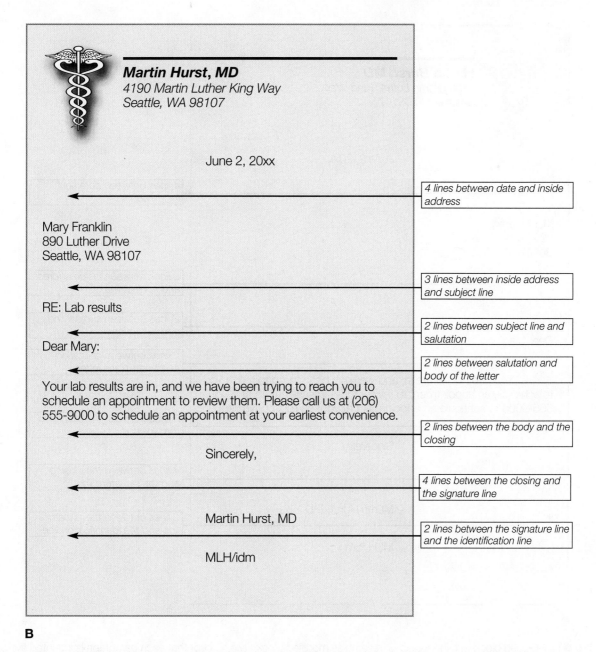

Martin Hurst, MD
4190 Martin Luther King Way
Seattle, WA 98107

June 2, 20xx

4 lines between date and inside address

Mary Franklin
890 Luther Drive
Seattle, WA 98107

3 lines between inside address and subject line

RE: Lab results

2 lines between subject line and salutation

Dear Mary:

2 lines between salutation and body of the letter

Your lab results are in, and we have been trying to reach you to schedule an appointment to review them. Please call us at (206) 555-9000 to schedule an appointment at your earliest convenience.

2 lines between the body and the closing

Sincerely,

4 lines between the closing and the signature line

Martin Hurst, MD

2 lines between the signature line and the identification line

MLH/idm

B

Figure 7-6 ■ B. Modified block style: date, closing, signature, and identification lines center, all other lines are flush left.

Using Fonts in Typed Communication

All word-processing software comes with a set of **fonts**, which are different styles of type. Professional letters should appear in 10- to 12-point formal fonts, like Times New Roman, Garamond, or Arial (**Figure 7-7** ■). While informal fonts may function for things like interoffice informational sheets, they are considered inappropriate for professional business letters.

Sending Letters to Patients

Medical offices send letters to patients for a number of reasons, including to communicate changes in office policy or procedure. Personalized letters serve to notify patients they need or have missed appointments. Whatever the reasons they are sent, patient letters should be professional and accurate. Copies of all written patient correspondence should be included in the patients' medical records.

Proofreading

As discussed earlier, while most word-processing software can check spelling and grammar, such programs are neither failsafe nor complete substitutes for manual error-checking processes. Software that checks spelling may not contain medical terminology; therefore, the medical assistant will need to check other sources if unsure how to spell a particular medical term. Because most documents today are composed electronically, medical assistants can proofread and correct those documents before printing. **Proofreading** is the process of

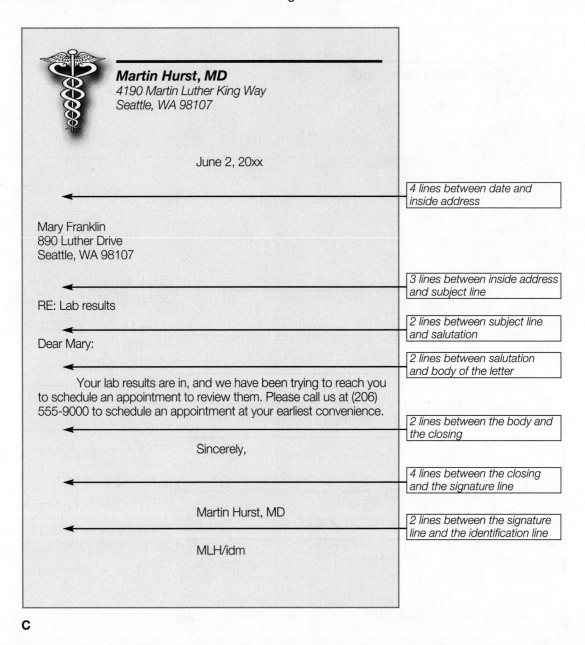

Martin Hurst, MD
4190 Martin Luther King Way
Seattle, WA 98107

June 2, 20xx

4 lines between date and inside address

Mary Franklin
890 Luther Drive
Seattle, WA 98107

3 lines between inside address and subject line

RE: Lab results

2 lines between subject line and salutation

Dear Mary:

2 lines between salutation and body of the letter

Your lab results are in, and we have been trying to reach you to schedule an appointment to review them. Please call us at (206) 555-9000 to schedule an appointment at your earliest convenience.

2 lines between the body and the closing

Sincerely,

4 lines between the closing and the signature line

Martin Hurst, MD

2 lines between the signature line and the identification line

MLH/idm

C

Figure 7-6 ■ C. Modified block with indentations: resembles modified block style, except that each paragraph is indented five spaces.

Arial 10-point font	Arial 12-point font
Garamond 10-point font	Garamond 12-point font
Times New Roman 10-point font	Times New Roman 12-point font

Figure 7-7 ■ Sample fonts.

checking written information for spelling or other errors. Sometimes, proofreading includes modifying a letter's style (e.g., line format) to make the letter more appealing on paper.

Proofreading requires medical assistants to read documents slowly and check that the documents are clear and logically organized. To indicate needed changes, medical assistants place **proofreader's marks** on printed documents (**Figure 7-8** ■).

To catch all errors, medical assistants should read all letters at least twice. A final version of the document should be printed only after it has been proofread. Once documents are printed, medical assistants should proofread them one last time to determine if format changes, like more or less space between lines, would make the documents more attractive.

Photocopying in the Medical Office

Though many medical offices today operate with an electronic health record, documents must still often be photocopied for the patient or for the patient's chart. Examples of items that must be photocopied for the patients' medical records would be

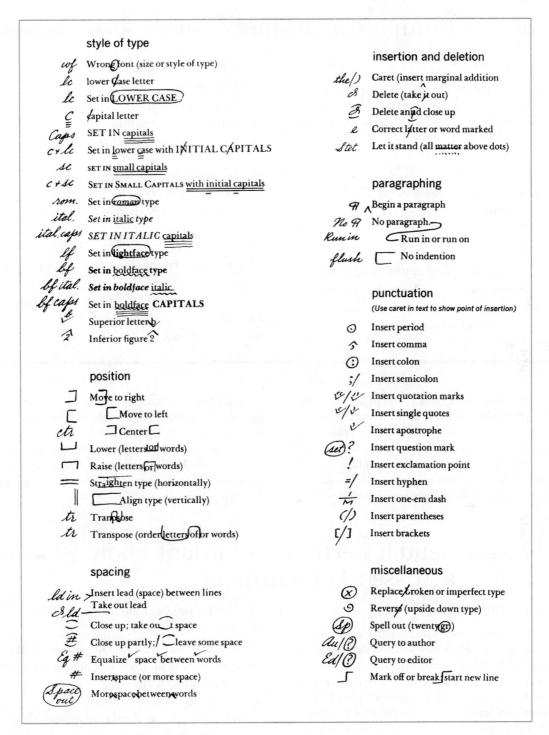

Figure 7-8 ■ Proofreader's marks.

reports or notes from other physicians or clinics, or laboratory results from outside agencies. The photocopier should be located in an area of the office that patients do not frequent because the items being photocopied may be sensitive in nature, and patients should not view any material that does not pertain to them. Though photocopiers vary in style, size, and features, most have similar services for use. Some photocopiers have a fax feature, and some are capable of collating and sorting material. More complex copiers are capable of printing on two sides of a sheet of paper or enlarging or reducing the size of a copy.

Working with Accepted Abbreviations

Abbreviations are common in medical terminology. For all members of the health care team, however, it is essential to use only accepted abbreviations in office communication. The Joint Commission (**TJC**), formerly known as The Joint Commission on the Accreditation of Healthcare Organizations, JCAHO has identified the standard abbreviations its members are required

PROCEDURE 7-1 Compose a Business Letter

Theory and Rationale

Administrative medical assistants often compose business letters from physicians. Because these letters directly reflect the physicians, they must be professional, grammatically correct, and free of typographical errors.

Materials

- Computer with word-processing software
- Information for the letter

Competency

1. Determine the recipient and content of the letter.
2. Using the word-processing software, type the date of the letter.
3. Type the recipient of the letter.
4. Type the subject line.
5. Type the greeting of the letter.
6. Type the body of the letter.
7. Type the salutation.
8. Indicate enclosures, if any.
9. Indicate if a copy of the letter will be sent to another party.
10. Enter the initials of the letter's author, followed by your initials as the typist.
11. Perform complete electronic spelling and grammar checks.
12. Print the letter.
13. On paper, perform manual spelling and grammar checks.
14. Give the letter to the physician for her signature.
15. Address an envelope.
16. Send the letter.

to use and those it should avoid. Table 7-7 on page 136 lists the latter. TJC prepared this list due to the growing concern that the use of more than one abbreviation for the same medical term created a situation where confusion, misdiagnosis, or even injury to the patient could occur. In the medical office, lists like these help staff maintain consistent terminology and avoid confusion and errors. Medical offices might have differing versions

of the accepted medical abbreviations that are used in that facility. For example, one office might use the abbreviation "BS" to indicate a patient's breath sounds, whereas another medical office may use the same abbreviation to indicate a patient's bowel sounds. Medical assistants who are unsure about abbreviations should always err on the side of caution and spell out the corresponding words.

PROCEDURE 7-2 Send a Letter to a Patient about a Missed Appointment

Theory and Rationale

Administrative medical assistants regularly write professional letters to patients. These letters may be sent for a variety of reasons when the physician wishes to communicate in writing with the patient, such as when the patient misses an appointment. Often, written communication is used when the physician desires written proof of what was said to the patient. Strict attention to detail helps avoid miscommunication between the patient and the medical office.

Materials

- Computer with word-processing software
- Patient medical record

Competency

1. Using the word-processing software, type the date at the top of the letter.
2. Type the patient's name and mailing address.
3. Type the salutation.
4. For the subject line, type "RE: Missed Appointment."
5. In the body of the letter, describe the appointment that was missed, including its date.
6. Per the physician's instructions or office policy, list the reasons the patient should call to reschedule the missed appointment.
7. Type the closing and the physician's name.
8. Obtain the signature of the letter's author (yours or the physician's).
9. Copy the letter for the patient's file.
10. Send the patient the original letter.

PROCEDURE 7-3 Proofread Written Documents

Theory and Rationale

Proofreading skills are imperative to the administrative medical assistant, because the composition of written documents is a large part of administrative medical assisting. Documents sent out without proofreading can confuse the recipient, or even lead to possible misdiagnosis or treatment of a patient.

Materials

- Computer document to be proofread
- Computer with word-processing software

Competency

1. Open the document using the word-processing software.

2. Use the word processor's spelling and grammar checking functions.
3. Save any changes.
4. Starting at the top, read the entire document to verify that all spelling, punctuation, and grammatical errors were corrected.
5. Save any changes.
6. Print the document.
7. Review the entire document to verify that all spelling, punctuation, and grammatical errors were corrected. If changes were made, reprint the document
8. Give the document to the physician for signature.

Creating Memos for the Office

A **memo** is a type of intraoffice correspondence. Memos are a quick and efficient means of communication. They require no postage and are designed to have clear messages. Office managers might compose memos to communicate with their entire staff, or staff members may write memos to communicate with other staff.

Most memos begin with the word "MEMO" or "MEMORANDUM" at the top. Below that, typically the date, recipient, and author appear (**Figure 7-9** ■). Many medical offices preprint memo paper, but some print memo paper on an as-needed basis.

Aside from the use of memos for interoffice communications, many offices have an electronic means for this purpose. The office staff may send e-mails to one another, or the electronic health record may have a mechanism for sending messages from one staff member to another.

Mailing Written Communication

Standard paper size is $8\frac{1}{2}'' \times 11''$, while standard business envelope size is $4\frac{1}{8}'' \times 9\frac{1}{2}''$. Professional business letters should be mailed in business-sized or "Size 10" envelopes. Such envelopes easily accommodate business letters that are folded in thirds (**Figure 7-10** ■).

PROCEDURE 7-4 Prepare a Document for Photocopying

Theory and Rationale

Many documents in the medical office will need to be photocopied. Often, originals are sent to the patient and copies are kept in the patient's file. The medical assistant must be familiar with how the photocopier works and the steps to correctly copy needed documents. Depending on the type and functions of the photocopier, the steps in this procedure may be modified.

Materials

- Photocopier
- Document to be copied
- Envelope
- Patient medical record

Competency

1. Turn the photocopy machine on and allow time for it to warm up.

2. Place the document to be copied face down on the glass surface of the photocopier, following the diagram on the photocopier.
3. Indicate the number of copies needed by entering the number in the appropriate place on the photocopier.
4. Press the "copy" button on the photocopier.
5. Once the copy has been made, remove the original.
6. Place the original document into an envelope to be mailed to the patient.
7. Place the photocopy of the document into the patient's file.

MEMORANDUM

Date: _____

To: _____

From: _____

Figure 7-9 ■ Sample opening of an intraoffice memo.

	TABLE 7-7 Medical Abbreviations to Avoid	
Abbreviation	**Potential Problem**	**Preferred Replacement(s)**
U (unit)	Mistaken for "0" (zero), the number "4" (four), or "cc"	"unit"
IU (International Unit)	Mistaken for IV (intravenous) or the number 10 (ten)	"International Unit"
Q.D., QD, q.d., qd (daily); Q.O.D., QOD, q.o.d., qod (every other day)	Mistaken for each other. The period after the Q is mistaken for "I" and the "O" is mistaken for "I" (q.i.d. is four times a day dosing)	"daily" or "every other day"
Trailing zero (X.0 mg) Lack of leading zero (.X)	Decimal point is missed	X mg or 0.X mg
MS	Can mean morphine sulfate or magnesium sulfate	"morphine sulfate"
MS04 and MgS04	Confused for one another	"magnesium sulfate"

Source: The Joint Commission.

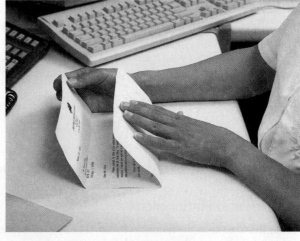

Figure 7-10 ■ When folded into thirds, the letter will easily fit within the standard business envelope.

Source: Pearson Education/PH College. Photographer: Michal Heron.

The envelope's upper left corner should carry the office's address (**Figure 7-11** ■). Many offices buy envelopes pre-printed with this information. The recipient's name and address should appear in the envelope's center and the stamp or postage-meter mark in the far upper right. When mail is personal, the word "Personal" or "Confidential" should appear below the recipient's address.

Some medical offices place their required registration forms on their Web site. By directing patients to access the

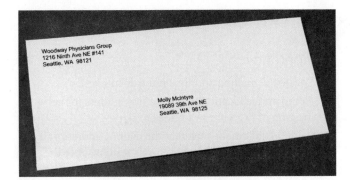

Figure 7-11 ■ Example of a properly addressed business envelope.
Source: Pearson Education/PH College. Photographer: Dylan Malone.

Web site to download, print, and fill out the needed forms, the medical office saves the cost of printing the packets and mailing them to the patient ahead of time.

Window Envelopes

For certain types of mail, like insurance billing forms or patient billing statements, medical offices often use window envelopes. Before such envelopes are sealed, however, medical assistants should ensure that addresses appear in the window (**Figure 7-12** ■).

HIPAA Compliance

Regardless of size or type, for personal patient information medical offices must use security envelopes. Security envelopes have internal patterns that keep the contents of documents obscured. **Figure 7-13** ■ shows a security envelope.

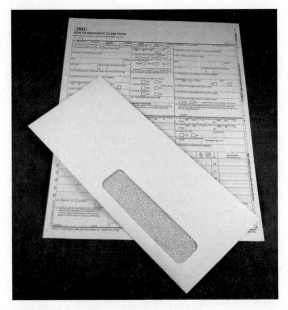

Figure 7-12 ■ Example of a window envelope.
Source: Pearson Education/PH College. Photographer: Dylan Malone.

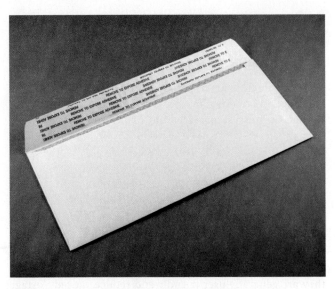

Figure 7-13 ■ Example of a security envelope.
Source: Pearson Education/PH College. Photographer: Dylan Malone.

Postage Meters in the Medical Office

Many medical clinics have **postage meters**, which weigh mail pieces, determine correct postage and print postage on envelopes or labels (**Figure 7-14** ■). Basic models simply weigh pieces of mail and print postage, while advanced versions accept stacks of mail, insert documents into envelopes, seal envelopes, and affix proper postage. Postage meters are extremely useful to the medical office because

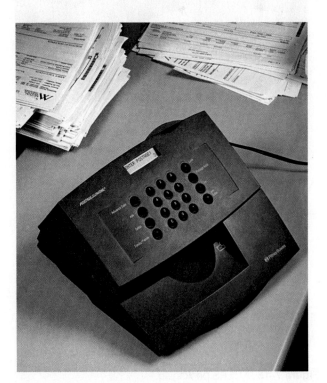

Figure 7-14 ■ An electronic postage meter.
Source: PhotoEdit, Inc./ Photographer: Spencer Grant.

PROCEDURE 7-5 Fold Documents for Window Envelopes

Theory and Rationale

When documents are folded properly before they are placed in window envelopes, post-office machinery can read addresses correctly and deliver mail in a timely manner.

Materials

- Document to be mailed
- Window envelope

Competency

1. Locate the mailing address on the document.
2. Compare the location of the mailing address to the location of the window on the envelope.
3. Fold the document such that the mailing address will be viewable through the envelope's window once the document has been inserted in the envelope.
4. Insert the document in the envelope.
5. Verify that the address is viewable through the window.
6. Seal the envelope.

---

they are generally user friendly and reduce wasted postage as well as time spent at the post office.

Most medical offices lease their postage meters from companies that supply the meters as well as corresponding supplies (e.g., ink cartridges, ribbons, labels). Once an office has arranged payment for its postage, the medical assistant facilitates meter use by calling the postage company's customer service department and providing the office's user identification number, office password, and meter serial number and access code.

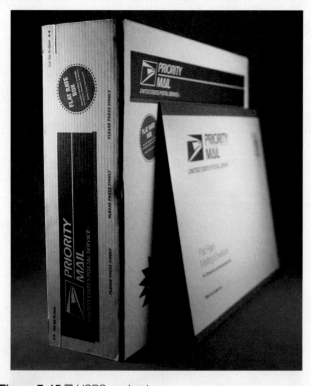

Figure 7-15 ■ USPS packaging.
Source: Pearson Education/PH College. Photographer: Dylan Malone.

Classifying Mail, Size Requirements, and Postage

The United States Postal Service (**USPS**) offers various services for mailing letters and packages according to urgency and value (**Figure 7-15** ■). A standard postage stamp facilitates first-class mail service, which is available for items weighing no more than 13 ounces. Mail that weighs over 13 ounces must be sent via Priority Mail or Parcel Post.

▸▸▸ Pulse Points

Choosing the Type of Mail Service to Use

Use This Service	When …
First Class Mail	Letters need not be received before 3 to 5 days and weigh no more than 13 ounces.
Priority Mail	Letters weigh more than 13 ounces, or packages have a maximum combined length, width, and depth of 108 inches, and must arrive within 2 to 3 days.
Priority Mail Flat Rate	Heavy items must arrive within 2 to 3 days and can fit into USPS Flat Rate envelopes or boxes.
Express Mail	Items must arrive by the next day.
Media or Standard Mail	Printed or bound materials (e.g., books or magazines, CDs or DVDs) must be sent.

After Express Mail, which is the fastest USPS service (with guaranteed next-day delivery 7 days a week), Priority Mail is the U.S. government's fastest mail service. For most destinations in the U.S., Priority Mail arrives within 2 to 3 days. However, Priority Mail items must weigh no more than 70 pounds, and packages cannot exceed a combined length, width, and depth of 108 inches. The USPS charges one flat rate to use their flat rate envelopes and boxes, regardless of where the item is being shipped within the United States or how much it weighs. When senders use envelopes and packages provided by USPS that clearly state "Flat Rate," Priority Mail is available at a flat rate.

Media Mail, or Standard Mail, is strictly for printed or bound materials such as books or magazines, sound recordings, videotapes, or CDs and DVDs. This service is more economical than the other services, but it tends to take longer, usually 2 to 10 days. Advertising cannot be sent by Media Mail.

In addition to its base services, the USPS offers a variety of optional services for an additional cost. Using certified mail, for example, provides a mailing receipt and a record of the mailing at the local post office, but it is available only for First-Class and Priority Mail packages and letters. Confirmation receipts are another, added service (**Figure 7-16** ■). Delivery confirmation allows senders and receivers to track pieces of mail or packages online. Registered mail, another option available for only First-Class and Priority Mail, offers the ability to purchase insurance for the value of the item, up to $25,000. A return receipt can also be added to this service. Insurance can be purchased for any item shipped via the USPS, but the cost of the insurance rises with the value of the item.

Buying Postage Online

The USPS now sells postage online to any consumer with a computer and a printer. This service is available for both domestic and international shipments and includes such options as insurance (up to a $500 value) and delivery confirmation.

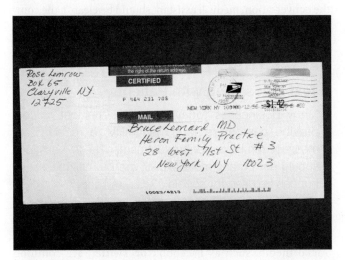

Figure 7-16 ■ Important items should be sent via certified mail.
Source: Pearson Education/PH College. Photographer: Michal Heron.

Using Multiline Optical Character Readers

The USPS uses multiline optical character readers (**MLOCRs**), with optical character recognition (**OCR**) to determine how to route mail through its systems. MLOCRs captures the image of the front of a piece of mail, looks up postal codes, prints barcodes, and performs mail sorts.

MLOCRs cannot read all mail, however. Some handwriting is hard to read and addresses might sometimes appear in incorrect locations. This type of mail is either sent to another, more powerful computer for scanning or to a human operator.

"ZIP + 4" Codes

The ZIP code is the USPS system of using five digits to indicate mail's intended destination. Since 1983, the USPS has been using "ZIP + 4" codes to expedite postal service by directing mail to more precise locations. These codes, which, as their name suggests, extend traditional ZIP codes by four digits, appear on the USPS Web site at http://zip4.usps.com/zip4/welcome.jsp.

USPS-Approved Abbreviations in Addresses

Mail that follows USPS recommendations reaches its destination far more quickly than mail that does not. Some of these recommendations—approved abbreviations for mailing addresses—appear in Table 7-8.

Restricted Materials

The USPS will mail no item that is outwardly or of its own force dangerous or injurious to life, health, or property. Similarly, it will not transport most hazardous material. The following items are also subject to certain restrictions:

- Intoxicating liquors
- Firearms
- Knives or other sharp instruments
- Odor-producing chemicals
- Liquids and powders
- Controlled substances

When in doubt about whether an item can be mailed, the medical assistant should call or visit the USPS.

Other Delivery Options

Some services compete with the USPS by offering package tracking, insurance, and delivery services; these services include Federal Express, United Parcel Service (**UPS**), and

TABLE 7-8 USPS-Approved Abbreviations

For Streets and Towns

Alley	ALY	Hill	HL
Annex	ANX	Island	IS
Avenue	AVE	Junction	JCT
Boulevard	BLVD	Lake	LK
Bridge	BRG	Lane	LN
Brook	BRK	Manor	MNR
Bypass	BYP	Meadow	MDW
Canyon	CYN	Mountain	MTN
Cape	CPE	Orchard	ORCH
Causeway	CSWY	Parkway	PKWY
Center	CTR	Place	PL
Circle	CIR	Plaza	PLZ
Cliff	CLF	Point	PT
Club	CLB	Port	PRT
Common	CMN	Ridge	RDG
Corner	COR	River	RIV
Court	CRT	Road	RD
Cove	CV	Route	RTE
Creek	CRK	Shore	SHR
Crossing	XING	Spring	SPG
Drive	DR	Square	SQ
Estate	EST	Station	STA
Expressway	EXPY	Street	ST
Forest	FRST	Terrace	TER
Freeway	FWY	Throughway	TRWY
Garden	GDN	Trail	TRL
Gateway	GTWY	Tunnel	TUNL
Grove	GRV	Turnpike	TPKE
Harbor	HBR	Valley	VLY
Heights	HTS	View	VW
Highway	HWY	Village	VLG

For Secondary Unit Designators

Apartment	APT	Office	OFC
Basement	BSMT	Penthouse	PH
Building	BLDG	Room	RM
Department	DEPT	Space	SPC
Floor	FL	Suite	STE
Front	FRNT	Trailer	TRLR
Lobby	LBBY	Upper	UPPR
Lower	LOWR		

DHL. Federal Express (FedEx) offers overnight courier, ground delivery, heavy freight delivery, and document copying services. FedEx services are available both to home and business customers, and FedEx offers shipping via its Express, Ground, Freight, and International services. The United Parcel Service (UPS), much like FedEx, offers shipping services both within the United States and worldwide via various shipping speeds and methods. Both of these companies offer package pickup, which alleviates the need to take a package to a FedEx or UPS retail location. The Deutsche Post World Net (DHL) offers shipping services worldwide at a variety of shipping speeds. In 2003,

DHL purchased Airborne Express—then the third largest private express delivery company in the United States.

Using E-Mail to Communicate

Electronic mail, or e-mail, is an electronic means of communication. Many medical offices use e-mail to communicate with patients. As a general rule, patients who give medical offices their e-mail addresses authorize those offices to send them e-mail. However, it is crucial that medical staff remember that e-mail is far from secure. For example, e-mail addresses can be misspelled, causing incorrect parties to receive messages. Also, employers have the right to view any e-mail their employees send on company systems. Because confidentiality is not guaranteed, all medical staff, including the medical assistant, should only use e-mail to send patients such nonconfidential information as appointment reminders. Many medical offices today have instituted an encrypted e-mail system so that it can be used for communication with patients.

Medical office managers will likely have a policy in place for when an e-mail is appropriate to send to a patient. Sending sensitive patient information, for example, will likely be forbidden in the policy. Even sending patient appointment reminders may be against the office policy for an e-mail.

Many medical offices provide patients with the e-mail addresses of providers, or even staff. These e-mail addresses may be listed on the clinic's website. In the event a patient sends an e-mail to the office, the medical assistant must respond in a manner that maintains the patient's privacy. For example, if the patient were to send an e-mail asking for the results of her laboratory work or other sensitive information, the assistant should respond with a telephone number the patient may call to receive those results directly.

E-mails from patients should be responded to in a timely manner. Typically, that means within one business day of receipt. E-mail etiquette dictates that one refrain from typing in all caps, as that is seen as "shouting" in written form. Because written communication, including e-mail messages, can be misunderstood due to the lack of being face-to-face in the conversation, medical assistant should be clear in the communication so that no misunderstanding occurs.

▶▶▶ Pulse Points

Text Messaging with Patients

Many businesses today, including medical offices, provide customers with the ability to receive text message reminders for appointments. These messages should not be any more explicit than e-mail messages but can be used for appointment reminders.

Social Media in Communications

Social media, such as Facebook or Twitter, are common means of communication today. Many medical offices maintain social media sites as a form of marketing and advertising to the community. Occasionally, patients may post messages to the clinic's social media site that contain personal information. Members of the medical office staff should not engage in conversations that violate the patient's HIPAA-mandated privacy, even when the patient is the one who first posts on the topic. In the event a patient posts something of this nature to a social media site, the proper way to respond, if a response is called for, is to contact the patient directly via telephone.

Managing Mail and Correspondence

Administrative medical assistants are typically in charge of sorting and distributing the medical office's incoming mail (**Figure 7-17 ■**). Because many such items, such as pathology reports or consultation letters, are time sensitive, assistants should sort and distribute incoming mail daily.

Often, the person who sorts and distributes the mail is also asked to stamp the date the mail was received. Many offices also require the person sorting the mail to open each piece so recipients can easily access the contents. Items marked "personal" or "confidential" should be left unopened, however.

To avoid confusion, each office should have a mail sorting and distribution policy that includes a list of the items each staff member should receive. For example, the physician may receive all communications or reports regarding patients, any professional journals, and literature from professional organizations. The office manager, by contrast, may receive all bills, advertisements for services or supplies, and samples from drug or supply companies.

HIPAA Compliance

Because many items sent to the medical office contain private patient information, mail should never be left where other people can access it, even when unopened.

Annotation

To abbreviate their reviews of the information they receive, some physicians charge their administrative medical assistants with **annotation**, a process that involves reading, highlighting, and summarizing information. Medical assistants who annotate should clarify the information physicians consider pertinent before they undertake the task (**Figure 7-18 ■**). Typically, the physician will ask the medical assistant to highlight the patient's name, any pertinent information about the patient, such as a diagnosis or treatment plan, and the name of the sender of the letter.

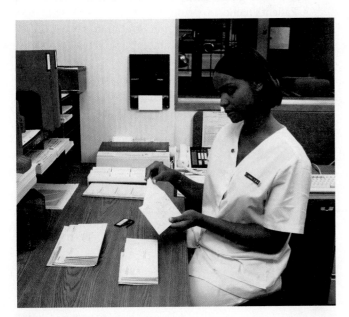

Figure 7-17 ■ The medical assistant is commonly the person to open and sort the mail.
Source: Pearson Education/PH College. Photographer: Michal Heron.

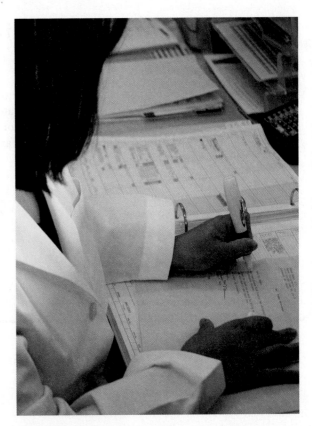

Figure 7-18 ■ The medical assistant may be asked to open and annotate portions of the physician's incoming mail.
Source: Pearson Education/PH College. Photographer: Dylan Malone.

PROCEDURE 7-6 Open and Sort Mail

Theory and Rationale

The medical office receives various kinds of mail daily. Some mail contains important, private patient information, whereas other is considered "junk." The medical assistant will likely need to learn to sort mail properly.

Materials

- A stack of incoming mail, including payments from insurance companies and patients, advertisements, drug samples, magazines, professional journals, bills for office services, a letter to the physician marked "Personal and Confidential," and consultation reports from other physicians
- Date stamp
- Letter opener

Competency

1. Using a date stamp, stamp the date on each received item.

2. Sort the mail into the appropriate files according to the following:
   - **Physician**— correspondence from other physicians, hospitals, or laboratories, as well as any professional journals
   - **Office manager**— bills for office services, drug samples, advertisements for supplies or services
   - **Receptionist**— magazines
   - **Billing office**— payments from patients or insurance companies, correspondence from insurance companies
3. Open each piece of mail, except for the piece marked "Personal and Confidential."
4. Distribute the mail appropriately. Leave the mail piece marked "Personal and Confidential" on the physician's desk.

PROCEDURE 7-7 Annotate Written Correspondence

Theory and Rationale

In a busy medical office, the physician may want to save time by having the medical assistant scan and annotate medical reports. Medical assistants who know what information to look for save time for the physician and can point out key pieces of information.

Material

- Written correspondence
- Highlighter pen
- Letter opener

Competency

1. Open the envelope with the document to be annotated.

2. Read the document once in its entirety.
3. Using the highlighter pen, review the document again, highlighting such pertinent information as:
   - Patient's name
   - Findings of any examination or laboratory work
   - Dates for followup appointments
   - Diagnosis
4. Read the document a third time to ensure all pertinent information has been noted.
5. Place the annotated document on the physician's desk for review.

REVIEW

Chapter Summary

- Proper grammar, spelling, and punctuation are all paramount to a medical office's positive image.
- Medical assistants should follow a defined process when composing letters to patients and other members of the health care team.
- Medical assistants must be familiar with the use of a medical dictionary.
- The proofreading of business letters, which involves attention to detail as well as a solid understanding of English essentials, is a means by which the medical assistant can help support a positive professional image for the office.
- In all correspondence, medical assistants should use only abbreviations that are accepted in the health care industry.
- Memos are one vehicle health care staff can use to communicate with other team members.
- The U.S. mail system is governed by a set of rules and restrictions the medical assistant should be familiar with to function as part of the health care team.
- E-mail is governed by its own unique set of rules and policies.
- The medical assistant is responsible for managing incoming mail and correspondence according to office policy.
- The medical assistant may be called upon to annotate the physician's mail correspondence.

Chapter Review

Multiple Choice

1. Which of the following USPS mail types is appropriate for mailing a DVD?
   a. Media
   b. Priority
   c. Express
   d. Ground
   e. Overnight

2. Which of the following mail types is appropriate for sending a letter that must arrive the next day?
   a. Media
   b. Priority
   c. Express
   d. Ground
   e. Transit

3. A piece of mail marked _____ should be left unopened and given directly to the intended recipient.
   a. "Open Immediately"
   b. "Personal"
   c. "Important"
   d. a and b
   e. a, b, and c

4. Which of the following substances is prohibited by the USPS for mailing?
   a. Alcoholic beverages
   b. Firearms
   c. Flammable material
   d. a and b
   e. a, b and c

5. In the medical office, it is appropriate to use a memo when the:
   a. Office manager wishes to notify staff of a holiday party
   b. Medical assistant must notify a patient of a missed appointment
   c. Physician would like to contact a patient with test results
   d. Physician would like to publish a column in the local newspaper
   e. Nurse would like to make a notation in a patient's chart

True/False

T F **1.** Any written correspondence in the medical office reflects on the physician and the office.

T F **2.** As a general rule, numbers from one to ten should be written out when writing letters.

T F **3.** The physician is responsible for managing incoming mail and correspondence.

T F **4.** "Miss" is the appropriate title to use when addressing a woman of unknown marital status.

T F **5.** The most common salutation in professional letters is "Yours Truly."

T F **6.** E-mail is a secure way to send patients test results.

Short Answer

1. What is the purpose of the subject line in a professional letter?
2. What is a typical closing in a professional letter?
3. What are the reference initials for Mark S. Stevens, MD, who authors a letter, and medical assistant Sarah Ellen Parker, who types it?

4. Which three fonts appear most often in a business letter?
5. Explain the process of annotation.
6. Describe the function of spell-check software.
7. Give several examples of words in English that sound the same yet have different meanings.
8. What is a logo, and why is it used?

Research

1. What classes could you take at your local community college to help improve your written communication skills?
2. Looking at the USPS Web site, how would you calculate postage to various locations throughout the United States? Outside the United States?
3. Review the Web sites for both FedEx and UPS. Compare their services. Does either offer a service the other does not?

Practicum Application Experience

When Dr. Yi asks office manager Marnie Glaser, CMA (AAMA), to open and distribute the day's mail, Marnie accidentally opens a piece to Dr. Yi marked "Personal." What is the proper way to handle this situation?

Resource Guide

United States Postal Service
Phone: (800) 275-8777
www.usps.com

Federal Express
Phone: (800) GO-FEDEX
www.fedex.com

United Parcel Service
Phone: (800) PICK-UPS
www.ups.com

DHL
Phone: (800) CALL-DHL
www.dhl-usa.com

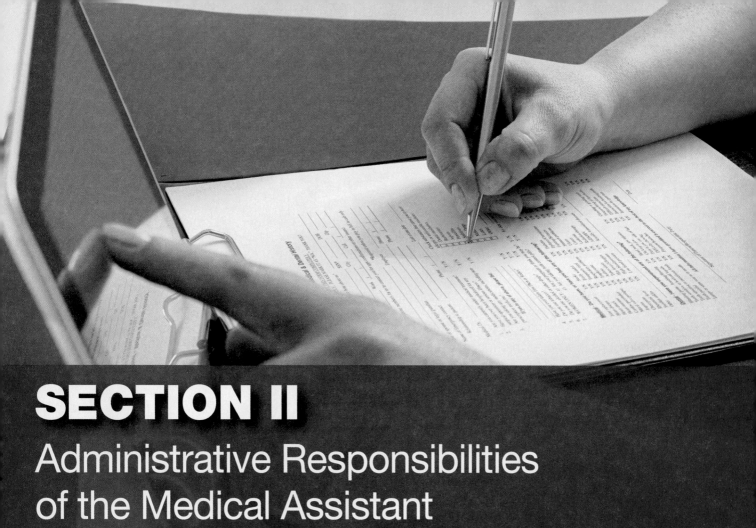

SECTION II
Administrative Responsibilities of the Medical Assistant

My name is Alicia Hayward, and I am employed as an administrative medical assistant at a women's care and family planning clinic. Each day, I am responsible for multiple tasks, including opening and closing the medical office, front desk reception, corresponding with patients on the telephone, and scheduling patients.

Administrative medical assistants must have professional telephone skills, since the telephone is very often the first contact the patient will have with the medical office. I find that handling all telephone calls courteously and efficiently is the best way to make a good first impression on our patients.

A high level of professional service on the telephone should carry over to the reception area, front desk, and back to the clinical and treatment areas. When a patient arrives to the office, I stop what I am doing and welcome her to the office. It is also important to ensure that the reception area is clean, tidy, and suitable for our patients. When I open the office in the morning, I check the reception area for cleanliness and safety prior to patients' entering, as the presentation of the reception area as well as the manners of the health care staff greatly impact a patient's first impression of our office. Each day, I strive to treat all of our patients with a high level of customer service.

8

Telephone Procedures

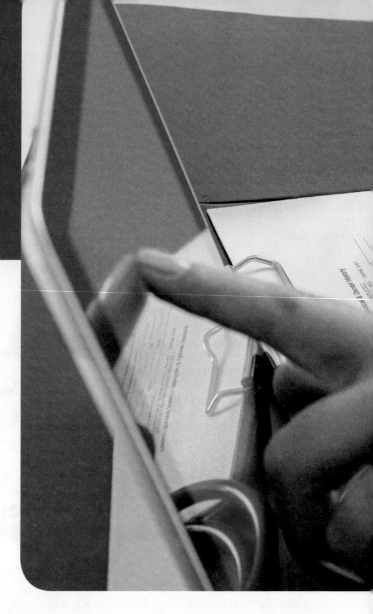

Case Study

Read the following case study and answer the critical thinking questions presented throughout the chapter.

Martha Hagen, one of the medical office's established patients, calls to notify the medical assistant that she is having chest pains. Martha is not sure if she should make an appointment to come into the office or if she should go to the emergency room. She tells the assistant that she would rather not go to the hospital as she doesn't believe she is having a heart attack.

Objectives

After completing this chapter, you should be able to:

8.1 Define and spell the key terminology in this chapter.

8.2 Describe the main features of telephone systems.

8.3 Outline the benefits of an answering service.

8.4 Discus patient telephone use in the medical office.

8.5 Answer the telephone in a professional manner.

8.6 Explain how to perform telephone triage, including a list of the steps to take when triaging patients this way.

8.7 Describe how to handle emergency calls and calls with difficult patients.

8.8 Outline the procedure for taking a proper telephone message.

8.9 Respond to telephone prescription requests.

8.10 Describe the steps to take when contacting patients and other facilities via telephone.

8.11 Use a telephone directory effectively.

8.12 Factor in time zones when making long-distance calls.

8.13 Discuss how the medical assistant can protect patient confidentiality when using the telephone.

Competency Skills Performance

1. Answer the telephone in a professional manner.
2. Take a telephone message.
3. Call a pharmacy with prescription orders.

Key Terminology

automatic dialer—telephone feature that dials numbers programmed into the system using codes; see also *speed dial*

automatic routing unit—telephone equipment that allows callers to self-select their call destinations via an automated, electronic prompt system

call forwarding—telephone feature that forwards incoming calls to other numbers

conference call—telephone feature that allows parties in different locations to participate in one call

direct telephone lines—telephone number that reaches a person directly rather than an operator or a receptionist

established patient—patient whom the medical office has seen previously

generic message—telephone answering message that fails to identify the receiver specifically

hands-free telephone device—headset or headphones with a speaker and microphone that allow users to participate in calls without picking up the telephone's receiver

hold feature—telephone feature that allows the user to place one call on hold and take another

last number redial—telephone feature that dials the last number dialed from that telephone

route—to direct telephone calls to other numbers

speaker phone—telephone feature that broadcasts the speaker's voice

speed dial—telephone feature that dials numbers programmed into the system using codes; see also *automatic dialer*

triage notebook—notebook the administrative medical assistant uses to properly handle calls from patients with potentially life-threatening conditions

triaging—process of prioritizing patients based on need

web chat—a system that allows users to communicate in real time using an Internet interface

Abbreviations

ADA—Americans with Disabilities Act

HIPAA—Health Insurance Portability and Accountability Act

TTY—teletypewriter system

Certification Exam Coverage

AAMA (CMA) Exam Coverage:
- Telephone techniques
  - Incoming calls management criteria
    1) Screening
    2) Maintaining confidentiality
    3) Gathering data
    4) Multiple-line competency
    5) Transferring appropriate calls
    6) Identifying caller, office, and self
    7) Taking messages
    8) Ending calls
  - Monitoring special calls
    1) Problem calls (e.g., unidentified caller, angry patient, family member)
    2) Emergency calls
- Appointment protocol
  - Emergency/acutely ill

AMT (CMAS) Exam Coverage:
- Communication
  - Address and process incoming telephone calls from outside providers, pharmacies, and vendors

- Employ appropriate telephone etiquette when screening patient calls and addressing office business
- Recognize and employ proper protocols for telephone emergencies

AMT (RMA) Exam Coverage:
- Oral and written communication
  - Employ appropriate telephone etiquette
  - Instruct patients via telephone
  - Inform patients of test results per physician's instruction
  - Receive, process, and document results received from outside provider

NCCT (NCMA) Exam Coverage:
- General office procedures
  - Patient instruction
  - Oral and written communication skills

AAMA (CMA) certification exam topics are reprinted with permission of the American Association of Medical Assistants.

AMT (CMAS) certification exam topics are reprinted with permission of American Medical Technologists.

AMT (RMA) certification exam topics are reprinted with permission of American Medical Technologists.

NCCT (NCMA) certification exam topics © 2013 National Center for Competency Testing. Reprinted with permission of NCCT.

Introduction

Professional telephone skills are essential for the administrative medical assistant. Often, the telephone is the first contact a patient has with the physician's office, and it can set the tone of the patient's relationship with the clinic. Allowing the telephone to ring too long before answering or placing a patient on hold for extended periods are two examples of poor telephone procedure. One disadvantage to using the telephone is that neither party can use nonverbal communication to determine the attitude or sincerity of the other party. For this reason, it is important for a medical assistant to keep his voice pleasant, polite, and professional while on the telephone. Handling telephone calls courteously and efficiently is the best way to make a good first impression on callers.

Telephone System Features

Today's telephone systems are sophisticated, multifeature units that require training for new administrative employees, including medical assistants.

Making Calls with Hands-Free Devices

For staff who answer telephone calls often throughout the day, **hands-free telephone devices** not only free the hands, they place little stress on the body. Wireless versions of these devices also allow medical assistants to conduct calls away from the telephone system, a feature that is particularly helpful when patient files must be pulled or assistants must move to different workstations (**Figure 8-1** ■). Assistants can wear wireless headsets all day throughout the office.

Dialing Numbers Automatically

Many telephone systems today have **automatic dialer** or **speed dial** functions that allow medical assistants to dial up to 100 programmed numbers with the push of a few buttons instead of several (**Figure 8-2** ■). Such features save medical assistants a great deal of time when contacting insurance companies, pharmacies, hospitals, laboratories, and physicians via the phone.

Redialing Last Numbers Called

The **last number redial** telephone feature, common today in home and office systems, dials with one button the last number called from the phone. Some systems offer a feature

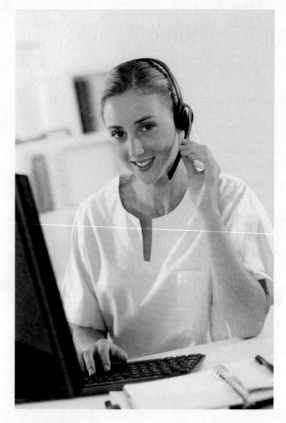

Figure 8-1 ■ Using a hands-free headset makes the medical assistant's job easier.
Source: Fotolia © goodluz.

that will redial the last number called until there is an answer.

Making Conference Calls

The **conference call** feature allows two or more parties to speak on the same phone line at once. Conversation flows more easily and misunderstandings between parties diminish

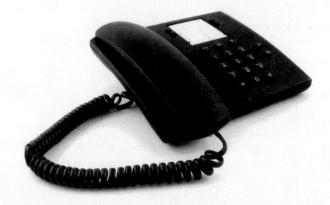

Figure 8-2 ■ Most telephone systems in the medical facility have features such as speed dial.
Source: Fotolia © .schock

when all parties involved are on the line at the same time. In the medical office, the physician may use this feature to speak with a patient and another member of the health care team, like the physical therapist.

As the number of parties to a conversation increases, however, so does the potential for confusion. Therefore, when conference calls have more than three parties, all parties should identify themselves before commenting.

Conversing via Speaker Telephone

The **speaker phone** feature, which broadcasts the speaker's voice from the unit, helps when more than one party at the same location wishes to participate in a telephone conversation. In the medical office, the physician may use this feature to broadcast the voice of another health care professional while a patient is in the office, for example. Medical professionals can work hands free, which means they can do things like write in patients' charts while taking part in the conversation. Whenever the speaker phone feature is used, however, it is important and courteous to advise speakers that they are being broadcast and to advise them of all other listeners in the room.

HIPAA Compliance

Patient confidentiality is an important part of Health Insurance Portability and Accountability Act (**HIPAA**) compliance. The speaker-phone feature can be used to discuss confidential patient information only when parties unauthorized to have the patient's information are unable to overhear the conversation.

Call Forwarding

Call forwarding automatically routes incoming calls to other telephone numbers. In the medical office, this feature is most commonly used after business hours to direct incoming calls to an answering service.

Recording Telephone Calls

The medical office, like other businesses, may wish to record incoming calls. Recorded calls support both quality-assurance efforts and training initiatives. For legal reasons, callers must be notified that their call may be recorded, and be given the option to refuse such a recording. Recording telephone calls without the callers' consent is illegal. Medical offices that wish to record calls should do one of the following:

- Prerecord a message that plays before the medical assistant takes the line. Such a recording may say, "This call may be recorded to maintain quality customer service."

- Have the medical assistant advise callers that calls may be recorded.

Callers can choose to avoid participating in recorded calls. When they do, medical offices cannot record calls.

Direct Telephone Lines

Many medical offices use **direct telephone lines** that **route** to selected members of the staff. Patients can call the billing department, for example, or staff in charge of appointment scheduling. While direct lines can eliminate the need for hold times, they require patients to have multiple telephone numbers for the office.

Automatic Routing Units

In many medical offices, callers can use **automatic routing units** to choose the parties they wish to reach by dialing the main line and choosing extensions. Routing units prompt the caller to choose from a list of options and key enter or speak their choice into the telephone. In some cases, callers may be able to access a directory where they will hear a list of options to choose from. Automated instructions direct callers to the parties they wish to reach. While such systems can be beneficial, they can also have drawbacks. For example, such systems may impose long wait periods on callers or require multiple steps to reach desired extensions.

Placing Callers on Hold

The **hold feature** of telephone systems places callers on hold so users can complete other tasks. With this feature, staff can juggle multiple telephone lines or handle calls while assisting patients in person. Callers cannot see who is in the medical office when they call, however, so medical assistants must use the hold feature judiciously. Improper use can extend wait times and give the impression that the patient on hold is not important. Medical assistants should verify that callers have only nonemergency issues before placing those callers on hold. In general, all members of the health care team should use the hold function in such a way that minimizes wait times and treats all patients equally. The medical assistant must be aware that long hold times are seen as unprofessional, and patients may choose to seek care with another facility if the patient finds they are spending lengthy times on hold when calling the office.

Even the simplest telephone systems can play music or recorded information during hold times. The most rudimentary systems connect the telephone system to a radio, while more advanced units allow callers to choose the type of information they will hear. Many medical offices record or buy messages for this purpose. Such messages can be specific to the practice, such as messages about well-child checkups for pediatric offices, or informative, like those about seasonal allergies for allergists' offices. Some physicians use **generic messages** and some will even record their own messages in their own voices. Messages like these add a personal touch that can both reassure patients and fortify their trust in the practice. However, only physicians with warm, pleasant-sounding, and clear voices should record messages like these. As mentioned earlier, the telephone is usually the patient's first contact with the medical office. Unpleasant-sounding physicians may unnerve new patients. Medical assistants with proper speaking voices can sometimes record such messages effectively.

Like the recorded information that is played during hold periods, hold music should be used with some stipulations. First, the music must be clear and generally pleasant. Callers are a captive audience that may become irritated by music that is broken by static or considered offensive. Religious music, for example, should be avoided, because it could offend followers of different faiths. So that they might better understand their callers' experiences, it is good practice for medical assistants periodically to call the offices where they work and assess the offices' recordings.

▸▸▸ Pulse Points

Placing Callers on Hold

Never place a caller on hold without first asking for and receiving permission. When callers agree to hold, they should wait no more than 20 to 30 seconds before a member of the health care team checks in with an update. Long periods of hold time give the impression that patients are forgotten or unvalued when callers should instead feel that the medical office values them and their time.

Critical Thinking Question 8-1

Referring to the case study at the beginning of the chapter, if the medical office uses an automated system where callers are greeted by a recording, how can the office set up a system so patients can bypass the recorded greeting in the event of a possible emergency?

Using the Voicemail Feature

Most medical offices use voicemail, often at each employee's personal extension. When a patient calls the office after hours via the main office telephone line, the patient will typically reach an answering service. If the call comes through to an internal extension within the medical office—for example, the billing office—a voicemail might be reached after hours.

In their outgoing message, employees should provide their name, their department name, and other pertinent information to let the caller know when a return telephone call should be expected. An example might be: "This is Debra Meyers in the billing office at Martha Lake Family Practice. I am away from my phone right now. If you will leave me a message, including your name and telephone number, I will return your call within one business day."

Other Special Features

Large medical offices might have the funds to purchase special telephone features, such as programs that call patients with electronic appointment reminders or requests. Automatic redial in reverse, which prevents long wait periods, is another such feature. With this feature, a patient calls the medical office and chooses a number for the type of service he needs, such as "1 to schedule an appointment." The patient then records his name, enters his telephone number, and hangs up. When a medical assistant becomes available, the system automatically redials the patient and connects the call. The patient is free to go about other tasks, and office staff need not retrieve messages. Some medical offices might use a telephone system that tells callers how long they can expect to wait before their call is answered or how many calls are ahead of the caller. These special features can make the time on hold less frustrating.

Using Web Chat

Many Internet interfaces are available that allow callers to communicate over the Internet in real time. These **web chat** services allow users to use the camera and microphone connected to their computer to record audio and visual images as they communicate with others on the call. Services such as Skype and Collaborate are examples of those that supply web chat capability.

Using an Answering Service

When closed, perhaps during lunch or after business hours, most medical offices use professional answering services to handle their calls. These services forward calls to appropriate parties and thereby eliminate the need for the call-forwarding feature mentioned earlier. Some telephone systems are designed to forward any calls not answered by the fourth ring to an answering service.

To ensure patients always receive high quality customer service, medical offices should only use answering services experienced in health care. In addition, answering services should always have the contact information for the physicians on call. This way, the service can reach the physicians in the event of patient emergency. To retrieve messages the service has taken, the medical office usually must call the service once the office reopens. Some answering services send messages via fax or e-mail.

Pulse Points

Disclosing Personal Information About Coworkers

Never give callers the personal telephone numbers of physicians or other members of the health care team. When physicians are unavailable and callers express an urgent need to speak with them, the medical assistant should take the caller's name, number, and purpose of the call, and call the physician with the information. Disclosing personal information about coworkers without the coworker's permission is unprofessional.

Patient Telephone Use

Some medical offices provide telephones for patient use, often in the reception area or at the front desk, although increasing cell phone use is eroding this practice. Offices that do provide patient phones will typically install a separate line that does not interfere with incoming calls, and they will restrict the phone to local calls only.

In Practice

Established patient Josie Welton often arrives early for her appointments. While she waits in the reception area, Josie uses her cell phone to make a call during which she details her health care problems and other personal information. The other patients in the reception area overhear the entire conversation. How should the medical assistant address this situation?

Answering the Telephone

Answering calls professionally is an art form that medical assistants should master, because telephone work is a large part of medical assisting. Before answering any calls, the medical assistant should obtain a pen and paper and prepare a cheerful yet professional greeting. Many assistants find practicing before a mirror, or even placing a "smile" symbol near the telephone, to be helpful when preparing for telephone work.

When medical assistants answer calls, they should speak clearly as they identify their office and themselves. Some offices identify themselves by physician names, while others use the names of their offices. Some offices even use original greetings, such as, "It's a great day at Mountain View Clinic. This is Sara."

As customer-service representatives are trained to do, medical assistants should answer calls within two to three rings. Any longer gives a negative impression—perhaps that staffing in the office is inadequate or the office is overburdened. Once the caller begins speaking, the medical assistant should try to match their rate of speech, although the assistant should always strive for a moderate pace.

As soon as the caller gives her name, the assistant should write the name down. Throughout the call, the medical assistant should refer to the caller by name, reinforcing that the caller is important. When the call is complete, the medical assistant should always say goodbye and allow the caller to hang up first. This reinforces the impression that the caller remains important and that the medical assistant is in no hurry to move on. In offices using an electronic health record, the medical assistant should look up the patient name as she speaks with the patient. This allows access to patient information so the medical assistant is fully prepared for the call.

In terms of call content, medical assistants should be familiar enough with their office location to be able to give most callers directions, as well as information about parking fees and availability. In addition to office location, the medical assistant should be familiar with the insurance plans her office participates in so she is prepared to answer patient questions in that arena. Printed lists near the phone serve as good reference. The following are some behaviors the medical assistant should avoid while on the phone:

- Acting with no authority or out of the scope of training (e.g., reducing fees, agreeing to refill prescriptions without the physician's consent, making diagnoses)
- Arguing with callers. Medical assistants must remain professional and calm.
- Violating patient confidentiality. Medical assistants must never release any patient information without the patient's permission, including the fact that the patient patronizes the medical office.
- Answering telephone calls where other patients can hear them.
- Taking inaccurate or incomplete messages.
- Eating or drinking while using the telephone.
- Allowing callers to wait on hold for more than 30 seconds with no contact.

Screening Telephone Calls

As part of his telephone duties, the medical assistant is charged with screening calls, which involves determining a call's purpose and whether that purpose is an emergency. The medical assistant should listen clearly to the caller's needs to properly handle or transfer the call. To give the assistant solid guidelines, every medical office should have a written policy for screening calls. To screen calls, the medical assistant should ask the caller for his or her name and the reason for the call. If the call is regarding a patient, the medical assistant should ask for the patient's date of birth. Once that information is given to the physician or other staff member, the assistant may be asked to take a message or to transfer the call to the intended recipient.

Directing Patient Calls to Physicians

Often, the calls medical assistants take are from parties who ask to speak with the physician directly. As a result, physicians should outline criteria for when they will accept patient calls (**Figure 8-3** ■). In addition to meeting physicians' needs and desires, such policies give medical assistants guidelines for telephone use. Many physicians accept no telephone calls, even when not with patients. Situations where physicians might take a telephone call during patient care hours could be when the caller is another physician calling about a mutual patient, the caller is a member of the physician's immediate family, or the lab is calling with stat lab results.

When a patient asks that a physician return his call, the medical assistant should place the message with the patient's chart on the physician's desk. In an office using an electronic health record, this message may be routed electronically to the physician. In offices with several physicians, typically only one physician will be "on call" after hours, a role the physicians

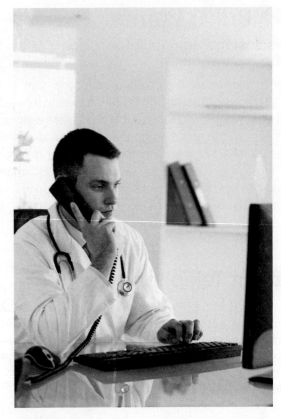

Figure 8-3 ■ A physician takes a telephone call at his desk.
Source: Fotolia © WavebreakmediaMicro.

 PROCEDURE 8-1 Answer the Telephone in a Professional Manner

Theory and Rationale

One of the administrative medical assistant's main duties, and one that is critical to the medical office, is to answer the office telephone. To complete this task, the assistant must have attention to detail, as well as the ability to multitask.

Materials

- Pen
- Paper
- Telephone

Competency

1. Answer the telephone between the second and third rings.
2. State the office's name, followed by your name.
3. If the caller fails to provide her name, ask for it and write it down.
4. Determine the reason for the call.
5. If the caller is having a medical emergency, ask if someone in the medical office might come to the phone to speak to the caller about it. If not, motion a coworker to dial for emergency services while keeping the patient on the line.
6. If the patient is calling to speak with another member of the health care team, transfer the call to that person if available.
7. When a requested party is unavailable, record a message. Include the name of the caller, the date and time of the call, the telephone number where the caller can be reached, the reason for the call, and the name of the person the caller wishes to reach.
8. When taking a message, inform the caller when the call will likely be returned.
9. Clarify information (e.g., appointment time) as appropriate.
10. Allow the caller to hang up before hanging up.
11. Route any message to the proper staff member.
12. Chart any health care-related information into the patient's chart as appropriate.

❑ **Line 1:** A mother is calling to schedule her 4-month-old child for a well-child checkup and vaccines. The office has not seen this child as a patient previously.

❑ **Line 2:** An equipment salesperson wants to speak with someone about equipping the office with new billing software.

❑ **Line 3:** An extremely angry patient states that she has been placed on hold twice by the "billing person" and has been disconnected both times.

❑ **Line 4:** A patient is calling to confirm the preoperative instructions he was given last week. His surgery appointment is for tomorrow morning.

❑ **Line 5:** A patient is calling for the results of her laboratory work done yesterday.

The medical assistant should address Line 3 first, because the patient is very angry. To minimize the damage, the medical assistant should apologize for the patient's inconvenience, secure the patient's return number, and advise the patient to expect a return call within an hour. The assistant should contact the billing department immediately upon handling all other calls and make the request for a return call.

After the angry caller, the callers on Lines 4 and 5 take priority. The assistant should route both to a clinical medical assistant or the nurse on staff. Line 2 is the next call in priority order. The medical assistant should route this call to the office manager, and then turn to the caller on Line 1. The Line 1 caller comes last in this situation, because a new-patient call takes the longest to resolve.

Figure 8-4 ■ Prioritization of telephone calls.

serve on a rotating basis. Any physician who is on call after hours must have some way of being reached. Due to the nature of the occupation, physicians must be available at all times, whether by telephone or pager. In addition to being readily available to the medical assistant, such numbers must be readily available to the office's answering service. When physicians do accept calls, the medical assistant should gather a caller's name and reason for calling before transferring the call to the physician.

Prioritizing Telephone Calls

In general, it is most efficient to address short telephone calls before longer ones. Short calls include those that simply need to be routed to staff or that derive from **established patients** needing to make appointments. Long, time-consuming calls include those from new patients or patients with elaborate questions. Calls from angry or agitated patients take precedence above all others, however. Hold periods, even short ones, could worsen the situation. The sooner medical assistants provide for patient needs, the happier patients are. **Figure 8-4** ■ outlines some common call scenarios.

Telephone Triage

The ability to **triage** patient telephone calls, or place them in priority order, is important not only for patient safety and well-being, but also because it cultivates a positive office image. To triage calls properly, the medical assistant must know the types of complaints considered emergencies and, of those, which demand immediate attention. Calls from patients with potentially life-threatening emergencies must be handled before all other calls. Potentially life-threatening emergencies include, but are not limited to:

● Complaints of chest pain
● Complaints of heavy bleeding due to an injury
● Bleeding in a pregnant woman

- High fever in an infant or child
- Severe asthma attack
- Severe shortness of breath
- Possible poisoning or allergic reaction
- Obvious broken bone
- Sudden confusion, loss of consciousness, or change in mental status
- Mention of suicide or harm to themselves or others.

When triaging calls, a **triage notebook** at the front desk is invaluable (**Figure 8-5** ■). The triage notebook is typically a three-ring binder with sections for call and emergency types. Physicians should participate in the construction of these notebooks so that they can dictate the actions medical assistants and other staff must take. **Figure 8-6** ■ explains how a triage notebook might be used.

Critical Thinking Question 8-2

If the medical office mentioned in the case study at the beginning of the chapter lacks a triage notebook, how should the medical assistant go about creating one? Who would be involved in creating such a notebook? What type of conditions would best be addressed in such a notebook?

Taking Emergency Telephone Calls

When patients need immediate transport to the hospital, the medical assistant might be asked to call for emergency services. If the emergency has occurred in the medical office, the medical assistant will need to direct emergency

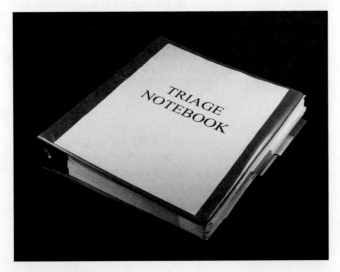

Figure 8-5 ■ A triage notebook.
Source: Pearson Education/PH College. Photographer: Dylan Malone.

services to the office to pick up the patient (**Figure 8-7** ■). The medical assistant should have the patient's name, age, and gender before making the call, as well as the problem type and type of care the physician is requesting. The medical assistant will need to be sure to give any specific directions, such as the office or suite number, and then advise the physician of the estimated time of arrival of the emergency services team.

▶▶▶ Pulse Points

Emergency Phone Numbers

Every medical office should keep a list of emergency telephone numbers near every office telephone. This list should include the numbers for police nonemergency services, the sheriff's department, and poison control, among others.

Being Professional on the Telephone

When using the telephone, the medical assistant must be professional. Professionalism includes never chewing gum or eating while using the telephone and being careful to pronounce words, including names, correctly. Assistants should avoid using unfamiliar words or slang, especially when speaking to people who use English as a second language. The medical assistant's voice should be calm and pleasant and its tone polite and warm. Callers should feel they have the medical assistant's complete attention.

In addition to using proper words and a soothing voice, medical assistants must be organized and prepared to answer the telephone properly. They should have a pen or pencil and paper ready before picking up the line. Never should assistants be rushed or anxious to end patient calls. When the time a caller needs exceeds the time the medical assistant has, the assistant should take the caller's name and number and get permission to call back. In the event the medical assistant is unable to assist the caller, the assistant might need to transfer the caller to another person in the medical office, or take a message for the coworker to return the call.

Especially over the telephone, many people get into the habit of using phrases or terminology that don't work in health care. The following list provides some examples with proposed improvements:

- When a caller asks for a staff member who is not in the office, inappropriate phrases include, "He isn't in yet," "She's in the restroom right now," or "I don't know where she is." An appropriate substitution is, "He's unavailable at the moment. May I take a message?"
- When a caller requests information or help with something, improper phrases include, "That isn't my job," "The

Scenario: A patient calls the office complaining of chest pain.

Action:

❑ Parents or legal guardians may consent for a child or dependent adult to become an organ donor. The next of kin may provide consent as well.

❑ The medical assistant turns to the page in the triage notebook labeled "Chest Pain."

❑ The medical assistant asks the patient to describe the pain.

Situation 1: The patient states the pain is radiating down the arm.

Action:

❑ The medical assistant asks the patient to verify their present address. When the physician is in the office, the medical assistant asks a coworker to notify the physician of the emergency call. The physician will typically take the call when in the office.

❑ If the physician is not in the office, the medical assistant motions for a coworker to call for emergency services on another line.

❑ The medical assistant keeps the patient on the line while giving the second medical assistant the information to give to emergency medical service personnel.

❑ The medical assistant lets the patient know that emergency help is on the way and remains on the line with the patient until emergency services arrive.

❑ The medical assistant charts the entire situation in the patient's medical chart and gives the chart to the physician for review.

Situation 2: The patient indicates some pain in the chest and stomach that has persisted for the past week but remained at a steady intensity.

Action:

❑ The medical assistant schedules the patient to see the physician.

❑ The medical assistant confirms the time and date of the appointment with the patient.

Figure 8-6 ■ Sample triage notebook use.

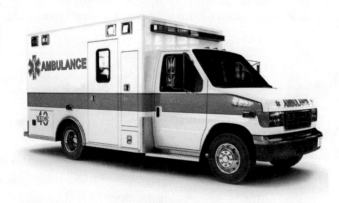

Figure 8-7 ■ In the event of a medical emergency, an ambulance may be called to the medical office to transport the patient to the hospital.
Source: Fotolia © storm.

computer is down," or "You'll need to talk with someone in billing." Instead, the medical assistant should take the caller's name and number, commit to checking with another member of the health care team, and promise to call the patient with the desired information.

● When a new patient calls to schedule an appointment, the medical assistant should not say things like, "We don't accept that insurance," "We don't take patients with your condition," or "I've never heard of the doctor who referred you." Instead, it is appropriate to say, "We are not preferred with your insurance plan, but let me find out who is and call you back," or "Our office doesn't specialize in conditions such as yours, but let me check with the doctor to see who she would refer you to and call you back." Another appropriate response is, "Will you please spell the referring doctor's last name, and do you have that office telephone number?" These statements are unlikely to offend the caller.

- The habit of asking patients, "How are you?" is an undesired one. Although common in American culture as a generic opener, some patients take the question literally and provide personal information. As has been discussed before, personal patient information must be guarded, especially at an office's busy front desk.

- Medical assistants should anticipate how terms might be interpreted. For example, the term *waiting room* implies an area where patients wait, but a more positive term is *reception room*, because it means patients are received into the office.

Communicating with Hard-to-Understand Callers

An integral part of acting like a professional includes listening to patients speak without interruption. When a patient has a speech impediment or speaks English that is unclear, the medical assistant might have to ask the patient to repeat himself. When confusion persists, the medical assistant should try repeating what she heard to verify that the patient's message was understood correctly.

Handling Difficult Callers

Occasionally, patients call the office while very upset. With calls like these, the most important thing the medical assistant can do is to remain calm and professional and avoid attacking the patient personally and taking the patient's emotions personally. Medical assistants must always speak politely and courteously, whatever the caller's attitude. While the medical assistant's job is not to take verbal abuse, most angry callers will calm quickly when the medical assistant remains calm and polite. Any calls like this, however, must be documented in patients' files.

To resolve matters involving difficult callers, the medical assistant should apologize for whatever the patient is angry about and determine how to correct the situation. Though the medical assistant should not allow abuse from the caller, it is often easy to calm the upset caller by apologizing for their issue and asking how the caller might be assisted. Any calls from patients that cannot be resolved must be brought to the physician's attention. The physician may choose to call the patient in the hope of finding resolution.

Receiving Calls from Emotional Patients

Emotional patients, such as those who are grieving or have been in accidents, will likely need more of the medical assistant's time. If the patient is emotional and calling to schedule an appointment, the medical assistant will need to determine if the patient needs to be seen right away. In a situation like this, the medical assistant should chart in the patient's medical record what happened during the telephone call and bring the situation to the physician's attention. It may be appropriate for the physician to call the patient back.

Documenting Calls from Patients

While not all patient calls must be documented in the patients' chart, any related to the patient's health care should be charted. Every medical office should have a policy about when and how to chart telephone calls, and medical assistants should be familiar with their office's policies. In most offices, the administrative medical assistant makes the entry in the patient's chart and places the chart on the physician's desk for review or possible followup action. In an office using an electronic health record, this process is done electronically.

Calls That Typically Must Appear in Patients' Charts

The following patient calls typically must appear in patient's charts:

- Patients who cancel appointments and fail to reschedule
- Patients who say they are in the hospital
- Relatives of patients who say the patient has died
- Patients who indicate they are not returning to the office for care
- Patients who contend they cannot afford to keep their appointments, fill their prescriptions, or see specialists

Calls That Typically Require No Charting

The following calls typically do not require charting:

- Patients confirming appointment times
- Patients rescheduling appointments
- Patients complaining about their bills

Taking Telephone Messages

Taking a telephone message properly saves time for the member of the health care team who is returning the call. Most offices have message pads for this purpose (**Figure 8-8** ■). These pads, which serve as reminders to the medical assistant, have spaces for all the information needed from patients. Many offices with

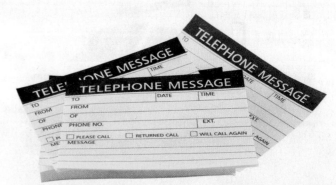

Figure 8-8 ■ Telephone message pads should be located near every office telephone in the administrative portion of the medical office.

Source: Shutterstock © kerrati.

PROCEDURE 8-2 Take a Telephone Message

Theory and Rationale

Administrative medical assistants often take telephone messages for other members of the health care team. In this task, accuracy is paramount. A simple numeric transposition, for example, can make a message useless. With accurate information, the intended recipient of the call is able to return the call with the correct information in a timely manner.

Materials

* Pen
* Telephone message pad or electronic message system
* Telephone

Competency

1. Answer the telephone call by the second ring.
2. Once the caller identifies the desired party, reach for the message pad.
3. Ask for the caller's full name, verify the spelling, and document it on the pad.
4. Verify the name of the party the caller is trying to reach, and document it manually or electronically.
5. Ask for the reason for the call, and document it manually or electronically.
6. Ask for the caller's telephone number, including area code, and document it manually or electronically.
7. Repeat the telephone number to the caller to verify it was documented correctly.
8. Document the date and time of the call manually or electronically.
9. Document your name or initials manually or electronically
10. Tell the caller when to expect a return call.
11. Bid goodbye to the caller, and allow the caller to hang up first.
12. Route the message to its intended recipient.

an electronic health record have an electronic means for sending telephone messages to the intended recipient.

When taking a telephone message, it is important to obtain the following information, and to document your name on the message:

* Date and time of telephone call
* Name of person with whom the caller wishes to speak
* Name of the caller (verify the spelling when unsure)
* Telephone number, including area code, where the caller can be reached
* Nature or reason for the call

Advise the caller when to expect a return call. If, for example, the caller is calling for Jane in the billing department but Jane is out, tell the caller when to expect a return call. This way, the caller can avoid wasting time waiting for the call. Also, be sure to route messages to appropriate parties in a timely manner.

Calling in Prescriptions and Refill Requests

Guidelines for prescription refills vary from one office to another. Generally, most offices require at least 24 hours' notice to refill prescriptions. Medical assistants should forward these calls, which may come from patients or pharmacists, to the clinical medical assistant or nurse. Many prescription refill requests come to the medical office via fax. These faxed refill requests are to be forwarded to the clinical medical assistant or nurse.

Alternatively, the medical assistant can check with the physician to see if the physician wishes to see the patient before allowing the refill. When office policy requires the medical assistant to check with the physician on all prescription refill requests but the physician is unavailable when the call comes in, the assistant must take the patient's name; the medication requested, including dosage; and the number where the patient or pharmacist can be reached. The medical assistant must then pull the patient's file and place it, with the corresponding message, on the physician's desk (**Figure 8-9** ■). In an office using an electronic health record, this process is done electronically by bringing up the patient's chart in the electronic health record. Once the assistant has verified that he has the correct patient, the assistant will then enter the prescription refill request, including the medication, the dosage, and the pharmacy where the patient would like the prescription filled. The assistant will then route the prescription refill request electronically to the physician for a response.

Calling Patients

Before making telephone calls, medical assistants should have all materials and information at hand, including the patient's medical chart. In an office using an electronic health record, the medical assistant should have the patient's chart open on the computer prior to making the call. Assistants who are calling patients to schedule appointments should be well versed in the time each procedure takes, as well as any special patient instructions, such as not eating for 12 hours before a particular visit. Any patient calls that are medically relevant must be charted in the patients' charts.

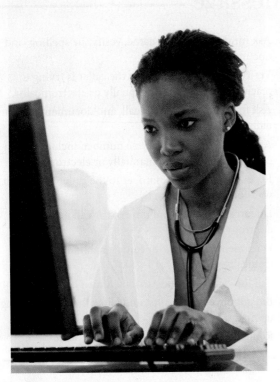

Figure 8-9 ■ When prescription refill requests come into the office, the medical assistant should look up the patient's medical record and send the prescription refill to the physician to approve.

Source: Shuttterstock.com/©wavebreakmedia.

Leaving Messages

To remain HIPAA compliant, medical assistants must maintain confidentiality at all times, including while on the telephone. When leaving messages, for example, assistants must remember that the people taking those messages, such as the patient's spouse or parents of minors seeking treatment for pregnancy, sexually transmitted diseases, mental illness, or drug and alcohol counseling, might not have the patient's permission to know the nature of the call.

When the medical assistant must leave a message for a patient, the assistant should leave her name, the physician's name, and the appropriate telephone numbers. When an office's name identifies the nature of its practice, such as "Marysville Oncology Specialists" or "Monroe Women's Care and Family Planning Clinic," the medical assistant should not leave the office's name, because doing so discloses some of the patient's confidential information. Instead, the medical assistant should leave the name of the physician only, as in, "This is Christine calling from Dr. Wilson's office. I'm leaving a message for Jose. Please call me at 555-123-4567."

Calling Other Health Care Facilities

Medical assistants often will be asked to call other health care facilities involved in the care of mutual patients, whether to schedule appointments with specialists or obtain information from patients' primary care providers. Whatever the reason for the call, the medical assistant will need to maintain patient confidentiality at all times. This means disclosing only absolutely

 PROCEDURE 8-3 Call a Pharmacy with Prescription Orders

Theory and Rationale

As part of their duties in the medical office, administrative medical assistants often call pharmacies with new or refill prescriptions. To complete this task properly and ensure patient safety, assistants must demonstrate strict attention to detail.

Materials

- Telephone
- Patient's chart
- Pen
- Prescription information
- Pharmacy telephone number

Competency

1. Carefully read the prescription the physician has ordered.

2. Ask the physician any questions about the prescription if needed.

3. Call the pharmacy where the patient would like the prescription filled.

4. Give the pharmacist the patient's name, and verify the spelling.

5. Give the pharmacist the patient's birthdate.

6. Give the pharmacist the name of the medication, dosage, and directions per the physician. Alert the pharmacist to any drug allergies the patient has.

7. Ask the pharmacist to repeat the information for verification, and inform the pharmacist if the patient is en route to the pharmacy.

8. Document the prescription, including pharmacy name and telephone number, on the medication record in the patient's medical chart.

necessary information to the other office staff when placing the call. If the medical assistant is scheduling a patient with a specialist, for example, that assistant will need to provide the patient's contact and insurance information. Other private patient information, like lifestyle habits and payment history, should remain undisclosed. Review the following tips on patient-related exchanges via telephone:

- If your physician is running behind schedule on appointments or has been delayed getting to the office, call patients who will be impacted. Offer to reschedule when a delay is unacceptable.

- When the physician cannot do so, have the medical assistant make followup calls to patients after surgical procedures. When patients report anything unusual, transfer the call to the physician.

- Give new patients all administrative information, such as parking and preferred manner of dress, and medications and foods to avoid for certain tests and procedures.

- Advise patients of important policies (e.g., pay at the time services are rendered) before they visit the office.

- Remind all patients to bring necessary information to visits (e.g., insurance cards or lists of medications).

- Stagger staff lunch hours so a person always answers the telephone.

Using a Telephone Directory

In the past, a *telephone directory* usually meant a *telephone book*, but today several different companies produce telephone books. The medical office might have one book for white pages and one for yellow pages, for example. When a medical office is in a large metropolitan area, it might have several books to cover its surrounding areas. Listings in the white pages are listed alphabetically by the person's name; in the yellow pages they are listed alphabetically by business type. Most telephone books create sublistings for business types, as well. For example, under the directory for physicians may be an alphabetical listing of physicians by type, such as pediatrician.

Most telephone directories are color-coded for ease of use. Many precede their white pages with business sections in different colors. Directories typically have listings for local ZIP codes at their beginnings and a government section that includes listings for federal, local, and state agencies. These pages are typically colored differently, sometimes blue.

Using an Online Directory

Many medical offices today use the Internet to look up telephone numbers. Web sites like www.Yahoo.com, www.anywho.com, www.dexknows.com, www.yellowpages.com, www.superpages.com, and www.bigbook.com, search for both local and national telephone numbers for personal and business information.

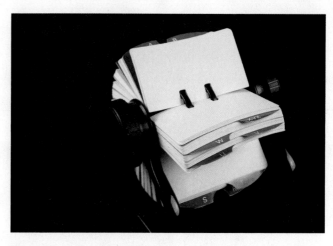

Figure 8-10 ■ A Rolodex card system next to the telephone allows the administrative medical assistant to quickly locate commonly called numbers.
Source: Fotolia © Albert Lozano Nieto.

Using a Rolodex System

Every medical office should keep a directory of commonly called telephone numbers on the computer or in a Rolodex card file (**Figure 8-10** ■). These tools make it easier to locate the number for the cardiac specialist the physician refers patients to, for example.

Long Distance or Toll-Free Calls

The medical assistant may frequently make long-distance telephone calls on behalf of the medical office. Some offices require staff to log any long-distance telephone calls with the call's purpose, as well as the name and number of the party being called. To comply with such requests, the medical assistants should familiarize himself with the office's policies.

Factor in time zones before making long-distance calls (**Figure 8-11** ■). When calling California from New York, for example, the medical office must take into consideration that the time in California is three hours earlier than it is in New York.

Most suppliers and businesses the medical office buys from will have toll-free telephone numbers, which typically begin with 1-800, 1-888, or 1-866, and which impose no charges on callers.

Patient Confidentiality

Maintaining patient confidentiality is extremely important. Violations of patient privacy are serious offenses punishable by fines under HIPAA. Patients must know that their private information will be kept confidential. One of the best ways to do this is for the medical assistant to refrain from discussing any patient information within hearing distance of other patients. When patients hear office staff discussing other

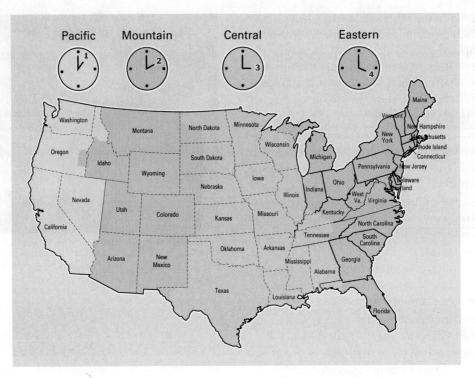

Figure 8-11 ■ A time zone map.

patients, they may assume that their private information is similarly discussed. Keeping conversations professional and never resorting to gossip about other staff members or patients is one way to reinforce to patients that the medical assistant is trustworthy and professional.

HIPAA Compliance

The medical office must treat all callers requesting patient information cautiously. Because a caller's identity cannot be determined via telephone, the office should disclose no confidential information over the telephone. Instead, members of the health care team should advise the callers to send any requests via fax or mail and to accompany those requests with a signed authorization from the patient or a court order.

Personal Telephone Calls

Studies on businesses across America have found that the average employee spends 65 hours per year on personal calls while at work. Because personal calls are very expensive for employers, they are generally frowned upon. Some employers feel that employees who spend time on personal telephone calls during work hours are stealing from them.

To avoid ill will, medical assistants should review and abide by their offices' policies for personal telephone use. Making or receiving personal telephone calls is unprofessional, and it ties up a business's telephone line (**Figure 8-12** ■). Most offices allow employees to receive only emergency telephone

calls during work hours. When medical assistants must make personal calls, they should do so on break or during lunch and out of patients' hearing range.

The Medical Assistant and Cell Phone Use

Because it is considered unprofessional, the medical assistant should not have his or her cell phone out and in use during patient care hours. When patients see the medical assistant

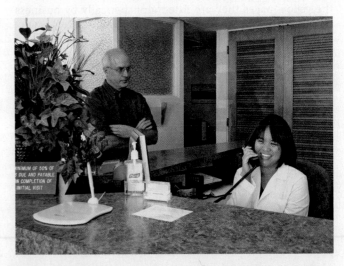

Figure 8-12 ■ Making or receiving personal telephone calls is unprofessional. When medical assistants must take personal calls, they should do so on break and out of patients' hearing.
Source: Pearson Education/PH College. Photographer: Dylan Malone.

using his or her cell phone for calls, texts, or Internet browsing, the patient gets the impression that the medical assistant is ignoring work that needs to be done. Any use of cell phones should be outlined in the office policy and should take place during break times and outside areas that patients frequent.

Even when making personal calls or texts during break or lunch periods, the medical assistant should be aware of patients who may be able to see or hear the call. Any calls that may be considered highly personal in nature should not be overheard by passing patients.

Telecommunication Relay Services

Patients who are hearing or speech impaired may use a telecommunication relay system to contact the medical office. The Americans with Disabilities Act (**ADA**) requires that telephone companies have telecommunication relay systems available 24 hours per day, 365 days per year. A telecommunication relay system works in the following manner:

1. The caller types a message into a special telephone.
2. The message transmits to the relay service.
3. An operator calls the medical office.
4. When the medical assistant answers, the operator self-identifies and identifies the caller.
5. The operator mediates between the medical assistant and the caller, reading messages to the assistant and typing responses to the caller.

When the call is complete, the medical assistant bids the patient goodbye, awaits the interpreter's response, and then hangs up.

A medical office with a large number of hearing-impaired patients, perhaps an audiology practice, might

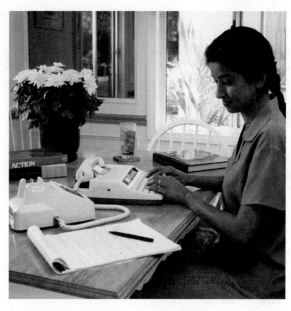

Figure 8-13 ■ A patient using a teletypewriter (TTY) system.
Source: PhotoEdit Inc., Photographer: Michael Newman.

have a teletypewriter (**TTY**) system (**Figure 8-13** ■). TTY systems connect to the telephone, allowing both parties to the call to type their responses and thereby eliminate the need for a telecommunication relay service.

When using services like these, it is important to note that conversations should be aimed at the caller, not the operator. The operator is charged with typing every spoken word, not serving as the call's recipient. In other words, the medical assistant should not say, "Tell Sharon the physician can see her at 10 A.M." Instead, the assistant should say, "Sharon, the physician can see you at 10 A.M. Will that time work?"

As with all equipment that may contain personal patient information, the TTY system should be located out of the patient area.

REVIEW

Chapter Summary

- Like the medical assistant, an answering service serves a crucial role in handling telephone calls efficiently and professionally.
- To triage the medical office's incoming calls properly, medical assistants need a distinct skill set, including a good understanding of the time requirements of any procedure.
- Emergency calls require special telephone attention, as do callers who are angry or otherwise upset.

- When answering calls in the medical office, the medical assistant should follow all office policies for taking messages properly.
- Prescription requests must be made using proper, professional telephone procedure.
- When calling patients on behalf of the medical office, it is crucial that medical assistants remain calm and professional at all times.

- Telephone directories, both electronic and conventional hard-copy versions, are helpful tools in the office's search for telephone numbers.
- While conducting telephone procedures in the medical office, the medical assistant's most crucial task is to maintain patient confidentiality.

- A medical office with a large number of hearing-impaired patients, perhaps an audiology practice, may have a teletypewriter (TTY) system.

Chapter Review

Multiple Choice

1. Which of the following telephone features dials a number with the push of just one button?
   a. Last number redial
   b. Speed dialer
   c. Automatic dialer
   d. Placing a caller on hold
   e. a, b, and c

2. Which of the following pieces of information need NOT be included when taking a message?
   a. Caller's name
   b. Call date
   c. Patient's insurance information
   d. Medical assistant's name
   e. The reason for the call

3. Which of the following is an appropriate way to handle an angry caller?
   a. Hang up the phone
   b. Remain calm
   c. Use the hold feature
   d. Tell the patient to calm down
   e. Respond with anger toward the patient

4. Which of the following calls should be handled first?
   a. Patient calling for lab results
   b. Doctor's college roommate calling for the doctor
   c. Patient complaining of shortness of breath
   d. Patient confirming an appointment time
   e. Vendor offering to demonstrate a new piece of medical equipment

5. Which of the following is the best choice for patients on hold?
   a. Generic message thanking callers for holding
   b. Local news station with slight static
   c. Physician's gruff voice
   d. a and b
   e. b and c

6. For a caller with a life-threatening emergency who needs emergency medical services, the medical assistant should:
   a. Ask the caller to hold while dialing emergency medical services on another line
   b. Ask the caller to hang up and immediately dial 9-1-1

   c. Ask the caller to hold while transferring the call to a clinical medical assistant
   d. Hang up on the caller and dial 9-1-1
   e. Place the patient on hold while trying to locate the patient's next of kin

7. To find the telephone number for a medical supplier, the medical assistant could:
   a. Use an Internet directory
   b. Check a telephone book
   c. Search Rolodex card file
   d. a and b
   e. a, b, and c

True/False

T F **1.** Telephone triage is the ability to transfer calls to voicemail.

T F **2.** When a patient calls to cancel an appointment but fails to reschedule, the call should be charted in the patient's medical chart.

T F **3.** When leaving messages for a patient, it is acceptable to tell the patient's spouse the purpose for the patient's visit.

T F **4.** When calling other health care facilities to schedule an appointment for a patient, the medical assistant should disclose only needed patient information.

T F **5.** Before answering the office telephone, the medical assistant should know the insurance plans the office participates with.

T F **6.** Because medical terminology is unfamiliar to most patients, layman's terms are best when speaking with patients.

T F **7.** Unidentified callers should be routed directly to the physician.

Short Answer

1. Why is it important to speak clearly on the telephone?
2. Explain why taking personal telephone calls during office hours is problematic.
3. Explain how a telephone relay system works.
4. What is the purpose of a telephone triage notebook?

5. Explain how a medical office can legally record patient telephone calls.
6. Differentiate between screening and prioritizing telephone calls.

Research

1. Look online for companies that sell multiline telephone systems. What kind of features do they offer?

2. What local companies can you find in your area that offer answering services to medical offices? What services do they offer?
3. How many local telephone directories are there in your local area? Why would a person choose one over another?

Practicum Application Experience

When Sofie Pouillon calls the office, she says that she wants to cancel her upcoming appointment because she is very unhappy with the physician. What can the medical assistant say to this patient? What is the proper way to chart this call and notify the physician?

Resource Guide

Amateur Radio Research and Development Corporation
Telecommunications for the Deaf
Post Office Drawer 6148
McLean, VA 22106-6148
www.amrad.org

Online Yellow Pages
http://www.yellowpages.com

SkillPath Seminars
"The Secrets to Being a Front Desk Superstar" Seminar
P.O. Box 2768
Mission, KS 66201-2768
Phone: (800) 873-7545
Fax: (913) 362-4241
http://www.skillpath.com

Online white pages telephone directory
www.whitepages.com

Reverse telephone number lookup
www.anywho.com

Contact information for people and businesses
www.411.com

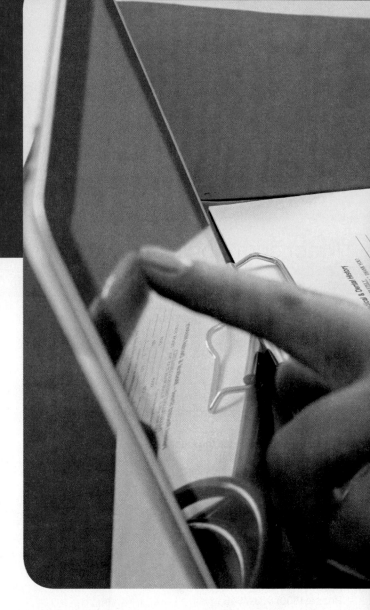

9

Front Desk Reception

Case Study

Read the following case study and answer the critical thinking questions presented throughout the chapter.

When Marilyn Peterson enters the medical office for a new patient appointment, the medical assistant greets her and gives her paperwork to complete. In response, Marilyn frowns and says, "I don't want to fill all of that out. I'm only here to see the doctor about a sore throat. I don't have time for paperwork."

Objectives

After completing this chapter, you should be able to:

9.1 Define and spell the key terminology in this chapter.

9.2 Describe characteristics of the front office receptionist.

9.3 List the steps to open the office efficiently.

9.4 List the steps to prepare files for patient arrivals.

9.5 Describe appropriate ways to greet and register both new and established patients.

9.6 Communicate with patients regarding scheduling delays and cancellations.

9.7 Collect payments at the front desk.

9.8 Properly escort patients to the examination room.

9.9 Manage difficult patients effectively in the reception room.

9.10 List the types of patients who should not be left in the reception room.

9.11 Discuss how to maintain a safe and pleasant reception-room environment.

9.12 List the steps the medical assistant should take with the patient as the patient leaves the office.

9.13 Describe the steps involved in closing the office.

Competency Skills Performance

1. Open the office.
2. Greet and register patients.
3. Collect payments at the front desk.
4. Close the office.

Key Terminology

Americans with Disabilities Act (ADA)—federal law that outlines appropriate treatment or accommodations for patients or employees with disabilities

checklist—list of activities or steps to take to perform a task

copayment—the established dollar amount per visit or service that patients are responsible for according to their insurance plan contracts

front desk—place in a medical office where the receptionist welcomes patients as they enter

hazard—something that is dangerous or possibly dangerous

office policy—agreed upon standard for handling a situation or procedure in the office

reception area—waiting area for patients in the medical office

receptionist—medical staff member who greets patients, answers the telephone, and directs office flow

service animal—animal that has been trained to assist a person with a handicap

sign-in sheet—paper or electronic document on which patients sign their names upon entering the office

Abbreviations

ADA—Americans with Disabilities Act

HIPAA—Health Insurance Portability and Accountability Act

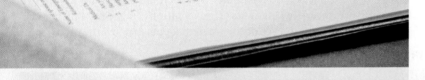

Certification Exam Coverage

AAMA (CMA) Exam Coverage:
- Receiving, organizing, and transmitting information
  - Modalities for incoming and outgoing data (e.g., mail, fax, telephone, computer)
  - Prioritizing incoming and outgoing data (e.g., importance, urgency, recipient availability)
- Appointment protocol
  - Cancellations/no-shows
  - Physician delay/unavailability

AMT (CMAS) Exam Coverage:
- Appointment management and scheduling
  - Address cancellations and missed appointments
  - Prepare information for referrals and preauthorizations
  - Arrange hospital admissions and surgery, and schedule patients for outpatient diagnostic tests
  - Manage recall system and file
- Reception
  - Receive and process patients and visitors
  - Screen visitors and vendors requesting to see physician
  - Coordinate patient flow into examining rooms
  - Format business documents and correspondence appropriately
  - Process incoming and outgoing mail

- Patient information and community resources
- Order and organize patient information materials

AMT (RMA) Exam Coverage:
- Medical receptionist/secretarial/clerical
  - Understand and correctly apply terminology associated with medical receptionist and secretarial duties
  - Employ appropriate communication skills when receiving and greeting patients
  - Understand basic emergency triage in coordinating patient arrivals
  - Screen visitors and sales persons arriving at the office
  - Obtain patient demographics and information
  - Understand and maintain patient confidentiality during check-in procedures
  - Prepare patient record
  - Assist patients into examination rooms
  - Employ effective written communication skills adhering to ethics and laws of confidentiality

NCCT (NCMA) Exam Coverage:
- General office procedures
  - Patient instruction
  - Cultural awareness

Introduction

The adage "There is no second chance to make a good first impression" holds as true for the medical office as it does for any other business. In the medical office, the person who answers the telephone, often the administrative medical assistant, plays a substantial role in a patient's first impressions. Because poor impressions can prompt patients to seek care in other facilities, the medical assistant who is serving as **receptionist** at the **front desk** must treat all patients with a high level of customer service. That level of service should carry through from the telephone, into the **reception area** when patients arrive, and beyond into the clinical and treatment areas. The visual impressions made by the presentation of the reception area, in conjunction with the appearances and professional manners of the health care staff, greatly impact a patient's first impression of the office.

Characteristics of the Front Desk Receptionist

While people can learn the skills they need to be adequate front desk receptionists, they must exhibit positive personality traits to excel at the job. When receptionists excel, they can positively impact the medical office's bottom line. Studies have shown that patients will continue to seek treatment with physicians they do not really like just because they feel well cared for by the rest of the health care team. Conversely, many patients will not return to the office when they feel the staff don't care about their needs (**Figure 9-1** ■).

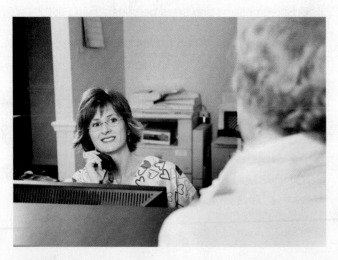

Figure 9-1 ■ The front desk receptionist must be kind and professional with all patients.
Source: Fotolia © Lisa F. Young.

In short, front desk receptionists should really enjoy interacting with people. Successful front desk receptionists remember patients' names. Remarkable receptionists remember the names of patients' children or spouses. Superior front-desk receptionists also remain calm, even with the rudest of patients or in the busiest of circumstances. Because receptionists can rarely start and finish their tasks without interruption, they must be open to constantly shifting their focus. The best front desk receptionists are happy, kind people who genuinely care about patients and who have the utmost faith in the clinical staff and physicians on their health care teams.

The front desk receptionist must be adept at providing outstanding customer service to the patient. This includes both interactions on the telephone as well as in person. Outstanding customer service includes being friendly, calm, and helpful, no matter what situation the receptionist is presented with.

Medical assistants throughout the office setting must be alert to the possibility that their conversations may be overheard by patients. Conversations between staff members should never occur where patients may overhear.

Critical Thinking Question 9-1

Refer back to the case study at the beginning of the chapter. How can the medical assistant demonstrate caring and concern to Marilyn?

Opening the Office

The task of opening and closing the medical office usually falls to the front desk receptionist. A policy that outlines the steps to opening and closing the office helps train new staff and ensures that other established staff can follow the proper procedures when serving in a cross-functional capacity. A printed **checklist** helps ensure that all staff follow all necessary steps.

While opening and closing procedures vary from office to office, most offices follow some basic steps. In general, to ensure the facility is ready for business, staff should arrive at the office 30 minutes before patients are expected to arrive. Scrambling to find supplies or searching for files while patients are in the office is unprofessional and gives the impression that the health care team is unprepared. This arrival time may vary from one health care organization to another.

Upon entering the office, the receptionist should turn on the lights and disarm the alarm system. Next, the receptionist should check the office answering system to identify patients who need visits that day or who have canceled their appointments. Calls should be handled in order of importance.

After making necessary calls, the front desk receptionist should ensure that the reception room is ready to receive patients. This means making sure the room is tidy and free of litter. When the office provides coffee or water, the receptionist should ensure that related supplies are adequate.

PROCEDURE 9-1 Open the Office

Theory and Rationale

When a medical office documents its standard opening procedures in a list, that list can help ensure that all members of the health care team have the tools to perform those procedures fully, accurately, and consistently.

Materials

- Checklist of office opening procedures

Competency

1. Arrive in the office at least 30 minutes before the first patient appointment.

2. Turn off the office alarm system.

3. Turn on all appropriate lights and equipment.

4. Retrieve messages from the office answering system, and return telephone calls as appropriate.

5. Verify that all patient charts needed for the morning were pulled the night before and that all needed information is attached to those charts.

6. Check the office for safety and cleanliness. For example, be sure all garbage cans are empty.

7. When the office is ready, unlock the door for patients to enter.

Preparing Patient Files

Before the office closes for the night, staff should pull all patient files needed for the next morning. Any new patient files should be started, which means inserting all appropriate paperwork. **Figure 9-2** ■ depicts a new patient file folder with various paperwork the patient and health care professionals will fill out. The amount and type of paperwork contained within the patient file depends upon the type of practice and the policies regarding necessary forms in that particular facility. **Figure 9-3** ■ is an example of a new patient history form. These forms may be

purchased from a variety of medical office supply retailers, though many medical facilities create their own. **Figure 9-4** ■ shows an example of a HIPAA authorization agreement. This form is necessary in any medical setting where private patient information will be gathered and kept on file.

In a medical office using an electronic health record, paper charts will not be pulled the night before, but necessary forms for the next day will be gathered. In some health care facilities, all patient paperwork is done electronically. In these facilities, patients may be instructed to a computerized kiosk to complete entry forms after they check in with the front desk receptionist.

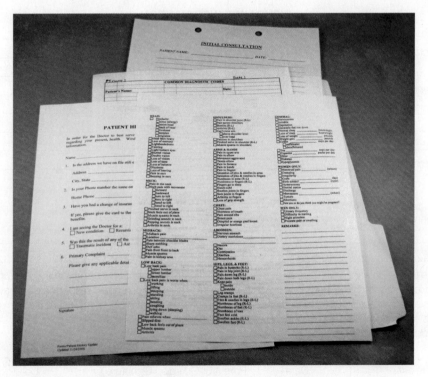

Figure 9-2 ■ A new patient medical record with various forms.

Source: Pearson Education/PH College. Photographer: Dylan Malone.

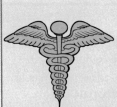

Victory Medical Center
4100 SW Highway 6
Victorville, WA 12345
(509) 555-9832

Patient Name: _____
             Last Name   First Name   Middle Initial

Address: _____
           Street   City   State   Zip

Home Phone: _____ Work Phone: _____

Mobile Phone: _____ Birthdate: _____

Social Security Number: _____ Age: _____

Sex: _____ Marital Status: S M D W Children: _____

How do you prefer to be addressed? _____

Spouse's Name: _____

Primary Care Physician: _____ Phone No.: _____

Name of Person Responsible for Bill: _____

Relationship to Patient: _____ Phone No.: _____

Address of Person Responsible for Bill: _____

Patient's Employer: _____ Phone No.: _____

Occupation: _____

Spouse's Employer: _____ Phone No.: _____

Occupation: _____

INSURANCE INFORMATION

Primary Insurance: _____ Policy No.: _____

Name of Policyholder: _____ Birthdate: _____

SS#: _____ Relationship to Insured: _____

Secondary Insurance: _____ Policy No.: _____

Name of Policyholder: _____ Birthdate: _____

If Injured: Date: _____ Place: _____

Claim Number: _____ Nature or Cause of Injury: _____

Employer at Time of Injury: _____ Phone No.: _____

EMERGENCY INFORMATION

In case of emergency, local friend or relative to be notified (not living at same address)

Name: _____ Relationship to Patient: _____

Address: _____ Phone No.: _____

I hereby authorize the health care professionals in this clinic to diagnose and treat my condition. I clearly understand and agree that all services rendered me are charged directly to me and that I am personally responsible for payment. I agree that I am responsible for all bills incurred at this clinic. I hereby authorize assignment of my insurance rights and benefits directly to the provider for services rendered. I also authorize the health care professionals to discuss my care with other health care providers who I am currently treating with.

_____   _____
Patient's Signature   Date   Parent or Guardian Signature   Date

Figure 9-3 ■ Sample new patient history form.

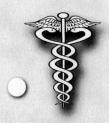

Martin Country Medical Clinic
2413 NW Greenlake Ave.
Westford, CA 12745

AUTHORIZATION TO RELEASE INFORMATION

ACKNOWLEDGMENT OF RECEIPT of the Notice of Privacy Practices of the Martin County Medical Clinic (MCMC)

I acknowledge that I have received or been offered the Notice of Privacy Practices of the Martin County Medical Clinic. I understand that the Notice describes the uses and disclosures of my protected health information by the Covered Entities and informs me of my rights with respect to my protected health information.

_____

Name of Patient

_____

Patient Date of Birth

_____

Signature of Patient or Personal Representative

_____

Printed Name of Patient or Personal Representative

_____

Date

If Personal Representative, indicate relationship:

_____

Declinations

_____ The Individual declined to accept a copy of the Notice of Privacy Practices.

_____ The Individual received a copy of the Notice of Privacy Practices but declined to sign an Acknowledgment of Receipt.

_____

Signature of MCMC Health Care Representative

_____

Name of MCMC Health Care Representative

Figure 9-4 ■ Sample HIPAA authorization form.

Some patients may not be comfortable with using a computer to enter their data. In this event, the medical assistant should offer to assist the patient in completing the necessary information.

When patients' first visits are scheduled at least a week after those patients call to schedule, administrative medical assistants may mail those patients new patient history forms to complete before arriving at the office. This system has one potential drawback, however: patients might forget to bring their paperwork to their first visit. Many medical offices today have their required forms uploaded to their Web sites. When patients call to schedule an appointment, the receptionist can let the patient know where to access the necessary forms to complete, either on paper or electronically, prior to their visit in the office.

Critical Thinking Question 9-2

Thinking back to the case study at the beginning of the chapter, how can the medical assistant explain to the physician or office manager that sending new patient history forms before a patient's first visit will in fact benefit the patient.

HIPAA Compliance

There are some patients who will refuse to sign the HIPAA authorization agreement form in the medical office. This is an infrequent event. When this happens, the medical assistant should simply write "refused to sign" where the patient's signature is indicated, along with the date. The fact that the patient has refused to sign the form should be brought to the physician's attention and the form, with the medical assistant's notation, should be filed in the patient's medical record.

Before patients arrive, the receptionist must verify that all patient files have all necessary paperwork, such as laboratory results reports (outlining the findings of a patient's blood tests, urine tests, or analysis of secretions taken from the patient) and pathology reports (a report outlining the findings of any gross or microscopic tissue examination). When the billing office asks to see patients about their accounts, notes should be placed on the patients' files so those patients can be routed to the billing office before seeing the physician. To ensure patient confidentiality, all patient files must be kept out of sight of nonessential staff and other patients.

Critical Thinking Question 9-3

Referring back to the case study at the beginning of the chapter, if the patient refuses to sign the HIPAA authorization form, what can the medical assistant do? How could this be handled in a HIPAA-compliant manner?

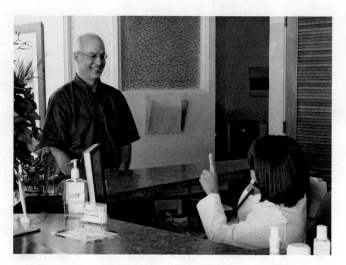

Figure 9-5 ■ If the receptionist is on the telephone when a patient comes in, she should look up and make eye contact with the patient immediately.
Source: Pearson Education/PH College. Photographer: Dylan Malone.

Greeting and Registering Patients

The front desk receptionist is the host or hostess of the medical office. As such, the receptionist should welcome all patients upon arrival, even when busy with other tasks. If, for example, the receptionist is on the telephone when a patient arrives, the receptionist should look up and smile at the patient and hold up an index finger to indicate a slight delay in service (**Figure 9-5** ■).

Years ago, a window separated the receptionist's desk and the reception room to keep conversations behind the front desk private. Today, most medical offices have adopted a friendlier, more open system in the reception room (**Figure 9-6** ■). Now

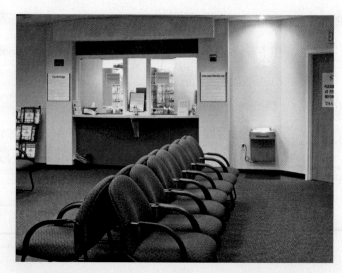

Figure 9-6 ■ Many reception rooms in medical offices today have adopted a friendlier, more open system.
Source: Fotolia © Sheri Armstrong.

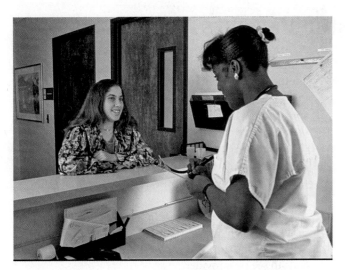

Figure 9-7 ■ The receptionist must maintain patient confidentiality at the front desk by keeping her voice low.
Source: PhotoEdit Inc., Photographer: Michael Newman.

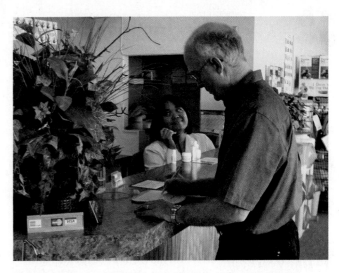

Figure 9-8 ■ A patient signs an electronic sign-in sheet.
Source: Pearson Education/PH College. Photographer: Dylan Malone.

when medical assistants must have private conversations with patients, they must either lower their voices or move the patients to private areas of the office. In modern times, the window is seen as a barrier to effective customer service.

As part of greeting new patients, medical assistants should orient patients to the office with such information as the locations of the restroom and coat rack and where to find reading materials. When greeting established patients, assistants should confirm that all information on file (e.g., address, telephone number, and insurance carrier) remains the same as since the last visit. When a patient's insurance information has changed, the medical assistant should photocopy both sides of new insurance cards.

Patient confidentiality at the front desk is essential to the medical office. Whenever the medical assistant must discuss confidential health or financial information with a patient, all exchanges must occur out of the hearing range of other patients (**Figure 9-7 ■**).

HIPPA Compliance

HIPAA legislation does not demand that the medical office keep patients from seeing one another in the reception room. Patients should not be asked to mention or discuss the reason for their visit within the hearing range of other patients or visitors.

Using Sign-in Sheets Effectively

Some medical offices require patients to sign in upon arrival. Before the Health Insurance Portability and Accountability Act (**HIPAA**) was enacted, **sign-in sheets** were typically sheets of paper that patients signed when entering the office. These sheets alerted the medical assistant to a patient's arrival and served as proof of the patient's visit. Today, many medical offices have replaced paper sign-in sheets with electronic methods for patients to sign in. One convenient method stores patient signatures electronically, much like department stores do (**Figure 9-8 ■**). Another method keeps individual sign-in sheets in patients' files.

Administering Patient Paperwork

When a patient arrives at the office, the medical assistant must give her any necessary forms to complete and identify any important portions of the forms, such as where signatures are needed. At this time, the assistant should also copy the new patient's identification and insurance cards.

The patient registration form (Figure 9-3) is one of the medical office's most important forms, because it contains all information needed to bill for patient care. To ensure billing processes remain up to date, this form should be verified at every visit but no more than once every month. When working with patient paperwork, medical assistants must keep all information confidential. For example, assistants should ask a patient to verify his birthdate or address only when other patients cannot overhear. Similarly, the reasons for a patient's visits should be disclosed only when other patients cannot overhear.

Sometimes, patients will refuse to disclose certain information. Patients most commonly hesitate to provide their Social Security number and birthdate, often because they fear identity theft. When a medical assistant encounters a patient like this, she should gently remind the patient that all information in medical files is confidential and is only released with the patient's written consent or a court order. When these facts fail to persuade a patient, the medical assistant should note on the patient's chart the information that the patient refused to give and give the chart to the clinical staff. Ultimately, the physician must decide whether to accept the patient for treatment.

PROCEDURE 9-2 Greet and Register Patients

Theory and Rationale

As patients enter the medical office, each needs to be greeted by the administrative medical assistant and then registered according to his or her needs.

Materials

- Patient history form
- Pen
- Clipboard

Competency

1. As the patient arrives at the front desk, look up and make eye contact right away. If you are on the telephone, make a motion to the patient with your index finger to indicate you will be with the patient in one moment. If you are not on the telephone, smile and ask the patient for his or her name.

2. Once you have obtained the patient's name, check the appointment schedule to verify the patient is there at the right time and to verify the type of appointment the patient is scheduled to have.

3. If the patient is new to the office, give him or her the appropriate new patient forms to fill out on a clipboard, along with a pen.

4. Ask the patient to take a seat in the reception area and provide the patient with an approximate amount of time he or she can expect to wait before being taken back to see the provider.

5. Alert the clinical medical assistant to the patient's arrival.

▸▸ Pulse Points

Helping the Patient Complete the History Form

Medical assistants must sometimes help patients complete their patient history forms. To maintain patient confidentiality, assistants should provide all such assistance out of the hearing range of other patients. Before asking any personal history questions, for example, the medical assistant should escort the patient to a private area away from the reception room. When the medical assistant has completed the patient forms for the patient, he must sign those forms and note why the patient could not complete the forms herself. Some patients cannot complete patient history forms due to disability, pain, illiteracy, or other factors. For these patients, medical assistants should enlist administrative support.

▸▸ Pulse Points

Obtaining Birthdates from Patients

Because insurance carriers use birthdates to help identify their members, they will not process claims when that information is missing. When a patient refuses to disclose his birthdate, he might have to forego insurance coverage and instead self-fund the charges.

Notifying Patients of Delays

Once a patient has completed all necessary paperwork, the medical assistant must notify the clinical staff of that patient's arrival. Delays happen in the medical office regularly, often due to unforeseen circumstances with emergencies or competing priorities. When delays occur, it is important for the assistant to keep patients apprised. Such consideration demonstrates sound customer service, because it lets patients know that the medical assistant and the physician value patients' time.

Some offices use electronic signs at the front desk to broadcast physicians' schedules, but such signs are only as good as the staff updating them. Therefore, whenever electronic signs are used, the medical assistant must ensure they accurately depict wait times. Whatever system is used, when delays start to exceed 20 minutes, the medical assistant should try to reach patients before they arrive at the office and suggest that they visit the office later or even reschedule.

Collecting Payments at the Front Desk

Part of greeting patients at the front desk includes collecting patients' **copayments** as those patients register. Most offices have signs at their front desks that state, "Copayments are due at the time of service." Patient files should clearly list any copays that are expected. For patients' convenience, the medical office should accept multiple forms of payment (e.g., cash, personal check, credit/debit card). To ensure payments are procured, offices should have policies for addressing patients who cannot pay their copayments at the time of service. Some offices allow patients to mail their copayments or to discuss payment with the billing office.

To track fees, most offices use preprinted fee slips, also called encounter forms or superbills. Fee slips follow patients through the office. The physician and/or clinical medical assistant circles the services or procedures that were performed, as well as any diagnoses the physician

PROCEDURE 9-3 Collect Payments at the Front Desk

Theory and Rationale

Most medical insurance plans today require the patient to pay an out-of-pocket amount at the time of each visit. This payment, known as a copay, should be collected from the patient upon arrival in the medical office. The copayment is a set dollar amount, which is the same no matter what services the patient is provided. Coinsurance, on the other hand, is a percentage of the allowed amount of the cost of the visit. Coinsurance is not collected at the time of service.

Materials

- Pen
- Cash receipt book
- Credit card machine
- Check endorsement stamp

Competency

1. As the patient arrives at the front desk, check the computer or chart to verify the patient's copayment amount.
2. After registering the patient, let the patient know the amount of the expected payment.
3. Ask the patient if he or she would prefer to make the payment via cash, check, or credit card.
4. If the patient pays via cash, write a receipt from the cash receipt book.
5. If the patient pays via check, endorse the check with the bank endorsement stamp. Ask the patient if he or she would like a written receipt. If so, write a receipt from the cash receipt book.
6. If the patient pays via credit card, process the card on the credit card machine, have the patient sign the slip, and provide the patient with his portion as a receipt.

---

assigns to the patient. While medical office supply companies sell standard fee slips, many medical offices customize fee slips to include the diagnoses and procedures they commonly use. Because procedural and diagnosis codes change every year, fee slips should be reviewed for accuracy annually and reprinted as needed.

Typically, the medical assistant who is working at the front desk when the patient arrives prepares the patient's fee slip for that date of service. The medical assistant attaches the slip to the patient's file and routes the file to the clinical medical assistant.

Escorting Patients

Almost always, an administrative medical assistant or clinical medical assistant should escort the patient to the examination room after verifying the patient's identity. The medical assistant should call the patient by his or her formal name, such as Mrs. Bueller. Once in the back office area, the assistant should confirm the patient's birthdate using the patient's file.

Because patients may sometimes have the same first and last names, medical assistants must verify files for all patients. Patient birthdate is one way to differentiate files. The medical assistant should ask the patient for his birthdate, rather than stating the birthdate and asking the patient if the date stated is correct.

Working with Special Needs Patients in the Reception Area

Patients with special needs may need accommodations in the reception area. Patients with disabilities or those who are sight or hearing impaired may arrive with an escort, for example. In

the event the patient arrives with an escort or guardian, the medical assistant should speak to both the patient and the escort to ensure communication is understood by the patient and the medical assistant collecting the information.

Managing Difficult Patients in the Reception Area

As the hub of the reception area, the front desk is on display for the rest of the office. Occasionally, the front desk receptionist must manage difficult patients in the reception area. Many difficulties can be avoided by keeping patients apprised of expected delay times. Medical assistants who remain calm and professional are best equipped to function in and defuse patient interactions.

Patients may be angry for a variety of reasons. The best practice is to keep patients from becoming angry in the first place. This is done mainly through communication, such as communicating wait times and delays in the schedule. Other preventative measures include communicating costs to the patient, so that bills do not come as a surprise. Some patients become angry or upset because they do not feel well or they are under stress due to their medical condition. It is important for the medical assistant to remember that the angry patient is not angry at the medical assistant, so the assistant should not take the anger personally.

Critical Thinking Question 9-4

Referring to the case study at the beginning of the chapter, what should the medical assistant do if the patient becomes angry and begins to shout about not wanting to fill out the paperwork?

When the medical assistant encounters a difficult patient in the reception area, the first goal is to remove the patient from the area. Patients who are out of the sight and hearing range of other patients tend to have less leverage. Once an angry patient is in another location, the medical assistant should work to address the patient's issue or find someone who can. The medical assistant should apologize to the patient for the cause of the irritation, even though the medical assistant is not personally at fault. A general statement such as, "I can see that you are upset. I am sorry this has happened to you; please let me help you" is often all the patient needs to hear to become calmer. It is important for the medical assistant to remember that arguing with the patient is not appropriate. This tactic will not only not solve the problem, it might escalate it further. Part of being a professional medical assistant is providing excellent customer service, and that includes working to resolve difficulties with patients.

Critical Thinking Question 9-5

Referring to the case study at the beginning of the chapter, how should the medical assistant respond to Marilyn? What is appropriate for facial expression and tone of voice?

Keeping Only Appropriate Patients in the Reception Area

In general, patients visit their physicians when they are ill. Depending on the type of practice, medical assistants may help support patients with contagious diseases or life-threatening conditions. As a rule, any patients with contagious conditions should not be left in the reception room. This includes children suspected of having chicken pox, and anyone with a high fever. In addition, any patient who is exhibiting signs of a condition that might make other patients in the reception room uncomfortable should also be removed. Moving these patients out of the reception room addresses their comfort, as well as the comfort of the other patients. Patients with obvious respiratory illnesses should be offered a mask to wear while in the office. Any emergency patient must be brought back to see the physician right away.

The following are examples of patients who should not be kept waiting in the reception area:

- A patient who is bleeding
- A patient who is visibly ill
- A patient who has broken out in a contagious rash, such as chicken pox
- A patient who states that he feels he might vomit
- A patient who is complaining of shortness of breath
- A patient who is complaining of chest pain
- A patient who states she is feeling very dizzy or lightheaded

Maintaining the Reception Room

The reception room should be quiet and peaceful. Patients who are waiting for appointments should be able to sit calmly, undisturbed by loud noises and other distractions. In addition to being quiet, the reception room must be kept clean and free of **hazards**. To attain this goal, medical assistants must check the reception room throughout the day to remove any garbage and retrieve any lost or forgotten items. To keep control of the room, the assistant must do things like ask children to be quiet and instruct patients to take food outside. Many offices play relaxing music in the reception area or have a television playing as a form of entertainment for those waiting. In some offices, a PowerPoint presentation may be playing as an educational tool for certain health care conditions or treatments offered in that facility.

Most people today have a cell phone, smart phone, or other electronic device they will use while waiting in the physician's reception room. To keep noise at a minimum, the medical office should have a sign posted asking patients to limit or restrict cell phone use.

Providing Adequate Seating and Decoration

To ensure patient comfort, the reception room should have an adequate amount of comfortable, easy-to-clean furniture. Experts in medical office space planning believe medical offices should have enough seating to accommodate at least one hour's worth of patients per physician, as well as the friends or relatives who accompany those patients. The furniture should be at a level from which most patients can rise easily and without assistance. Many offices have coat racks for patients' coats or umbrellas.

Practice type dictates the reception room's décor. A pediatric practice has a very different reception room than a women's health care practice, for example. A pediatric practice should have videos and toys, whereas a practice that caters to geriatric patients might have a fish tank or other soothing decorations (**Figure 9-9** ■).

Choosing Reading Material for the Reception Room

Like décor, reading material in the reception area is dictated by practice type. Reading material that is current and tailored to office clientele is a nice customer service touch. For example, a practice that specializes in prostate problems might have magazines about fishing, hunting, or sports activities, while a practice that specializes in women's breast surgery might have magazines about women's fashion (**Figure 9-10** ■).

Managing Children in the Reception Room

Pediatric offices or family practices often have reception areas geared toward children. In offices where children are not the primary patient population, reception areas may have small areas devoted to children. All child-geared areas should have toys and books and other items of interest to children. In all cases, child-geared reception areas and materials must be safe and clean. For example, toys must be checked regularly to confirm they are safe and in good working order. Young children might place small items, including toys, in their mouths. Most states have laws that dictate how to clean toys for public settings. In Washington State, for example, the law dictates that toys must be cleaned with a 10 percent bleach solution after every use.

At no time, including when parents see physicians, should children be left unattended in the reception room. Medical assistants who allow children to be unattended give unspoken consent and assume responsibility for those children on behalf of the office. To ensure their safety, children must remain with their parents throughout the parents' office visits. To be proactive, medical assistants might speak with parents before scheduling those parents' next appointments. To underscore the message, an office might post a sign in the reception area that states, "Children May Not Be Left Unattended in the Reception Area."

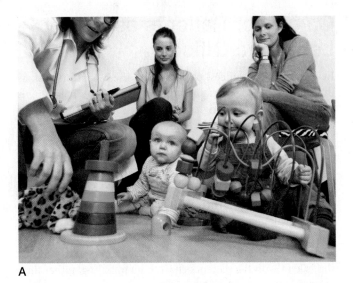

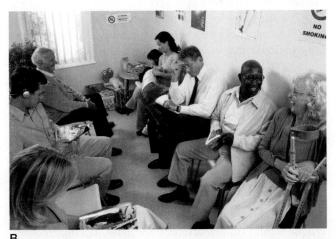

Figure 9-9 ■ (A) A pediatric reception room will typically have child-size furniture and toys; (B) a family practice reception room will cater to patients of all ages.
Source: PhotoEdit Inc. Photographer: Michael Newman.

In Practice

The small physician's office where Jenny works as a front desk medical assistant is on the first floor of a building where cars are parked outside the door. When Marion Wilson arrives for her appointment, she approaches the front desk and tells Jenny that she is going to leave her 2-year-old son sleeping in his car seat because Jenny can see the car from her desk. How should Jenny respond to Marion? What are some appropriate suggestions?

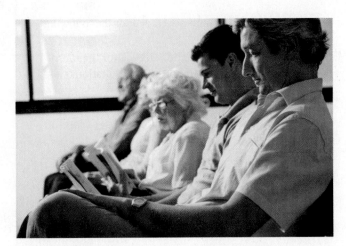

Figure 9-10 ■ Having educational materials available to the patients in the reception area is very common.
Source: Fotolia © Tyler Olsen.

Accommodating Patients with Disabilities

The **Americans with Disabilities Act (ADA)** stipulates that patients with disabilities must be able to access all public buildings, including medical facilities. Medical offices must therefore be able to accommodate people who are in wheelchairs or otherwise unable to use stairs. Ramps and elevators can render medical offices accessible.

Entrance doors must be at least 36 inches wide to accommodate a wheelchair. Interior doors, such as to a restroom or treatment room, must also be accessible by wheelchair. Carpeting in the facility must be no more than one half inch high, because wheelchair users find deeper carpeting difficult to navigate. In addition, all wheelchair-accessible restrooms must be clearly marked and all doorknobs operational with a closed fist (such as with a patient with arthritis who cannot open his or her hand).

Serving Patients with Service Animals

Service animals, usually easily identifiable by their collars or harnesses, must accompany their owners throughout the owners' office visits. Service animals of all kinds assist their owners by doing such things as:

- Pulling wheelchairs
- Carrying or picking up items
- Alerting to hazards

While dogs most often serve as service animals, some patients enlist cats, monkeys, or even ferrets in this role. The Americans with Disabilities Act prohibits excluding the service animal from accompanying the patient, except under certain circumstances. The medical assistant may ask the patient if the animal is a service animal, and what service the animal provides. The medical assistant may not ask the patient about his or her disability, nor ask for any proof that the animal has been formally trained. Service animals may be excluded from entering the building if the animal is thought to be a danger to others, and the owner does not appear to be in complete control of the animal. Another reason for excluding the animal is if the animal is not housebroken.

Caring for Patients as They Leave the Office

In most medical offices, patients pass the reception desk as they exit. Offices are designed this way to ensure that patients complete any final activities, such as scheduling followup appointments. In some large offices, staff in the back office might schedule followup appointments. In small offices, the front desk receptionist makes such appointments. In all cases, whether in a large or small medical office, all exiting patients should be instructed to give the receptionist their superbills or fee slips. On these forms, the physicians should have noted any followup appointments they would like scheduled. Only with this information in hand should the front desk receptionist schedule the followup appointment. In some offices, the fee slip is kept with the patient's chart to go to billing, rather than carried to the front desk by the patient.

The receptionist should bid goodbye to all patients exiting the office, even those who need no followup. This small act not only reinforces that the office staff care about their patients, it promotes a friendly, warm environment.

Closing the Office

To ensure the medical office is closed consistently, properly, and completely, offices should document their desired procedures in **office policies**. Any member of the health care team who is charged with closing the office should complete such tasks as pulling charts for patients scheduled for the following morning, transferring telephone lines to the office answering system, turning off all machinery and lights, locking the doors, and enabling the office alarm system.

 PROCEDURE 9-4 Close the Office

Theory and Rationale

Medical assistants are often tasked with closing the medical office. Just as it supports the office-opening procedure, a checklist helps ensure that medical staff complete this procedure correctly.

Materials

- Checklist of office closing procedures

Competency

1. Ensure all patients have exited the office. Check treatment rooms and restrooms.
2. Verify that all the day's patient files have been routed to the appropriate area (e.g., billing, physician, clinical medical assistant).

3. Pull all files for patients scheduled for the following morning.
4. Confirm that all information needed for the morning's patients (e.g., lab reports or consultations) is available.
5. Attach needed information to patient files.
6. Call to confirm any patient appointments made prior to three days ago.
7. Forward the telephones over to the answering system.
8. Turn off all appropriate equipment and lights.
9. Activate the alarm and lock the doors when leaving the building.

REVIEW

Chapter Summary

- Office policies are invaluable tools for ensuring medical offices are closed and opened properly by all members of the health care team.
- When patients arrive, office staff should be prepared with all necessary information and paperwork.
- Both new and established patients deserve the highest level of customer service from the medical office.
- It is paramount that the entire health care team safeguard patient confidentiality at the front desk and throughout the medical office.
- Medical assistants should learn to professionally persuade patients to provide necessary information and to handle unavoidable delays in nondisruptive ways.

- When patients are difficult, medical assistants must strive to remain calm and diffuse the situation.
- Medical assistants should ensure that the reception area is used only for patients who may be left alone and is always in a condition that is appropriate both for the patients and the overall image and goals of the office.
- When patients have special needs, medical assistants should strive to provide them appropriate care.
- It is particularly important that children and other unique populations receive the care and attention that is appropriate for their needs.

Chapter Review

Multiple Choice

1. Staff members should arrive in the office _____ minutes before the first patient appointment.
   a. 10
   b. 15
   c. 30
   d. 40
   e. 45

2. Which of the following patients should not be left alone in the reception room?
   a. Child with symptoms of chicken pox
   b. Adult with HIV
   c. Patient with eczema
   d. Patient with a sight impairment
   e. a and b

3. When a physician is running 30 minutes behind schedule, the medical assistant should:
   a. Notify patients of the delay as they enter the office
   b. Avoid eye contact with patients in the waiting area
   c. Ask a clinical medical assistant to notify the patients in the reception area
   d. Have the physician come to the reception room to chat with the patients who are waiting
   e. Offer patients a magazine, but do not tell them of the delay

True/False

T F **1.** Studies have shown that patients will stay with physicians they do not really like when they feel the rest of the staff care about their needs.

T F **2.** A window between the reception room and the receptionist's desk is the best way to keep patients from overhearing the receptionist's conversations.

T F **3.** Copayments should never be collected at the front desk.

T F **4.** An electric sign that relays the physician's scheduling delays relieves staff of having to communicate those delays verbally.

T F **5.** HIPAA prevents staff from calling patients' names in the reception room.

T F **6.** When patients refuse to disclose all necessary information, medical assistants should ask them to leave.

T F **7.** Patients who are bleeding visibly should not be left in the reception room.

T F **8.** Reading materials in the reception room should be geared toward the type of patients receiving services.

T F **9.** Educational materials that are specific to the type of practice make good reading materials for the reception room.

Short Answer

1. Describe how, while on the telephone, the front desk receptionist should greet patients entering the office.
2. Explain how to render a sign-in sheet HIPAA compliant.

3. Why is it important to notify patients of any delays in the office?
4. What does it mean to escort a patient?
5. Why might patients become irritable in the reception room?
6. What is the best way to handle a loud, angry patient in the reception room?
7. Why is it important regularly to inspect children's toys in the reception room?
8. Why is it important to have a policy that states no children may be left unattended in the reception room?

Research

1. What classes could you take at your local community college that would help you to communicate better with patients at the front desk?
2. What are the laws in your state that pertain to how often toys in the office must be cleaned?
3. Interview someone who works in a medical office. Ask the person how their reception staff deal with difficult patients.

Practicum Application Experience

When Mrs. Rundholz calls to make an appointment for a complete physical examination, she says she can make the appointment but will not have child care for her 2-year-old and 6-month-old children. She asks if she can bring her children to her hour-long appointment. How should the medical assistant respond to Mrs. Rundholz? What are some appropriate suggestions?

Resource Guide

The Americans with Disabilities Act (ADA) Homepage
www.ada.gov

Microsoft Office Online
Work Essentials
http://office.microsoft.com/en-us/workessentials/

Healthcare Design Magazine
http://www.healthcaredesignmagazine.com

10

Scheduling

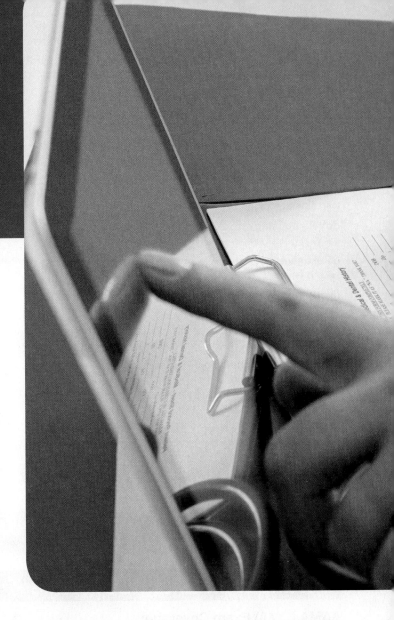

Case Study

Read the following case study and answer the critical thinking questions presented throughout the chapter.

When Glenn Jenson calls the office to set up an appointment, he says he has never been in to see the physician before. When the registered medical assistant asks him why he must see the physician, he responds, "I'd rather not go into that with you. I'll tell the doctor when I see her." The RMA will need to obtain critical pieces of information from the patient to properly schedule his office visit.

Objectives

After completing this chapter, you should be able to:

10.1 Define and spell the key terminology in this chapter.

10.2 Create guidelines for scheduling patient appointments.

10.3 Differentiate between paper and electronic scheduling systems.

10.4 Discuss the various methods of appointment scheduling.

10.5 Explain how to correct the appointment schedule.

10.6 Chart patient no-shows accurately, and follow up with patients who miss their appointments.

10.7 Manage the physician's professional schedule.

10.8 Schedule patients for hospital services and admissions.

10.9 Arrange for interpreters for non-English-speaking patients.

10.10 Arrange for patient transportation.

10.11 Discuss how the office can achieve efficiency in scheduling.

Competency Skills Performance

1. Establish an appointment matrix.
2. Schedule a new patient appointment.
3. Schedule an established patient appointment.
4. Use patient reminder cards.
5. Reschedule a missed patient appointment.
6. Manage the physician's professional schedule and travel.
7. Schedule a hospital procedure.
8. Schedule an inpatient admission.

Key Terminology

buffer time—an appointment scheduling method of leaving certain times of day open to accommodate situations such as patients who call for same-day appointments or physicians who need to catch up on charting

cluster scheduling—scheduling method that groups patients with similar appointments around the same time of day

double booking—scheduling more than one patient for the same appointment time

established patient—patient whom the medical office has seen previously

fixed-appointment scheduling—scheduling system that assigns every patient a specific appointment time

matrix—process of blocking out times in the appointment schedule when the provider is unavailable or out of the office

modified wave scheduling—a scheduling system where two or three patients are scheduled at the beginning of each hour, followed by single patient appointments every 10 to 20 minutes for the rest of that hour

new patient—patient whom no provider of the same specialty in the office has seen for three or more years

new patient checklist—list of information new patients must provide when calling to schedule appointments

office brochure—pamphlet outlining an office's staff and services

open hours—scheduling method that allows patients to seek treatment without appointment times

preapprovals—the process of calling a patient's insurance carrier prior to a service in order to obtain pre-approval or authorization for the service to be performed

slack time—an appointment scheduling method of leaving certain times of day open to accommodate situations such as when patients call for same-day appointments or physicians who need to catch up on charting

triage notebook—notebook kept near the administrative medical assistant answering incoming telephone calls that outlines questions and steps to follow in the event a caller has a potentially life-threatening condition

virtual appointment—a medical appointment conducted via e-mail, telephone, or video, rather than in person

wave scheduling—a scheduling system where patients are scheduled only during the first half of each hour.

Abbreviations

ECG—Electrocardiogram

Certification Exam Coverage

AAMA (CMA) Exam Coverage:

- Utilizing appointment schedules/types
  - Stream
  - Wave/modified wave
  - Open booking
  - Categorization
- Appointment guidelines
  - Appointment schedule matrix
  - Legal aspects
  - New/established patient
  - Patient needs/preference
  - Physician preference/habits
  - Facilities/equipment requirements
- Appointment protocol
  - Followup visits
  - Emergency/acutely ill
  - Physician referrals

- Cancellations/no-shows
- Physician delay/unavailability
- Outside services (e.g., lab, X-ray, surgery)
- Reminders/recalls
  1) Appointment cards
  2) Phone calls

AMT (CMAS) Exam Coverage:

- Appointment management and scheduling
  - Schedule and monitor patient and visitor appointments
  - Address cancellations and missed appointments
  - Prepare information for referrals and preauthorizations
  - Arrange hospital admissions and surgery, and schedule patients for outpatient diagnostic tests
  - Manage recall system and file

AAMA (CMA) certification exam topics are reprinted with permission of the American Association of Medical Assistants.

AMT (CMAS) certification exam topics are reprinted with permission of American Medical Technologists.

AMT (RMA) Exam Coverage:
- Scheduling
  - Employ appointment scheduling system
    1) Identify and employ various scheduling styles (wave, open, etc.)
  - Employ proper procedure for cancellations and missed appointments
  - Understand referral and authorization process

- Understand and manage patient recall system
- Schedule non-office appointments (hospital admissions, diagnostic tests, surgeries)

NCCT (NCMA) Exam Coverage:
- General office procedures
  - Patient instruction

Introduction

While the specifics of appointment scheduling vary from one medical office to another, the basic concepts remain the same. Patients may call to schedule their first visit or routine followup appointments. They may also call with medical emergencies. Administrative medical assistants must know how to best handle each of these situations. In many medical offices today, patients are able to book their own appointments online, through the medical office's Web site. Still other medical organizations offer **virtual appointments**, which are appointments that do not require the patient to come into the office in person. Some of these virtual appointments are in the form of telephone calls between the patients and the medical office staff or physician; others are in the form of electronic communication, such as e-mails or through a secure electronic connection between the patient and the medical office. Over the past couple of years, companies offering video medical visits have been gaining in popularity. These companies allow the patient to consult an RN, or medical provider, via video chat, regarding the medical question or concern. Patients who are referred by another physician may have their appointments scheduled by the staff in the referring physician's office. In these cases, the medical assistant taking the call will be speaking with a medical assistant from the referring physician's office, working together to schedule the patient appointment.

Scheduling New Patient Appointments

When a **new patient** calls the medical office to schedule an appointment, it is important to collect specific patient information while remaining professional, objective, and consistent.

A patient's financial information should not command special attention from the medical assistant and should not be the first question the medical assistant asks of the caller. A **new patient checklist** can help ensure that medical assistants ask appropriate questions, cover all bases, and gather information from all new patients consistently. The following items are typically included on a patient checklist:

- Full name, correctly spelled
- Home telephone number
- Correct address for the patient, if mailing paperwork for completion before the appointment.
- Work telephone number
- Mobile telephone number
- Reason for the visit
- Length of condition
- Type of insurance
- Name of the referring physician, when applicable
- Appointment date and time
- Treating physician
- Directions provided or not

Critical Thinking Question 10-1

Refer back to the case study at the beginning of the chapter. If Glenn fails to state his reason for requesting a physician visit, how can the medical assistant determine the time to allot for the appointment?

Because most health care providers are members of several managed care plans as preferred providers, it is important that medical assistants ask for patients' insurance information before scheduling appointments. When a patient refuses to provide this information, the assistant should let the patient know that this information is needed for the patient to receive the highest benefits from her plans, and that the patient might need to pay in full for her visit if the physician is not participating with her plan. Some medical offices decline to accept patients who have health insurance plans that the clinic is not contracted with. If the medical office accepts a patient with a plan outside of a contract, the medical assistant will need to alert the patient to the costs that will be associated with the visit. When the medical office requires payment at the time of the visit, the medical assistant must also apprise patients of this policy.

Many patients today have high deductible—high out-of-pocket costs associated with the plan. These patients are often concerned with the costs associated with seeking medical care and will ask the medical assistant to give a range of costs over the telephone, prior to scheduling. While the medical assistant might not know the exact costs, particularly when scheduling a patient who might need a variety of services during the visit, the assistant should have a range of charges that can be provided to the patient.

Critical Thinking Question 10-2

Referring back to the case study presented at the beginning of the chapter, how should the medical assistant respond if Glenn refuses to disclose his insurance information?

In addition to obtaining information, the medical assistant might need to provide the patient with information. Patients sometimes need directions to the office or information regarding bus routes that reach the office. Preprinted directions near the office telephone can serve as clear guides. The medical assistant will also need to inform patients of any special parking arrangements and costs.

Critical Thinking Question 10-3

Refer back to the case study presented at the beginning of this chapter. Assume that the patient, Glenn, will be taking the bus to the office. What steps can the medical assistant take to ensure Glenn obtains correct route information?

Many offices choose to mail information to new patients before the patients' first visit. This practice is especially beneficial when patients must complete several forms. As added information, offices should expand their mailings to include their **office brochure** and information about the physician's or office's policies (**Figure 10-1** ■).

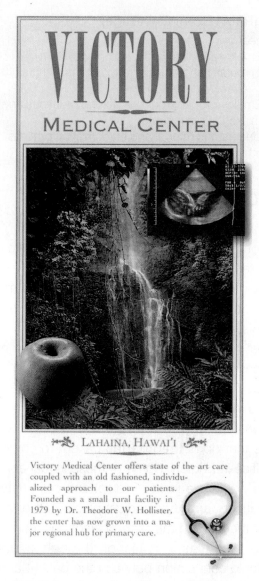

Figure 10-1 ■ Sample medical office brochure.

When the medical assistant will be mailing forms to a patient, he must advise the patient that the forms are coming and that the patient should complete them before arriving for the first appointment. When offices do not send forms as a practice, the assistant will need to ask the patient to arrive early for the appointment so that the patient can complete the paperwork before seeing the physician. The number of forms drives how much time patients will need for this task, but in general, 10 to 20 minutes will suffice. Many medical offices have on their Web site copies of the forms patients will be required to fill out. Patients can be directed to the Web site and asked to download and fill out the forms, and to bring those forms at the time of their visit. In some medical clinics, patients can fill out the forms online, without having to print or bring in any paper versions. When another health care provider has referred a new patient to the office, the medical assistant may want to ask the patient to bring the referral form and any other relevant materials (e.g., X-rays or laboratory reports) to the visit. Sometimes, however, referring providers send such information separately.

New and Established Patients

Medical offices have varying policies on what constitutes *new* and *established* patients. In general, a new patient has not been seen in the medical office by any of the health care providers of the same specialty within the past three years. Conversely, an **established patient** has seen one of the health care providers of the same specialty in the medical office within the past three years. This rule especially applies when billing a patient's health insurance plan. When a patient has been seen in the medical office by a provider of the same specialty, that patient is considered *established* by their insurance carriers. For physicians who see patients in the hospital setting, the new patient rule still applies to that setting. In other words, if a patient sees a physician in the hospital, then comes in to that physician's office to see the same physician, or a partner of the same specialty within three years of the hospital visit, that patient is considered an established patient. It does not matter what the patient's health concern is, or if the two visits are for entirely different concerns; having been seen within three years classifies that patient as an established patient.

Patients who have been involved in accidents, such as car accidents or on-the-job injuries, may be considered *new* when seeking care for related injuries because they will likely need to provide accidental-injury information and undergo evaluations as if the office had never seen them before. Therefore, it is important for the medical assistant to know his office's policies for new and established patients and to follow those policies consistently.

▶▶▶ Pulse Points

Accidental Injury Files

Keep a patient's accidental injury files separate from her general medical files. Then when insurance companies request copies of the patient's medical records due to the accidental injury, the copying task is far easier.

Allowing Appointments Adequate Time

The time patient appointments require depends on the type of practice and the preferences of the health care providers. Table 10-1 lists examples of general appointment types and times allowed; however, appointment times may vary for each provider. In typical offices, new patients are seen for longer periods than established ones. For example, a new patient appointment may be scheduled for 30 minutes, whereas an established patient appointment might extend only 10 or 15

TABLE 10-1 Time Allotted for Patient Appointments

Appointment Type	Allotted Time (in Minutes)
New patient	30
Physical exam	60
Routine checkup	15
Well-child checkup	15
Blood pressure check	5

minutes. Each medical office should document its policy for allotting appointment time and review it regularly to ensure it continues to be appropriate for patients and physicians.

Many physicians prefer to limit certain types of appointments in any given day. For example, a pediatrician might only want to see one or two sports physicals in a day. An OB/GYN physician might only want to see one or two new maternity patients in a day. Again, documented policies are beneficial, because they can clarify the physician's preferences and help the medical assistant schedule appointments properly. If, for example, the pediatrician will only allow two sports physicals a day, the office may schedule those appointments for 10 A.M. and 3 P.M. Once those appointments are filled, the medical assistant can easily see that the schedule will support no more sports physicals that day.

Creating an Appointment Matrix

The process of scheduling medical office appointments begins with an appointment **matrix**. An appointment matrix, which can be applied to paper and computerized appointment schedules alike, depicts the appointment times available in the medical office. Medical assistants block out the times on the matrix when physicians are unavailable due to hospital rounds, vacations, or holidays. When appointment matrices are paired with appointment systems, medical assistants can also block times for certain pieces of equipment so conflicts for the use of equipment do not arise.

Depending on the type of practice or the specialties of the physicians, medical assistants use certain abbreviations in their matrix notations. Within an office, however, these abbreviations must be standard so that all members of the health care team can interpret the abbreviations accurately. For example, an office may use the abbreviation "NP" for a new patient.

Even in one-physician practices, different columns of the appointment book may be used for different procedures. For example, all new patients might be scheduled in the far left column and all followup appointments in the far right one. In some offices, appointment types are highlighted in different colors to indicate type of patient or procedure. For example, patients undergoing laboratory work might be highlighted in orange while patients having X-rays might be highlighted in blue. Each office devises a system that works for it. When using an electronic scheduling system, each provider will have

PROCEDURE 10-1 Establish an Appointment Matrix

Theory and Rationale

With an appointment matrix, the administrative medical assistant is able to create time slots for the various appointment types in the medical office. Using this method, the medical assistant is better able to accurately schedule patients for the necessary amount of time and facilitate efficient flow in the office.

Materials

- Pen
- Paper or electronic appointment schedule

Competency

1. Determine the amount of time the providers want patients to have for each appointment type.

2. Within the appointment book, block out the time when the providers will be out of the office for lunch or other appointments. If using an electronic scheduling system, block out the time in the electronic appointment schedule.

3. Highlight or create blocks of time in the appointment book for appointments the provider specifies as those he or she would like only a limited number of, such as physical exams. If using an electronic appointment system, use the features contained within the program to accomplish this task.

4. Go over the created appointment matrix with the providers to determine where any adjustments need to be made.

---

his or her own schedule, with the medical assistant having the ability to see more than one schedule at once.

Balancing Patient and Office Needs in Scheduling

When medical assistants schedule appointments, they must pay attention to patients' needs. For example, assistants should schedule patients who need fasting blood draws at the beginning of the day. Just as assistants should heed patient needs, they should factor in what is appropriate for the office. For example, if the office has only one electrocardiogram (**ECG**) machine, it would be inappropriate for the medical assistant to schedule two patients who need the machine at once. When only one staff member performs a certain procedure or test, the medical assistant must keep that person's availability in mind when scheduling appointments.

▶▶▶ Pulse Points

Considering Patient Requirements

Every office has a few patients who need extended appointment times due to disability or complex health issues. Staff should note these unique requirements on the patients' paper or electronic health records so that the medical assistant who is scheduling appointments can allot appropriate amounts of time.

Electronic Scheduling

Today, most large medical offices use computer software to manage their patient appointments (**Figure 10-2** ■). Computerized systems vary depending on the specific needs of the

medical practice. Some practices may need scheduling software only, while other larger practices might contract with a commercial appointment-scheduling service. For those practices that purchase scheduling software, the software companies often provide installation, training, and support services to the practice's administrative staff.

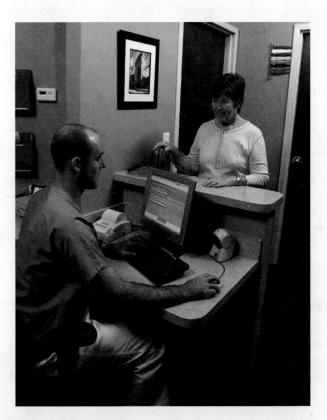

Figure 10-2 ■ Scheduling appointments on the computer saves time over using a manual scheduling system.

Electronic appointment scheduling offers many advantages, some of which include the following:

- With computerized systems, several staff members can access the appointment schedule at once and from different locations in the office. Physicians are also able to view future appointments from any remote location at any time.

- Administrative assistants have the ability to schedule multiple physicians at the same time, from any computer in the medical office.

- Assistants can print out detailed patient information for physicians, such as detailed histories, prior to the patient's visit.

- Some computerized systems allow staff and/or physicians to access the appointment schedule from outside the office.

- Computer appointment scheduling is faster and easier than paper scheduling for those staff members experienced with the software. Some software allows the medical assistant to search for available appointment times by doctor, by first available appointment, by day of the week, or by month, by time, and so on.

- The administrative medical assistant is able to print multiple copies of the appointment schedule for distribution in the office.

- Various screens provide such information as last patient appointment, next appointment scheduled, and current prescriptions.

- The practice may choose to work with technology companies that can access the practice's appointment list and place automated calls to patients reminding them of their appointments. Several electronic scheduling systems are marketed to medical offices today. Some of these programs are incorporated into the electronic health record, allowing the user to link the patient's appointment to the medical record.

Offices that use paper appointment books should choose books that support their number of physicians and patients. In multiphysician practices, appointment books, whether paper or electronic, might be color-coded by the provider (**Figure 10-3 ■**). This offers the medical assistant an easy-to-see schedule, with a different color for each provider in the office.

HIPAA Compliance

The appointment book, whether paper or electronic, is considered a legal document. Paper appointment books, like all hard-copy medical records, must be kept in a safe location. Computerized appointment schedules must be protected just like any other item that contains private patient information. Computerized schedules are protected through secure computer systems and password use by all administrative staff. At the end of the day, any printouts of the computerized system should be shredded to protect patient confidentiality.

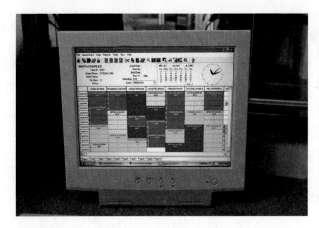

Figure 10-3 ■ Using a color-coded scheme is easier in a multi-specialty practice.

Methods of Appointment Scheduling

Ambulatory health care uses several different methods to schedule patient appointments. Practice type and physician preference determine which method is used.

Cluster Scheduling

Cluster scheduling is a system of booking several patients around the same block of time. This method is normally used when the patients all need the same type of service, such as laboratory work or consultations. By clustering similar appointments, the office can serve patients most efficiently. Cluster scheduling is also used for physicians whose schedule might not be filled entirely. The physician may prefer to see all of his morning patients in the first hour of the day, leaving the remainder of the morning schedule open for other office projects, such as marketing to other physicians in the area. **Figure 10-4 ■** is an example of cluster scheduling.

Double Booking

Double booking is done when two or more patients are scheduled to see the same health care provider at once. This method serves when an emergency patient must be seen that day, or it may be used to accommodate patients who need added services while in the office. For example, if the medical office has two patients who are both going to need laboratory work, the medical assistant might schedule both patients for the same appointment time. This option works, because the clinical medical assistant can perform laboratory work with one patient while the physician sees the other. This system uses the treatment rooms as well as the clinical staff's time effectively.

Fixed Appointment Scheduling

The most common method of scheduling patients is **fixed appointment scheduling**. In this method, the office gives

PROCEDURE 10-2 Schedule a New Patient Appointment

Theory and Rationale

Most patients who schedule appointments at a medical office do so over the telephone. The administrative medical assistant must know what information is needed from each new patient and be able to answer any questions professionally.

Materials

- Telephone
- Blue or black pen
- Paper or electronic appointment book
- New patient checklist

Competency

1. Using a professional, friendly voice, answer the telephone by the second ring.
2. State the office name followed by your name.
3. When the caller does not self-identify as a new patient, ask the caller the date of his or her last visit in the office. If the patient states he or she has not been seen previously, the medical assistant may proceed with scheduling the patient as a new patient.
4. Ask the patient to spell his or her first and last names.
5. Write the patient's full name on the checklist.
6. Ask the patient for work and home telephone numbers, and home address.
7. Ask the patient how he or she was referred to the office.
8. Ask the patient to identify the type of health insurance he or she will be using.

9. Confirm that your physician participates in the patient's health care plan.
10. If the physician does not participate in the patient's health care plan, advise the patient that he or she might fail to receive preferred benefits or might need to pay in full for services.
11. Ask the patient to state the condition prompting the visit.
12. Ask the patient to define the length of the condition.
13. Offer the patient appointment times to see the physician.
14. Schedule the patient.
15. If mailing paperwork to the patient to complete before the appointment, direct the patient to complete the paperwork before the visit.
16. If the patient will need to complete the paperwork at the first visit, direct him or her to arrive 15 minutes before the appointment's scheduled start time. In offices that keep electronic versions of their medical forms online, assistants will direct patients on how to fill out the paperwork prior to their visit.
17. Document the patient's information in the manual or electronic appointment schedule.
18. Ask the patient if directions to the office are needed.
19. Give the patient any needed parking information.
20. Confirm the appointment's date and time with the patient.
21. Allow the patient to hang up the telephone before hanging up yourself.

PROCEDURE 10-3 Schedule an Established Patient Appointment

Theory and Rationale

Patient scheduling, which constitutes a large portion of the administrative medical assistant's job, is vital to proper time management in the medical office. Therefore, the assistant must be properly trained to perform this task. When scheduling an established patient, the assistant will not need to collect as much information from the patient prior to scheduling the appointment as for a new patient. Demographics, such as birthdate, that do not change over time, do not need to be collected from the established patient.

Materials

- Paper or electronic appointment book
- Blue or black pen
- Patient's chart

Competency

1. Locate the chart of the patient to be scheduled.
2. Determine the type of appointment that is needed.
3. Determine the patient's schedule.
4. Determine the physician's schedule.
5. Enter the patient in the appointment schedule.
6. Restate the appointment date and time to the patient. If the patient is in the office, provide a written reminder card. Remind the patient to bring any needed items to the appointment or to follow any procedures (e.g., fasting before the visit).

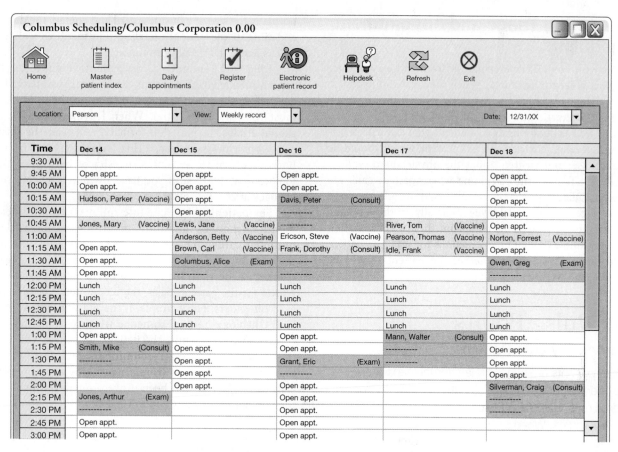

Figure 10-4 ■ In this example, all immunizations are scheduled for morning appointments.

each patient a specific appointment time. Patients are asked to arrive at their appointed time, and the physician and medical assistant can prepare for the patients and conditions they will treat that day, knowing how much time is allotted to each.

Scheduling with Open Hours

The **open hours** scheduling method works for patients who do not need specific appointment times. This system is used in walk-in clinics, laboratories, and X-ray facilities where patients are normally seen on a first-come, first-served basis. The drawback to this type of schedule is that many patients might arrive at the same time and might have to wait to be seen. Another drawback, on the other hand, is that there can be times in the day when no patients are seen, and the medical office is staffed with medical personnel who do not have clinical work to do for a period of time.

Wave Scheduling

Medical clinics with large numbers of procedure rooms and clinical staff may use a method called **wave scheduling**. In wave scheduling, patients are scheduled only for the first half of each hour. The first patient to arrive is seen first. If two or more patients arrive at once, the clinical medical assistant will need to triage the patients to make the decision on whom to

take first. This type of scheduling can be beneficial to the medical office in that the patients with needs that take little time to address are seen quickly, while patients with more complicated needs remain in the clinic.

Modified Wave Scheduling

The **modified wave scheduling** method is a variation on the wave method just discussed. With modified wave scheduling, two or three patients are scheduled at the beginning of each hour, followed by single patient appointments every 10 to 20 minutes for the rest of that hour. Complicated cases are generally scheduled at the beginning of the hour, while minor cases are usually scheduled toward the end.

Leaving Slack or Buffer Time

Most medical offices that use scheduling systems for patient appointments leave certain times of day open to accommodate things like patients who call for same-day appointments or physicians who need to catch up on charting. These open periods, called **slack time** or **buffer time**, are generally 15- to 30-minute slots at the end of the morning and the end of the afternoon or evening. These buffer times may be used for the scheduling of urgent patients, should the need arise.

Conducting Triage and Appointment Scheduling

Patients with medical emergencies will sometimes call their physician's office for assistance. When they do, administrative medical assistants should have clearly written protocols for handling the situation. A **triage notebook** outlines these protocols, as well as questions to ask patients who call with possible medical emergencies. Such a notebook, which should be clear, concise, and written under the physician's direction, should be left near the telephone where patient calls are answered. Offices using an electronic health record may have such a triage system available electronically. In these offices, the assistant can type in the complaint the patient is calling about and follow the online instructions for what the patient should be told, including whether the patient should be directed to the emergency room for care.

▶▶▶ Pulse Points

Chronically Late Patients

When patients are habitually late for their appointments, the medical office should give those patients appointment times that precede scheduled appointment times by 15 minutes. When a chronically late patient is scheduled for a 2:15 P.M. appointment, for example, the office should advise the patient to arrive at 2:00 P.M.

Using Appointment Reminder Systems

Typically, patients are given appointment reminder cards as they leave the office (**Figure 10-5** ■). These reminder cards are

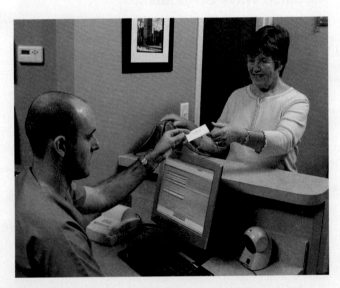

Figure 10-5 ■ Typically, patients are given appointment reminder cards when they leave the office.

normally the size of a business card and contain the date, day, and time of the patient's next appointment, as well as the office's name and telephone number.

Even with reminder cards, patients might forget their appointments. For this reason, many offices call patients the day before their appointment to remind them. Such calls must remain confidential. When leaving messages, staff should disclose no patient information. Instead, the assistant can leave a message like, "This is Jared calling from Dr. Barker's office to remind Kaneesha of her appointment tomorrow at 2:00 P.M. If you have any questions, please call me back at 201-555-6000."

For patients who schedule followup appointments a month or more in the future, many offices choose to send reminder cards. These cards can be postcards only when they contain no personal patient information such as the reason for the visit. If the name of the office discloses the reason for the patient's visit, the office should not use postcard reminders. For example, if the office is called "Woodland Oncology Center," someone who sees a postcard with this name might assume the patient has cancer. Offices like these should either mail appointment reminders in envelopes or call patients with reminders. The use of reminder calls or phone calls has been proven to reduce dramatically the number of no-show appointments.

▶▶▶ Pulse Points

Automated Telephone Reminder Systems

Many medical offices today use automated telephone reminder systems to remind patients of their upcoming appointments. These systems, typically paired with computerized appointment systems, automatically dial a patient's contact telephone number and play a recorded reminder message.

Correcting the Appointment Schedule

As with patients' medical records, white correction fluid is disallowed from the paper appointment book. When an appointment is changed in the appointment book, it should not be obliterated or erased or blacked out with a marker. Instead, the medical assistant should draw one line through the patient's name and note why the patient failed to keep the appointment (**Figure 10-6** ■). Some medical offices use color-coded systems to indicate schedule changes. For example, a red "X" next to a patient's name might indicate an appointment cancellation. Electronic schedules accept notations, cancellations, and rescheduled or missed appointments.

PROCEDURE 10-4 Use Patient Reminder Cards

Theory and Rationale

Many patients, as they leave the medical office, will require a followup appointment. The medical assistant will need to schedule that appointment for the patient and provide the patient with a reminder card.

Materials

- Pen
- Paper or electronic appointment book
- Appointment reminder card

Competency

1. As the patient arrives at the reception desk, look at the fee slip to verify when the provider wants the patient to return for an appointment.

2. Ask the patient if there is a day or time that works best for her schedule for the appointment.

3. Check the appointment book to find an appointment time that fits with the patient's schedule.

4. After verifying that the appointment will work with the patient's schedule, write or type the appointment into the appointment schedule.

5. Write the patient's appointment on a reminder card and give the card to the patient.

Documenting No-Show Appointments

Patients who fail to arrive for their appointment and who do not call to reschedule are considered *no-shows*. The medical office must try to reach all no-shows. Typically, this is done via telephone 15 to 30 minutes after a patient's appointed time. When the medical assistant reaches the patient, she should try to reschedule the appointment. When she cannot reach the patient, however, she should leave a message requesting a return call to reschedule. When the assistant can neither reach the patient nor leave a message, she may mail a note requesting rescheduling.

Following Up on No-Show Appointments

Patient appointments that are missed for whatever reason must be documented in the patient's medical record. Any steps the medical office staff takes to try to reschedule the patient must be documented as well. When a patient refuses to reschedule or remains unreachable, the medical assistant must make notes to that effect in the patient's medical record and submit the record to the physician for review.

Well-documented patient medical records become particularly important when a patient experiences an adverse outcome due to a missed appointment. Medical offices with clear, comprehensive patient records are better able to defend against malpractice suits. Some offices take the extra step of sending the patient a certified letter when the patient misses an important followup appointment, such as a postoperative appointment. Proof of the patient's receipt of such letters demonstrates the office took every step possible to encourage the patient to obtain needed care.

Many medical offices charge patients for no-show appointments. In these offices, the patient must be informed of this policy and that the fee will be the patient's responsibility at the time the appointment is scheduled. Office policy will dictate whether a fee is charged for the first missed appointment or if the fee is assessed only after missing two or three appointments. Medical offices may dismiss a patient from care for multiple missed appointments, after notifying the patient of such a policy. No matter what policy the medical office chooses, that policy must be enforced uniformly, without making exceptions for certain patients.

Medical offices are legally able to dismiss patients from care if those patients do not routinely make their scheduled appointments. In cases such as these, the medical office staff will need to alert the patient via a certified letter that the physician–patient relationship is being severed, and offer to refer the patient to another provider in the area.

◦ In Practice

Dr. Brosnan performed a vasectomy on William Grissom and asked him, as he asks all patients who have undergone this procedure, to have a followup evaluation and laboratory work done to determine the procedure's effectiveness. Mr. Grissom, however, failed to show for his followup appointment. Three months later, Dr. Brosnan received a notice that Mr. Grissom has filed a malpractice suit. According to the notice, Mr. Grissom is alleging that Dr. Brosnan was negligent because Mr. Grissom's wife is newly pregnant. How could Dr. Brosnan's office have protected itself against this situation?

		SERV.	COLL.	R/S		SERV.	COLL.	R/S		SERV.	COLL.	R/S		SERV.	COLL.
9	Clarisa Hansen New patient (509) 555-1264														
9¹⁵															
9³⁰	Quinn Thuh BP check														
9⁴⁵	Maryann Jones Well child ck														
10	Rory McIntyre Physical exam														
10¹⁵															
10³⁰															
10⁴⁵															
11	~~Jose Rodriquez~~ ear ache	Rescheduled to 1/10													
11¹⁵	Monica Reiman New patient (509) 555-9926														
11³⁰															
11⁴⁵	Staff Meeting														

AM

Figure 10-6 ■ Sample appointment book indicating a patient who has changed his appointment time.

PROCEDURE 10-5 Reschedule a Missed Patient Appointment

Theory and Rationale

The medical office must follow up on all missed patient appointments. The medical assistant must call the patient to attempt to reschedule the missed appointment.

Materials

- Paper or electronic appointment schedule
- Pen
- Patient's chart

Competency

1. Fifteen minutes after the patient's appointment time, call the patient's home telephone number.
2. If the patient answers:
   - Point out the missed appointment time and ask for an appropriate time to reschedule.
   - If the patient reschedules the appointment, document the new appointment in the paper or electronic appointment book as well as the patient's chart. Also chart that the patient missed the originally scheduled appointment.
   - If the patient does not wish to reschedule, politely state that you will inform the physician. Chart the missed appointment and refusal to reschedule in the patient's chart, and give the chart to the physician.
3. If the patient fails to answer:
   - Leave a message on voicemail or with the person who answers. Be certain to disclose no confidential patient information. An appropriate message is, "This is Juan at Dr. Saunders's office. I'm calling for Mrs. Banfield. We had you scheduled for an appointment today at 9:00 A.M., and I'm calling to reschedule. Please call me back at 715-555-6789."
   - In the patient's chart, document the missed appointment and the message.

Managing the Physician's Professional Schedule

Many physicians attend professional meetings outside the office. These range from lunches with colleagues to traveling to out-of-state seminars. In many medical offices, the administrative medical assistant manages the physician's professional schedule. At minimum, this task includes blocking out times in the appointment schedule when the physician is unavailable for patient appointments. The assistant may also be asked to book flights or hotel rooms, or to reserve seats at conferences.

To ensure accuracy and efficiency, medical assistants should clearly write all information on the physician's travel plans, including any confirmation numbers (**Figure 10-7** ■).

A copy of all such information should remain in the office to keep the rest of the health care team apprised of the physician's schedule. The physician can retain any original documents. When the physician attends a seminar or conference

- Leaving on United Airlines Flight #12 at 7:10 P.M. Thursday.
- Arriving in Chicago at 10:02 P.M.
- Reservations with Hertz car rental, Confirmation #1298745.
- Reservations at the Red Lion hotel, Confirmation #LEN987.
- Seminar starts in the Capital Boardroom at 9 A.M. Friday.
- Return on United Airlines Flight #81 at 9:10 A.M. Sunday.

Figure 10-7 ■ Sample physician's travel schedule.

that awards continuing-education credits, the medical assistant should track that information, as well.

Scheduling Hospital Services and Admissions

Many physicians care for or perform procedures on patients in hospital settings as well as in ambulatory clinics. For this reason, administrative medical assistants must be well-versed in the procedures for scheduling patients for hospital services.

To facilitate the hospital scheduling process, the medical office should keep all hospital and related telephone numbers near the telephone, or program them into speed dial. Most health insurance plans require physicians to obtain **preapprovals** for surgical procedures. Unless the procedure is an emergency, the medical assistant should call the patient's insurance carrier to obtain authorization for the procedure before scheduling the patient. Whenever possible, the medical assistant should schedule the patient for hospital services while the patient is in the office. With the patient present, the assistant is better able to coordinate the patient's schedule.

Every office should have guidelines for scheduling patients for hospital services. These guidelines should list the type of procedure, the physician, the time the physician needs, and any information that must be relayed to the patient, such as fasting presurgery. The medical office should also have preprinted information forms from the hospital or outpatient facility that give such specifics as directions to the facility and check-in procedures. Patients should receive such forms before they leave the office.

PROCEDURE 10-6 Manage the Physician's Professional Schedule and Travel

Theory and Rationale

Many physicians travel out of town for speaking engagements or seminars while gaining continuing education credits for relicensure. The medical assistant will often be asked to coordinate the physician's schedule and make all necessary travel arrangements for these trips.

Materials

- A telephone
- A list of the physician's travel needs, including dates and times of the meeting or seminar, place of the seminar, and the physician's preference for airline and hotel arrangements.
- Paper and pen

Competency

1. Call the physician's preferred airline and book the appropriate flight.

2. Make a note of the date, time, airline, and flight number for the departure time and arrival time for both the outgoing flight and the return flight.

3. Call the physician's preferred hotel and book the appropriate room.

4. Make a note of the confirmation number for the hotel room.

5. Arrange for any necessary transportation to or from the hotel and airport.

6. Create a list of all arrangements made and give the list to the physician.

7. Give a copy of the list of arrangements to the office manager and to the receptionist.

8. Verify the receptionist has blocked out the dates the physician will be away, if applicable.

Specialty Referral Appointments

Many patients in the medical office will need to be scheduled for an appointment with a specialist. When this happens, the physician will notify the medical assistant of the patient's need for a specialty referral. The physician will also state the name of the specialist the patient is to be referred to, information regarding the condition for which the patient needs to be seen, and a time frame within which the appointment should be made.

Depending upon the policy in the medical clinic, the medical assistant may call to schedule the referral for the patient directly. In other offices, the medical assistant may supply the information about the referral to the patient and the patient will make the telephone call directly. Either way, the medical assistant must supply the patient with the information that is needed for the additional appointment.

▸▸▸ Pulse Points

Preparing the Patient for the Medical Procedure

Medical procedures make many patients nervous. Medical assistants can help make the patient's experience a positive one by letting her know exactly what to expect before, during, and after the procedure. The assistant should include information about any dietary or activity restrictions before or after the procedure, and should specify how long the procedure is expected to take.

Arranging for Language Interpreters

Occasionally, the medical office will treat patients who are not fluent in English or who cannot communicate due to a disability. Typically, these patients visit the office with family members or friends who can translate for them. When patients cannot arrange for interpreters, the medical office must arrange interpreter services. Many states offer translation services for their Medicaid-covered patients. When translation services are needed, offices should keep interpreters' telephone numbers at the front desk. When using a translator, the medical assistant must document the name and contact information of the translator in the patient's chart.

To bring translation services in house, many medical offices, especially those in communities with large non-English-speaking populations, seek employees who are fluent in other languages. Members of the health care team who can translate for patients are valuable assets to the medical office.

Arranging Transportation for Patients

Many medical offices treat patients who cannot drive themselves to the office. Patients might have disabilities, or offices might be in challenging locations. As a courtesy to patients, the administrative medical assistant should keep a telephone

PROCEDURE 10-7 Schedule a Hospital Procedure

Theory and Rationale

When procedures cannot be performed in the medical office or patients would be better served in hospitals, physicians ask the medical assistant to schedule patients for hospital procedures.

Materials

- Patient's chart
- Hospital/surgery scheduling form
- Scheduling guidelines
- Calendar
- Telephone
- Notepad
- Pen

Competency

1. Obtain information from the physician or clinical medical assistant about the needed surgery or procedure and the desired hospital.
2. Call the patient's insurance carrier to obtain preauthorization for the procedure.
3. Document the preauthorization number in the patient's chart along with the name of the customer service representative spoken to at the insurance company.
4. If the patient is in the clinic, ask what date or time would be most convenient for the procedure. If the patient is not in the clinic, call the patient to determine scheduling needs.
5. Call the hospital to communicate the procedure the physician has planned, the amount of time needed for the procedure, and the date preferred for the procedure.
6. Provide the hospital staff the patient's information, including name, birthdate, address, telephone number, insurance information, and preauthorization number. Also relay all pertinent health information, such as allergies or disabilities.
7. After agreeing on a date and time, give the information to the patient and enter it in the physician's appointment schedule.
8. Advise the patient that the hospital will likely call to provide instructions and verify the check-in date and time.
9. Schedule the patient for a postoperative appointment in the physician's office, if needed.
10. Chart all information in the patient's medical record, and give the chart to the physician for review.

 PROCEDURE 10-8 Schedule an Inpatient Admission

Theory and Rationale

When a patient requires an inpatient procedure or observation, the physician will ask the medical assistant to schedule the patient for inpatient hospitalization. The medical assistant who knows the proper procedure helps to ensure that the scheduling process goes smoothly.

Materials

- Patient's chart
- Inpatient scheduling guidelines
- Calendar
- Telephone
- Notepad
- Pen

Competency

1. Call the patient's insurance carrier to obtain preauthorization for the procedure, the needed followup, and the allowable number of hospital days.
2. Document the preauthorization number in the patient's chart along with the name of the customer service representative spoken to at the insurance company.
3. Call the hospital admissions office with the patient's name, physician's name, and reason for admission.
4. Let the admissions office know when the physician would like the patient to be admitted.
5. Give the admissions office the patient's contact information, birthdate, insurance information, and preauthorization number.
6. Instruct the patient when to arrive at the hospital and where to go once there.
7. Give the patient any specifics on what to bring (or not) to the hospital.
8. Chart all information in the patient's medical record, and give the chart to the physician for review.

list of transportation services. Such lists should include taxicab services as well as local services for the elderly or disabled.

Achieving Efficiency in Scheduling

All medical offices at some point realize that their appointment scheduling procedures could be improved. Physicians might routinely exceed scheduled appointment times, or extended delays might regularly irritate patients. When flaws like these become apparent, it is important for the health care team as a whole to re-evaluate how the office schedules appointments. Every member of the team should participate in improvement efforts, because scheduling affects every staff member (**Figure 10-8** ■).

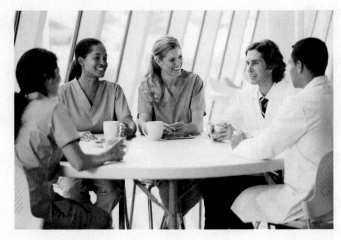

Figure 10-8 ■ Regular staff meetings keep the lines of communication open in the medical office.
Source: Shutterstock © Monkey Business Images.

REVIEW

Chapter Summary

- Guidelines for scheduling patient appointments are invaluable tools for medical offices intent on providing effective, efficient patient service.
- Today, medical offices can choose between paper and electronic scheduling systems.
- Both paper and electronic scheduling systems accommodate patient no-shows, which always must be documented properly for legal and other purposes.
- When patients miss their appointments, the medical assistant should follow up to attempt rescheduling.

- The physician's professional schedule, which includes travel, is part of a medical office's overall scheduling scheme.
- Like the physician's travel, the medical assistant must be able to accommodate the patient's hospital appointments in the office's scheduling system.
- Effective medical assistants arrange appropriate transportation services or language interpreters for patients in need.

Chapter Review

Multiple Choice

1. At _____ minutes after a patient has missed an appointment, the medical assistant should call to reschedule.
   a. 5
   b. 10
   c. 15
   d. 60
   e. 90

2. A new patient is defined as someone who has:
   a. Not been seen in the medical office for more than one year
   b. Not been seen by any physician in the office for more than three years
   c. Been seen by another physician in the office within the last year but is now seeing a new provider in the office
   d. a and b
   e. a, b, and c

3. A new-patient checklist is worthwhile when scheduling new patient appointments to ensure the medical assistant:
   a. Gathers all necessary information from the new patient
   b. Provides directions to the office, if needed
   c. Gives information on parking arrangements
   d. a and b
   e. a, b, and c

4. The medical office should ask new patients to arrive _____ minutes before their scheduled appointment to complete new patient paperwork.
   a. 5
   b. 15
   c. 25
   d. 35
   e. 60

5. Which of the following scheduling methods books several patients around the same time?
   a. Cluster booking
   b. Stream scheduling
   c. Set appointment time scheduling
   d. Open appointment hours
   e. Wave scheduling

True/False

T F 1. The time allowed for patient appointments remains constant from practitioner to practitioner.

T F 2. The appointment book is a legal document.

T F 3. Double booking is the process of allowing patients to arrive for appointments at their leisure.

T F 4. It is appropriate to tell a chronically late patient that his appointment begins 15 minutes before the time scheduled in the appointment book.

T F 5. It is unnecessary to chart a no-show appointment in a patient's chart.

T F 6. Charting a patient's missed appointments can help the medical office avoid losing malpractice lawsuits.

T F 7. When scheduling a patient for a procedure, it is important to disclose everything to expect.

T F 8. Administrative medical assistants do not arrange transportation services.

T F 9. A medical office's appointment scheduling system should be reviewed periodically to determine its efficiency.

Short Answer

1. What is one way to prepare the appointment schedule to allow appointments for patients who call and want same-day appointments?
2. Describe a triage notebook and its role in the medical office.
3. How can the administrative medical assistant help patients remember their appointments?
4. What is meant by a *no-show* appointment?
5. What can the medical assistant do when he finds that patients are waiting long periods for appointments?
6. Describe how an appointment matrix is used in the medical office.

Research

1. Research online for companies that sell medical office appointment scheduling software. How do these companies compare to one another?
2. Interview someone who works in a medical office. Do the physicians in this office travel for out-of-town events related to their practice? If so, who in the office handles the scheduling arrangements?
3. What local resources are available in your area for arranging for medical language interpreters?

Practicum Application Experience

When Shawn Guthmein calls to schedule a new patient appointment with Dr. Gootkind, he mentions that he will be bringing his service animal to his appointment because he is legally blind. Because Shawn is a new patient, he will need to complete several forms once he is in the clinic. How can the medical assistant best handle this patient?

Resource Guide

MicroWiz Medical Appointment Scheduling Software
http://www.microwize.com/ohpro.htm

MedStar Medical Appointment Scheduling Software
http://www.medstarsystems.com

NewMedia Medicine Medical Appointment Scheduling Software
http://www.newmediamedicine.com/

ScheduleView Medical Appointment Software
http://www.scheduleview.com/

11

Medical Records Management

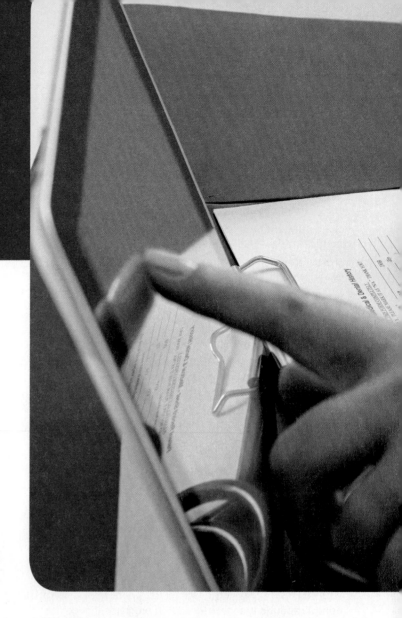

Case Study

Read the following case study and answer the critical thinking questions presented throughout the chapter.

When Melissa begins working for Dr. Kingsley, Caroline, one of the physician's longtime certified medical assistants, is charged with training her. One day, as Caroline looks up charts in the electronic health record system for patients scheduled for that afternoon, she finds an alert that comes up in Robert Olson's chart that reads, "Problem Patient." Caroline explains that the note alerts the certified medical assistants and the physician to patients who are "hard to work with." She says these patients complain, are late to their appointments, or are just generally unpleasant.

Objectives

After completing this chapter, you should be able to:

11.1 Define and spell the key terminology in this chapter.

11.2 List information contained in the medical record.

11.3 Describe the purpose of the medical record.

11.4 Discuss the importance of signing off on the medical record.

11.5 Explain various charting styles.

11.6 Explain why it is important for facilities to use a standard list of abbreviations in charting.

11.7 Describe how to correct an error in a patient chart.

11.8 Describe the steps to take when adding to the medical record.

11.9 Describe how to chart conflicting orders.

11.10 Discuss how to chart patient communication.

11.11 Describe the different types of filing systems used in medical facilities, and why each would be used.

11.12 List and describe the common types of file storage systems.

11.13 Differentiate between active, inactive, and closed patient files.

11.14 Describe the steps to take when converting paper records to electronic records.

11.15 Discuss guidelines pertaining to the retention of medical records.

11.16 Understand ownership of the medical record, and list the steps to take when patients want to make changes to their medical record.

11.17 Document prescription refill requests.

11.18 Describe the process used for releasing medical records in various situations.

11.19 Explain the importance of documenting medical research in the patient's medical record.

Key Terminology

active patient files—files for patients who have appointments or who have been in to see the physician recently

advance directives—documents that outline patients' wishes regarding health care should those patients be unable to speak for themselves

chief complaint—main reason a patient seeks care

closed patient files—files for patients who will not be returning to the clinic

cross-referencing—method of tracking and finding patient files for patients with multiple last names

electronic signature—electronic version of a person's signature to be used in electronic health records

financial information—data on payment record or ledger, health insurance identification numbers, and policy numbers

flow charts—graphs in patient medical records that track such things as weight gain or newborn growth

inactive patient files—files for patients who have not seen the physician for extended periods

indecipherable—unreadable

medical information—information on a patient's medical care and history

medical record—legal document consisting of medical information obtained from the patient via consultations, examinations, and tests

medical research program—research conducted to determine the effectiveness or harm of certain medications or medical treatments

narrative—type of medical charting in which the health care provider writes a narrative version of patient contact

nontherapeutic research—research programs that do not benefit the study's patients

obliterate—to make unreadable or unrecognizable

patient information—the information contained within the patient's medical record

personal information—information such as patient's name, birthdate, gender, marital status, occupation, next of kin, and any other items collected for personal identification

problem-oriented medical record charting—type of medical record charting that focuses on patients' health care problems and addresses those problems at each visit

progress notes—notes in a patient's medical chart outlining the patient's progress or complaints

purge—to remove closed or inactive patient medical records from the medical office

SOAP note charting—type of charting that considers the patient's subjective and objective findings, the provider's assessment of the patient's condition, and the prescribed plan of action for treatment

social information—information about a patient's social habits, such as tobacco, drug, or alcohol use

source-oriented medical record—type of charting that groups similar sections together

standard of care—legal term that describes the type of care a reasonable health care provider is expected to provide under the same situation

statute of limitations—period within which a patient must file a lawsuit after an injury

subpoena—court order demanding that a party appear in court or that copies of the medical record be sent to a third party

Abbreviations

EDP—electronic data processing

FDA—Food and Drug Administration

HIPAA—Health Insurance Portability and Accountability Act

NKA—no known allergies

PHI—protected health information

POMR—problem-oriented medical record

SOAP—subjective, objective, assessment, and plan

SOMR—source-oriented medical record

Certification Exam Coverage

AAMA (CMA) Exam Coverage:

- Documentation/reporting
  - Medical records
    1) Patient activity
    2) Patient care
    3) Patient confidentiality
    4) Ownership

AAMA (CMA) certification exam topics are reprinted with permission of the American Association of Medical Assistants.

- Releasing medical information
  - Consent
    1) Patient written authorization
    2) Federal codes
       a) Right to privacy
       b) Drug and alcohol rehabilitation records
       c) Public health and welfare disclosures
       d) HIV-related issues
  - Rescinding authorization for release

- Needs, purposes, and terminology of filing systems
  - Basic filing systems
    1) Alphabetic
    2) Numeric/terminal digit
    3) Subject
  - Special filing systems
    1) Color code
    2) Electronic data processing (**EDP**)
    3) Cross-reference/master file
- Filing guidelines
  1) Storing
  2) Protecting/safekeeping
  3) Transferring
- Medical records (paper/electronic)
  - Organization of patient's medical record
  - Types
    1) Problem-oriented
    2) Source-oriented
  - Collecting information
  - Making corrections
  - Retaining and purging
    1) Statute of limitations
- Documentation guidelines

AMT (CMAS) Exam Coverage:

- Systems
  - Demonstrate knowledge of, and manage patient medical records systems
  - Manage documents and patient charts using paper methods
- Procedures
  - File records alphabetically, numerically, by subject, and by color
  - Employ rules of indexing
  - Arrange contents of patients' charts in appropriate order
  - Document and file laboratory results and patient communication in charts
  - Perform corrections and additions to records
  - Store, protect, retain, and destroy records appropriately
  - Transfer files
  - Perform daily chart management
  - Prepare charts for external review and audits

- Confidentiality
  - Observe and maintain confidentiality of records, charts, and test results
  - Observe special regulations regarding the confidentiality of protected information

AMT (RMA) Exam Coverage:

- Documentation
  - Understand and utilize proper documentation of patient encounters and instruction
- Records and chart management
  - Manage patient medical record system
  - Record diagnostic test results in patient chart
  - File patient and physician communication in chart
    1) File materials according to proper system
    2) Chronological
    3) Alphabetical
    4) Problem-oriented medical records (POMR)
    5) Subject
  - Protect, store, and retain medical records according to proper conventions and HIPAA privacy regulations
  - Prepare and release private health information as required, adhering to state and federal guidelines
  - Identify and employ proper documentation procedures adhering to standard charting guidelines

NCCT (NCMA) Exam Coverage:

- General office procedures
  - Organizational skills
  - Medical record keeping

Competency Skills Performance

1. Prepare the medical chart.
2. Chart patient telephone calls.
3. File documents using the alphabetic filing system.
4. File manually using a subject filing system.
5. File documents in patient medical records.
6. Use the numeric system to file medical records.
7. Correct errors in the patient medical record.

Introduction

Medical records play an important role in health care delivery, so they must be accurate and complete. Health care providers rely on patients' medical records as accurate depictions of patients. With the patient's consent, medical records are often sent between physicians and hospitals to give physicians a complete picture of a patient's medical history.

As legal documents, medical records are often the single most important tools health care providers can use to defend against medical malpractice lawsuits. Risk management and quality improvement programs rely on medical records to catch errors in patient care. Insurance companies often request copies of patient medical records to determine the appropriateness of billing codes and reimbursement levels. Medical records that are incomplete or **indecipherable** may cause problems in patient care.

Medical offices have been moving from paper medical records to electronic health records since a government mandate to do so by 2015 was enacted. This mandate included financial incentives to health care providers and facilities in the form of higher reimbursement to those using electronic health records, instead of paper charts. This penalty is a 1 percent reduction in Medicare reimbursement for 2015, and the penalty increases by 1 percent every year beyond that if the provider does not move to electronic health records. Because some smaller medical offices continue to use paper medical charts, their use is covered in this chapter. Even when moving to electronic health records, many items continue to come into the medical facility in paper form. These items include reports from other physicians, copies of laboratory work, and letters from insurance companies, as examples. Medical assistants need to know how to address these paper items, either with a paper medical record, or an electronic one.

Information Contained in the Medical Record

Medical records include four types of **patient information**: (1) **personal information**, (2) **financial information**, (3) **medical information**, and (4) **social information**. Personal information is the information patients supply when first seeing the physician for care. Such information includes a patient's name, birthdate, gender, marital status, occupation, next of kin, and any other items collected for personal identification. Personal information may also include any comments the medical assistant might write in the patient's file regarding the patient's language or cultural background, if such information pertains to the patient's health care, and any accommodations that might be needed to provide that patient with care.

A patient's financial information includes a patient's ledger and insurance information, which includes policy and identification numbers and insurance-plan contact information, as well as any other information needed to bill the insurance company for the patient's care. In many medical offices, some portion of the patient's financial information is kept in a separate file from medical information. Financial information also includes copies of insurance company correspondence, and signed authorizations from the patient allowing the medical provider to release information to the insurance company.

Medical information includes the **chief complaint**, or the main reason a person seeks care; any family medical history; the patient's medical history; the results of examinations; the physical examination form; the prescribed course of treatment, including any medications or referrals; immunization records; and the patient's diagnoses, progress notes, operative reports, radiology reports, laboratory reports, and any other reports or information that pertains to the patient's health care (**Figure 11-1 ▪**).

Social information is any personal information on the patient, such as race and ethnicity, hobbies, and regular sports participation. Social information also includes such lifestyle choices as smoking, alcohol consumption, drug use, and sexual habits.

In addition to personal, financial, medical, and social information, other documents are routinely part of the patient's medical record. These documents include the **HIPAA** understanding form, which indicates the patient has been notified of the office's privacy policies; the HIPAA release form which authorizes the medical provider to discuss the patient's care with other parties; documents from hospitalizations; and any items the patient brings to the appointment, such as a list of current medications or copies of information from other medical providers' files.

▶▶▶ Pulse Points

Obtaining Sensitive Patient Information

Patients sometimes refuse to divulge such private information as Social Security number or birthdate or such lifestyle information as smoking, drinking, or drug habits. Let these patients know that anything in their medical records is confidential and cannot be released to anyone without the patients' written consent or a court order. When patients remain uneasy, notify the physician. Notification gives physicians an opportunity to discuss issues with patients and decide if they wish to treat those patients—if those patients continue to refuse to provide the requested information.

OPERATION DATE: 8/11/xx

PATIENT: ADAM PARCHER

SURGEON: MARIA FERNANDEZ-RAUL, MD

PREOPERATIVE DIAGNOSIS;
Congenital external nasal deformity.

POSTOPERATIVE DIAGNOSIS:
Congenital external nasal deformity.

PROCEDURE:
Aesthetic rhinoplasty

DESCRIPTION OF PROCEDURE:
The patient is a 33-year-old male who presented with concerns for nasal airway obstruction and discontent with the external appearance of his nose. Examination confirms the above-noted concerns with a widened nasal base, palpable and visible dorsal cartilage and nasal bones.

Correction of the external deformity by open rhinoplasty, lowering of the dorsum, lowering of the cartilaginous dorsum, narrowing of the nasal bones, resection and narrowing of the nasal tip, excision of caudal septum and nasal spine were discussed. The nature of the procedures and risks, including bleeding, hematoma, infection, poor wound healing, scarring, asymmetry, airway difficulties, palpable or visible nasal structures and possible need for secondary procedures were all discussed. The patient understands and wishes to proceed as outlined.

FINDINGS:
The patient underwent open rhinoplasty through a columellar chevron incision. The nose was copiously infiltrated with 1% lidocaine with epinephrine prior to incision. The chevron incision was incised and carried to bilateral rim incisions. The nasal skin was then degloved using sharp dissecting scissors. This was opened over the nose up to the root of the nose to allow full exposure. The irregular nasal bones were initially smoothed with a rasp. Excision of the dorsal nasal bone was then carried out using a straight guarded osteotome. Approximately 1 mm thickness of bone was removed. After osteotomy was completed from a low to high position, infracture of the nasal bones was carried out. This provided good narrowing of the nasal base. A small piece of septal cartilage was crushed and flattened using the cartilage crusher and this was placed over the nasal dorsum. Hemostasis was assured. The skin was redraped and closure was carried out using interrupted 6-0 Prolene for the columellar and stab incisions. Interrupted 5-0 plain gut sutures were used to close the rim incisions and the septal transfixion incision. Xeroform packs were removed and nasal splints were placed. A second set of Xeroform packs was placed lateral to the nasal splints. The dorsum of the nose was taped and a dorsal thermoplast splint was also placed. The procedure was well tolerated. The posterior throat was suctioned and a throat pack that had been placed at the beginning of the procedure was removed. The patient was awakened and extubated and discharged to the recovery room in stable condition.

Maria Fernandez-Raul, MD

Figure 11-1 ■ Sample operative report.

The Purpose of the Medical Record

A patient's medical record documents a patient's treatment plan and goals, whether the record is in paper or electronic form. The medical record must contain a full account of all patient treatment, including what treatment was given and why it was given, or if treatment was withheld and why.

In whatever form, medical records must be complete, accurate, organized, concise, timely, and factual. They should never contain opinions or judgments about patients. Whenever medical records are **subpoenaed** for trials, physicians might have to explain notations. A jury who thinks a physician is judgmental or unkind could hand down an unfavorable verdict. In addition, unprofessional notations might predispose other health care professionals to treat patients differently. The best way to keep medical charting professional is to always write as if the patient will be reading the comments. Anything the medical assistant would not say to the patient should remain out of the patient's medical record.

Critical Thinking Question 11-1

Recall the case study at the beginning of this chapter. How could typing "Problem Patient" in the patient's chart work against the physician's office? How might information like this be documented in the chart?

Risk management departments use medical records to determine if the **standard of care** has been met. The standard of care states that a health care provider must use reasonable and necessary skill when caring for patients, the same care another provider with the same training would use in the same circumstances. The best defense against malpractice claims is a well-kept, accurate medical record. Some civil cases have held health care providers liable for their failure to maintain proper records.

Some health care providers might review patient medical records as part of consultation visits or "second opinions." Others will review medical records when patients transfer to other offices.

When a patient has completed an **advance directive**, a copy of that document should be placed in the patient's medical record. Advance directives outline the patient's wishes should he be unable to speak or make sound decisions for himself. Examples include a do-not-resuscitate order, or a health care power of attorney.

Medical records are frequently used to determine reimbursement. The coding professionals who work in the medical office will often review the medical record in order to determine the proper code to use for billing purposes. This is another reason why proper documentation in the medical record is so important.

Signing Off on Medical Records

Any entry in a patient's medical record must have an identifying mark indicating the person who made the entry. Policies on this will vary from one medical office to the next, but the minimum should be no less than the initials and credentials of the person making the entry. Some medical offices require a complete signature along with credentials; others allow a first initial, last name, and credentials (**Figure 11-2** ■). In medical offices where the initials or partial signature of the medical

staff is allowed in charting, the office needs to keep documentation on file of the full name of the person who is using her initials or partial signature.

Any time a medical record contains a signature with initials rather than the full name, the medical office must keep a permanent record of the signer. In Figure 11-2, for example, Sara Mendoza's full signature must be on file in the administrative office so that her initials "SPM" or partial name "S. Mendoza" can be easily mapped to Sara Mendoza.

An office that uses electronic health records may use an **electronic signature**. In offices where medical notes are dictated and printed for patient files, an electronic signature or rubber-stamp signature may replace handwritten signatures. Again, a permanent record of the signer, as well as an original version of the signature, must be on file.

▶▶▶ Pulse Points

Documenting the Patient's Medical Record

The phrase in health care that states, "If it wasn't charted, it wasn't done," means that, as far as the law is concerned, anything that is not documented in a patient's medical record did not happen. Similarly, anything that is charted in a record did happen from a legal standpoint. Therefore, the medical assistant must ensure medical records are comprehensive and accurate, because even the smallest omission or incorrect statement can cause a host of problems, including malpractice lawsuits, incorrect patient care, patient injury, and miscommunication between health care providers.

Forms of Charting

Just as medical offices vary, so, too, do the methods of inserting information into medical records. Preference in style may be dictated by the type of practice, or may depend on whether the office is using paper or electronic health records.

Medical charting must adhere to the following "Five Cs rule," which state that patient charts must be:

- **Concise**—Patient charts must be to the point and contain no entries that fail to relate to the patient's health care in some way.
- **Complete**—Medical records must be complete and objective. All pertinent information must be included while opinions and judgments are excluded.
- **Clear**—Handwritten patient information should be printed, not written in cursive, and delivered in a clear, easy-to-read manner.
- **Correct**—Medical records must be error free. Errors include both improper additions and omissions. When errors are made, they must corrected by their creator as soon as possible.
- **Chronologic**—Medical records should be in chronologic order, with the latest entries on top.

Initials only—*SPM, CMA (AAMA)*
Full signature—*Sara P. Mendoza, CMA (AAMA)*
Variation—*S. Mendoza, CMA (AAMA)*

Figure 11-2 ■ Sample sign-off signatures.

PROCEDURE 11-1 Prepare the Medical Chart

Theory and Rationale

Every patient in the medical office must have a medical chart. In many ambulatory clinics today, electronic health charts are more common than paper versions. Until paper charts become obsolete, administrative medical assistants must be aware of how to prepare them.

Materials

- Medical chart
- Metal file clips
- Medication record sheet
- Progress notes record
- Color-coded alphabet stickers
- File label
- Two-hole punch
- Patient's name

Competency

1. Print the patient's name on a file label, with the last name followed by first name and middle initial. For example, print "Smith, John R." on the file label.
2. Verify the spelling of the patient's name.

3. Using the color-coded alphabet stickers, place the first two letters of the patient's last name on the file near the file label. In the preceding example, "SM" stickers would appear near the file label.
4. One space after the stickers in the preceding step, place a color-coded alphabet sticker for the first letter of the patient's first name. Building on the preceding example for John R. Smith, the file stickers would read "SM [space] J."
5. Add metal file clips to both sides of the file.
6. Using the two-hole punch, punch holes in the top of the documents to be filed in the patient's chart. These documents include the patient's history form, the Health Insurance Portability and Accountability Act (HIPAA) notification form, and the patient's consent to be examined.
7. Place the medication record sheet on one side of the chart.
8. Place the progress report sheet on the other side of the chart.
9. On the front of the chart in red ink, note any of the patient's known allergies. When the patient has no known allergies, write "**NKA**" (i.e., no known allergies) on the front of the chart.

The Narrative Style

Narrative notes are simply descriptions of patients' visits that are written out, rather than entered into sections or noted on forms or in boxes. As one of the oldest forms of medical charting, narratives are chronological. Findings of the visit appear with the doctor's instructions or prescriptions. Many physicians dictate their narrative notes about patient care, which are then transcribed and placed in the patients' files, although narratives can be manual or electronic (**Figure 11-3** ■). In some offices, physicians underline or outline certain terms in narrative notes to add emphasis.

Charting with SOAP

SOAP note charting is a method that tracks the subjective, objective, assessment, and plan (**SOAP**) for a patient's visit. Subjective findings include patient statements, including any information about the chief complaint. This section would include any quotes the patient makes about his condition ("My back feels as if I have a heavy weight on it"), and any other information provided by the patient regarding the duration and intensity of the complaint.

Objective findings are observations by the medical assistant and the health care provider, examination findings, and patient vital signs. This section would include the results of

any tests performed, such as orthopedic or neurological tests, and any visual examination findings made by the physician, such as rashes the patient is exhibiting or the fact that the patient winces when the physician touches a certain body part.

The assessment of the patient is the doctor's diagnosis, possible diagnosis, or the diagnosis that the physician wishes to rule out for that visit. If the physician can make the diagnosis at the time of the visit, the assessment will include that information. An example would be an assessment of "eczema" when the physician can clearly see this condition on the patient. If the physician must access certain test results before she can make a definitive diagnosis, the assessment might list "possible pneumonia" while the physician waits to see the patient's chest X-ray to make a definitive diagnosis.

The plan is the health care provider's prescribed plan of action, which includes any prescriptions, tests, instructions, or referrals to other providers or therapies. This section will include any information about both prescription and over-the-counter medications, herbal remedies, or diet plans the physician has recommended for the patient.

The SOAP method of charting is extremely popular and easy to use. By clearly identifying the four areas in the SOAP format, anyone reading the notes can easily locate information within the patient medical record notes (**Figure 11-4** ■).

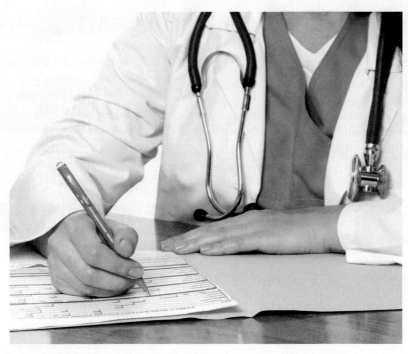

Figure 11-3 ■ Physician documenting in a handwritten chart note.
Source: Fotolia © shefkate.

Problem-Oriented Medical Record Charting

Problem-oriented medical record charting (POMR) tracks a patient's problems throughout his or her medical care. This charting system was originally designed by Dr. Lawrence Weed and is sometimes called the Weed System. Each problem is assigned a number, and that number is referenced when the patient comes in for care. Advocates for POMR charting believe that charting according to patients' problems renders

PROGRESS NOTES									
Patient's name: Jessica Lopez								Page: 1	
Date	Problem Number	**S**	**O**	**A**	**P**	S = Subjective	O = Objective	A = Assessment	P = Plan
3/12/xx	1	"I'm having dizzy spells and have not been taking my BP med."							
			BP 170/110 both arms, lying down, sitting & standing; WT. 202#						
				Hypertension					
					Rx for Norvasc 5mg daily; to monitor BP and return in 1 week				
					for BP check; placed on 1200 calorie diet to lose 20#				

Figure 11-4 ■ Sample SOAP note charting.

NAME		AGE	
OCCUPATION		SOC. SEC.#	

	BLOOD PRESSURE	VISION Without Glasses	Diagnostic Tests	Results
Height _____	**Sitting**	Far R^{20}/ L^{20}/		
Weight _____	R / :L /	Near R / L /		
Build _____	**With Glasses**			
(Sm.Med.Lg.Obese.)	**Standing**	Far R^{20}/ L^{20}/		
Pulse _____	R / :L /	Near R / L /		
Resp. _____		**Tonometry** R ___ L ___		
Temp. _____	**Lying**	**Colorvision** _____ (Ishihara plates missed)		
	R / :L /	**Peripheral Fields** R ___ L ___		

AUDIOMETRIC TESTING	250 500 1000 2000 4000 8000
	R ___ ___ ___ ___ ___ ___
	L ___ ___ ___ ___ ___ ___
	Gross Hearing _____

PULMONARY FUNCTION

Initial Problem List

_____

_____

_____

_____

_____

_____

_____

_____

_____

_____

_____

_____

_____

_____

_____

_____

_____

_____

Employment status _____	Physician's signature _____
	DATE _____

Figure 11-5 ■ Sample medical history sheet used by the physician to list patient problems.

health care providers less likely to overlook previous problems. For example, assume Horatio Black arrives for an initial appointment with Dr. Stella Bartlett. When Horatio arrives, he mentions he has had trouble with back pain for the past year or so. He also states that he has been diagnosed as "borderline diabetic." The main reason for today's visit, however, is for Horatio to discuss problems with depression and sleeplessness.

Using the POMR method of charting, Dr. Bartlett would assign a number to each of the problems Horatio mentioned. She might assign the main reason for the visit, depression and sleeplessness, the number 1, Horatio's back pain number 2, and possible diabetes number 3. Each of these problems would have its own page in the medical chart so Dr. Bartlett can easily reference the problems at each visit. Once a condition is resolved, a notation is made so the doctor need not reference the problem on subsequent visits. As new problems arise, new numbers are assigned, and new pages are allotted for tracking the problems.

Figure 11-5 ■ is an example of a medical history sheet used by physicians to list patient problems.

Source-Oriented Medical Record Charting

Source-oriented medical records keep material together by subject matter. In this type of charting, all laboratory results, medication records, and operative reports would be kept together, and all progress notes would be similarly placed together in the chart. Information within the chart is kept in reverse chronological order, with the most recent additions to the chart found on top, or first in that section.

CHEDDAR Form of Charting

CHEDDAR is an acronym for medical personnel to follow in charting patient information. The acronym is as follows:

C: Chief Complaint—This is the main reason the patient is currently seeking care.

H—History of the present illness. This pertains to any history the patient has with the chief complaint.

E—Examination findings by the physician.

D—Details of any further problems or complaints the patient might be experiencing.

D—Drugs and dosages the patient might be on, to include both prescription medications and those purchased over the counter.

A—Assessment of the patient, to include diagnosis made by the physician.

R—Return visit information regarding the physician's advice for followup care.

Indexing in the Medical Record

Regardless of the format of charting used in the medical record, many medical offices use indexing within the medical record. This is the process of separating items or materials into different sections within the chart. Indexing may be used in facilities where more than one physician is seeing the same patient, using the same chart. Each physician may have his information on the patient indexed into a separate section from the other physician's information. In a paper chart, this may be done using a tabbed divider to separate items. Within an electronic health record, the data may be kept under separate tabs in the medical chart.

Inserting Flow Charts in Medical Records

Flow charts are visual tools that help track certain information in patients' medical records. An example is the growth of children. Each time the physician sees an infant, the clinical medical assistant will measure the child's weight, length, and head circumference and make notations on a flow chart that the physician can then use when discussing any concerns with the child's parent or guardian (**Figure 11-6 ■**). Using these charts, physicians are able to project the expected adult height of the child.

Progress Notes

Progress notes are daily chart notes made during patient visits that document a patient's progress or status with certain conditions. Assume a patient arrives for an appointment complaining of fatigue. On the patient's subsequent visits, progress notes would outline the patient's current condition, any treatment recommendations, and outcomes. Depending on the office, progress notes may be made in SOAP, **SOMR**, POMR, CHEDDAR, or narrative format. The notes may also be handwritten or electronic.

Transcription in Charting

Many medical offices today use electronic health records for charting patient care. With most electronic health records, the user can either type patient information using abbreviations or drop-down menus, or use speech recognition software that translates the spoken word into written form.

Transcription of the spoken word or the handwritten word is done in some medical offices. With these systems, someone other than the physician types what the physician says into the audio dictation system, or what the physician hand writes, into the patient's chart. Because the person who transcribes the dictation or notes does not need to be onsite, transcriptionists may work from home—materials are faxed or sent via electronic means to the transcriptionist—or they might be located outside the United States. Performing medical transcription for American health care organizations is a large business in countries such as India and the Philippines.

Using Abbreviations in Charting

Given that abbreviations can lead to confusion in health care, or even errors in patient care, medical assistants must be extremely careful when using abbreviations in patients' charts and ensure that the abbreviations are accepted by their facilities. Because different facilities may use different abbreviations for medical terms, when in doubt, assistants should write out rather than abbreviate words. For example, one office might use the abbreviation "cx" to mean appointment cancellation. Another office might use the same abbreviation to indicate a cancer diagnosis.

Confusion among abbreviations can be avoided with a standard list of abbreviations between facilities. With the goal of patient safety in mind, The Joint Commission (TJC) publishes a list of abbreviations that should never be used, so that miscommunication is minimized.

Table 11-1 lists common medical abbreviations.

Critical Thinking Question 11-2

What are the potential implications of abbreviations for "problem" patients? How does this approach compare to full notes on patient charts, as described in the chapter-opening case study?

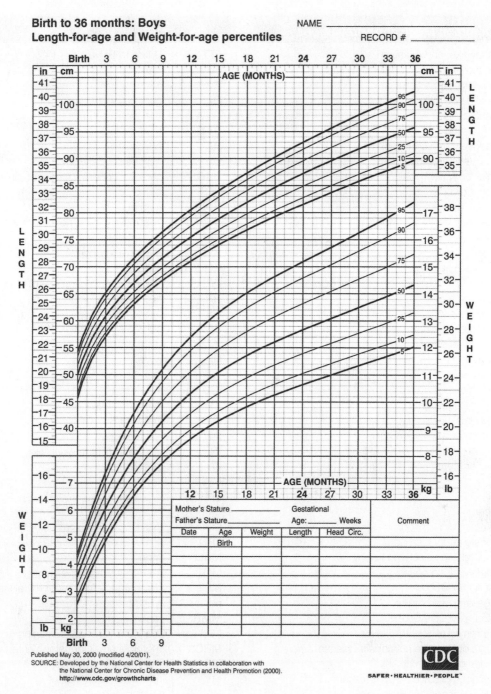

Birth to 36 months: Boys
Length-for-age and Weight-for-age percentiles

NAME _____

RECORD # _____

Published May 30, 2000 (modified 4/20/01).
SOURCE: Developed by the National Center for Health Statistics in collaboration with
the National Center for Chronic Disease Prevention and Health Promotion (2000).
http://www.cdc.gov/growthcharts

Figure 11-6 ■ Sample growth chart.
Source: ww.cdc.gov

Correcting Medical Records

Medical records must be corrected lawfully, or it might appear that the medical office is trying to conceal an error in patient care. When errors do happen, they must be corrected as soon as possible. The correct way to address an error is to draw one line through the error, initial and date the correction, and write the correct information above or beside the inserted line (**Figure 11-7** ■).

When an error is an entire line or several lines in the patient chart, the entire portion of the entry that is in error should be struck with a line. When an entire entry is in error, which can happen if the medical assistant accidentally charts in the wrong patient's chart, the assistant should draw a line through the entire entry, make a notation such as "wrong patient's chart," and include the date and the medical assistant's initials and credentials. Only the person who made the error should correct the medical chart (**Figure 11-8** ■).

TABLE 11-1 Common Medical Abbreviations

AAO	alert, awake, and oriented	FTT	failure to thrive
A&O	alert and oriented	FU	followup
ABD	abdomen	Fx	fracture
ABG	arterial blood gas	GI	gastrointestinal
abs	absent	GSW	gunshot wound
AC	before eating	GTT	glucose tolerance test
ACLS	advanced cardiac life support	HA	headache
ADH	anti-diuretic hormone	HBP	high blood pressure
adm	admission	HCG	human chorionic gonadotropin
ADR	adverse drug reaction	HCT	hematocrit
ad lib	as much as needed	HDL	high density lipoprotein
AFP	alpha-fetoprotein	HEENT	head, eyes, ears, nose, throat
amb	ambulatory	Hgb	hemoglobin
amt	amount	HIV	human immunodeficiency virus
ant	anterior	HO	history of
ante	before	H&P	history and physical examination
AOB	alcohol on breath	HR	heart rate
AP	anteroposterior	HS	at bedtime
ASAP	as soon as possible	HSV	herpes simplex virus
BCP	birth control pills	HTN	hypertension
BE	barium enema	Hx	history
bid	twice a day	I&D	incision and drainage
BM	bowel movement	ICU	intensive care unit
BMR	basal metabolic rate	ID	infectious disease
BP	blood pressure	IG	immunoglobulin
BPH	benign prostatic hypertrophy	IM	intramuscular
BPM	beats per minute	INF	intravenous nutritional fluid
BS	bowel or breath sounds	IV	intravenous
BX	biopsy	L	left
c	with	LLL	left lower lobe
CA	cancer	LMP	last menstrual period
Ca	calcium	LOC	loss of consciousness or level of consciousness
CAD	coronary artery disease	LPN	licensed practical nurse
CAT	computerized axial tomography	MAO	monoamine oxidase
CBC	complete blood count	MBT	maternal blood type
CC	chief complaint	MI	myocardial infarction or mitral insufficiency
CHF	congestive heart failure	mL	milliliter
CNS	central nervous system	MMR	measles, mumps, rubella
C/O	complaining of	MRI	magnetic resonance imaging
COPD	chronic obstructive pulmonary disease	MRSA	methicillin resistant staph aureus
CP	cerebral palsy	MS	multiple sclerosis
CPAP	continuous positive airway pressure	MVA	motor vehicle accident
CPR	cardiopulmonary resuscitation	NG	nasogastric
CT	computerized tomography	NKA	no known allergies
CVA	cerebrovascular accident	NKDA	no known drug allergies
CXR	chest X-ray	NMR	nuclear magnetic resonance
DC	discontinue or discharge	NPO	nothing by mouth
DNR	do not resuscitate	NSAID	nonsteroidal anti-inflammatory drugs
DOA	dead on arrival	NSR	normal sinus rhythm
DTR	deep tendon reflexes	OB	obstetrics
DVT	deep venous thrombosis	OPV	oral polio vaccine
DX	diagnosis	OR	operating room
ECG	electrocardiogram	PA	posteroanterior
EMG	electromyogram	PC	after eating
ENT	ears, nose, and throat	PDR	*Physician's Desk Reference*
FBS	fasting blood sugar	PE	physical exam

(continued)

TABLE 11-1 Common Medical Abbreviations (*continued*)

PKU	phenylketonuria	TB	tuberculosis
PMH	previous medical history	tid	three times a day
PO	by mouth	TIG	tetanus immune globulin
PR	by rectum	TMJ	temporo mandibular joint
PRN	as needed	TNTC	too numerous to count
PT	prothrombin time, or physical therapy	TO	telephone order
Pt	patient	TPN	total parenteral nutrition
PTT	partial thromboplastin time	TSH	thyroid stimulating hormone
PUD	peptic ulcer disease	TT	thrombin time
q	every (e.g., q6h = every 6 hours)	Tx	treatment
qd	every day	UA	urinalysis
qh	every hour	UAO	upper airway obstruction
qid	four times a day	UBD	universal blood donor
qod	every other day	URI	upper respiratory infection
R	right	US	ultrasound
RA	rheumatoid arthritis	UTI	urinary tract infection
RBC	red blood cell	VO	verbal order
R/O	rule out	WBC	white blood cell
ROM	range of motion	WD	well developed
ROS	review of systems	WF	white female
RTC	return to clinic	WM	white male
s	without	WNL	within normal limits
SOAP	subjective, objective, assessment, plan	WO	written order
SOB	shortness of breath	yo	years old
SQ	subcutaneous	YOB	year of birth
STAT	immediately	yr	year
Sx	symptoms	ytd	year to date
T&C	type and cross		

Errors in medical charts should never be **obliterated**, scribbled out, or covered with correction fluid, because records with such effects are viewed as an attempt to hide the truth or cover wrongdoing. One line through an incorrect entry leaves no doubt as to the information being corrected.

Critical Thinking Question 11-3

Refer back to the case study at the beginning of the chapter. Imagine that the medical office has decided to discontinue notes like "Problem Patient" in patient charts. How should the office go about removing such notes from patient files?

Adding to Medical Records

When an error in a medical chart is one of omission, information may be added to the medical record after the fact by beginning the entry with the date the addition is being added, followed by the words "Late Entry," the date of the visit the late entry pertains to, the notes that were originally omitted, and the signature of the person making the entry. When a correction exceeds the space where the error is, the medical assistant can insert an addendum to the medical record. This insertion should read "ADDENDUM to [date of the visit]" just before the entry. The use of all capitals is significant in such entries. Table 11-2 provides examples.

> 1/10/xx CMJ, CMA (AAMA)
> 1/10/xx Patient complains of pain in her ~~left~~ right hand, constant for the past 2 days.
> C. Jones, CMA (AAMA)

Figure 11-7 ■ Sample correction of a charting error.

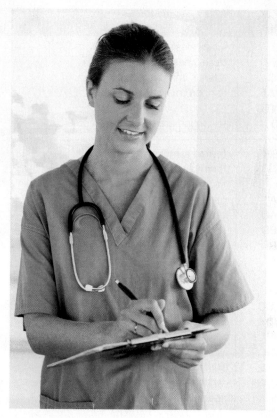

Figure 11-8 ■ The medical assistant must chart accurately.
Source: Shutterstock © wavebreakmedia.

TABLE 11-2 Additions to the Medical Record

Addition Type	Example
Late entry	Oct. 3, 2014 LATE ENTRY for Sept. 25, 2014: Patient stated she was unable to fill her prescription due to cost. *S. Nguyen*, CMA
Addendum	Oct. 2, 2014 ADDENDUM for Sept. 25, 2014: Ms. Manfredo stated she had been involved in an automobile accident on Sept. 24, 2014. She was seen in the emergency room of Brattleboro Community Hospital. Ms. Manfredo stated, "The pain in my right arm was so bad I could not put on my jacket." *S. Nguyen*, CMA

why the orders will not cause patient injury, the medical assistant should chart the events, including the fact that she questioned the doctor as to the accuracy of the orders. She should also include the physician's response.

Charting Patient Communication

Communications with a patient outside of office visits must be documented in the patient's chart when that communication is medically relevant. Such communication includes telephone calls or e-mails from the patient that relate to the patient's medical care, to missed or cancelled appointments, or to requests from pharmacies to refill prescriptions. It is important to accurately chart all such exchanges in a patient's medical records. Each office should have a policy regarding the type of communication that requires charting, and all members of the health care team should closely follow that policy.

Charting Conflicting Orders

Every member of the health care team is obligated to take reasonable action to ensure patient safety. The medical assistant should follow no orders she feels might harm a patient. Instead, she should consult the physician out of the range of the patient's hearing. When the physician insists that the orders be followed according to instructions, and explains

 PROCEDURE 11-2 Correct Errors in the Patient Medical Record

Theory and Rationale

Medical assistants regularly make notations and entries in patients' medical records. When assistants make errors, they must follow legal protocol to correct those errors.

Materials

- Patient medical record
- Blue or black ink pen

Competency

1. Locate the error in the patient's medical record.

2. Draw a straight line through the error.
3. Initial and place the date above the line.
4. When the corrected entry will fit above the line, write the correction there. Include the date of the new entry and your initials. When the corrected entry will not fit above the line, add a new entry to the progress notes with the day's date and the word "ADDENDUM" in all capitals. Include the date of the addendum, enter the corrected entry, and initial the entry.

PROCEDURE 11-3 Chart Patient Telephone Calls

Theory and Rationale

Patient telephone calls are frequently noted in patients' medical records. Chart notes such as these help to safeguard the medical office from malpractice claims and/or misunderstandings. Medical offices should have clear policies for charting patient calls, and medical assistants should understand their offices' policies.

Materials

- Notepad and pen
- Paper or electronic patient medical record

Competency

1. While answering an incoming patient call, determine if the call is medically relevant to the patient's care in the office.
2. When the call is medically relevant to the patient's care, note the call's time and date, the patient's complete

name and telephone number, and the nature of the message.

3. When the call ends, bring up the chart electronically in the electronic health record, or pull the patient's chart.
4. In the progress notes section of the patient's chart, note the current date and time.
5. Enter the medically relevant portion of the call in the patient's medical record, using quotation marks to indicate any direct quotes from the patient.
6. Sign or enter your name and credentials at the end of the chart entry.
7. When the call requires the physician's attention, leave the paper chart on the physician's desk or forward the electronic message to the physician in the electronic health record. When the call does not require the physician's attention, file or close the chart.
8. After transferring all relevant information to the chart, shred any notes from the call that contain personal patient information.

Such chart notes help to safeguard the medical office from malpractice claims or misunderstandings.

While thoroughness is important, not all patient conversations merit charting. Medical assistants should use their best judgment to determine if conversations are medically relevant. Calls from patients questioning their medical bill, for example, are not considered medically relevant. Calls from patients stating they will not return for care because they cannot afford to pay, as an example, are medically relevant and should be documented in the patient's chart, as well as brought to the physician's attention.

 ## In Practice

Dylan McElvaney, RMA, has taken a telephone call from Lynn Kinney, a patient in the office. Lynn states she is very unhappy with the office because she has been waiting for three days for her laboratory results to be conveyed to her. She says she won't be coming back to the office and will be calling to have copies of her medical file sent to another facility. What should Dylan say to Lynn? How should Dylan chart this telephone call in Lynn's medical record?

Filing Systems

Most medical offices use one of two types of filing systems: 1) alphabetic or 2) numeric. While alphabetic is far more common overall, numeric filing is more common in facilities where patient treatment records must be kept extremely

confidential, such as in facilities specializing in mental health, **HIV** or AIDS treatment, or reproductive health care.

Alphabetic Filing

In alphabetic filing, patient information is filed alphabetically by last name. In order to easily identify if a patient chart is filed incorrectly, offices using alphabetic filing of paper charts will use color-coded alphabetic stickers on the outside of patients' charts (**Figure 11-9** ■). Color coding causes misfiled charts to stand out. Some offices file according to the first two letters of the patient's last name. With this system, a patient named Shannon Nelson would have alphabetic stickers "NE" on the chart. Other offices use the patient's first and last name initials. In that system, Shannon Nelson's chart would contain alphabetic stickers "SN." Still other offices use a portion of the patient's last name and the first initial of the first name. In this system, Shannon Nelson's chart might have the alphabetic stickers "NE" and "SH" to indicate the first two letters of her first and last names.

Patients with hyphenated last names can confuse filing practices in medical offices. When a patient's last name is Morris-Davidson, for example, some staff might file the patient's chart under the first part of the hyphenated name, Morris, while other staff might file according to the latter part, which is Davidson. To avoid confusion, medical offices should have clear policies for filing the charts of patients with hyphenated names and strictly follow those policies.

Unfortunately, even with clear policies, hyphenated names can still be confusing. A patient with the last name Morris-Davidson may go by Morris on some occasions yet use Morris-Davidson or even Davidson at others. **Cross-referencing**

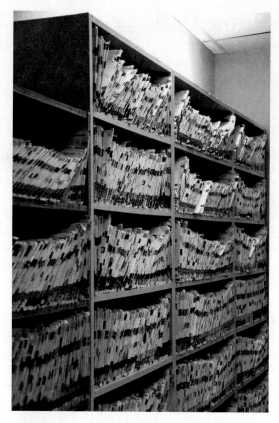

Figure 11-9 ■ Using color-coded labels enables the medical assistant to quickly locate a misfiled chart.
Source: Shutterstock © Elena Elisseeva.

files with cards that direct staff to proper files can help address such variations. In the case of Morris-Davidson, for example, the patient's original medical record would be filed under the correct full name of Morris-Davidson, and a blank patient file labeled with the name's other combinations would be filed under Morris and Davidson. Under this system, if the patient called and identified herself as "Mrs. Ann Davidson," the medical assistant would look in the "Davidson" file and find a

blank file that said "Ann Morris-Davidson's file is under Morris-Davidson."

Numeric Filing

Some patient files, such as those in offices devoted to HIV or AIDS–related care, mental health, pregnancy or family planning, or alcohol and drug rehabilitation, may demand a higher level of security. Numeric filing is often used in these types of offices. In a numeric filing system, patient charts are assigned a number and filed by that number, rather than by the patient's name. For example, the chart for Jeff Mooney might have been assigned numeric file number 22490. Jeff's chart would be filed numerically under the number 22490. Because the numeric system masks the identity of patients, it is difficult to retrieve filed information without the proper number. Someone searching for Jeff Mooney's chart would not likely find it without knowing the numeric file number assigned to his chart. In offices that file with numeric systems, lists of patient names and corresponding numbers must be kept in a secure location for the systems to work.

Terminal Digit Filing System

In a terminal digit filing system, medical charts are assigned a numerical code and are filed according to that code. Most terminal digit filing systems consist of four numbers, each grouped into sets of two. The biggest disadvantage of using a terminal digit filing system is that users need to become accustomed to searching for and filing charts in reverse order, right to left, in groups of two digits. Files are ordered by the last two digits, then the first two digits. For example, the following three numbers would be filed as shown below. Example numbers: 3524, 6524, and 5424.

These numbers would be filed as 3524, 5424, then 6524.

Like numeric filing systems, terminal digit filing systems are typically used in facilities where the identity of the patient is highly guarded. An advantage to using a terminal digit filing system is that a misfiled chart stands out easily, just as a misfiled chart in an alphabetic system stands out.

 PROCEDURE 11-4 File Documents Using the Alphabetic Filing System

Theory and Rationale

Most medical facilities use the alphabetic method for filing patient medical record files. The medical assistant must pay close attention to detail and be certain files are filed accurately in order to ensure the file will be easily found when needed. Color coding helps misfiled charts stand out.

Materials

- Patient medical records
- Color-coded alphabetic file letter stickers

Competency

1. Using the color-coded alphabetic file letter stickers, apply stickers to each medical record using the patient's first two letters from the last name.

2. Arrange the medical records in alphabetical order by last name.

3. File the medical records accurately in the filing cabinet.

PROCEDURE 11-5 File Manually Using a Subject Filing System

Theory and Rationale

Medical facilities will often keep documents relating to various diseases or illnesses on file in the office. These documents may be given to patients as part of the education process.

Materials

- Documents to be filed by subject
- Alphabetic card file
- Index card listing subjects

Competency

1. Organize the documents by subject matter.
2. Match the subject of the document to the appropriate category on the index cards.
3. Underline the subject title on the document.
4. File the document under the appropriate category.
5. If the document fits into more than one category, create an index card as a cross-reference listing the name of the document and the category under which it is filed.

PROCEDURE 11-6 File Documents in Patient Medical Records

Theory and Rationale

A patient's medical record expands as new documents, test results, and consultations from other health care facilities are added to it. Often, the administrative medical assistant is responsible for filing documents in patients' medical records.

Materials

- Patient medical record
- Documents to be filed
- Two-hole punch

Competency

1. Using the two-hole punch, punch holes in the top of each document to be filed.
2. Verify that the physician has viewed any report to be filed (e.g., laboratory or pathology report) by locating the physician's initials on the report.
3. Verify that the patient file matches the name on the documents to be filed.
4. Using the metal clips in the file, place the documents in the patient medical record with the most recent documents on top.
5. Fasten the metal clips.

PROCEDURE 11-7 Use the Numeric System to File Medical Records

Theory and Rationale

Some medical facilities use the numeric method for filing patient medical record files. These facilities are typically ones where the patient medical information is considered to be of a highly sensitive nature. The medical assistant must pay close attention to detail and be certain files are filed accurately in order to ensure the file will be easily found when needed.

Materials

- Patient medical records
- Color-coded numeric file stickers

Competency

1. Using the color-coded numeric file stickers, attach the first two numbers of the patient's medical record number to the patient's medical record.
2. After verifying that the patient's identification number is accurately recorded on a master sheet kept away from the patient files, organize the records in numerical order.
3. File the medical records in numerical order into the medical records filing cabinet.

File Storage Systems

Most medical office filing systems consist of metal cabinets that hold paper patient charts in alphabetical order. Old-style filing cabinets were designed in a tower shape, with drawers that pulled out to reveal the files within. Other styles of freestanding filing cabinets have drawers that pull out to reveal the sides of files. These cabinets are useful for identifying files by their color-coded alphabetic or numeric tabs (**Figure 11-10** ◾).

Large medical offices often require large file storage systems. These offices use filing systems that allow the entire filing cabinet to move to access files. These types of filing systems take up less space than stationary models and are ideal for large facilities that must accommodate large numbers of paper files.

▸▸▸ Pulse Points

Misfiled Medical Information

When medical records are misplaced, look first under the patients' first names instead of their last. When the file for Krystle Shawger is not filed under "S" for "Shawger," for example, look under "K" for Krystle. If the file is not there, next determine when Krystle was last in the office. Identify the other patients who were in the office at the same time, and determine if Krystle's file was accidentally filed with one of those patient's files. Apply the same method to misfiled medical information. If, for example, Krystle's lab results are missing, check the files of patients who had lab work around the same time.

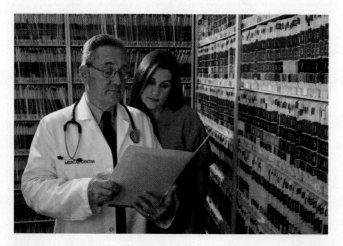

Figure 11-10 ◾ A medical office filing system.
Source: Shutterstock © Condor36.

Active, Inactive, and Closed Patient Files

Paper medical charts take up a lot of space, especially in large offices or offices where physicians have been in practice for long periods. Keeping all patient charts in the same filing system can be overwhelming and increases the time it takes to find a patient's file. For these reasons, many clinics **purge** inactive or closed patient files. This process entails moving medical files to other locations or perhaps scanning the documents in the files and then digitally storing the data on microfilm, microfiche, CD, DVD, or another electronic storage system. Once this process is done, the paper medical records can be destroyed. To purge properly, however, a clear policy on what constitutes a closed or inactive file must be written.

Most offices would agree that files for patients who actively have appointments or who have been in to see the physician recently are considered **active patient files**. **Inactive patient files** are normally those for patients who have not been in to see the physician for a period between two and five years depending on the type of practice, the number of files the practice must store, and the office policy. Removing inactive patient files leaves room for new patient files and makes finding active patient files easier.

The term *closed* is normally reserved for the files of patients who have moved and will not be continuing to treat with the physician or facility. It is also used to describe files for patients who are deceased or files for patients who have stated they will be discontinuing treatment in that facility. **Closed patient files** are normally moved to other storage systems, leaving the space available for active patient files. Patient files fluctuate among active, inactive, and closed status. A file that is considered active today may be closed tomorrow if the patient contacts the office to report an out-of-state move. That same file may return to active status if the patient moves back and resumes care in the medical office.

Converting Paper Records to Electronic Storage

Paper records can be converted to an electronic format for long-term storage. When this happens, the paper records are typically no longer needed. Paper records that are no longer needed must be destroyed so their information cannot be related to patients. Typically, paper records are shredded after copying or scanning (**Figure 11-11** ◾). All medical offices should have paper shredders to destroy confidential information. Shredding companies can complete large projects. These companies will shred documents and provide certifying notices to the medical office.

Even when medical offices use an electronic health record, papers containing sensitive patient information still remain. Patients will often bring in copies of paper records, for

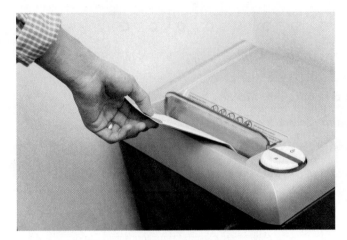

Figure 11-11 ■ Using a paper shredder ensures patient confidentiality.
Source: Shutterstock © sixninepixels.

example. Larger medical offices will use outside shredding companies to shred sensitive documents. These outside companies will provide secure bins for the gathering of sensitive documents needing to be shredded. At regular intervals, the company will send a truck to pick up the sensitive documents and shred them (**Figure 11-12** ■).

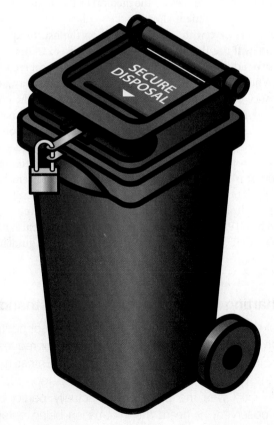

Figure 11-12 ■ A locked secure bin for collecting documents to be shredded.
Source: Shutterstock © Zern Liew.

Retaining Medical Records

State and federal regulations dictate how long medical records must be kept. To comply with those regulations, medical assistants should know the **statute of limitations** in the state where they practice and help their offices keep medical records at least as long as those statutes require. Patients can bring malpractice lawsuits during the statute of limitations, which typically begins when the injury occurs. In many states, however, the discovery rule can greatly alter the statute of limitations. The discovery rule states that the statute of limitations starts on the day the injury was discovered or should have been discovered. Take a patient who has had surgery during which the surgeon leaves a surgical sponge in the surgical site. This patient might fail to realize the medical error for some time. In states where the discovery rule applies, the statute of limitations would begin when the injury, the sponge in this case, is discovered, even if it is many years later. This rule can also apply to minors by beginning the statute of limitations on the day the minor child turns 18.

Medicare guidelines state that medical records must be retained for at least five years. Because the statute of limitations may exceed five years in some states, and because medical records are an extremely important part of defending any claim of medical negligence, it is a good idea to keep medical records for as long as possible. Once an office has no more storage space for medical record files, records can be scanned and kept on CDs, DVDs, microfilm, or in any other safe electronic format. In all forms, medical records must be stored in a secure environment, safe from any water or fire damage, and easily accessible by the health care team as needed.

HIPAA Compliance

HIPAA states that medical records must be kept confidential. A record can only be disclosed with a patient's consent or a court order. When it is determined appropriate to destroy a medical record, HIPAA dictates that the record must be shredded beyond recognition. It cannot be in a condition that allows it to be put back together to reveal personal patient information.

Ownership of the Medical Record

Medical records belong to the physicians or facilities where they are created. The information inside, however, belongs to the patients. Patients have a right to access their medical records and to correct those records when they feel errors have been made. Patients should not, however, be left alone to peruse their chart. When patients request corrections to their medical records, the health care team must determine whether

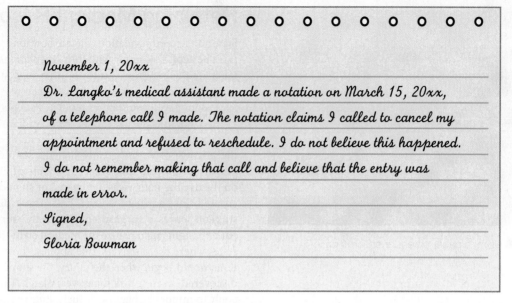

November 1, 20xx

Dr. Langko's medical assistant made a notation on March 15, 20xx, of a telephone call I made. The notation claims I called to cancel my appointment and refused to reschedule. I do not believe this happened. I do not remember making that call and believe that the entry was made in error.

Signed,

Gloria Bowman

Figure 11-13 ■ Sample addition to the medical record from the patient.

errors exist. If the physician agrees an error has been made, the correction should be made as described earlier in this chapter. If the physician feels the entry was not in error, the physician cannot be forced to treat the entry as an error. In this case, patients must be allowed to create their own version of the event, and copies of those written statements must be placed in the medical records (**Figure 11-13** ■). Such statements become permanent parts of the patients' medical records.

Documenting Prescription Refill Requests

Pharmacies call in prescription refill requests to the medical office. Each medical office should have a policy that requires at least 24 hours for refill requests so physicians have time to review patients' files.

When a pharmacy calls with a prescription request, the medical assistant must pull the patient's file and place the request and patient file on the physician's desk for review. If the physician feels the patient should be seen in the office before a prescription refill, the medical assistant should first call the pharmacy to notify them of the physician's request, and then call the patient to schedule an appointment. If the physician authorizes the refill request, the medical assistant should call the pharmacy back with the appropriate information. All information about the refill request, authorized or not, must be charted in the patient's medical record.

Releasing Medical Records

Requests for copies of the patient's medical record are common. These requests may come from insurance companies, other health care facilities, or from the patient. Any request for copies of the patient's medical record must be accompanied by a signed authorization from the patient or a court order.

Copies of the medical record cannot be released to anyone, including the patient's spouse, without the patient's consent. HIPAA legislation allows for the medical facility to obtain a signature from the patient allowing the medical office to discuss the patient's care with anyone named on the list. Frequently, patients will use this form to indicate they wish to have their spouse or adult child be given access to their medical record.

When copies of the chart are needed right away, some insurance companies or other entities may request the copies be faxed. It is important to note that faxing personal patient information should never be done unless it is absolutely necessary as use of the fax in this manner is not considered to be an appropriate way to safeguard patient confidential information. It is important for the medical assistant to remember that any data in the patient's medical record that identifies the patient or links the patient to the type of care received is protected by HIPAA legislation. A patient's protected health information (**PHI**) is specifically covered under HIPAA guidelines.

▸▸▸ Pulse Points

Charting Only What You Know Firsthand

Make entries to patient charts only after direct contract with patients. Do not chart what is shared or requested by other members of the health care team. Entries made in the patient's chart indicate that the person making the entry was the person who actually participated in, observed, or heard the information being entered. Medical assistants may be held responsible for entries made, and must be sure to only enter that information that they learn or observe firsthand.

Releasing Information When a Medical Practice Closes

When a medical practice closes and no other facility takes responsibility for the patient's medical records, notices must be sent to all patients with medical files at the facility. These notices should give patients a reasonable timeline within which to contact the office to request file transfers. Whether transfer requests are made or not, the physician or the physician's estate will be responsible for the original files for the period outlined by the state's statute of limitations.

Medical Records Used in Research

When patients participate in **medical research programs**, their medical records must be kept indefinitely. If adverse effects arise, even in subsequent generations, the medical office must be able to prove the physician had the patient's consent to participate in the research. Medical research involves patients taking experimental medication or their being involved in **nontherapeutic research**.

In nontherapeutic research, a pharmaceutical company develops a new drug to combat a certain disease or disorder. Before that company can market the drug, however, it must receive approval from the Food and Drug Administration (**FDA**). The FDA requires extensive testing before drugs are considered safe and effective enough to be released. Part of FDA testing usually includes a nontherapeutic research trial in which companies pay physicians to dispense the drug to healthy patients who do not have the disease or disorder the drug is targeting so as to identify any side effects. Patients in these types of research programs must be fully aware of the risks and must sign consent forms to that effect.

REVIEW

Chapter Summary

- Medical records are an integral piece in the health care process, so it is crucial that they are complete, accurate, and effective.
- The medical assistant must be aware of how to sign off on the medical record in order to properly indicate that he is the author of any notations he made in the record.
- Several different charting styles are found in health care, including alphabetic, numeric, and terminal digit. Each facility will mandate the type of charting to be used.
- Having a standard list of medical abbreviations in the medical office helps prevent errors in patient care.
- Medical offices should have systems in place to find missing files.
- Color-coded filing systems are one efficient way for offices to find patient information.
- Offices desiring a high level of security might choose a numeric filing system, as it masks patient identity.
- Depending on their size and intent, medical offices may choose varying file storage systems.
- Patient files fluctuate between active, inactive, and closed status as patients traverse the health care system.
- Medical records are often separated into different locations, based on whether the file is that of an active patient, an inactive patient, or a closed patient record. Each medical facility will have a definition of each of those categories for medical assistants to follow.
- Medical offices should correct errors in patient charts according to accepted protocol.
- Patients must be allowed to add corrections to their individual medical records in the event the patient feels there is an error in the chart.
- Prescription refills must be documented to indicate the patient's name, the medication name and dosage, frequency of dosing, and the pharmacy where the prescription was to be filled.
- Once a paper medical record has been converted into an electronic form, the paper record must be disposed of properly in order to maintain patient confidentiality.
- At times, physicians will participate in medical research and will use their patient files for this purpose. When a patient is on an experimental medication, or participating in any kind of medical research program, that information must be carefully documented in the patients' file.

Chapter Review

Multiple Choice

1. Which of the following is NOT one of the four types of patient information contained in medical records?
   a. Personal information
   b. Social information
   c. Geographic information
   d. Medical information
   e. a and b

2. Which of the following describes the patient's chief complaint?
   a. The main reason the patient is seeking care that day
   b. The most significant finding on the patient's exam
   c. The highest level diagnosis code assigned to the patient
   d. The most noticeable symptom the patient has
   e. The issue that takes the longest for the physician to resolve

3. Which of the following describes a reason a "late entry" might be made in a patient's chart?
   a. The medical assistant realizes he forgot to add a relevant fact into the patient's medical chart. He makes that entry the following day
   b. The patient asks the medical assistant to make a correction in the medical record
   c. The medical assistant realizes she has charted something in the wrong patient's file
   d. The medical assistant doesn't chart in the patient's chart until the end of her shift
   e. The physician asks the medical assistant to make an additional appointment for the patient

4. Which of the following type of medical record keeping is the oldest form of medical charting?
   a. SOAP format
   b. POMR
   c. Narrative style
   d. SOMR
   e. Progress notes

True/False

T F **1.** Flow charts are used to note a patient's progress relative to others in the population.

T F **2.** Numeric filing systems are more secure than alphabetic filing systems.

T F **3.** All medical facilities use the same medical abbreviations.

T F **4.** Nontherapeutic studies do not benefit the patient/subject.

T F **5.** Inactive patient files are typically those patients who have not been in to see the physician for a period of two to five years.

T F **6.** Health care facilities in all states must keep patient medical records on file for the same period of time.

T F **7.** The term *closed patient file* typically describes the file of patients who have moved or will not be continuing treatment with the physician or facility.

Short Answer

1. What is the most common reason for a cross-referencing system in the medical office?
2. Medical records should be faxed only under what circumstances?
3. What does the acronym POMR stand for?
4. Describe how a prescription refill request should be handled.
5. What are the "Five Cs" of medical charting?
6. What does the acronym SOAP stand for?
7. What information in the medical record is considered personal information?
8. Describe how a late entry should be charted in a patient's medical chart.
9. Outline the steps to take to locate a missing patient chart.

Research

1. Interview a person who works in a medical office. How does that office file patient files? Alphabetically or numerically? How are the files labeled? Are color-coded labels used?
2. Research online for local companies that offer shredding services. How much do they charge for their services? How do they guarantee confidentiality?
3. Look online for companies that sell filing systems to medical offices. What type of systems can you find? What type of system is more expensive?

Practicum Application Experience

Sylvia Bissey, a patient of Dr. Borshack's for over 20 years, tells the medical assistant that she would like to get a copy of her husband's current lab results. The medical assistant explains that she will need a signed authorization from Mr. Bissey in order to release the information to his wife. Sylvia becomes upset and says, "I have *always* been given copies of his lab results in the past." How should the medical assistant respond to Sylvia?

Resource Guide

Health Insurance Portability and Accountability Act (HIPAA) Web site
http://www.hhs.gov/ocr/hipaa/

The Institute of Medicine
http://www.iom.edu

iHealth Record Web site
http://www.ihealthrecord.org/
This Web site allows users/consumers to house their medical records online.

12

Electronic Health Records

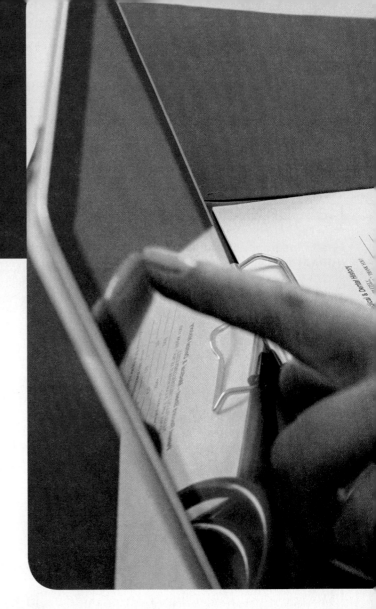

Case Study

Read the following case study and answer the critical thinking questions presented throughout the chapter.

Walter Reardon is a patient in Dr. Rand's office. Dr. Rand has recently converted his patient files from paper medical records to electronic health records. David is Dr. Rand's registered medical assistant. David escorts Mr. Reardon to the examination room and then begins to perform his initial assessment using the electronic health record he accesses from the computer in the examination room. When Mr. Reardon notices this, he becomes upset, saying he doesn't trust computers and doesn't want his private medical information "out there for everyone to see."

Objectives

After completing this chapter, you should be able to:

12.1 Define and spell the key terminology in this chapter.

12.2 Describe the function and uses of electronic health record (EHR) software.

12.3 Distinguish between the steps taken in the medical office to chart on paper versus those taken to chart electronically.

12.4 Describe how to convert from paper to electronic health records.

12.5 Discuss HIPAA compliance with regard to the use of electronic health records.

12.6 Describe the use of personal digital assistants with electronic health records.

12.7 List the benefits of using electronic health records.

12.8 Describe the steps to correct a mistake in the electronic health record.

Competency Skills Performance

1. Correct an electronic health record.

Key Terminology

electronic health record—medical record kept via computer; refers to a patient's entire medical history in electronic form

electronic signature—electronic version of a person's signature to be used in electronic health records

indecipherable—unreadable

meaningful use—an incentive program put in place by the Centers for Medicare and Medicaid Services (CMS) to promote the use of electronic health records in medical facilities

Abbreviations

CMS—Centers for Medicare and Medicaid Services

EHR—electronic health record

EMR—electronic medical record

HIPAA—Health Insurance Portability and Accountability Act

HITECH Act—Health Information Technology for Economic and Clinical Health Act

Certification Exam Coverage

AAMA (CMA) Exam Coverage:
- Medical records (paper/electronic)
  - Organization of patient's medical record
  - Collecting information
  - Making corrections

AMT (CMAS) Exam Coverage:
- Medical records management
  - Systems
    1) Demonstrate knowledge of and manage patient medical records systems
    2) Manage documents and patient charts using computerized methods
  - Procedures
    1) Perform corrections and additions to records
  - Confidentiality
    1) Observe and maintain confidentiality of records, charts, and test results
    2) Observe special regulations regarding the confidentiality of protected information

AMT (RMA) Exam Coverage:
- Documentation
  - Understand and utilize proper documentation of patient encounters and instruction
- Records and chart management
  - Manage patient medical record system
  - Record diagnostic test results in patient chart
  - File patient and physician communication in chart
  - Protect, store, and retain medical records according to proper conventions and HIPAA privacy regulations
  - Prepare and release private health information as required, adhering to state and federal guidelines
  - Identify and employ proper documentation procedures adhering to standard charting guidelines

NCCT (NCMA) Exam Coverage:
- General office procedures
  - Computers
  - Medical record keeping

Introduction

Electronic health records (EHRs) are part of health care's future. Although electronic health records have been around since the Mayo Clinic began using them in the 1960s, the technology has been slow to move into ambulatory care. As today's health care providers strive to make health care safer and allow for efficient team communication, electronic records are playing a more prominent role.

In his 2004 State of the Union address, President George W. Bush stated, "By computerizing health records, we can avoid dangerous medical mistakes, reduce costs, and improve care." Shortly after this speech, President Bush outlined a plan to ensure that most Americans have electronic health

AAMA (CMA) certification exam topics are reprinted with permission of the American Association of Medical Assistants.

AMT (CMAS) certification exam topics are reprinted with permission of American Medical Technologists.

AMT (RMA) certification exam topics are reprinted with permission of American Medical Technologists.

NCCT (NCMA) certification exam topics © 2013 National Center for Competency Testing. Reprinted with permission of NCCT.

records by 2014. According to the Centers for Disease Control and Prevention, as of 2012, 72 percent of office-based physicians were using electronic health records; this was up from 48 percent in 2009.

Electronic Health Records

Electronic health records are simply the portions of patients' medical records that are kept on a computer's hard drive or a medical office's computer network rather than on paper (**Figure 12-1** ■). While physicians must retrieve paper files from separate and often large rooms, electronic records are easily accessible on a computer. In large offices where patients may see several different providers, electronic health records allow physicians to easily locate patients' laboratory results, consultations, X-rays, and examination findings from other providers. The term *electronic health record* refers to a patient's entire medical history in electronic form. *Electronic medical record* (EMR) is the term used to describe just the medical information collected on the patient in one particular physician's office.

Using electronic health records (EHRs), medical offices are able to access any one patient's file from more than one networked computer in the office. For example, the billing office might have the patient's medical record open on a computer screen while accessing information needed for coding a specific procedure. At the same time, the physician might have the same patient's file open on a separate computer screen while she inputs treatment notes.

Charting patient information, such as telephone calls, is easily done within the electronic health record. Typically the software will contain a section for adding information, such as telephone calls or personal conversations that are related to the patient's medical care.

Many medical offices have computer terminals in each examination room, allowing the medical personnel to add information to the patient's electronic health record, download test results, or research past medication records while the patient is in the room. In some offices, the physician or medical assistant uses a portable electronic tablet to enter patient data into the computer system (**Figure 12-2** ■).

How Does Paper Charting Differ from Electronic Charting?

With paper charting, the patient's chart is only available to one staff member at a time. The following example illustrates the steps an office using paper charting might take:

1. The patient telephones the medical office and schedules an appointment to see the physician. The receptionist writes down the information the patient gives her, such as the patient's name, address, telephone numbers, insurance information, and the patient's current complaint.

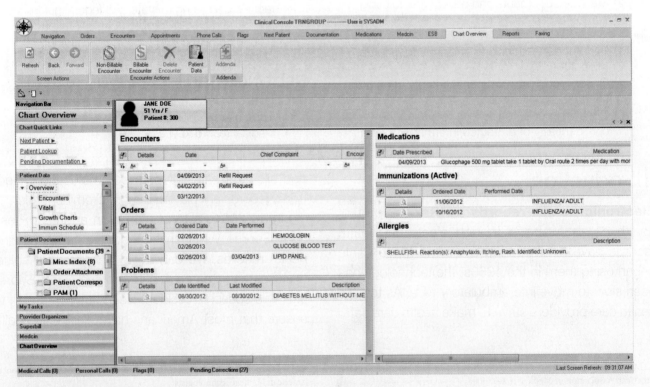

Figure 12-1 ■ An example of one screen within an electronic health care record.
Source: Success EHS. Used with permission.

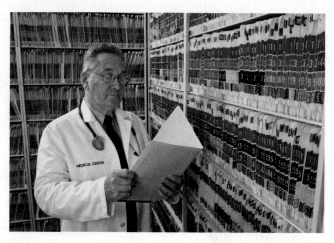

Figure 12-3 ■ The physician will pull the patient's paper medical chart to review the results of tests.
Source: Shutterstock © Condor.

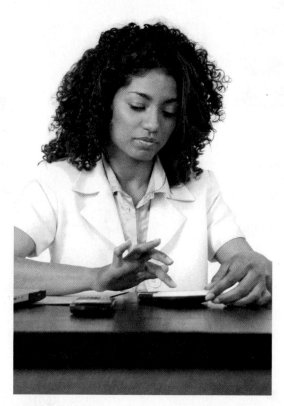

Figure 12-2 ■ A physician uses a TabletPC to enter patient data into the medical record.
Source: Shutterstock © Tyler Olsen.

2. Sometime before the patient's appointment, the receptionist or the billing office may call the patient's insurance carrier to verify the patient's benefits.

3. The day before the patient's appointment, the receptionist may call the patient to remind him of his appointment for the next day.

4. The day before the patient's appointment, the receptionist will prepare the new patient's chart. This is typically done by gathering a paper file folder, color-coded labels to identify the patient's last name, and any other paper forms the patient and the medical staff will fill out on that first visit.

5. When the patient arrives for his visit, the receptionist will give the patient the necessary papers to fill out.

6. When the patient is taken back to the examination room, the clinical medical assistant will begin taking vital signs, such as blood pressure, pulse, and temperature, and begin noting this information by writing in the patient's paper medical chart.

7. When the physician sees the patient, she will review the information the patient has filled out, along with the information the medical assistant has filled out, and begin making notes of her own into the patient's paper chart. If the physician writes a prescription, she will make a note of this in the patient's chart, along with writing the actual prescription on a paper for the patient to take to the pharmacy. In some offices, the physician does not make written notes in the patient's chart and instead dictates her findings into a tape recorder. Those notes will be transcribed by an assistant or a transcription service, then added to the patient's paper chart.

8. If the physician orders X-rays or laboratory tests, the patient's paper chart will be pulled once those reports are returned to the office in order for the physician to review the results along with the patient's chart (**Figure 12-3** ■). **Figure 12-4** ■ shows the workflow in a medical office using paper charts.

In contrast, here are the steps an office using electronic charting might take:

1. A patient calls the office to schedule a new appointment. The receptionist begins an electronic chart while she has the patient on the telephone, adding information about telephone numbers, insurance information, and symptoms into the software program.

2. Sometime before the patient's appointment, the electronic health record system may be used to confirm electronically the patient's health insurance coverage.

3. The day before the patient's appointment, the electronic health record system may be used to call and remind the patient of his appointment the next day. If not, the system may send a reminder for office personnel to make this phone call.

4. When the patient arrives in the office, he may be escorted to an examination room, where a medical assistant will fill out the patient information form on the computer while the patient is present to answer any questions.

5. The medical assistant will then take the patient's vital signs, entering all gathered information into the electronic health record as she goes.

6. When the physician comes into the room, he will review the patient's information in the electronic health record and make his own notes there while interviewing and

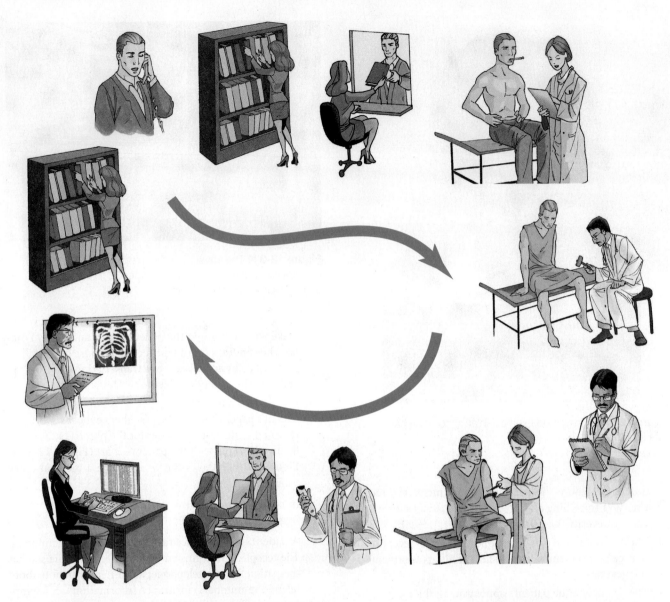

Figure 12-4 ■ Workflow in a medical office using paper charts.

examining the patient. If a prescription is written, the physician will fill this information out in the electronic health record, including faxing the prescription to the pharmacy the patient chooses. If any laboratory work or X-rays are ordered, the physician or medical assistant will fill this out within the electronic health record. If the physician wishes to give the patient any educational materials, such as information on reducing cholesterol, this information may be quickly printed from within the computer system, and a notation can be made in the patient's electronic health record that the information was given.

7. If laboratory work or X-rays are ordered, the physician need only review the patient's electronic health record on the computer, which may be done from any computer terminal within the clinic (**Figure 12-5** ■). **Figure 12-6** ■ shows the workflow in a medical office using electronic health records.

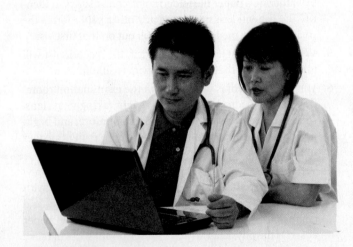

Figure 12-5 ■ A physician uses a computer to access a patient's electronic health record.

Source: Shutterstock © William Casey.

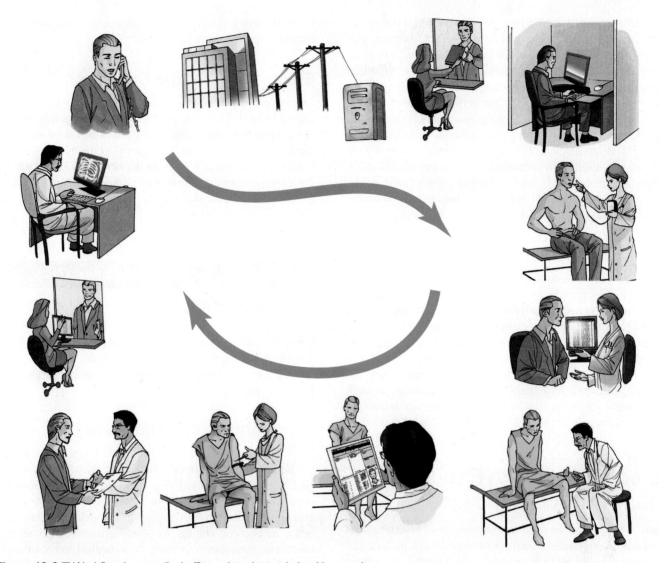

Figure 12-6 ■ Workflow in a medical office using electronic health records.

Making the Conversion from Paper to Electronic Health Records

Though many health care providers and clinical support staff find that the process of changing from paper to electronic health records format is time consuming, most would agree that once the **EHR** has been implemented, using the computer rather than writing in the patient's chart by hand saves a great deal of time.

The conversion from paper to electronic health record format is typically done over a period of time. Some clinics are able to use a scanner to scan documents from the patient's paper medical record to the electronic record. Other clinics might need to enter information from the paper chart to the electronic record manually. The process depends on the type of electronic health record software being used and the preferences of the medical staff (**Figure 12-7** ■).

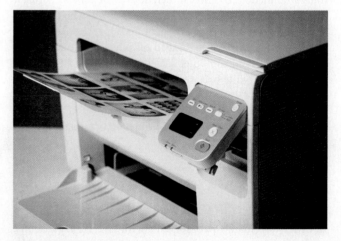

Figure 12-7 ■ In many clinics, a scanner is used to copy documents from the patient's paper medical record into the electronic health record.

Source: Shutterstock © Marco Prati.

Once the information from the paper medical record has been transferred to the electronic health record, the clinic staff may choose to destroy the paper record. This must be done by shredding the documents contained in the medical record. In some offices, the staff chooses to simply store the paper record in a secure location rather than destroy the file. Some medical offices choose to hire outside companies who will store paper medical records securely once the office has converted from paper to electronic records. When documents such as written reports or consultations from other facilities come into the office, these documents are typically added to the electronic health record using a scanner. If the original document is no longer needed, it can be shredded in order to protect patient privacy.

Training

Any software company that sells electronic health records software should supply the medical office with a certain amount of training for the staff to learn to use the equipment. This training should be attended by anyone in the office who will be using the software, including the physicians. In addition, a training manual should be supplied for use in training future staff members. Software companies that sell electronic health record software should also supply the office with contact information to reach a technical support person in the event a question or concern with the new software should arise in the medical clinic.

Electronic Health Records and HIPAA Compliance

Just as with paper medical records, electronic health records must be kept private. In order to ensure patient privacy and compliance with **HIPAA** legislation, all computer users must have their own password to access the patient medical records. With each person having login information, the software can track who made each entry or deletion. With paper records, it is not always obvious who last had a record and who made the latest changes if the user is not identified.

Each station must be logged off when the user is away from her desk, and computer screens must not be viewable by other patients while private patient information is displayed on the screen. Given the regulations in HIPAA legislation, computerized medical records are just as safe, if not more so, than paper medical records with regard to possible improper disclosure of information.

Backing Up Computers and Electronic Health Records

In order to remain in compliance with HIPAA regulations, medical offices must use data backup systems to safeguard the information contained on the office computer systems, including patient medical records. This is typically done on a daily basis, and in most offices the computer backup system is set to work automatically. By having daily backup files, the medical office will not likely lose computer data, even if the entire computer system goes down.

Electronic Storage Systems

Several companies offer electronic off-site storage of electronic patient records. These companies typically charge a fee to host the data on their own computer systems in a location other than the physician's office. The benefits to the office using this type of service is that it frees up the needed storage space on the office's computers. This may be helpful, especially in a smaller medical practice. Another benefit is that the information is stored in a secure, off-site location, where it cannot be accessed should someone break into the physician's office.

Critical Thinking Question 12-1

Recall the case study at the beginning of this chapter. What should David, the registered medical assistant, tell Mr. Reardon about the safety of the private patient information contained within the electronic health record? How can David reassure the patient that his information isn't at any risk?

Meaningful Use Objectives

In 2009, Congress passed the Health Information Technology for Economic and Clinical Health Act, also known as the **HITECH Act**. This legislation provided access to incentive payments to physicians, with the goal of increasing the use of electronic health record systems in physician practices. In order to become eligible for these incentives, physicians needed to prove they were using their medical record in a way that would provide the safest care and best outcomes for the patients. This method of measuring for the incentives was referred to as the **meaningful use** objectives. Meaningful use is being implemented in three stages:

● Stage 1—2011–2012 Data capture and sharing
● Stage 2—2014 Advance clinical processes
● Stage 3—2016 Improved outcomes

In order to qualify for the incentives for providing an electronic health record under this legislation, the electronic health record used by physicians had to meet specific meaningful use objectives. The Stage 1 core objectives are:

● Computerized provider order entry system for medications
● Drug-to-drug contraindications and drug allergy interaction checks
● Generation and transmission of permissible prescriptions electronically
● Record patient demographics
● Maintain an up-to-date problem list of current and active diagnoses
● Maintain an active medication list

- Maintain an active medication allergy list
- Vital signs
- Smoking status
- Implement one clinical decision support rule and the ability to track the patient's compliance with that rule
- Calculate and transmit Centers for Medicare and Medicaid Services (**CMS**) quality measure
- Electronic copy of health information
- Clinical summaries
- Exchange key clinical information
- Privacy and security

Additional criteria exist for Stages 2 and 3 and can be found at the following sites:

http://www.cms.gov/Regulations-and-Guidance/Legislation/EHRIncentivePrograms/Meaningful_Use.html

http://www.healthit.gov/providers-professionals/how-attain-meaningful-use

▶▶▶ Pulse Points

Protecting Electronic Health Records

Electronic health records must be protected—both the information and the computer systems. Computers must be password-protected and safeguards must be in place to limit access to protected information.

Benefits of Electronic Health Records

Depending on the program, electronic records are available via keyboard connected to a computer system or stylus tapped on a notebook computer, or on a personal digital assistant (PDA). These devices have many of the same functions as a full-size computer and have the added benefit of being small enough for physicians to carry with them from patient to patient. Some of these devices use a stylus pen to make choices on the screen; others are used simply with one's fingertip. Most electronic health records systems can be configured to work according to an office's specific needs. The following is a list of the functions many of these systems provide:

- Time-stamp recordings in the EHR
- Prescriptions printed or faxed to the pharmacy
- Printed patient education information that directly relates to the patient's care
- Search for a certain type of condition or certain age or geographic location of a group of patients
- Digital photos or X-rays attached in the patient's EHR
- Electronically ordered lab results, imaging items, or medical tests
- Electronic graphs of lab results of height, weight, or blood pressure data

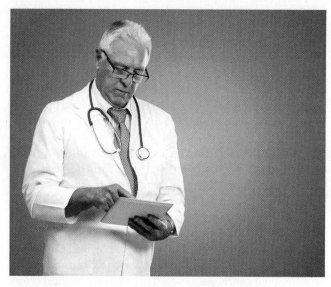

Figure 12-8 ■ A physician uses a handheld electronic notepad to make notes in a patient's medical record.
Source: Shutterstock © Aaron Amat.

- Letters to patients
- Electronic data transmission to other health care providers

One of the many benefits of such systems is the ability to access medical record information from many locations in the health care facility and to quickly search for and retrieve information in the patient's medical record (**Figure 12-8** ■). These devices are often helpful for physicians who see patients in different settings, such as in the hospital, a skilled nursing facility, or even in the patient's home. Using the handheld electronic device, the physician can access and document in the patient's electronic health record, even when she is nowhere near a desktop computer.

▶ In Practice

Dr. Jonas runs a private practice and makes rounds in two local hospitals. He uses one type of electronic health records software in his private office and two other packages in the two hospitals. Not only must Dr. Jonas learn three software systems, he may at times be unable to move patient information between those systems due to incompatibility. What might Dr. Jonas do to address these issues?

There are additional benefits to using electronic health records, which are discussed in the following sections.

Electronic Signatures

An office that uses electronic health records may use an **electronic signature**. In offices where medical notes are dictated and printed for patient files, an electronic signature or rubber-stamp signature may replace handwritten signatures. In these offices, there must be a permanent record of the signer, as well as an original version of the signature on file.

Avoiding Medical Mistakes

Electronic health records can be used to alert health care providers to possible medication reactions. This is especially helpful when treating patients who are co-treating with several specialists. The EHR software will typically have a safeguard mechanism built in that alerts the prescribing physician to any contraindicated medications a particular patient might be taking.

One of the most convincing arguments for converting paper medical records to an electronic format is based on patient safety. In 1999, the Institute of Medicine published a report called "To Err Is Human: Building a Safer Health System." This report stated, "At least 44,000 people, and perhaps as many as 98,000 people, die in hospitals every year as a result of medical errors that could have been prevented." One of the institute's recommendations was to move to electronic health records. Their conclusions suggested that some medical errors are caused by **indecipherable** handwriting, a problem that would be eliminated if providers made their entries electronically rather than in handwritten form.

Some states have enacted legislation to address the issue of illegible handwriting and medical errors. In March 2006, Washington State passed a law that requires all prescriptions written by physicians to be submitted electronically to pharmacists or to be printed rather than written in cursive.

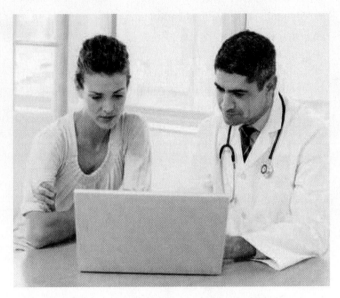

Figure 12-9 ■ Physicians can save time and improve patient communication by using the electronic health record in patient education.
Source: Shutterstock © Monkey Business Images.

Critical Thinking Question 12-2

Recall the case study at the beginning of this chapter. What might David, the medical assistant, say to Mr. Reardon to convince him the change from paper to electronic health records is in his best interest?

Saving Time

The time saved by using electronic health records can be better invested in patient care. Many health care providers believe they spend a great deal of time charting, far more time than they spend on actual patient care. With the cost of health care rising, it makes sense to free up the health care provider's time while decreasing avoidable patient injuries (**Figure 12-9** ■).

Most electronic health records programs have drop-down menus that allow the user to choose information or symptoms from a preprogrammed list. For example, when the user inserts a diagnosis of diabetes, the software might display a list of possible symptoms the patient could be having, such as excessive thirst or frequent urination. Many EHR programs also include lists of possible diagnoses for the physician to choose from, based on the symptoms the patient lists. For example, if the patient complains of excessive thirst and frequent urination, the program might offer diabetes as a possible diagnosis for the physician to choose from.

Electronic health records allow medical staff to easily transmit patient information to a patient's health insurance companies when requested, rather than having to photocopy the paper records and send them via the postal service. It is just as important to follow HIPAA guidelines for releasing medical records electronically as it is for releasing photocopies of the patient's paper medical record.

Health Maintenance

Many medical offices send reminder cards or letters to patients regarding the need for upcoming services. These are typically used to remind patients of the need for a dental exam, a mammogram, a yearly physical, immunizations, or well-child checkups. Using electronic health records, the administrative medical assistant can have the software program print these reminders.

Using Electronic Health Records with Diagnostic Equipment

With electronic health records software, the medical office is able to perform many tests in the office and have the results show immediately in the electronic health record. The same can be done with digital X-rays, Holter monitors, spirometers, and a number of laboratory tests on blood and urine samples (**Figure 12-10** ■).

Critical Thinking Question 12-3

Referring back to the case study at the beginning of the chapter, what sort of health maintenance reminders do you think a patient such as Mr. Reardon might benefit from receiving?

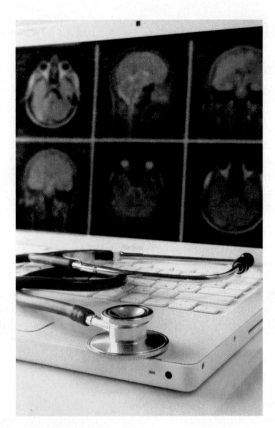

Figure 12-10 ■ Digital images appear immediately in the electronic health record.
Source: Shuttertstock © lenetstan.

Marketing Purposes

Many medical clinics send information flyers to patients on a regular basis. For example, a flyer might be sent during flu season describing the signs and symptoms of the flu, along with prevention tips. One of the prevention tips might encourage readers to come into the physician's office for a flu vaccine.

With electronic health records, the administrative staff is also able to create a list of patients according to specific parameters. For example, if the office has recently welcomed a physician who specializes in allergies, the administrative staff can create a list of patients who have been treated for allergies and use that list to send a letter stating that the new physician is available.

Communicating Between Staff Members

Sometimes one staff member needs to communicate with another staff member about a particular patient—for example, a patient who has an outstanding balance owing in the medical office. The billing staff member might need to see the patient when he comes into the office for his visit

with the physician. Using the electronic health record, the billing staff member can post an alert that will be seen by the receptionist when she checks the patient in. The alert allows the billing staff member to have the receptionist direct the patient to the billing office prior to his visit with the physician.

Putting Medical Records Online

Some clinics, like The Everett Clinic in Washington State, allow patients to look up portions of their electronic health records via the Internet. Using this password-protected system, patients can access a company's network or intranet for their lab results, dates of immunizations, or medication levels, which can help when patients travel or need to seek emergency care with someone other than their primary care provider. Several Internet-based businesses now offer individuals online storage of medical information, such as immunizations, medications, and surgeries, as well as the ability to schedule appointments and pay medical bills online

Critical Thinking Question 12-4

Recall the case study at the beginning of this chapter. How might David convince Mr. Reardon that having access to his medical records online might be helpful to him?

Making Corrections in the Electronic Health Record

Just as with paper medical records, medical staff entering data into the electronic health record might make mistakes in their entries. When this happens, the mistake must be corrected as soon as possible. With electronic health records, the steps involved in making the correction will depend upon the software. Most often, the user will make the correction by crossing out the error and entering the correct information. The original entry will still be viewable, though it might show on a separate screen or it might show as having a line drawn through the entry (**Figure 12-11** ■).

Patient complains of ~~right~~ left leg pain.

Figure 12-11 ■ Mistakes in the electronic health record must be corrected as soon as possible. Most often, the user will cross out the error and enter the correct information, as shown in this example.

PROCEDURE 12-1 Correct an Electronic Health Record

Theory and Rationale

Mistakes can be made in an electronic health record just as they can in a paper medical record. The medical assistant must be aware of how to make appropriate corrections to the electronic health record in an accurate manner. Corrections must be made in an accurate manner to avoid lawsuits or other legal issues.

Materials

● Computer with electronic patient medical record

Competency

1. Identify the correct patient electronic health record where the error was made.
2. Locate the error within the record.
3. Using the rules associated with the software you are using, make the appropriate correction within the medical record.
4. Sign off on the changes as necessary, according to the steps required within the software program.
5. Verify that the change is correct before closing the patient's electronic health record.

REVIEW

Chapter Summary

● Electronic health records are the portions of a patient's medical record that are kept on a computer's hard drive or a medical office's computer network rather than on paper.

● Electronic health records are gaining popularity over conventional paper files because they offer enhanced ease, efficiency, and accessibility.

● With paper charting, the patient's chart is only available to one staff member at a time. Electronic health records make the patient's chart available to many health care team members at the same time.

● The conversion from paper to electronic health record format is typically done over time. Once paper

medical records are converted to electronic versions, those paper records must be appropriately destroyed.

● Medical offices should correct errors in a patient chart according to accepted protocol.

● By using electronic health records, a medical office is more easily able to perform tasks such as sending reminder post cards than with paper medical records.

● Other benefits of electronic health records include using electronic signatures, avoiding medical mistakes, saving time, and communicating between staff members.

● *Meaningful use* is an incentive program put in place by the CMS to promote the use of electronic health records in medical facilities.

Chapter Review

Multiple Choice

1. A PDA is often used in the medical office. What does PDA stand for?
   a. Professional desk assistant
   b. Personal digital assistant
   c. Progressive digital assistant
   d. Programmable download alternative
   e. Program delay assistant

2. Which of the following is a reason the medical office would send postcard reminders to patients?
   a. Yearly physical examination
   b. Mammogram
   c. Immunizations
   d. a and b
   e. a, b, and c

3. Using EHR software, the medical staff will typically be able to do which of the following?
   a. Locate possible contraindications with prescribed medications
   b. Allow two or more staff members to access the same patient file at the same time
   c. Fax medical records to other medical offices
   d. Schedule patients for appointments in other facilities
   e. a, b, and c

4. Which of the following is a reason a patient might want to access her own medical records online?
   a. View her current medications
   b. View the date of her vaccination
   c. Read a current lab report
   d. Send an e-mail to her physician
   e. All of the above

True/False

T F **1.** Electronic health records do not have to comply with HIPAA regulations.

T F **2.** Electronic health records are the same thing as electronic medical records.

T F **3.** Converting from paper to electronic health records is a quick and easy process.

T F **4.** Correcting charting errors in an electronic health record is much the same as correcting an error in a paper chart.

T F **5.** Electronic health records allow one staff member to communicate with another staff member via electronic notes.

T F **6.** Using PDAs, physicians can transfer data about their patients from one computer system to another.

Short Answer

1. Explain how the use of EHRs can help avoid medication prescription errors.
2. Why would it be important for all staff members, even those with extensive computer experience, to attend a training session for new electronic health records software?
3. Explain how a medical office might enter a letter from an outside medical facility into a patient's electronic health record.
4. How would a medical office use the information contained in their electronic health records software for marketing purposes?
5. Who said, "By computerizing health records, we can avoid dangerous medical mistakes, reduce costs, and improve care"?
6. Explain how an electronic signature is used.
7. What is a drop-down menu?
8. How would using electronic health records save time over using paper medical records?
9. What was the first medical clinic to begin using electronic health records?
10. Why should a medical office shred papers that contain patient information once those records have been entered into an electronic format?

Research

1. Interview a person who works in a medical office that is using electronic health records. How does that person feel about working with the electronic health record as opposed to using paper records?
2. Research the various personal digital assistants (PDAs) that are available for medical personnel to purchase. What kinds of features do they offer?
3. Search the Internet for companies that offer an electronic health record. How do the services compare?

Practicum Application Experience

Dr. Shelley Fredrich is works in a busy family practice clinic. When the office begins the conversion from paper to electronic health records, Dr. Fredrich says she does not think she needs to attend the orientation and training session scheduled for the remainder of the staff. She believes that she is "computer-savvy" and that the training session will be a waste of her time. How could Dr. Fredrich be convinced to attend the training session?

Resource Guide

Epic electronic health record system
http://www.epic.com

NextGen computerized electronic health record system
www.nextgen.com

CureMD electronic health record system
www.curemd.com

Health Insurance Portability and Accountability Act (HIPAA) Web site
http://www.hhs.gov/ocr/hipaa/

The Institute of Medicine
http://www.iom.edu

PowerMed computerized electronic health record system
http://www.powermed.com/

13

Computers in the Medical Office

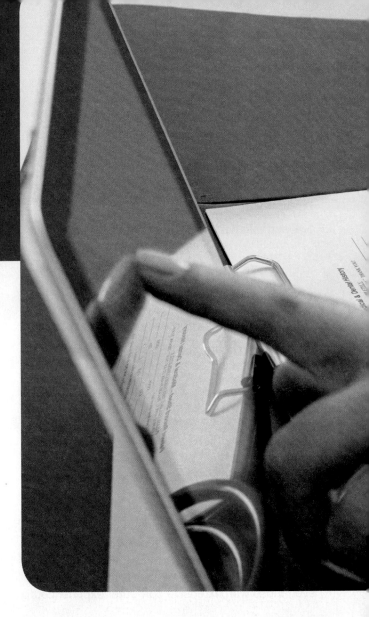

Case Study

Read the following case study and answer the critical thinking questions presented throughout the chapter.

Dr. Crates has asked the certified medical assistant to research options for adding a new computer terminal to the office. The physician wants to ensure that the chosen system can run all the latest software in addition to the practice management and electronic health record software used in the office. Dr. Crates would like the medical assistant to investigate whether an electronic tablet system would be useful in their clinic.

Objectives

After completing this chapter, you should be able to:

13.1 Define and spell the key terminology in this chapter.

13.2 Describe the functions and uses of computers in the medical office.

13.3 Describe the components of a computer system.

13.4 List and describe different types of computer peripherals.

13.5 Explain how to properly maintain computer equipment.

13.6 List and describe the functions of medical software.

13.7 Describe ways to secure office computers.

13.8 Use the Internet to search for information.

13.9 Discuss the importance of having a medical office policy that outlines personal computer use in the medical office.

13.10 Discuss safe practices for purchasing medications online.

13.11 Describe a personal digital assistant and smart phone, and how they work with computers.

13.12 Explain the basic principles of computer ergonomics.

Competency Skills Performance

1. Use computer software to maintain office systems.

2. Use an Internet search engine.

3. Use the computer to verify preferred provider status on an insurance company Web site.

Key Terminology

bar-code scanner—device that scans or views bar codes for transfer to attached computers

battery backup system—system that protects computers in the event of power surges or power outages

computer peripherals—devices that connect to computers to add function or use

computer virus—program written to disrupt computer function

electronic sign-in sheet—computer program that displays the names of those who sign in

ergonomic—designed for proper body posture

flash drive—small, external data storage device; see *thumb drive*

health-related calculator—computer program that quantifies health-related conditions (e.g., target body weight)

Internet search engine—Web site that searches the Internet for information based on set criteria

malware—computer software that can destroy or disable computer programs

medical management software—software medical offices use to perform day-to-day functions (e.g., billing, appointment scheduling)

personal digital assistant (PDA)—small, portable device that stores and transmits data

scanner—device that copies documents or pictures for transfer to computer systems

smart phone—cellular phone that has features for browsing the Internet or composing word-processed documents

thumb drive—small, external data storage device; see *flash drive*

Abbreviations

AMA—American Medical Association

CD—compact disc

CDC—Centers for Disease Control and Prevention

CPU—central processing unit

DPI—dots per square inch

DVD—digital versatile/video disc

FDA—Food and Drug Administration

HIPAA—Health Insurance Portability and Accountability Act

PDA—personal digital assistant

PHI—protected health information

RAM—random access memory

ROM—read-only memory

URL—universal resource locator

USB—universal system bus

VIPPS—Verified Internet Pharmacy Practice Site

Certification Exam Coverage

AAMA (CMA) Exam Coverage:

- Keyboard fundamentals and functions
  - Alpha, numeric, and symbol keys
  - Tabulation
- Computer components
  - Technology
  - Central processing unit (CPU)
  - Printer
  - Disk drive
  - Storage devices (e.g., hard drives, magnetic tapes, CD-ROMs, flash drives)
  - Operating systems
  - Basic commands
- Computer applications
  - Word processing
  - Database (e.g., menu, fields, records, files)
  - Spreadsheets, graphics

- Electronic mail
- Networks
- Security/password
- Medical management software
  1) Patient data
  2) Report generation
- Internet services

AMT (CMAS) Exam Coverage:

- Fundamentals of Computing
  - Possess fundamental knowledge of computing in the medical office including keyboarding, data entry, and retrieval
  - Possess fundamental knowledge of PC-based environment
  - Possess fundamental knowledge of word processing, spreadsheet, database, and presentation graphics applications

AAMA (CMA) certification exam topics are reprinted with permission of the American Association of Medical Assistants.

AMT (CMAS) certification exam topics are reprinted with permission of American Medical Technologists.

Certification Exam Coverage (continued)

- Employ procedures for ensuring the integrity and confidentiality of computer-stored information
- Medical Office Computer Applications
  - Employ medical office software applications
  - Use computer for billing and financial transactions
  - Employ e-mail applications

AMT (RMA) Exam Coverage:
- Computer applications
  - Identify and understand hardware components
  - Identify and understand application of basic software and operating systems
  - Recognize software applications for patient record maintenance, bookkeeping, and patient accounting system

- Employ procedures for integrity of information and compliance with HIPAA Security and Privacy regulations
  1) Encryption
  2) Firewall software and hardware
  3) Personnel passwords
  4) Access restrictions
  5) Activity logs
- Maintain records of biohazardous waste and chemical disposal.

NCCT (NCMA) Exam Coverage:
- General office procedures
  - Computers

Introduction

Most medical offices use computer systems for some form of operations. From appointment scheduling to bookkeeping and electronic charting, computers have become integral to medical offices. To function most effectively, medical assistants should understand the components of the computer system, as well as how to maintain parts and update software. Computer systems and software programs advance quickly, so it is important to maintain skills and attend training classes as needed.

Components of the Computer System

Computer systems have three main components:

1. **Hardware**—the equipment itself
2. **Software**—programs in the system
3. **Peripherals**—extra devices that can attach to or be installed in the hardware

Each computer component is intricately intertwined with the others. An office can have the most powerful hardware available yet be limited by software. Similarly, an office can have top-of-the-line software that fails to work due to old,

outdated hardware. Table 13-1 discusses main computer-system types.

Computer Hardware

Computer hardware consists of several parts. All computers have a central processing unit (**CPU**), which is the computer's brain. The CPU enables the computer to process data and run software. All CPUs function in the same basic way but differ in speed and capabilities. Generally, the faster the CPU, the higher the computer's cost.

Virtually all computers have ports that serve as connections for a keyboard, monitor, mouse, printer, and speakers (**Figure 13-1** ■). Other ports may be used for such add-on items as scanners or backup drives.

TABLE 13-1 Main Computer System Types	
Supercomputers	Introduced in the 1960s; have the fastest processing capacity of today's computers
Mainframe computers	Used for large-volume applications (e.g., government statistics)
Minicomputers	Multiuser computers that fall between mainframe computers and microcomputers in size and capabilities
Microcomputers	Generally small, ranging from desktop models to handheld versions; commonly used in health care facilities

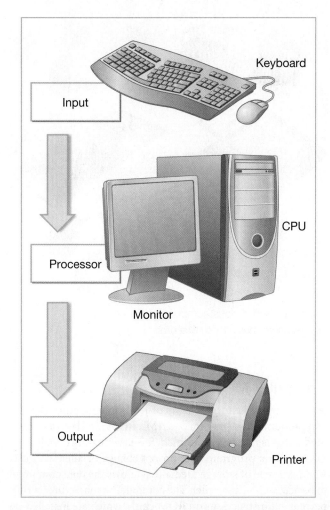

Figure 13-1 ■ Components of a computer system.

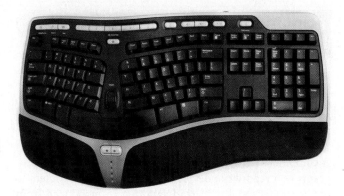

Figure 13-2 ■ Ergonomic keyboard.
Source: Fotolia © Creativa.

the top of the keyboard. These keys are designated by number, indicating the function each performs. Function keys exist for functions F1 through F12. Depending on the software system being used, function keys may be assigned to a variety of functions in that system. Though function keys might not be supported by all software programs, below is a list of how function keys are typically used with modern systems:

- F1—Used as a help key; will open a help window within the currently running program
- F2—Used to rename an icon, file, or folder
- F3—Used to open a search feature within the currently running program
- F4—Used to close the program window currently active
- F5—Used to refresh or reload the current page
- F6—Used to open an additional document in the Microsoft Word program
- F7—Used to perform spell check and grammar check within the currently active document
- F8—Used to access the Windows startup menu and Windows Safe Mode
- F9—Used to open Windows in a variety of software programs
- F10—Used to activate menu bars of open applications
- F11—Used to activate full screen mode in the currently running program
- F12—Used to open the "save as" window in the currently running program

The tab key on the keyboard is often used to navigate from one field to another within a fillable document. This key is also used to indent paragraphs, as when composing a letter.

The Monitor

Computer monitors come in various sizes and qualities. Monitor display is based on the number of dots per square inch (**DPI**). The higher a monitor's DPI, the clearer its picture. Much like with the CPU just discussed, cost increases as DPI increases.

Critical Thinking Question 13-1

Refer back to the case study presented at the beginning of this chapter. What must the medical assistant know about the medical office's computer needs? How does office need dictate computer choice?

The Keyboard

Computer keyboards may be standard or **ergonomic** (**Figure 13-2** ■). Ergonomic keyboards reduce typing stress by supporting the hands and wrists comfortably. Keyboards typically attach to computers via cords, but many offices now have wireless models that work from any spot within the computer's range, typically 15 to 30 feet.

Keyboards contain many functions, in addition to alpha and numeric characters. The computer keyboard allows the user to enter commands, information, and data by pressing various keys. The layout of the computer keyboard is called the QWERTY design—those are the characters on the top left row of letters. Keyboards contain function keys, which are across

Critical Thinking Question 13-2

Referring back to the case study at the beginning of the chapter, what factors would justifiably influence the medical office to fund a flat-screen monitor?

The Computer Hard Drive

A computer's hard drive houses the computer's files and programs as a read/write device. The term *read/write* refers to the computer's ability to read data that is introduced from other sources and its ability to write (save) data to its own hard drive. Because hard drives can fail, jeopardizing critical data, medical offices should regularly back up the data on their hard drives. This is typically done with a backup system, such as a separate computer to save data to or some form of external device designed to save the computer data. Again, the larger the hard drive, the more expensive the computer.

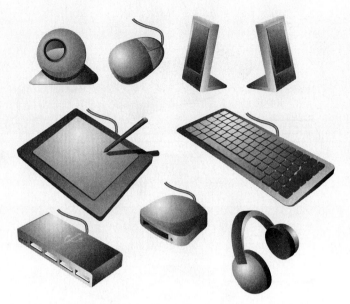

Figure 13-3 ■ Various computer peripherals.
Source: Shutterstock © Ken Guan Toh.

Types of Computer Drives

Computers have various types of drives. Most systems come with compact disc (**CD**) drives that allow computers to access files and programs on CDs. CDs are plastic discs used to store data or programs. Digital versatile disc (**DVD**) drives, an option for most contemporary computers, provide access to files on DVDs. DVDs, like CDs, are plastic discs that are used to store data or programs. DVDs can hold approximately six times the amount of information that a CD can hold.

Additional Computer Peripherals

Computer peripherals connect to computer systems to offer useful functions. Examples include keyboards and monitors, which were covered above, as well as printers, scanners, digital cameras, bar-code readers, and electronic sign-in sheets (**Figure 13-3** ■).

Flash drives are small memory devices with no moving parts. These devices, sometimes called **thumb drives**, vary in size from 8 gigabytes to 124 gigabytes and are used to store files for transport between computer systems. These drives are small enough to carry in a pocket; many attach to neck chains for convenience. Flash drives usually connect to computers via a universal system bus (**USB**) port. The USB port may be located on the back or side of the computer and is where the USB device plugs into the computer. Just as with other computer components, the greater the storage capability of a flash drive, the higher its price.

Like flash drives, Zip drives store data. These devices are slightly larger than floppy drives and hold much more data. Because they are portable, Zip drives can be used to transport data between computers. They are also commonly used for file backup.

Computer Memory

A computer's memory consists of read-only memory (**ROM**) and random access memory (**RAM**). ROM is a class of storage media that is not easily modified. It is used mainly to hold permanent data: programs that do not change or alter with use. RAM is a type of storage media that allows the data contained to be accessed in any order. The computer manufacturer writes permanent instructions on ROM chips, which are installed on the computer's motherboard. The amount of RAM, which varies according to users' needs, is also in chip form on the motherboard. Information stored in RAM erases when the computer shuts down or experiences a power failure. When a computer's RAM is insufficient, the computer typically runs more slowly.

The Printer

When a printer is attached to a computer, the user can print information housed on the computer. Printers come in various types, sizes, and speeds. Some, called inkjet printers, use liquid ink, whereas laser printers use toner to print. Offices might sometimes need to order printer supplies from manufacturers. Other printer supplies may be found at office supply stores. Because the cost of printing supplies can vary greatly, offices should factor in these costs when selecting printers.

Critical Thinking Question 13-3

Referring to the case study, what type of information can the certified medical assistant gather to give the physician an accurate idea of printer costs?

▸▸ Pulse Points

Surge Protection

Computers should be protected against damage caused by power outages or electrical surges. All computers in the medical office should be connected to an uninterruptible power supply or **battery backup systems**. All computer power supplies should also have surge protection to prevent voltage surges, which can be very damaging to computer components.

Scanners

Scanners are similar to photocopiers in that they copy documents. Unlike photocopiers, however, scanners can transfer electronic versions of documents or images to computers. Scanners are often part of larger equipment that can scan, photocopy, and fax documents.

Digital Cameras

Digital cameras take pictures without film. Images are stored electronically in the camera until the user downloads them to a computer. Typically, images are downloaded from the camera to the computer via a USB cable. Images can also be transferred from a camera to the computer by inserting the camera's memory card into the computer. Digital cameras range from inexpensive models designed for home use to expensive models capable of high-quality images. In the medical office, these cameras typically are used to document patient injuries, such as visible signs of abuse. Other medical offices might use these cameras to create office brochures or other marketing materials.

Bar-Code Readers

Many modern medical offices use bar coding to manage information. Some offices use bar codes to identify patient files or enter patient data into computers. Others use the technology to track inventory or supplies. **Bar-code scanners**, one type of reader, vary in size and type. Some models work via trigger, while others use what looks like an ink pen (**Figure 13-4 ■**).

Electronic Sign-in Sheets

Electronic sign-in sheets, which work like the devices department stores use for signing for credit card use at checkout, arose due to concern for patient privacy. Though paper sign-in sheets were not found to be in violation of HIPAA legislation, many medical offices found that moving to an electronic system eliminated paper and made the process more efficient. With **electronic sign-in sheets**, patients enter their names electronically on tablets or pads, and the sheets display the resulting signatures on receptionists' computer screens (**Figure 13-5 ■**).

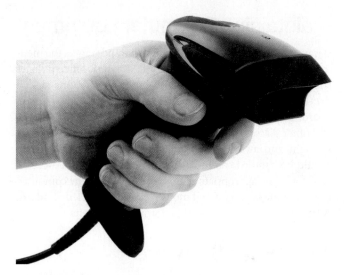

Figure 13-4 ■ A handheld barcode scanner.
Source: Shutterstock © Ruslan Kuzmenkov.

Electronic Pads and Tablets

Many medical offices have providers and staff using portable electronic pads or tablets while in the patient care area. These electronic devices allow the user to enter information into the patient's medical record without the need to be connected physically to the computer. In the case of a wireless or infrared transfer system, these electronic pads are synced with the main office computer system, and data is exchanged. In wired systems, the tablets must be connected, or docked with the main office computer to exchange data from the portable device to the main system.

Critical Thinking Question 13-4

Refer to the case study at the beginning of the chapter. What are some reasons for the medical office to incorporate the use of electronic pads or tablets into the office computer system? How might the use of these devices save time or space in the medical office?

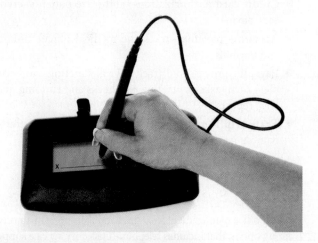

Figure 13-5 ■ Electronic signature pad.
Source: Shutterstock © glenda.

Maintaining Computer Equipment

Because computer equipment is expensive and fragile, the medical office should strive to maintain it. To start, office policies should disallow food and drink near computers. One spilled drink can irreversibly damage a computer or destroy a keyboard. In addition, computer systems, as well as CDs, DVDs, and other discs, should be kept in cool, dry places, out of direct sunlight and away from potentially damaging items. Discs should be handled carefully and cleaned only with static-free, soft cloths and appropriate chemicals. All parts of the computer, including the keyboard and mouse, should be dusted regularly. A trained professional should perform any maintenance.

Computer Software

Most medical offices use some form of **medical management software** that performs such functions as appointment scheduling, patient charting, electronic health record management, bookkeeping, insurance billing, and task and prescription managing. An office's needs determine which software it uses. Demonstrations by the software salesperson can help medical offices ensure that they buy programs that are appropriate for their needs. Following the trend in other areas of technology, feature-rich management software tends to cost more than simple programs. The following is a list of common features in medical management software:

- **Patient accounting**—enter patient charges and payments, and track accounts receivables
- **Coding**—choose codes for patients' procedures and diagnoses
- **Appointment scheduling**—track patient appointment times and send reminder cards
- **Insurance billing**—print medical insurance claims
- **Electronic billing**—submit medical insurance claims electronically
- **Verify insurance coverage**—verify patient's insurance benefits via insurance companies' Web sites
- **Credit card authorization**—authorize patients' credit-card payments
- **Accounts payable**—track the medical office's finances and pay bills
- **Payroll**—process and track payroll functions and complete such tasks as printing paychecks and running quarterly reports
- **Transcription**—transcribe documents via dictation equipment or voice recognition

Table 13-2 identifies medical software companies.

Training Staff on Medical Software

Medical office management software should come with an onsite training option that includes telephone customer service support and manuals or demos for future training needs. All staff who will be working with the software should attend training. Because

TABLE 13-2 Medical Software Companies	
AccuMedic Computer Systems, Inc.	www.accumedic.com
Advanced Data Systems (ADS)	www.adsc.com
Athena Health	www.athenahealth.com
Benchmark Systems	www.benchmark-systems.com
Epic	www.epic.com
Kareo Medical Practice Software	www.kareo.com
Lajolla Digital	www.lajolladigital.com
MediPro	www.medipro.com
Medisoft Practice Software	www.medisoft.com
MedStar	www.medstarsystems.com
Nuesoft Practice Software	www.nuesoft.com/
Practice Partner	www.mckessonpracticesolutions.com
TheraManager	www.theramanager.com
Waiting Room Solutions Medical Practice Software	www.waitingroomsolutions.com

such training might be costly, medical offices should explore that possibility before making any software purchases.

Types of Software Packages

Most medical offices use word-processing software, most commonly Microsoft Word. Using such software, medical assistants can type patient letters, print mailing lists, format documents and brochures, and create charts and forms. Word processing software is sometimes incorporated into the electronic health record, allowing the medical assistant to save a copy of a letter created in the word-processing software into the patient's electronic health record. Word processing software contains a spell check and grammar check feature, which enables the user to avoid spelling and grammatical errors in the documents created. Because many medical terms are not found in spell and grammar check functions, the medical assistant should read through all documents to verify accuracy before sending.

Spreadsheet software like Microsoft Excel® completes calculations statistics and creates corresponding graphs and charts. Medical offices can use spreadsheet software to track statistics on patient care and personnel management. Spreadsheet software can also be used to track supplies and equipment in the medical office, or used to take and maintain inventory. Any biohazardous materials kept in the medical office must be catalogued and documented in order to track their use. Spreadsheet software is commonly used for this task.

Presentation software like PowerPoint® helps when medical offices plan educational meetings or seminars for patients. Not only can presenters create slides for projection, they can print those slides as note-taking tools for attendees.

PROCEDURE 13-1 Use Computer Software to Maintain Office Systems

Theory and Rationale

The computer software used in the medical office is capable of performing a multitude of tasks. One such task is to maintain the office systems. An example of such a task would be to keep track of the equipment used in the medical office. By performing this task, the medical assistant can keep track of information pertaining to needed maintenance, such as the name of the company that performs the repairs, and the schedule for which the equipment must be maintained.

Materials

- Computer with spreadsheet software
- List of equipment to enter into the computer

Competency

1. Launch the spreadsheet software.
2. Using the list of equipment, enter each piece of equipment onto a separate line on the spreadsheet.
3. Enter the date each piece of equipment was purchased or leased by the medical office.
4. Enter the name of the manufacturer that supplied the piece of equipment.
5. Enter the type of maintenance the piece of equipment needs on a regular basis.
6. Enter information about the needed maintenance, such as the name of the company that performs the repairs, and the schedule for which the equipment must be maintained.

Several software programs currently on the market, such as Microsoft Outlook®, keep electronic calendars, which can be invaluable to medical offices trying to coordinate staff schedules. Many of these programs send e-mail invitations that recipients can add to their electronic calendars or print in daily, weekly, or monthly slices.

Computer Security

To safeguard computer systems, staff members should be required to use alphanumeric passwords to access them. To thwart hackers, users should choose unobvious passwords, taking care to avoid initials, birthdates, and telephone numbers. Users should also be careful to avoid sharing their passwords and leaving their passwords in plain view. In many offices, sharing passwords may be a violation of policy. Many organizations require users to change their passwords periodically, for example, every 90 days, in order to maintain a higher level of security. It is good practice for users to log off when leaving their computer workstations unattended. The following are HIPAA standards for safeguarding protected patient health information:

- Protected health information (**PHI**) must be backed up periodically.
- An audit trail must exist for backed-up data that leaves the medical facility.
- Access to backed-up data must be restricted to authorized parties.
- A backup plan and disaster recovery plan must be in place.
- Data must be retrievable, exact copy.
- All computers must be password protected.

HIPAA has a section known as the Security Rule, which requires that appropriate safeguards (administrative, physical, and technical) are in place to ensure the confidentiality, security, and integrity of electronic protected health information.

Backing Up Computer Systems

To avoid critical data loss, computers in the medical office should be backed up regularly. Offices can use the various tapes or drives discussed earlier in this chapter, or they can back up data from one computer system to another. Whatever backup system the medical office uses, the backup tape, drive, and computer should be housed in a location separate from the originating computer so fire, flood, or theft cannot threaten the data.

● HIPAA Compliance

Health Insurance Portability and Accountability Act (**HIPAA**) regulations require medical offices to prevent unauthorized users from accessing office computers. Virus-detection and elimination software, firewall technology (a software or hardware-based network security system that controls the incoming and outgoing network traffic by analyzing the data and determining whether they should be allowed through or not, based on a rule set), and intrusion-detection tools all serve this purpose by keeping unauthorized users from violating office computers and patient information.

Computer Viruses

Computer viruses are programs designed to perform mischievous functions. Viruses are often introduced to a computer system by way of a file that is downloaded by the user. These files might be attached to an email or be inadvertently downloaded from a Web site the user visits. **Malware**, a twist on the computer virus, is software designed to damage computer programs by infiltrating computers. Malware includes spyware, adware, Trojan horses, and worms. These programs can damage or corrupt hard drives, as well as infect other computers without users' knowledge. Because these types of programs exist, every computer in the medical office should have virus-protection software that is updated regularly. The two most commonly used antivirus software programs are made by McAfee and Norton.

Computer users can avoid introducing viruses or malware into their computers by avoiding certain risky activities, such as clicking on files or images attached to emails, keeping current with antivirus software, and being sure all computer users are aware of these safety techniques.

Internet Search Engines

Internet search engines use key words and phrases to retrieve information from the Internet. Popular search engines include Yahoo!, Google, Bing, Lycos, Dog Pile, and Ask.com. Contemporary health care providers often search the Internet for medical information. Medical offices often need source material for patient brochures or presentations, and the Internet can be a valuable resource.

In Practice

Dr. Victor is giving a presentation on a new procedure she is performing for scar-tissue removal. Dr. Victor has asked Jamie, her medical assistant, to use the Internet to find information on other, similar procedures for comparison. How should Jamie begin, and where? What key words would be appropriate for the search engine?

▶▶ Pulse Points

Using the Computer for Work-Related Purposes Only

Because the computer systems in a medical office belong to the physician or the office, they should only be used for private use when employers grant permission. Since employers own the computer systems, they have the right to inspect any personal documents or personal e-mails the computer is used for, even if such access is allowed and not done on work time. Even if permissible, staff should not download screen savers or other, similar files. Most computers get viruses and malware when users open malicious e-mails or visit certain Web sites. Therefore, to protect computers, medical assistants should open no attachments from unknown sources or Web sites.

Finding Appropriate Web Resources

When newly diagnosed with conditions or illnesses, patients often have many questions for their health care providers. Many such providers find it helpful to give patients lists of reputable Web sites for further information. When patients have long-term or chronic illnesses or conditions and might be seeking support groups, such lists can be especially beneficial.

▶▶ Pulse Points

Obtaining Physician Approval before Distributing Material to Patients

Before giving Web site information to patients, be sure to obtain the physician's permission. Give patients information from reputable Web sites only. Physicians may ask that information be emailed to patients. Once the patient has given consent for this way of receiving information, the medical assistant can send an email with the requested information. If the information is to be sent as an attachment, photos and brochures should be saved in a .pdf format.

Professional medical Web sites are the sites physicians visit when seeking up-to-date information on conditions, illnesses, or pharmaceuticals. Table 13-3 lists some reputable examples. Physicians use reputable sites for medical information because non-medical sites, for example, Wikipedia, might not contain completely accurate information. Many physicians subscribe to online journals that charge for access but offer the latest information on research, medications, and techniques. Seminars and conferences can be informative, but Web sites serve as ongoing resources as topics arise.

Many Web sites have **health-related calculators** that aid both patients and health care staff. These calculators address factors such as basal metabolic rate, body mass index, pregnancy due date, ovulation, target heart rate, children's adult height predictions, smoking costs, and seafood mercury intake.

Often, major health insurance carriers maintain their own, comprehensive Web sites that allow subscribers and physicians alike to access a wide span of information. Some sites even give physicians access to patients' benefit information, although direct contact with the insurance companies is often

TABLE 13-3 Medical Web Sites	
American Medical Association (**AMA**)	www.ama-assn.org
The Joint Commission	www.jointcommission.org
Centers for Disease Control and Prevention (**CDC**)	www.cdc.gov
WebMD	www.webmd.com
Mayo Clinic	www.mayoclinic.com
MedlinePlus	www.nlm.nih.gov/medlineplus/

PROCEDURE 13-2 Use an Internet Search Engine

Theory and Rationale

The Internet provides access to a vast amount of information the medical office can use to educate patients, research new technologies and equipment, and contact patients. Search engines can quickly locate desired information and resources.

Materials

- A computer with Internet access

Competency

1. Turn on the computer.
2. Launch an Internet browser.
3. Visit the uniform resource locator (**URL**) of the search engine.
4. Enter the search keywords.
5. Visit retrieved Web sites to obtain the desired information.
6. To refine the search, enter more or different key words.

---

still needed, especially when authorizations are required. Such sites are particularly helpful for offices wishing to verify that patients have active policies at the time of visit.

Buying Medications Online

Patients who lack prescription drug coverage may use the Internet as an economical way to obtain medications. Online medication purchase can be dangerous, however, so medical offices should encourage patients to use only sites certified by the Verified Internet Pharmacy Practice Site (**VIPPS**). VIPPS certification ensures that the National Association of Boards of Pharmacy has reviewed the online pharmacy for safety and compliance. Certified online pharmacies provide information on prescribed medications, including possible adverse reactions or side effects and any safety concerns.

Medical offices should advise patients never to purchase medications from Internet sites outside the United States. Staff should direct patients to the U.S. Food and Drug Administration (**FDA**) (www.fda.gov) Web site for tips on buying mediations online.

Personal Computer Use in the Office

All medical offices should write policies for personal use of office computers and ensure that all members of the health care team follow those policies strictly. Patients who feel office computers are being used for personal reasons may develop negative impressions of the office. As a result, some offices forbid all personal computer use, while others allow personal use during breaks or the periods before and after shifts. Policies should reflect an office's approach. For example, personal computer use may be allowed, but not within sight of patients.

Personal Digital Assistants and Smart Phones

Many physicians today use **personal digital assistants** (PDAs) and **smart phones** to quickly check medication dosages or

research drug interactions. *Personal digital assistant* is a term used to describe any small, mobile handheld device that provides computing and information storage retrieval capabilities for personal or business use, often for keeping schedule calendars and address book information handy. Outside the medical office, PDAs can be used to record a patient's hospital visit or the calls a physician takes while on call (**Figure 13-6** ■). Smart phones work not only as telephones; they also have features for browsing the Internet or composing word-processing documents.

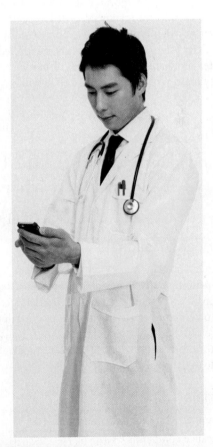

Figure 13-6 ■ A physician using his smart phone to verify a medication dosage for a patient.
Source: Shutterstock © Hans Kim.

When a physician's PDA or smart phone contains private patient information, it must be kept inaccessible to unauthorized parties. Passwords protect PDAs and smart phones, just as they do computers.

Because PDAs and smart phones can connect to computer systems, information can transfer between the two. For example, a physician can enter patient information into her PDA or smart phone and then later download that information to her desktop computer. PDAs and smart phones especially benefit physicians who wish to review patient charts outside the office. Rather than removing patient charts from the office, physicians can record the necessary information in their PDA or smart phone through a secure connection.

Computer Ergonomics

Ergonomics is the study of equipment and workspace design in order to determine the most comfortable positioning for users of the equipment and space. Paying attention to ergonomics allows organizations to reduce worker injury caused by stressful positioning or use of equipment. Long-term computer use has prompted a number of recommendations that help address health concerns. For example, members of the health care team can avoid eye strain by frequently looking away from the computer screen. Anti-glare screens are another option, as is placing the monitor at an angle to avoid glare. Carpal tunnel syndrome is associated with repeated use of the wrists, such as when typing on a keyboard. Many computer users find that the ergonomic keyboards mentioned earlier in this chapter alleviate the symptoms of carpal tunnel syndrome. Keyboard wrist supports are also helpful.

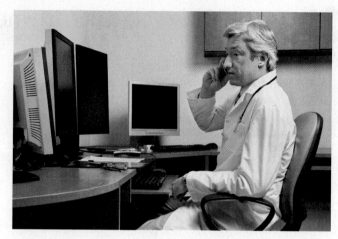

Figure 13-7 ■ Medical staff who spend long periods of time during the day at the computer need to have an ergonomically correct desk, chair, and keyboard.
Source: Shutterstock © Tyler Olsen.

Proper posture and equipment placement are crucial to avoiding computer-related injuries. Users should sit straight in chairs that support the lower back (**Figure 13-7** ■). Chairs should have armrests for use as comfortable by the user. Keyboards should be placed to allow a 90-degree angle at the elbows and should be close enough that users need not reach forward. Monitors should be at eye level, with a viewing angle of 5 to 30 degrees. Users should not have to twist to see their monitors. Feet should be flat on the floor, and legs should be uncrossed.

PROCEDURE 13-3 Use the Computer to Verify Preferred Provider Status on an Insurance Company Web Site

Theory and Rationale

Insurance company names can change when companies merge. Administrative medical assistants must keep abreast of the insurance plans their offices participate with. The ability to verify preferred provider status is a valuable function for both the physician and the patient because it allows access to information about the current medical coverage available to the patient.

Materials

- Computer with Internet connection
- Insurance company's URL
- Name of target physician

Competency

1. Using the computer, launch an Internet browser.
2. Enter the URL of the insurance company.
3. Navigate to the provider page or section.
4. In the search field, enter the provider's name and/or location.
5. Verify if the physician is preferred with the target insurance company.

REVIEW

Chapter Summary

- Computers serve varied functions and have many uses in the medical office, all of which the medical assistant should be familiar with.
- The purchase of a new computer system requires careful, informed research to ensure that the needs of the medical office are met.
- The components of a computer system include hardware, software, and peripherals.
- Office staff can take steps to maintain computer equipment, but repairs should be left to professionals.
- Security is an important part of office computing, because it helps ensure the confidentiality of patient information.

- The Internet can serve as a resource for nearly infinite medical information.
- Medical offices should instate clear policies for the use of their computers.
- Personal digital assistants and smart phones can help bridge the computing gap when physicians or other medical staff are out of the office.
- Ergonomically designed computer equipment helps ensure that all members of the health care team work safely.

Chapter Review

Multiple Choice

1. Computer peripherals include:
   a. Printers
   b. Scanners
   c. External hard drives
   d. a and b
   e. a, b, and c

2. Another term for flash drive is _____ drive.
   a. Star
   b. Thumb
   c. Media
   d. Small
   e. External

3. An electronic sign-in sheet is designed to:
   a. Maintain patient confidentiality
   b. Ensure HIPAA compliance
   c. Track patients in the office
   d. a and b
   e. a, b, and c

4. A medical office may use a scanner to:
   a. Copy photos into a patient's chart
   b. Photocopy documents to give to patients
   c. Track insurance correspondence
   d. Maintain patient confidentiality
   e. Make patient medical appointments

5. Which piece of computer equipment may help avoid carpal tunnel syndrome?
   a. Monitor
   b. Scanner
   c. Ergonomic keyboard
   d. Personal digital assistant
   e. Digital camera

True/False

T F 1. The CPU is considered the computer's brain.

T F 2. Flat-panel monitors are often used when desk space is at a premium.

T F 3. Computer passwords should be something easy to remember, such as a birthdate or an address.

T F 4. Medical management software companies should provide onsite training of staff.

T F 5. A trained professional should perform any maintenance on office computers.

T F 6. Bar-code scanners are used in health care to track supplies, among other things.

Short Answer

1. What is PowerPoint software used for?
2. What is the importance of an external battery backup system?
3. What is a thumb drive used for?
4. What is the difference between a computer virus and malware?
5. What is the main danger in downloading files to an office computer?

6. Name Internet search engines for finding information online.
7. Name some functions of a health-related calculator.
8. What is an ergonomically correct keyboard?
9. Describe the functions of medical practice management software.

Research

1. Search the Internet for computer retailers. What type of system do you think would be a typical set up for a medical office computer station? What components do you believe would be included?
2. Interview a person who works in a medical office. How does that facility back up its data? How often is the backup done?
3. Search online for information on computer ergonomics. What kind of information did you find about posture and working at a computer?

Practicum Application Experience

As Monica Friedenrich is training the medical assistant on the medical office's computer systems, she explains the HIPAA regulations for passwords, which include a unique password for every staff member. Monica then directs the medical assistant to use her own password during training. Should the medical assistant comply? If the assistant chooses to comply, what issues could result?

Resource Guide

Language Scientific
Medical Translation Services
www.languagescientific.com

CSGNetwork and Computer Support Group Health-Related Calculators
http://www.csgnetwork.com

Occupational Safety and Health Administration (OSHA)
www.osha.gov

14

Equipment, Maintenance, and Supply Inventory

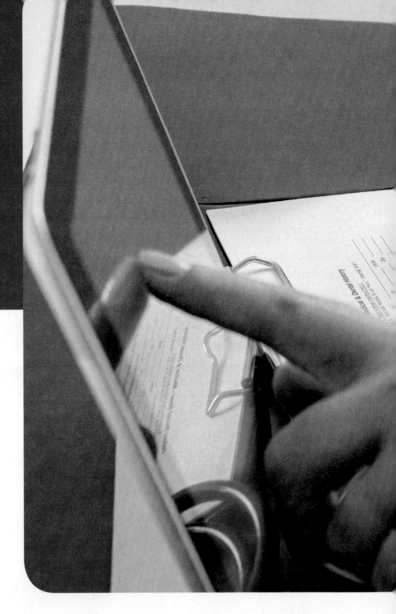

Case Study

Read the following case study and answer the critical thinking questions presented throughout the chapter.

During a medical office's weekly staff meeting, several staff members voice their frustration over frequently running out of clerical supplies before new supplies are received. As the person in charge of inventory and supply ordering in the administrative office, the registered medical assistant is asked to devise a system to address the situation.

Objectives

After completing this chapter, you should be able to:

14.1 Define and spell the key terminology in this chapter.

14.2 Discuss the importance and functions of a user manual and warranty.

14.3 List the information found in the medical office equipment maintenance log.

14.4 Describe the process the medical assistant should follow when replacing or buying medical equipment.

14.5 Explain the pros and cons of leasing and purchasing office equipment.

14.6 Maintain patient confidentiality while faxing.

14.7 Discuss factors the medical assistant should research prior to the purchase of a copy machine.

14.8 Describe the use of a 10-key adding machine in the medical office.

14.9 Discuss transcription practices in the medical office.

14.10 Maintain inventory of medical office supplies.

14.11 Explain the steps involved in receiving and logging drug samples.

14.12 Discuss how supplies are stocked in a medical office.

14.13 Explain how scanners are used in supply ordering.

Competency Skills Performance

1. Take inventory of administrative equipment.
2. Fax a document.
3. Perform routine maintenance of a computer printer.
4. Prepare a purchase order.
5. Receive a supply shipment.

Key Terminology

expiration date—date on which something loses full strength or validity

inventory—supplies on hand

maintained—kept in good working order

packing slip—list of supplies ordered and included in a shipment

scanner—device that copies documents or pictures for transfer to computer systems

transcribe—to type words as they are spoken

transcription machine—piece of equipment that allows the user to listen to and type recorded words

user manual—document that describes how something (e.g., equipment) is used

warranty—a guarantee from a vendor stating that certain defects or problems will be repaired for a predetermined period

Abbreviations

HIPAA—Health Insurance Portability and Accountability Act

OSHA—Occupational Safety and Health Administration

Certification Exam Coverage

AAMA (CMA) Exam Coverage:

- Equipment operation
  - Calculator
  - Photocopier
  - Computer
  - Fax machine
  - Scanners
- Maintenance and repairs
  - Contents of instruction manual
  - Routine maintenance
    1) Agreements
    2) Warranty
    3) Repair service
- Maintaining the office environment—physical environment
  - Arrangements of furniture, equipment, and supplies
  - Facilities and equipment
    1) Maintenance and repair
    2) Safety regulations
       a) Occupational Safety and Health Act (OSHA)
  - Equipment and supply inventory
    1) Inventory control
    2) Purchasing
  - Restocking supplies

AMT (CMAS) Exam Coverage:

- Supplies and equipment
  - Manage medical and office supply inventories and order supplies
  - Maintain office equipment and arrange for (and maintain records of) equipment maintenance and repair

AMT (RMA) Exam Coverage:

- Supplies and equipment management
  - Maintain inventory of medical/office supplies and equipment
  - Coordinate maintenance and repair of office equipment
  - Maintain equipment maintenance logs according to OSHA regulations

NCCT (NCMA) Exam Coverage:

- General office procedures
  - Equipment operation and maintenance

Introduction

In medical offices that run smoothly, equipment is well **maintained** and supplies and **inventory** are effectively managed. While some large offices track their supplies and inventories electronically, others opt for a manual process. Medical assistants who are adept at equipment use in the medical office are both efficient at their jobs and competitive in the job market.

Medical Office Equipment

Every piece of equipment a medical office buys or leases comes with a **user manual**. A new piece of equipment typically also comes with a **warranty**, a guarantee from the vendor that certain defects or problems will be repaired for a predetermined period. Many companies sell extended warranties that cover equipment for longer periods. To track warranty periods and expedite repairs or replacement, the date a piece of equipment was leased or purchased should be written on the equipment's user manual. When possible, any receipts should be included. User manuals should be kept in a central location, like a file cabinet, so they can quickly and easily be found when needed.

Training Employees to Use Medical Office Equipment

Every employee who is asked to use a piece of office equipment must be trained on that equipment's proper use and care. Many suppliers train employees when equipment is purchased, but often just once, which means staff who have been trained must document their training if future employees are to be trained as well.

Training manuals can be invaluable tools for documenting training content in the medical office. Manuals should devote one page to each piece of equipment. In addition to explaining how to use and maintain the equipment, each page should provide a place for employees to sign and date once properly trained (**Figure 14-1** ■). In addition to furthering training objectives, such manuals keep the medical office in compliance with Occupational Safety and Health Administration (**OSHA**) safety regulations. Part of keeping staff safe in the medical office is training on possible injury in using office equipment. Safety issues such as electrical injury or burn avoidance must be taught to all new users of equipment.

Keeping a Maintenance Log for Medical Office Equipment

For each piece of equipment that requires regular maintenance, the medical office should keep a log of the maintenance requirements, schedule, and responsible party. When equipment must be maintained by the manufacturer or another professional repairperson, the log should include the contact

Training Employees on the Use of the Photocopier
Familiarize employees with:
❑ On/off switch
❑ Paper placement on glass
❑ Paper replacement
❑ Use of enlarge/reduce feature
❑ Toner replacement
❑ Location of telephone number for repairs
❑ Location of telephone number for supplies
Signature of Employee: _____
Signature of Trainer: _____
Date: _____

Figure 14-1 ■ Sample page from an office equipment training manual.

information for that repairperson. Anyone who performs maintenance should sign and date the maintenance log. A complete maintenance log helps the medical office prove that its equipment has been well maintained, which can in turn help expedite warranty work (**Figure 14-2** ■).

Replacing or Buying Medical Office Equipment

When the time comes to replace or acquire equipment, the physician may ask the medical assistant to research options. For small, easy-to-transport pieces, assistants may ask sales representatives to bring samples to the office for review. Assistants may also research equipment online or visit stores where equipment is displayed. For high-dollar purchases, sales representatives should refer the medical assistant to other customers who are using the product. In turn, the assistant should take the time to call those references and poll them on customer service and the ease of use of the equipment.

When calling other medical offices for equipment references, the medical assistant should be sure to talk to the staff members who actually use the equipment. Those staff will accurately depict how that equipment works.

▶▶▶ Pulse Points

Equipment Malfunction

Medical office equipment might sometimes malfunction. When it does, report the malfunction to the office manager or physician immediately. Malfunctions in some equipment, especially clinical equipment, can injure patients or medical staff.

Office Equipment Maintenance Log				
Equipment name	Maintenance to be performed	Maintenance schedule	Name of person performing the maintenance	Signature and date
Photocopier	Clean spilled toner inside the machine	Once monthly	Louise Glaser, CMA (AAMA)	*L. Glaser, CMA (AAMA) 9/4/XX*

Figure 14-2 ■ Sample office equipment maintenance log.

Weighing Equipment Leasing Against Buying

Leasing and buying have distinct advantages when it comes to equipment. Leasing does not award ownership, but it typically requires no down payment. When leasing equipment, the medical office might pay a small or even no down payment and make monthly payments on the lease. In the event the equipment breaks or malfunctions, the manufacturer usually replaces or repairs it as part of the lease. With some leases, the equipment is returned at the end of the lease; with other leases, the equipment might have a purchase option at the end of the lease. Purchased equipment generally requires full funding up front or a down payment and financed balance. Buying, however, confers ownership. Once the equipment is paid for, the owner need only cover the costs associated with maintenance or repairs. Physician's preference, price, and intended use all help drive the lease/buy decision.

Fax Machines in the Medical Office

Facsimile or *fax* machines are common pieces of medical office equipment that come in varied sizes and prices (**Figure 14-3** ■). Via telephone lines, fax machines make it possible to send and receive printed documents anywhere in the world where other fax machines are located. Simple, relatively inexpensive models simply fax documents from one location to another. Higher end versions also serve as photocopiers and **scanners**.

 PROCEDURE 14-1 Take Inventory of Administrative Equipment

Theory and Rationale

An up-to-date list of a medical office's administrative equipment helps determine the equipment's age in the event the equipment needs repair, or replacement if fire, flood, or theft occurs.

Materials

- Paper
- Pen
- Computer with word-processing or spreadsheet software

Competency

1. Locate all administrative equipment in the medical office.

2. List each piece of equipment with manufacturer name, serial number, and date of purchase, when known.
3. Include information about the company maintaining the equipment.
4. Include information about the supplies needed to maintain the equipment, including where those supplies are purchased.
5. Using word-processing or spreadsheet software, create an inventory of all equipment information.
6. Update the inventory sheet as needed when new equipment is purchased or older equipment is replaced.

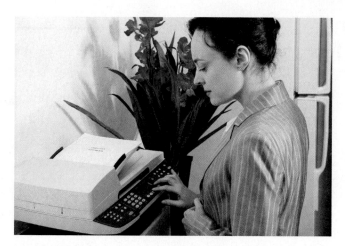

Figure 14-3 ■ The fax machine in a medical office must be located outside areas frequented by patients.
Source: Fotolia © Stephen Coburn.

To guard patient confidentiality, fax machines must be kept in areas of the office that are inaccessible to patients. These machines should not reside on the counter at the front desk or in a hallway, for example. While medical offices commonly use fax machines to send and receive confidential patient information, the Health Insurance Portability and Accountability Act (HIPAA) dictates that fax machines be used only when other modes of transmission fail to suffice. Therefore, when medical offices must transmit information on patients' behalf, medical assistants should use conventional mail when there is time. Some medical offices use courier services in lieu of faxing, especially for such highly confidential information as HIV status or reproductive health care decisions. Any faxed documents must be accompanied by a HIPAA-compliant fax cover sheet. Such cover sheets include disclaimers that the faxed information cannot be disclosed to any party without the patient's written consent or a court

order. Many electronic medical record programs offer the ability to fax information from the medical record to an outside fax recipient.

Copy Machines in the Medical Office

Copy machines, like fax machines, come in all sizes and at all price levels. Medical offices should have high-quality copiers that are maintained and serviced regularly. Because medical offices tend to use their copiers heavily, unreliable machines can severely impede office functioning. Like fax machines, office copiers should be placed where patients cannot access them. Copiers are best placed behind the front desk or near the billing office, as staff in those areas use copiers the most.

When researching copiers, medical offices should consider various factors. While price and warranty are of obvious concern, the cost of supplies is also an important consideration. Some copiers require difficult-to-find or expensive parts. When purchased, many pieces of equipment are accompanied by a service agreement that typically lasts for a set period of time. The service agreement is similar to a warranty in that it outlines the services and repairs that will be covered during the time of the service agreement contract. During the time of the service agreement or warranty, equipment is often repaired at no charge to the owner. Before purchasing a copier, the medical assistant will want to research these options in order to determine the best machine for the medical office.

Adding Machines

Upon hearing the words *adding machine*, many people envision 10-key calculators. Such calculators are normally electronic, and most have tape for printing (**Figure 14-4** ■). With

 PROCEDURE 14-2 Fax a Document

Theory and Rationale

Faxing documents from the medical office requires strict attention to HIPAA regulations for safeguarding private patient information. Medical assistants must take care that the information being faxed is only that which needs to be faxed and no more or less. The fax number being used must be verified so that accidental faxing to the wrong number does not occur. In addition, any fax that contains patient information must be accompanied by a HIPAA-compliant cover sheet.

Materials

- Document to be faxed
- HIPAA-compliant fax cover sheet
- Pen
- Fax machine

Competency

1. Complete the fax cover sheet with your own name, phone number, and clinic contact information.
2. Fill in the name and fax number of the fax recipient.
3. List the number of pages in the fax, including the cover sheet.
4. Properly orient the fax cover sheet and document to be faxed in the fax machine.
5. Dial the target fax number.
6. When the fax has fully transmitted, remove the documents and file them with the fax confirmation sheet in the patient's file.

PROCEDURE 14-3 Perform Routine Maintenance 📋 of a Computer Printer

Theory and Rationale

While most equipment in the medical office requires a trained technician to provide maintenance, the medical assistant performs basic maintenance on many pieces, such as the computer printer.

Materials

- Paper
- Pen
- Computer printer
- Maintenance logbook

Competency

1. Review the maintenance logbook and service agreement for the computer printer.
2. Following the manufacturer's directions, open the printer cover and remove the toner cartridge.
3. Using the manufacturer-provided cleaning tool, clean any dust and spilled toner from inside the printer.
4. Replace the cleaning tool and the toner cartridge.
5. Close the printer cover.
6. In the maintenance logbook, enter information about the maintenance, including the date and your signature.

regular use, most administrative staff in the medical office become proficient with 10-key calculators. This skill is especially helpful when adding long columns of numbers, like those on deposit slips, or when calculating a patient's copayment for medical service. Medical staff also often use handheld calculators. These come in all shapes and sizes, typically run on battery power, and are convenient when 10-key systems are impractical. Some handheld calculators are small enough to fit in the pocket of a clinic jacket. Many electronic health record programs, as well as numerous software programs on today's computers offer the same function as an electronic calculator. Many clinical medical assistants keep a small, handheld calculator in their clinic jacket to quickly calculate figures for things such as medication doses when away from a computer or electronic calculator.

Medical Transcription

In the past, **transcription machines** were common in medical offices. Physicians would dictate patient information into tape recorders and give the tapes to administrative staff, who would **transcribe** the information into printed form (**Figure 14-5** ■). The transcriber would use headphones to listen and foot pedals to control the tapes. Volume and speed buttons controlled

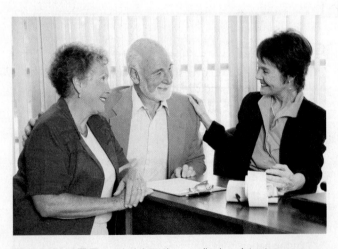

Figure 14-4 ■ The administrative medical assistant may use a 10-key calculator for tasks such as calculating a patient's copayment for medical services.
Source: Shutterstock © Lisa F. Young.

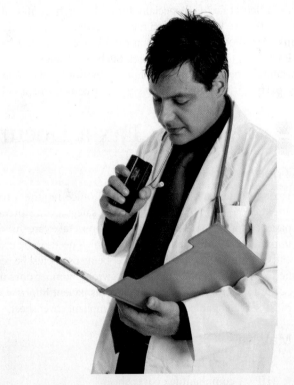

Figure 14-5 ■ A physician records his chart notes into a tape recorder for transcription.
Source: Fotolia © Leah-Anne Thompson.

those functions. Some physicians and medical facilities continue to use transcription services, though the service is often performed offsite by transcriptionists.

The physician who has dictated the information must review the transcript before the tape is erased in order to verify wording or correct errors. Once the physician has approved the transcript, the tape can be erased and reused. In health care today, transcription done onsite by transcription staff is less common than in years past. Physicians using an electronic medical record will typically type their own medical notes, using a series of shortcuts to populate their medical notes. Software programs such as Dragon Naturally Speaking allow users to speak into a microphone, and the software translates the spoken word into written form.

Finding Outside Transcription Services

Many medical offices today use outside transcription services. These services typically require physicians to call a recorded telephone line to dictate their information. The corresponding printed documents arrive via fax, e-mail, or postal service.

For a number of reasons, thorough research is important when choosing outside transcription services. Many transcription services are based outside the United States, where patient privacy laws can vary and fail to meet U.S. **HIPAA** regulations. Research should reveal a transcription company's reputation as well as its prices and services. While the Internet can be a valuable research tool, the best way to find an outside transcription service is to identify which services other medical offices in the area use. Medical assistants can then delve into the patient confidentiality policies, costs, and turnaround times of those companies. Armed with this type of information, medical assistants can give informed, comprehensive presentations to the physician on recommended services.

Logging Medical Office Supplies

To effectively manage office inventory and supplies, the medical office should create a master list of all regularly purchased items. This list should include all disposable supplies; separate lists should detail clinical and clerical supplies. All such lists should include the supply, the order or part number, the name of the company, and the typical quantity and frequency of ordering (**Figure 14-6 ▪**).

Inventorying Supplies

To ensure that the medical office remains fully functional, a designated member of the health care team should regularly inventory all supplies to ensure they remain in stock. Out-of-stock items force offices to reschedule procedures or incur high next-day reordering expenses. Offices use supplies at different rates, and their reorder schedules should reflect those differences. Most offices inventory supplies weekly, while others adhere to monthly or daily schedules. Because medical assistants' vacation schedules and days off vary, the inventory task works best when shared by more than one staff member.

Today, many medical facilities have electronic inventory systems for supplies. With these systems, supplies are scanned into the system, where they are then tracked for the purposes of billing and reordering. When multiple physicians or departments share the same supply room, these electronic systems allow the organization to properly allocate the expense of supplies used to the appropriate department.

Critical Thinking Question 14-1

Refer back to the case study presented at the beginning of this chapter. How does rotating the person in charge of inventory each week benefit the medical office's inventory process?

Inventory Supply Log				
Supply	**Order or Part Number**	**Supplier**	**Number in Order**	**Frequency of Order**
Fee slips	N/A	Minuteman Press (425) 555–9000	5,000	Twice annually
Fax toner cartridges	HP6545	Office Depot (800) 345-3000	2	Once monthly

Figure 14-6 ▪ Sample inventory supply log.

The key to effective supply management is to have enough supplies to efficiently run the office but not so much as to risk expiration or storage issues. Many of the supplies used in the clinical part of the office, such as laboratory collection containers or medications and vaccines, have expiration dates. Some supplies, especially medications, have expiration dates of no more than one year from the date of manufacture. A medical office might get a good price on gloves by ordering 500 boxes at once, for example, but if the staff will take two years to use those gloves and storage space is at a premium, the saving is not likely worth the inconvenience.

Many offices devise systems to remind themselves when certain supplies must be ordered. If, for example, staff knows to reorder gloves when only ten boxes are left in stock, a reorder reminder note can be attached to the tenth box of gloves. Using this process, the medical office will see a reduction in supply expenses, as there is less chance of duplication in supply ordering.

Reducing Office Supply Expenses

While keeping track of needed supplies and ordering supplies only as needed for use are mechanisms for reducing supply costs, there are other ways in which the medical office staff can reduce the cost of supplies. Because many companies produce and sell similar items, medical office staff are best able to reduce costs by comparing prices and quality between various companies. Companies that offer free shipping, for example, might be a better resource for supplies if the cost of the supplies is the same as a company that does not offer free shipping. Some medical supply companies offer free samples of their products to medical offices that use those supplies. These free supplies allow the medical office to determine if the supply is of appropriate quality for the purpose intended. This ability to try a product at no cost before committing to the purchase of that product is yet another method for reducing inventory costs.

▶▶▶ Pulse Points

Taking Office Supplies

Medical office staff must have a high level of integrity, which means office and medical supplies must stay in the office. Employees who take office pens, notepads, or even bandages without permission steal and place the office in jeopardy of running out of supplies sooner than expected, which can impede procedure scheduling. Taking office supplies without permission may result in termination or loss of trust in the offender.

Some medical offices use purchase orders for ordering supplies or equipment needed in the office. Purchase orders are written sales contracts that outline the items to be received, and the agreed upon price between the purchaser and the vendor. In some facilities, these purchase orders must be authorized by the office manager or the physician; in other facilities they are filled out by the person in charge of ordering supplies and sent directly by that person to the supplier.

In Practice

Before the medical assistant was hired, the medical office lacked a system for ordering supplies. Members of the health care team simply ordered supplies as they felt necessary. As a result, the office now has cupboards full of supplies that will expire in a month. As a new employee, the medical assistant is charged with devising a system for tracking office inventory. Where should the assistant start? What steps will help ensure all supplies are counted correctly?

Checking for the Next Day's Supplies

At the end of the workday, one member of the health care team should ensure that the office has enough supplies for all procedures scheduled the next day. Rescheduling due to supply deficiencies reflects poorly on the office and impedes efficient office operation. The medical office should develop a good relationship with other, nearby offices so that supplies can be borrowed in the event of unexpected shortages.

Storing Supplies upon Arrival

When supplies arrive in the medical office, one staff member must locate the **packing slip** and check to ensure all the supplies that were ordered are included. Usually, this slip is sealed in a clear plastic envelope and attached to the outside of the box, but it might be in the box with the supplies. The packing slip lists the supplies that were ordered and the supplies in the shipment. This slip might also serve as an invoice (**Figure 14-7** ■). If so, it must

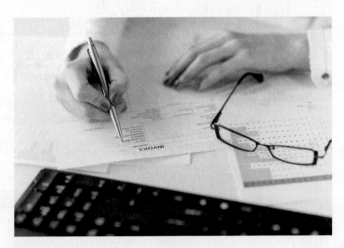

Figure 14-7 ■ Invoice for supplies received.
Source: Fotolia © Syda Productions.

PROCEDURE 14-4   Prepare a Purchase Order

Theory and Rationale

Purchase orders allow the medical office to accurately track the supplies that are needed and used in the clinic, as well as how often these supplies are being ordered.

Materials

- List of needed supplies
- Purchase order form
- Pen
- Fax machine or telephone

Competency

1. Review the list of needed supplies, grouping them according to the vendor they will be ordered from.
2. Fill in the name and fax number of the company the supplies are to be ordered from.
3. List each supply individually on the purchase order, taking care to note the quantity needed and the part number associated with each item.
4. If the physician's signature is required, obtain his or her signature. If it is not required, sign and date the form yourself.
5. If the purchase order can be faxed to the supplier, fax the document and make a note of the date and time the fax went through.
6. If the purchase order cannot be faxed to the supplier, call the supplier and place the order over the telephone. Document the name of the person you spoke to and the date and time of the call.
7. File the purchase order in a folder for pending orders.

---

be routed to the accounts payable office after the order is checked for completeness. When part of an order is missing or back-ordered, the medical assistant must make a notation and keep the packing slip until the remaining supplies arrive in the office.

Except for clerical supplies, all newly arrived medical office supplies should be stored behind older inventory so older supplies are used first. Because many medical supplies have **expiration dates**, this procedure helps eliminate waste.

In the event medications need to be discarded by the medical office, often due to expiration, the medical office must follow legal guidelines for this disposal. According to the U.S. Food and Drug Administration, the proper way to dispose of medication is to remove it from its container and mix it with an undesirable substance such as coffee grounds or cat litter. Once placed into a plastic bag with this substance, the medication should then be discarded in the trash.

Handling Drug Samples

Many medical offices welcome the pharmaceutical representatives who supply drug samples; these drug samples are normally small quantities of the drugs pharmaceutical companies sell. Usually, samples are name-brand, costly drugs that are new to the market. Companies give physicians drug samples in the hope that physicians will prescribe the drugs to their patients. Typically, physicians set aside short periods to meet with drug-company representatives. In most states, medical assistants may sign for the drug samples that sales representatives leave. Not all medical offices permit pharmaceutical representatives access to the physicians or other clinical staff.

In medical offices, drugs should be grouped according to type. Antibiotics should be kept together, for example, as should antidepressants or cough medicines. All medications, including drug samples, must be kept out of patient access areas. Medications, including drug samples, have expiration dates and must be discarded once those dates have passed. In some states, sample drugs must also be tracked. Medical offices should track samples even when the law does not require it. Tracking discourages staff from taking drugs and supplies for personal use.

Stocking Clerical Supplies

Clerical supplies are easier to stock than clinical supplies because most medical offices know how many envelopes, stamps, and forms they regularly use. In addition, clerical supplies do not expire and most such items (except for preprinted business cards or letterhead) are readily available at local supply stores. While an abundance of clerical supplies can present a storage problem, many suppliers offer volume discounts.

When storing clerical supplies, there is no need to place the newest products behind the older products. Products without expiration dates can be used at any time. Exceptions include a new piece of equipment or products that might become obsolete due to a service contract. For example, an office that has stocked multiple toner cartridges for a particular printer would find excess inventory on hand if that printer is replaced while toner stock remains.

Medical offices must keep enough supplies on hand to ensure there is never a shortage. On the other side of that goal, the medical office does not want to have an abundance of supplies that places a strain on the ability to store them. Supplies that are commonly used are typically stocked within the medical office. Supplies that might be used only infrequently may be ordered only when needed.

PROCEDURE 14-5 Receive a Supply Shipment

Theory and Rationale

Medical office supplies are ordered and received regularly. To ensure that all ordered supplies have been received, the medical assistant must carefully check the packing list that comes with the supplies.

Materials

- Box of supplies
- Packing slip
- Supply inventory logbook
- Pen

Competency

1. Open the box of supplies, and locate the packing slip.

2. Remove each item from the box, checking it on the packing slip.

3. On the packing slip, circle any missing supplies.

4. Put the supplies away, newer ones behind older ones.

5. Note in the supply log that the supplies have been received.

6. When any supplies on the packing slip are absent from the shipment, notify the supplier.

7. When any supplies on the packing slip are on back-order, retain the slip until the backordered supplies arrive.

8. When the packing slip also serves as an invoice, route it to the accounts payable department.

9. Discard packing materials appropriately.

Tracking Supplies with Computer Software

Many medical offices today use barcode-equipped computer software to ensure that they have adequate supplies. When members of the health care team take items from the supply room, they use the software to scan the bar code of those items and note the department using the supplies. When supplies drop below a preprogrammed level, the staff member in charge of ordering supplies is notified to order more of that supply. Software ordering systems are only as accurate as the staff members who use them, however. When supplies are scanned inaccurately, they cannot be tracked and supplies might not be adequately stocked.

In medical offices where electronic systems are not used, the medical staff might need to take inventory of supplies manually. This might be done daily, weekly, monthly, or even quarterly, depending upon the needs of the office. Some offices use a checklist of supplies, with a system that indicates at what level of supply the reorder should be made.

REVIEW

Chapter Summary

- For the medical office, an equipment maintenance manual serves to ensure all needed equipment is in working order and able to support business initiatives.

- At the physician's request, the medical assistant is often charged with researching the best options for buying supplies and equipment.

- Depending on factors like need, cost, and long-term objectives, medical offices may choose to lease or buy their business equipment.

- Fax machines are just one common piece of equipment that require all members of the health care team to remain vigilant to patient confidentiality.

- A photocopier in the medical office can provide copies of documents for patient and office use.

- Staff in the medical office often become adept at using 10-key calculators to manipulate numbers.

- Transcription machines, once widely used in health care, are still sometimes used to convert spoken words to written ones.

- When researching transcription services outside the medical office, the medical assistant should be conscious of such factors as location and cost.

- An inventory control manual helps a medical office ensure that it is always fully equipped with needed supplies.

- Medical supplies might have expiration dates and should be ordered with the goal of using all supplies before they expire.

- Drug samples must be tracked and notice must be taken of any expiration dates on these samples.

Chapter Review

Multiple Choice

1. When investigating options for replacing medical equipment, it is acceptable to:
   a. Have a salesperson bring the equipment to the office to demonstrate it
   b. Buy new equipment without investigating any other options
   c. Buy the least expensive piece of equipment, assuming it is the best bargain
   d. Buy the most expensive piece of equipment, assuming it is the highest quality
   e. Buy the equipment the salesperson tells you is the best

2. In the medical office, fax machines:
   a. Should be used to send patient information between offices because it saves postage
   b. Can be placed anywhere that is most convenient for office staff
   c. Come in all sizes and prices
   d. Do not need to be maintained regularly
   e. Use the same supplies regardless of the model of the machine

3. The best way to dispose of expired medications is to:
   a. Donate them to an agency that will use them outside the United States
   b. Give them to patients who might want them
   c. Sell them on eBay
   d. Wrap them in plastic and place them in the garbage
   e. Flush them down the toilet

4. It is important to keep a maintenance log for medical office equipment to:
   a. Prove the equipment has been maintained in the event warranty work is needed
   b. Be able to prove to the CDC that the equipment is safe for use
   c. Show to any inspectors that the equipment has been maintained
   d. Provide proof of maintenance when the time comes to sell the equipment for replacement
   e. Create a need for additional paperwork in the office

5. When looking to purchase a new copy machine for the medical office, staff should consider the:
   a. Cost of supplies
   b. Ease of use of the equipment
   c. Ability to borrow supplies from other offices
   d. Placement in the office
   e. Availability of videos online regarding the use of the equipment

True/False

T F **1.** It is always a good idea to call for references with any new supplier before making an expensive purchase.

T F **2.** Many transcription services use employees outside the United States.

T F **3.** Clinical inventory in the medical office should be taken weekly, whatever the practice type or patient load.

T F **4.** Taking office pens and paperclips for home use is stealing, and should not be done.

Short Answer

1. Give one advantage to leasing a piece of office equipment instead of buying it.
2. Name one advantage to buying a piece of office equipment instead of leasing it.
3. Explain the use of a scanner in the medical office.
4. When calling other medical offices to get references for supply companies, why speak with the staff who use the supplies or equipment?
5. Explain why the medical office should keep an employee training manual for office equipment.
6. What should be the medical office's main consideration when researching outside transcription services, and why?
7. Why separate the inventory list of clerical supplies from the list for clinical supplies?
8. Explain why expiration dates on medical supplies are important to track.
9. Why is it important to check the packing slip for supplies that have been received?
10. Why do pharmaceutical companies give medical offices free drug samples?
11. What clerical supplies are usually ordered with an office's name, address, and telephone number pre-printed?

Research

1. Interview a person who works in a medical office. How does that office keep track of the various supplies needed and used?
2. Research various office supply companies online for information about photocopiers. What type of machine do you think would be appropriate for a medical office?
3. Call a medical office-supply company. How quickly are orders typically shipped? Are there discounts offered for higher quantity purchases?

Practicum Application Experience

A package of medical office supplies arrives at the medical office. While checking off the supplies listed on the packing slip, the medical assistant notices five items on the packing slip are not in the box. How should the medical assistant handle the situation?

Resource Guide

Parker Inventory Management System
Manufactures bar code scanning software for inventory control management
http://www.parker.com

Decision Software Systems
Provides software solutions for accounting, inventory, and other information management problems
http://www.decisionsw.com

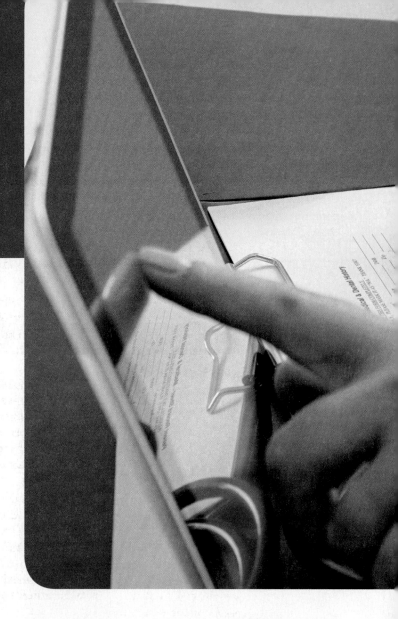

15

Office Policies and Procedures

Case Study

Read the following case study and answer the critical thinking questions presented throughout the chapter

Monte Taylor recently passed the registered medical assisting exam and has just obtained his first job as a registered medical assistant. Dr. Radcliff, an internist who shares her office space with several other physicians, has hired Monte. On Monte's first day, he asks the office manager if there is a manual that outlines office procedures. The office manager tells Monte that office staff have never taken the time to compose a procedures manual, and asks Monte if he would be willing to take on such a task.

Objectives

After completing this chapter, you should be able to:

15.1 Define and spell the key terminology in this chapter.

15.2 Create patient information pamphlets.

15.3 Develop a personnel manual.

15.4 Create a policies and procedures manual for the medical office.

Competency Skills Performance

1. Create an office brochure.

2. Create a procedure for the office procedure manual.

Key Terminology

brochure—document containing information about a topic

mission statement—summary of an organization's purpose or reason for existing

organizational chart—breakdown of the chain of command in a business

personnel manual—compilation of employment policies for an office; also called an *employee handbook*

policy—a rule by which an individual or organization is guided

procedure—steps to perform a task or project

Abbreviations

HIPAA—Health Insurance Portability and Accountability Act

OSHA—Occupational Safety and Health Administration

Certification Exam Coverage

AAMA (CMA) Exam Coverage:
- Resource information and community services
  - Patient advocate
    1) Services available
    2) Patient referrals
    3) Followup
- Office policies and procedures
  - Patient information booklet
  - Personnel manual
  - Policy and procedures manuals/protocols

AMT (CMAS) Exam Coverage:
- Human resources
  - Maintain office policy manual

AMT (RMA) Exam Coverage:
- Patient resource materials
  - Develop, assemble, and maintain appropriate patient brochures and information materials

Introduction

Every business needs written policies and procedures to ensure that employees know how to perform their jobs correctly, and health care is no exception. Policies and procedures are perhaps even more important in the medical field than in others because they contribute to patient safety and risk reduction. A **policy** is a statement of guidelines or rules on a given topic. A **procedure** describes how to perform a given task or project.

Patient Information Pamphlets

Every member of the health care team is responsible for educating patients. Much of the information physicians want patients to receive may be in written form. Many medical offices buy educational **brochures** to give to patients. These documents are available on a multitude of topics, including back pain, child immunizations, and menopause (**Figure 15-1 ■**).

For physicians who want to provide more detailed information, brochures may be created with the help of in-house staff or a professional printing company. However the office chooses to create patient educational pamphlets, those pamphlets must be professional. All printed material must be accurate and free of typographical errors. Depending on the cultural makeup of an office's patients, brochures may be printed in various languages.

Typical information in the office brochure includes the hours the office is open, any special treatments or type of care offered in the facility, and financial information regarding insurance coverage or required payment from the patient. Brochures may be mailed to patients, and they may be offered to patients in the office. Brochures are sometimes

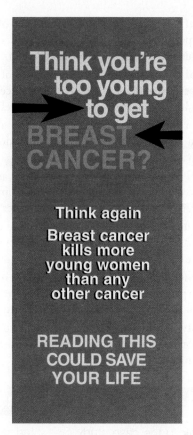

Figure 15-1 ■ A patient education pamphlet on breast cancer.

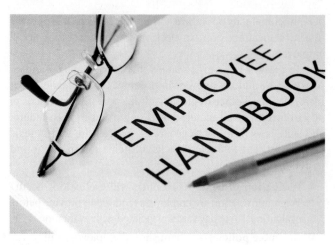

Figure 15-2 ■ The employee handbook should be updated on a regular basis and made available to each new employee.
Source: Fotolia © emiliezhang.

and direct patients to download the information. By keeping the information online, medical offices are able to update the information as needed, without having to reprint brochures or pamphlets.

The Personnel Manual

A **personnel manual**, also called an employee handbook lists the rules and regulations that apply to all staff in the medical office (**Figure 15-2** ■). In some organizations, the employees are asked to sign the employee handbook as an indication that it has been received. This manual also breaks down the office's benefits for health, life, and disability insurance, among others. Many offices give all new employees copies of their

used as marketing materials as well, mailed out to members of the community in an attempt to garner new patients to the facility.

In addition to creating materials that can be handed out to patients, many offices keep this material on their Web sites

PROCEDURE 15-1 Create an Office Brochure

Theory and Rationale
Office brochures are a useful way to educate patients on the physician's specific types of treatment or therapy. All office brochures must be professional, accurate, and free of typographical errors.

Materials
- Computer with word-processing and/or publishing software
- List of information the physician would like in an office brochure

Competency
1. Gather information on the brochure's subject.
2. Launch the word-processing and/or publishing software.

3. Create a title for the brochure, such as "Living with Diabetes."
4. Add information to the brochure in an easy-to-read format. Use simple terms rather than medical terminology.
5. Add information regarding where the patient can look for further resources, such as Web sites.
6. Include the office's name, address, and telephone number.
7. Check for typographical and grammatical errors.
8. Print the brochure, and give it to the physician for review before making copies for patients.

personnel manuals upon hire. Other offices keep single copies in central locations or in an electronic format accessible to all employees.

To create a personnel manual, the office manager and/or physician should list items of importance for the manual. For ideas, a medical office might consult the personnel manuals of other offices. For all material, it is important to keep federal and state laws in mind to ensure all policies are within legal boundaries. The following is a list of items commonly found in personnel manuals.

- **Evaluation process**—How often will evaluations occur? What information are employees required to provide before evaluations? Are pay raises associated with evaluations?
- **Absentee policies**—Whom should employees call in the event they must miss work? Are employees responsible for finding replacements when they must miss work? Is a doctor's note required in the event of illness?
- **Confidentiality policy**—What are the penalties for violating patient confidentiality? What constitutes a violation of patient confidentiality? How does the office require certain situations be handled, such as calling out the patient's name in the reception room?
- **Continuing education requirements**—Does the office require written verification of attendance or completion of continuing education? Does the office require more hours of continuing education than the employee needs for recertification/relicensure? Does the office require certain types of continuing education, such as clinical or administrative?
- **Grievance procedures**—How should employees handle situations in which they disagree with their supervisors?
- **Parking**—Are employees required to park in certain areas? Are employees required to pay for their own parking? Are there incentives for employees who carpool or take public transportation?
- **Pay**—What is the starting rate of pay? At what point are pay increases possible?
- **Health and dental benefits**—Are health and dental benefits available? At what point are employees eligible for these plans? Are employees able to add coverage for their spouses or children? Where can employees find information on benefits?
- **Staff meetings**—How often are staff meetings held? Are staff meetings compulsory (mandatory)? Where are staff meetings held? What type of information should employees bring to staff meetings?
- **Paid time off**—Are employees eligible for paid time off? Under what circumstances? How should requests for time off be handled?
- **Holiday compensation**—Are employees paid extra for working on holidays? If the office is closed on holidays, are employees compensated?
- **Sexual harassment**—What constitutes sexual harassment? How should employees handle incidences of sexual harassment?

- **Personal telephone use**—Is personal use of office telephones permitted? Under what circumstances? What are the penalties for excessive personal telephone use?
- **Personal computer use**—Is personal use of office computers permitted? Under what circumstances? What are the penalties for excessive personal computer use?
- **Vacation days**—Are employees eligible for paid or unpaid vacation days? At what intervals? How do employees request vacation days?
- **Severe weather or power outage**—What is the policy should severe weather prevent employees from traveling to the office? What is the policy should the office lose power?
- **Emergency fire procedures**—How are fire emergencies handled? Who is responsible for clearing patients from the office?
- **Emergency procedures for patient accidental injury**—How are patient injuries handled in the office? Under what circumstances are emergency personnel called to the office?
- **Jury duty**—How should employees notify the office that they are called for jury duty? Does the office pay employees during jury duty?

Critical Thinking Question 15-1

Refer back to the case study presented at the beginning of this chapter. What type of policies and procedures should Monte start identifying for his office?

Creating Policies and Procedures for the Medical Office

One of the most important reasons for having a medical office policy and procedure manual is to clarify rules and regulations and the physician's expectations for procedures. Strict adherence to policies as they are outlined achieves uniformity in the office and provides a fair method of treating staff.

The medical office's policy and procedures manual may contain both policies and procedures, or policies and procedures may be separated. Whatever the approach, each policy and procedure manual should contain the following items in separate sections:

- Mission statement
- Organizational chart
- Personnel policies
- Clinical procedures
- Administrative procedures

A table of contents should clearly direct readers to important pages. Per Occupational Safety and Health Administration (**OSHA**) regulations, infection control and quality improvement and risk management procedures must be kept in separate notebooks and reviewed and updated regularly.

Fitzsimmons Family Practice Organization Chart

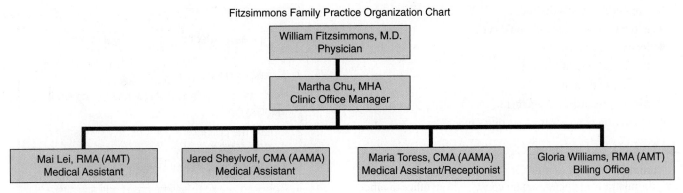

Figure 15-3 ■ Sample organizational chart for a medical office.

Writing a Mission Statement

The policy and procedures manual for a medical office should begin with an office **mission statement** that is concise and communicated to all staff. For example, a mission statement might read, "To care for all patients in a compassionate and dignified manner, with a focus on patient safety and satisfaction." Many medical offices frame and hang their mission statements for patients to see. The mission statement is important in that it outlines, in a short format, what the organization or clinic represents—their purpose for being in business.

Critical Thinking Question 15-2

Referring back to the case study at the beginning of the chapter, if Monte's office lacks a mission statement, how should he go about explaining its importance to the physician?

Preparing an Organizational Chart

In addition to the mission statement, the policy and procedures manual should break down the office's organizational structure in an **organizational chart** (**Figure 15-3** ■). Organizational charts diagram office hierarchies, from physicians to entry-level staff. Members of the health care team should be able to use these charts to identify their supervisors, as well as their supervisors' supervisors, all the way to the top of the chain of command. The chain of command is the reporting structure, from the employee to his supervisor, to his supervisor's manager and so on. In addition to reporting structure, an organizational chart might explain how employees can contact various health care staff. In a situation where an employee feels his concern lies with the actions of his direct supervisor, the employee may wish to seek out the guidance of the person his supervisor reports to. In an event such as this, access to an organizational chart would be helpful.

Outlining Clinical Procedures

Any clinical procedure that requires patient care should be documented for employee reference. Procedures should clearly list appropriate steps, as well as information on patient education, documentation, and infection control. The type of clinical procedures found in a policies and procedures manual varies according to the type of medical practice and the physician's specialty (**Figure 15-4** ■).

Outlining Administrative Procedures

Administrative procedures should be documented to include such topics as:

- Office opening and closing
- Inventory and supply ordering

Policy: Administering Injectable Medications

Purpose: To provide injectable medications to the patient per physician orders

1. Verify the five rights of medication.
   a. Verify the right patient identity by asking the patient his full name and birthdate.
   b. Verify the right route the medication is to be delivered by checking physician orders.
   c. Verify that the medication is right by checking physician orders and the label on the medication.
   d. Verify that the right dose of medication has been drawn by checking the physician orders.
   e. Verify that the right time of the medication administration is correct by checking the physician orders.
2. Administer the medication according to the physician's orders.
3. Discard the syringe in the sharps container.
4. Document the medication administered, including dose and route, in the patient's medical record.

Figure 15-4 ■ Sample clinical procedure.

- Appointment scheduling
- Patient accounting and bookkeeping
- Insurance processing
- Insurance benefit verification
- Release of patients' records
- Medical records management
- Operation of administrative office machinery

Like clinical procedures, administrative procedures vary according to the type of medical practice, but the vast majority of administrative policies remain constant from office to office (**Figure 15-5** ■).

Critical Thinking Question 15-3

Referring back to the case study at the beginning of the chapter, how should Monte determine which policies should appear in his office's policy manual?

Documenting Infection Control Procedures

Infection control procedures should be written for all of a medical office's applicable procedures, including:

- Biohazardous waste disposal
- Employee needlestick injuries
- Employee exposure to infectious materials
- Employee education for infection control
- OSHA-required documentation
- Local, state, and federal reporting requirements for infectious agents

---

Policy: Releasing Medical Records to a Patient

Purpose: To release medical records to the patient following legal guidelines

1. Verify the patient's identity by requesting photo identification.
2. Obtain the patient's signature on the release of records form.
3. Ensure the patient has dated the release form.
4. Check to see if the patient has made any alterations to the release form, such as restricting the records release to a limited date.
5. Check to see if the patient has checked the boxes allowing release of information regarding HIV/AIDS, reproductive health, mental health, or drug and alcohol rehabilitation.
6. Pull the patient's medical record.
7. Photocopy the appropriate parts of the medical record according to any limitations noted by the patient on the release form.
8. Send copies of the records to the patient.
9. Note in the patient's file when the records were released.
10. File the original signed release form.

Figure 15-5 ■ Sample administrative procedure.

As mandated by OSHA, infection control procedures must be part of the office's exposure control plan, which must be kept separate from other procedure manuals in the office and must be made available to an OSHA inspector if needed.

PROCEDURE 15-2 Create a Procedure for the Procedure Manual

Theory and Rationale

Medical offices need clearly written policies and procedures for all members of the health care team to understand how each task is performed.

Materials

- Computer with word-processing software

Competency

1. Determine the type of procedure to be created.
2. Gather the information on how this procedure is to be performed.

3. Title the procedure (e.g., "Policy: Sorting Incoming Mail"), and determine if it will be listed under administrative, clinical, infection control, personnel, or quality improvement and risk management.
4. Describe the policy's purpose (e.g., "Purpose: To describe the method of routing incoming mail to appropriate staff").
5. List each step in the procedure.
6. Print the procedure, and give it to the office manager for approval.
7. Once approved, place the procedure in the office procedure manual.

Policy: Patient Wait Time on the Telephone

Purpose: To keep patients from waiting on the telephone longer than 1 minute before call is taken

1. When patients call into the office, the call is sent to a queue for the next available receptionist.

2. Patient wait time is to be no longer than 1 minute in the call queue.

3. If a receptionist sees that there are more calls in the queue than the reception team can answer within 1 minute, she will alert the medical assistants to assist with answering calls.

Figure 15-6 ■ Sample quality improvement policy for reducing patient wait time on the telephone.

Policy: Escorting patients while in the medical office

Purpose: To keep patients from falling while in the medical office

1. When greeting the patient, visually determine if the patient is able to walk unassisted. If the patient is in a wheelchair, or using a device (walker or cane), or appears unsteady in their gait, offer to assist.

2. Assist any patient who needs help by gently taking the patient's arm.

3. Walk at the same pace as the patient and do not allow the patient to be out of your sight as you escort them.

Figure 15-7 ■ Sample risk management policy for escorting patients.

In Practice

Anka is a registered medical assistant working for Dr. Radcliff. While Anka is finishing a blood draw on a patient, she accidentally sticks herself with the contaminated needle. How will Anka know what to do now that this injury has happened?

Creating Quality Improvement and Risk Management Procedures

Quality improvement and risk management procedures are designed to reduce patient or staff injury in the medical office. These policies range from information on washing children's toys in the reception room to handling life-threatening patient events in the office. While quality improvement and risk management procedures policies vary according to office needs, the vast majority apply to all office types. Quality improvement (**Figure 15-6** ■) and risk management (**Figure 15-7** ■) procedures should be kept in a separate notebook that is clearly marked and updated regularly.

Writing Other Office Policies

To ensure ongoing compliance and relevance, all medical office policies should be reviewed and updated regularly. Many large medical offices separate their policy manuals into clinical and administrative sections. Some offices further divide their manuals according to position or department. Table 15-1 identifies policies that may be found in medical office policy and procedure manuals.

TABLE 15-1 Sample Policies and Procedures	
Policy or Procedure	**Purpose**
Emergency closure policy	Outlines the steps to take in the event the office closes due to emergency
Building lockup policy	Describes the steps to take to lock the building at the end of the day
Publications and distribution policy	Outlines the policy with regard to allowing publications or pamphlets to be distributed to patients and staff
Smoking policy	Describes the availability of smoking areas near the office
Personal relationships between office staff	Outlines the policy for personal relationships between coworkers
Personal relationships between staff and patients	Outlines the policy for personal relationships between office staff and patients
Termination policy	Describes the policy for terminating employment
Disciplinary policy	Describes the policy for disciplining of employees; includes an outline of the offenses justifying discipline
Grievance policy	Describes the process staff must follow to file grievances
Continuing education	Outlines the requirements for continuing education
Malpractice insurance	Describes the requirements for holding malpractice insurance
Reimbursement for seminars	Outlines the policy for reimbursing staff who attend medical-related seminars

(continued)

TABLE 15-1 Sample Policies and Procedures (continued)

Policy or Procedure	Purpose
Computers for personal use policy	Describes the policy for personal use of office computers
Petty cash funds	Describes the policy for using petty cash, including the type of expenses that qualify as petty cash and the amount to be kept as petty cash
Parking policy	Outlines where employees may park, as well as reimbursement for parking expenses
Dress code policy	Describes the dress code for each office position
Opening office policy	Outlines the steps to take to open the office at the beginning of the day
Disclosure of patient information policy	Describes the procedure for disclosing patient information, including the forms required and the Health Insurance Portability and Accountability Act (**HIPAA**) regulations
Job descriptions	Provides a job description for each office position
HIPAA privacy officer duties	Outlines the duties of the HIPAA privacy officer in the medical office
Calling patients from the reception room	Describes the procedure for calling patients from the reception room
Missed patient appointments	Describes the steps to take when patients miss their appointments; includes proper charting technique
Termination of the physician/patient relationship	Outlines the steps to legally terminate the physician/patient relationship
E-mail policy	Describes the conditions under which the medical office may e-mail information to patients or other facilities
Obtaining consent for a procedure	Describes the consent forms used in the medical office and outlines the process of witnessing patient signatures
Prescription refill requests	Outlines the policy for taking telephone calls for prescription refills, including documentation in the patient's medical record
Jury duty policy	Describes the policy for employees called for jury duty
Sick leave policy	Describes the policy for employees who take sick leave
Personal telephone calls	Describes the policy for employees making and receiving personal telephone calls

REVIEW

Chapter Summary

- Informational pamphlets are effective for educating patients.
- Office personnel manuals are needed to ensure all members of the health care team perform appropriately and to consistent standards.

- A policies and procedure manual in the medical office serves as written record of the legal, desired behavior of all health care staff.

Chapter Review

Multiple Choice

1. Any _____ procedure that requires patient intervention should be documented for patient reference.
   a. Clinical
   b. Appointment
   c. Purposeful
   d. Structural
   e. Random

2. Quality improvement and risk management procedures are designed to:
   a. Reduce the length of the patient appointment
   b. Increase the length of the patient appointment
   c. Avoid liability lawsuits
   d. Limit employee injury
   e. a, b, and c

3. A procedure for filing insurance claims would be found under which policies section of the office procedure manual?
   a. Clinical
   b. Infection control
   c. Risk management
   d. Administrative
   e. Management

4. Once a policy and procedure manual has been written, it should be updated:
   a. Once a month
   b. Once a year
   c. Once every five years
   d. As the policy or procedure changes
   e. Only if the physician retires

5. The office mission statement should be shared with:
   a. Administrative staff
   b. Clinical staff
   c. Patients
   d. Vendors
   e. a, b, and c

True/False

T F **1.** Only the office manager can compose a procedure for the office manual.

T F **2.** An organizational chart outlines the chain of command in the office.

T F **3.** By strictly following a policy and procedure manual, medical office management gives the impression that all staff members will be treated consistently.

T F **4.** Office policies for quality improvement and risk management must be kept in a separate notebook.

T F **5.** Compulsory means choosing to participate.

Short Answer

1. List the sections all policy and procedure manuals should include.
2. What is the purpose of an office mission statement?
3. Give five examples of an administrative policy.
4. Give five examples of a clinical policy.
5. Give five examples of a quality improvement or risk management policy.
6. Give five examples of an infection control policy.
7. Differentiate between a policy and a procedure.
8. Describe the steps to take to create an educational brochure.
9. Why might a medical office have separate policy and procedure manuals for its administrative and clinical areas?
10. Differentiate between a clinical policy and an administrative policy.

Research

1. Search online for policy and procedure manuals for medical facilities. Describe what each of these companies has in common with the others.
2. Call a local medical office. Ask the office manager if the office has a policy and procedure manual. How often is it updated? How are employees given access to the manual?
3. Search the Internet for companies that make office educational brochures. What type of information can you get ready-made pamphlets for?

Practicum Application Experience

Manuel is unsure how to handle a patient who refuses to schedule a followup appointment. He asks two other members of the health care team to explain the office policy for proceeding and receives two vastly different responses. Should Manuel follow the advice of one staff member over the other? How can he know how this situation is supposed to be handled?

Resource Guide

Sample personnel policies
http://www.info.com/sample personnel policies

Sample financial policies (American Academy of Pediatrics)
http://www.aap.org/en-us/professional-resources/practice-support/financing-and-payment/Billing-and-Payment/pages/Office-Financial-Policies.aspx

Sample medical office procedural manual
http://www.mybookezzz.net/medical-office-procedure-manual-sample/

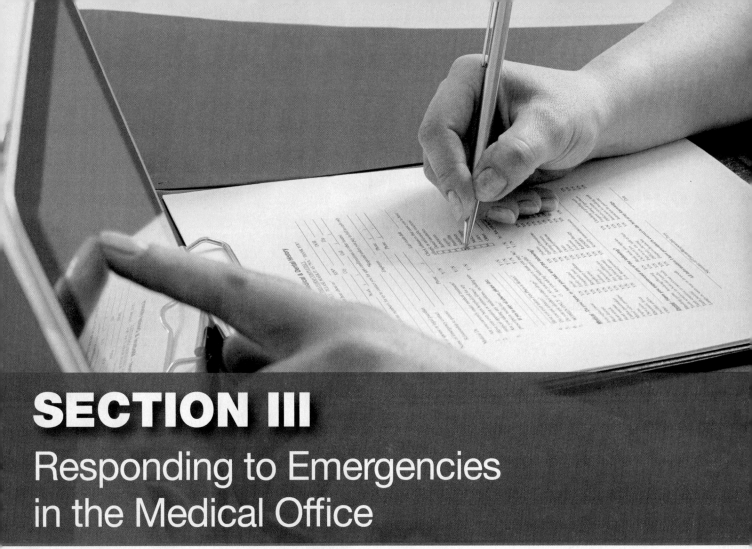

SECTION III
Responding to Emergencies in the Medical Office

My name is Maria Martinez, and I was recently hired as an administrative medical assistant at a busy family medical practice. I have current CPR certification as well as knowledge of first aid skills, which will enable me to respond appropriately to medical emergencies.

When emergencies occur, I may be the first member of the health care team to know and respond; therefore emergency preparedness is essential. Our medical office has a thorough policy and procedures manual that identifies the steps health care staff members should take in the event of an emergency.

My employer recommended that I participate in a mock environmental exposure event at our local community college. This was an invaluable experience that taught me how to help victims and provide assistance to other health care providers in the event of a disaster, such as a tornado. I would highly recommend that any medical assistant preparing for emergency situations research and partake in one of these courses, which may be available at community colleges, community organizations, and/or hospitals.

16 Handling Medical Office Emergencies

16

Handling Medical Office Emergencies

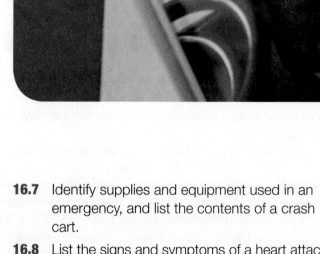

Case Study

Read the following case study and answer the critical thinking questions presented throughout the chapter.

Adrianna is a registered medical assistant working at the reception desk on a busy Monday morning. Mark Whitford, a 70-year-old patient, has just entered the office for his appointment with Dr. Hardy to discuss adjusting his Coumadin due to his history of multiply pulmonary emboli. As he approaches the reception desk, Mr. Whitford stumbles, loses his balance, and falls. During the fall, he strikes his head on a cabinet, loses consciousness, and sustains a gash on his forehead that is bleeding profusely.

Objectives

After completing this chapter, you should be able to:

16.1 Define and spell the key terminology in this chapter.

16.2 Describe the medical assistant's role in an emergency.

16.3 Understand how to prevent accidents and injuries in the medical office.

16.4 Prepare for and manage medical emergencies.

16.5 Describe the use of Hands-Only CPR.

16.6 Assist and monitor a patient who has fainted.

16.7 Identify supplies and equipment used in an emergency, and list the contents of a crash cart.

16.8 List the signs and symptoms of a heart attack.

16.9 List the signs and symptoms of choking.

16.10 Describe the steps to stop bleeding.

16.11 Assist a patient in shock.

16.12 Care for a patient with a fracture.

16.13 Assist a patient with burns.

16.14 Discuss the potential role(s) of the medical assistant in emergency preparedness.

Key Terminology

anaphylaxis—severe, life threatening, allergic reaction

CPR mouth barrier—disposable device used to prevent infection

crash cart—wheeled cart that contains emergency medical equipment

defibrillator—a device that delivers an electric shock to a patient

standard precautions—infection control techniques used by health care professionals that include proper hand hygiene, personal protective equipment, respiratory hygiene and cough etiquette, safe injection practices, and proper handling of potentially hazardous and contaminated materials

syncope—fainting; the sudden loss of consciousness

Abbreviations

AAMA—American Association of Medical Assistants

AED—automatic external defibrillator

AHA—American Heart Association

CAB—compressions, airway, breathing

CPR—cardiopulmonary resuscitation

ECC—Emergency Cardiovascular Care

EMS—Emergency Medical Services

FBOA—Foreign Body Obstructed Airway

FEMA—Federal Emergency Management Agency

HEPA—high efficiency particulate air filter

OSHA—Occupational Safety and Health Administration

PPE—personal protective equipment

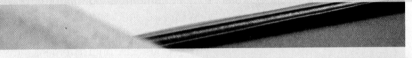

Certification Exam Coverage

AAMA (CMA) Exam Coverage:

- Principles of infection control
  - Disposal of biohazardous material
  - Standard precautions
- Emergency preparedness
- First aid—identifying and responding to:
  - Bleeding/pressure points
  - Cardiac and respiratory arrest/CPR
  - Choking/Heimlich maneuver
  - Diabetic coma/insulin shock
  - Poisoning
  - Seizures
  - Shock
  - Stroke
  - Syncope
  - Wounds

AMT (CMAS) Exam Coverage:

- Medical office emergencies
  - Recognize and respond to medical emergencies
  - Employ first aid and CPR appropriately
  - Report emergencies as required by law

- Safety
  - Maintain records of biohazardous waste, hazardous chemicals, and safety conditions
  - Comply with Occupational Safety and Health Act (**OSHA**) guidelines and regulations

AMT (RMA) Exam Coverage:

- First aid procedures
  - Identify criteria for and steps in performing CPR and the Heimlich maneuver
  - Maintain emergency (crash) cart
  - Identify injuries, recognize emergencies, and provide appropriate response
- Legal responsibilities
  - Understand scope of practice when providing First Aid

NCCT (NCMA) Exam Coverage:

- Infection and exposure control
  - Biohazardous waste disposal
  - Exposure control
  - Asepsis
  - Personal protective equipment
  - Universal precautions; blood and body fluids
  - Sanitation, sterilization, and disinfection
  - OSHA safety regulations

Competency Skills Performance

1. Maintain a current list of community resources for emergency preparedness.
2. Perform adult rescue breathing and one-rescuer cardiopulmonary resuscitation (CPR).
3. Care for a patient who has fainted.
4. Administer oxygen to a patient.
5. Use an automated external defibrillator (AED).
6. Respond to an adult with an airway obstruction.
7. Remove an airway obstruction in an infant.
8. Control bleeding.
9. Develop a safety plan for employees and patients: fire evacuation.
10. Develop an environmental safety plan.
11. Participate in a mock-environmental exposure: responding to an earthquake.

Introduction

Medical emergencies are rare in the medical office; however, when patients or members of the health care team become severely ill or injured in the medical office, medical assistants must be trained to respond appropriately. In fact, all members of the medical staff, including those who work in the administrative area, should have and maintain current CPR certification as well as knowledge of first aid skills. With proper first aid and/or cardiopulmonary resuscitation (**CPR**), patients may well recover completely. Instruction in CPR is offered through many medical assisting programs as a separate course. These courses can also be found through the American Red Cross, The American Heart Association (**AHA**) or through local fire departments or hospitals.

The Medical Assistant's Role in an Emergency

When emergencies occur in ambulatory care, administrative medical assistants might be the first members of the health care team to know. In fact, when emergencies arise in an office's reception area or hallways, the medical assistant might well be the first to respond. When emergencies arise in an office's clinical area, medical assistants might be asked to move patients to other areas, keep other patients or family members calm, or telephone for emergency services. To ensure that assistants are well prepared, medical assistants should maintain current, health care provider-level CPR certification. Though certification was previously required for recertification, in May of 2013, the American Association of Medical Assistants (**AAMA**) decided that current CPR certification would no longer be required for recertification of the medical assistant's CMA (AAMA) credential and that the medical assistant's employer should be responsible for maintaining CPR certification for the medical assistant. Today, maintaining current CPR certification is a requirement of many, if not all, employees of medical facilities.

▶▶▶ Pulse Points

Performing Within Scope of Practice

Medical assistants must remember to perform only those skills they have been trained to perform. In the event of a medical emergency, the medical assistant should quickly alert the physician and/or emergency medical services.

Preventing Accidents and Injuries

The key to avoiding injuries and accidents in the medical office is to be proactive. For example, administrative medical assistants are likely responsible for the reception and front desk areas, and should pick up fallen items before patients or other members of the health care team can trip and fall. Medical assistants must constantly look for potential trouble areas, such as wrinkled area rugs or outlets lacking childproof plugs.

Critical Thinking Question 16-1

Referring back to the case study at the beginning of the chapter, how does Mr. Whitford's history of hemophilia affect this medical emergency?

Preparing for Medical Emergencies

In the medical office, emergency preparedness can mean the difference between chaos and ordered, effective response. Medical offices should have well-written and complete policy and procedures manuals that identify the steps to take in the event of an office emergency. In addition to patient and staff injuries or life-threatening illnesses, office emergencies can also include severe storms, power outages, fires, and even acts of terrorism.

PROCEDURE 16-1 Maintain a List of Community Resources for Emergencies

Theory and Rationale

One of the main responsibilities of the medical assistant during an emergency is to help and assist patients as needed. One proactive way to help patients is to equip them with the many community resources that can serve as an aid both during and after the emergency. Inform patients that these lists are available in the office for their personal use. It might also be helpful to post the list of the community resources in a highly visible area, such as near the front desk.

Materials

- Notepad and pen
- Computer with word-processing software
- Internet connections with search engine availability
- Phonebook
- Printer
- Printer paper

Competency

1. Using a notepad and pen, compile a list of community resources that are available either during or after an emergency. Some resources you will want to include are:
   - Poison Control Center
   - Local fire and police departments—main numbers, not 9-1-1
   - Local chapter of the Red Cross
   - Federal Emergency Management Agency (**FEMA**)
   - Local food banks
   - Local housing shelters
   - Emergency medical facilities including hospitals and urgent care facilities
   - Other facilities that are unique to your area that can provide assistance during or after an emergency
2. Using an Internet search engine or a local telephone book, write down the contact telephone numbers and corresponding Web sites for each company and organization listed.
3. Open the word processing software on the computer.
4. Create a new document that clearly and neatly organizes this information. You may want to choose to create a brochure with a description of each agency, or you may choose to create a single sheet of information that displays the information in a table format.
5. After you have created the information in the Word document, review the information for accuracy.
6. Using the software tools, perform a spelling and grammar check making changes as necessary.
7. Review the document for a second time to check for information accuracy and perform a second spelling and grammar check.
8. Save the document in the appropriate file on the computer.
9. Print the document and show it to the office manager or physician for approval.
10. Once final approval is given, make multiple copies to have on hand to pass out to patients as necessary.

In most towns and cities, medical offices can reach their local emergency personnel by dialing 9-1-1. While medical offices should have all their local emergency service numbers readily available, they should also have the following numbers on hand:

- Poison Control Center (1-800-222-1222)
- Local fire department
- Local police department

Managing Medical Emergencies

When emergencies arise in the medical office, medical assistants must remember to stay calm so they can direct patients as needed. Patients look to medical assistants as authority figures.

Emergency intervention is called for in any situation that might be life-threatening (Table 16-1). The responder provides appropriate intervention and stays with the injured or ill person until more advanced care can be provided. Triage of emergency patients is a critical care issue.

Before assessing any patient, the medical assistant should don disposable gloves to prevent exposure to blood or other bodily fluids. The medical assistant must follow **standard precautions**, because in emergencies, all bodily fluids must be considered infectious. When the patient is nonresponsive, the medical assistant should shout for help and ask a coworker to notify the physician immediately while the medical assistant stays with the patient. When the physician is unavailable, the medical assistant should ask other members of the health care team to call for emergency personnel.

After securing assistance from the physician or emergency personnel, the medical assistant should determine if a nonresponsive patient is breathing.

Respiratory and cardiac arrest can be caused by an occluded airway, electrocution, shock, drowning, heart attack, trauma, **anaphylaxis**, drugs, poisoning, or traumatic head or chest injury. Intervention must be immediate if resuscitation is to be successful. For individuals experiencing acute chest pain, loss of consciousness, or respiratory arrest, follow CPR protocol.

TABLE 16-1 Emergency Intervention

Life-Threatening Condition	Not Life-Threatening: Immediate Intervention	Not Life-Threatening: Intervention as Soon as Possible
• Extreme shortness of breath (airway or breathing problems) • Cardiac arrest • Severe, uncontrolled bleeding • Head injuries • Poisoning • Open chest or abdominal wounds • Shock • Severe burns, including face, hands, feet, and genitals • Potential neck injuries	• Decreased levels of consciousness • Chest pain • Seizures • Major or multiple fractures • Neck injuries • Severe eye injuries • Burns not on face, hands, feet, or genitals	• Severe vomiting and diarrhea, especially in the very young and the elderly • Minor injuries • Sprains • Strains • Simple fractures

CPR guidelines are similar for respiratory arrest, cardiac arrest, and obstructed airway but vary somewhat according to age group. Table 16-2 lists the major differences in the performance of CPR-related skills as defined by the AHA. Early access to emergency medical services (**EMS**) is important. Access for the adult victim is initiated by calling 9-1-1 as soon as it has been determined that the victim is unconscious and not breathing. In general, the rule of thumb is to phone first for an unresponsive adult.

TABLE 16-2 Adult, Child, and Infant CPR Skills

CPR Skill	Adult: 8+ years	Child: 1 year–puberty (approximately 12–14 years)	Infant: under 1 year
EMS access by calling 9-1-1 and giving emergency information	If sudden collapse is witnessed, immediately activate EMS and get AED. If asphyxiation (e.g., drowning, injury, overdose) suspected, first perform 2 minutes of CPR (or 5 cycles), then activate EMS.	If sudden collapse is witnessed, immediately activate EMS and get AED. Otherwise perform 2 minutes of CPR (5 cycles), then activate EMS.	If sudden collapse is witnessed, immediately activate EMS. Otherwise perform 2 minutes of CPR (5 cycles), then activate EMS.
Assessment of unresponsiveness	Shout, asking for a response; tap or gently shake the shoulders.	Shout, asking for a response; tap or gently shake the shoulders.	Snap or poke the feet. Do *not* shake the shoulders.
Rescue breathing rate of 1 second long, normal breath until chest rises	10–12 breaths per minute or one breath every 5–6 seconds	12–20 breaths per minute or one breath every 3–5 seconds	12–20 breaths per minute or one breath every 3–5 seconds
Obstructed airway foreign-body	Abdominal thrusts	Abdominal thrusts	Back slaps and chest thrusts
Pulse check location	Carotid	Carotid	Brachial or femoral
Compression technique	One hand linked over second hand, with heel of second hand on sternum	Heel of one hand on sternum	Single rescuer: two fingertips on sternum Two rescuers: two thumbs touching on sternum and hand encircling chest and back technique
Compression landmarks	Center of chest, between nipples	Center of chest, between nipples	Center of chest, just below nipple line
Compression depth	At least 2"	1/2 to 1/3 depth of chest	At least 1/3- 1 ¼" depth of chest
Compression rate	At least 100 per minute	At least 100 per minute	At least 100 per minute
Compression ratio to rescue breathing	Single rescuer: 30:2 Two rescuers: 30:2	Single rescuer: 30:2 Two rescuers: 15:2	Single rescuer: 30:2 Two rescuers: 15:2

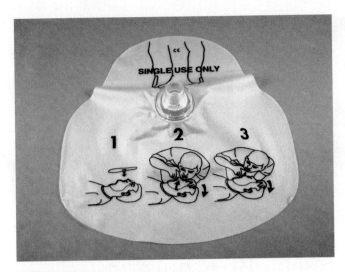

Figure 16-1 ◼ CPR mouth barrier.
Source: Pearson Education/PH College. Photographer: Dylan Malone.

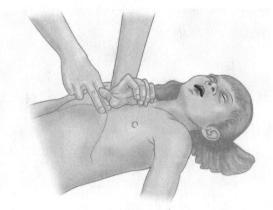

Figure 16-3 ◼ Compressions for a child.

With children and infants, EMS access is made after two minutes of CPR if there is only one rescuer. If more than one rescuer is available, one person should initiate CPR while the other rescuer contacts EMS. In general, the rule of thumb is to perform CPR first for unresponsive children and infants. In 2010, the AHA changed the CPR sequence. The original sequence of airway, breathing, and compressions has now been changed to compressions, airway, breathing (**CAB**). This sequence is thought to be more helpful as early compressions can help circulate oxygenated blood that is still in the blood stream. Defibrillation then follows breathing once the automated external defibrillator unit (**AED**) is made available.

From the crash cart or an emergency medical supply cabinet the medical assistant should secure pocket masks, also called **CPR mouth barriers** (**Figure 16**-1 ◼). The types and varieties of CPR mouth barriers will vary by office. Next, the medical assistant should check to see if the patient is breathing, taking no more than 10 seconds for breathing assessment. If the patient is not breathing, the medical assistant will immediately begin chest compressions, followed by rescue breaths. As stated in Table 16-2, the ratio of compressions to breaths is 30:2. This means after performing 30 compressions, the medical assistant will stop and administer two rescue breaths. When the patient has a pulse, the medical assistant should continue rescue breathing every 5–6 seconds for adults and every 3–5 seconds for children. If the patient does not have a pulse, an AED should be immediately used when it is available. Until the AED is available for use, the medical assistant should continue with compressions and rescue breaths. See **Figures 16-2** ◼, **16-3** ◼, and **16-4** ◼ for compressions for an infant, child, and adult, respectively.

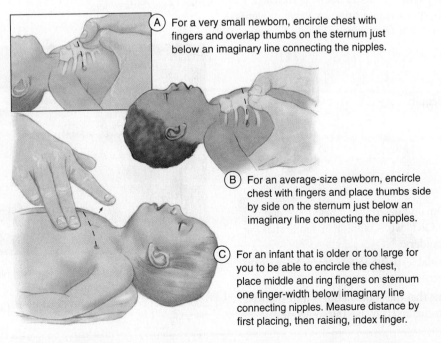

(A) For a very small newborn, encircle chest with fingers and overlap thumbs on the sternum just below an imaginary line connecting the nipples.

(B) For an average-size newborn, encircle chest with fingers and place thumbs side by side on the sternum just below an imaginary line connecting the nipples.

(C) For an infant that is older or too large for you to be able to encircle the chest, place middle and ring fingers on sternum one finger-width below imaginary line connecting nipples. Measure distance by first placing, then raising, index finger.

Figure 16-2 ◼ Compressions for an infant.

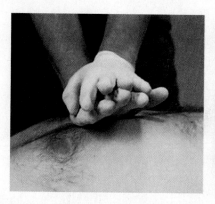
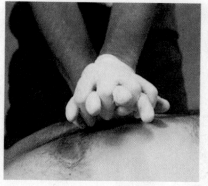
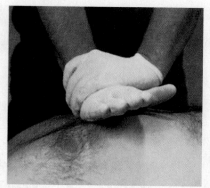

Figure 16-4 ■ Location and position of hands during chest compressions for an adult.

 PROCEDURE 16-2 Perform Adult Rescue Breathing 📋 and One-Rescuer CPR

Theory and Rationale

Chest compressions and rescue breathing are performed in adults that have no respiratory and cardiac function. The AHA recently revised guidelines for CPR and Emergency Cardiovascular Care (**ECC**) in an effort to simplify the process. The 2010 guidelines require health care providers to begin compressions first, followed by rescues breaths. Revised guidelines recommend a universal compression-to-ventilation of 30 to 2 for lone rescuers for victims of all ages (except newborns). Rescuers must provide compressions of adequate rate (at least 100 beats/minute) and depth (at least 2") for adult victims and allow adequate chest recoil with minimal interruptions in chest compressions. Additionally, actions for Foreign Body Obstructed Airway (**FBOA**) were simplified. The tongue-jaw lift is no longer taught and blind finger sweep should not be performed.

Using a mouth guard with a one-way valve prevents vomit or other body fluids from contaminating the rescuer's mouth.

Materials

- Approved mannequin
- Gloves
- Ventilator mask
- Mouth guard

Competency

1. Assess the victim and determine if help is needed. Shout "Are you OK?" while tapping or gently shaking the victim's shoulders.
2. If gloves are available, put them on. If you have a ventilator mask, place it on the victim.
3. If you determine that the adult victim is unresponsive, activate EMS immediately by having someone else call 9-1-1 and retrieve an AED if available. If you are alone, begin the rescue sequence for 1 minute and then attempt to call 9-1-1 yourself.
4. Check the carotid artery for a pulse and assess for breathing, taking no more than 10 seconds (**Figure 16-5** ■.)
5. If pulse is absent, position yourself and prepare for chest compressions: Kneel at the victim's side. Find the sternum and place the heel of one hand just below the nipple line.

    Place your other hand on top of the first hand, making sure to lift your fingers off the chest, using only the heels of your hands to administer compressions.
6. Using the full weight of your upper body, perform 30 compressions at a depth of at least 2 inches in 18 seconds or less.

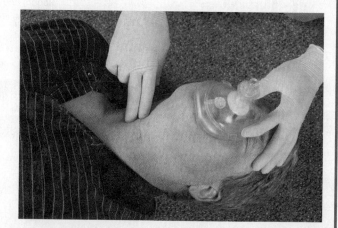

Figure 16-5 ■ Assess the patient's circulation by feeling for a pulse at the carotid artery.

Source: Pearson Education/PH College. Photographer: Michal Heron.

PROCEDURE 16-2 Perform Adult Rescue Breathing
and One-Rescuer CPR (continued)

7. Put on a mouth guard, perform the head tilt–chin lift and administer two rescue breaths (**Figure 16-6 ■**). If your breaths do not cause the chest to rise, look in the victim's mouth and remove any object you see. If no object is seen, make a second attempt to administer a rescue breath. If the breath still does not enter the chest, proceed to abdominal thrusts for unconscious victims.

8. Continue with chest compressions and rescue breaths at a 30:2 ratio. After five complete cycles, reassess the patient by checking for breathing and a pulse at the carotid artery. To check for breathing, remove the mask and place your ear near the patient's mouth to see if you can hear or feel breath, while at the same time observing the chest for rising and falling associated with breathing (**Figure 16-7 ■**).

9. If a pulse is present, continue with rescue breaths at a rate of 1 every 5–8 seconds, or about 10–12 per minute. After 1 minute of rescue breathing, reassess the patient for breathing and pulse.

10. If neither is present, continue with compressions and rescue breaths at a 30:2 ratio until an AED is made available or until emergency medical services arrive and you are relieved from performing CPR.

Patient Education

Advise the patient to follow up with his or her personal physician after release from the EMS.

Charting Example

08/05/XX 7:30 PM Patient found collapsed in bathroom and unresponsive. 911 call placed and CPR started. EMS arrived in approximately 10 minutes and took over care. Patient was transferred to Deaconess Medical Center. Vivian Nagle, CMAS (AMT)

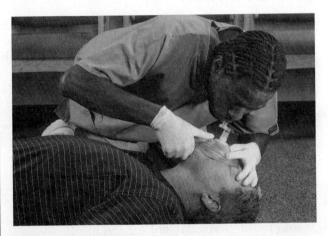

Figure 16-6 ■ Administer two rescue breaths with mouth guard in place.
Source: Pearson Education/PH College. Photographer: Michal Heron.

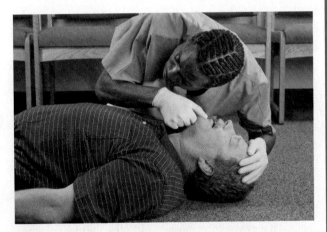

Figure 16-7 ■ Look and feel for breath and chest movements.
Source: Pearson Education/PH College. Photographer: Michal Heron.

Hands-Only CPR

Sometimes a patient will ask the medical assistant if and how they, the patient, should respond if they observe an emergency situation. In all circumstances, medical assistants must respond according to the office's policies and guidelines. However, as a result of changes to the American Heart Association's 2010 CPR Guidelines, "Hands-Only CPR" has been gaining wide popularity with non-trained rescuers. This emergency medical response teaching is designed for people who have very little or no training in CPR. The idea is that the non-trained rescuer will only administer chest compressions until emergency medical services arrive, the thought being that by eliminating the mouth-to-mouth breathing component, non-trained rescuers would be less intimidated and more willing to provide help. In 2012 the AHA launched the "Stayin' Alive— One Minute to Save a Life" campaign in which it encouraged non-trained individuals to save a life by delivering chest compressions to the musical beat of the song, *Stayin' Alive* by the Bee Gees. The song's rhythm is said to be near-perfect to the rhythm necessary for delivering effective chest compressions. It is important to note that this method of hands-only CPR is intended for teens and adult victims who are seen suddenly collapsing and are without pulse or breath.

Fainting (Syncope)

Many serious disorders cause unresponsiveness. Simple faint-ing, or **syncope**, occurs often in some people and almost never in others. The sudden loss of consciousness seems to be caused by a brief interruption in the body's ability to control blood circulation to the brain. The patient usually collapses and becomes totally unresponsive, but within a minute should awaken and return to normal function. Patients seldom become incontinent or have seizures as a result of simple fainting, but they might be injured in the course of a fall. The following is a list of some serious disorders that can produce fainting:

- Airway obstruction/apnea
- Assault
- Brain infection
- Brain tumor
- Cardiac arrest
- Cardiac rhythm disturbance
- Cerebral edema
- Diabetes
- Drugs or alcohol ingestion
- Electrolyte imbalance
- Epilepsy
- Head trauma
- Hypoglycemia

- Hyperglycemia
- Hypovolemia
- Hypoxia
- Metabolic disorders
- Overdose
- Poisoning
- Respiratory arrest
- Seizure
- Sepsis
- Shock (any kind)
- Stroke

Critical Thinking Question 16-2

Refer to the case study at the beginning of the chapter. When a patient loses consciousness after hitting his head, what should the medical assistant do?

Emergency Equipment and Supplies

Every medical office must have emergency equipment and supplies that include an appropriately stocked **crash cart** (**Figure 16-8** ■). Table 16-3 includes supplies that may be found on a crash cart in the ambulatory care setting.

PROCEDURE 16-3 Respond to a Patient Who Has Fainted

Theory and Rationale

Patients who are ill, pregnant, or who have just received upset-ting news might faint. Medical assistants must be properly trained to respond to these patients, since patients could be injured if they lose consciousness and fall in the medical office.

Materials

- Blanket
- Washcloths
- Footstool or box

Competency

1. If the patient says he is feeling faint, help him sit, bend forward, and place his head on his knees. If the patient collapses with no warning, do not move him. He might have sustained a neck or back injury.
2. Notify the physician immediately.
3. Loosen any tight clothing, and cover the patient with a blanket for warmth. If the patient has fainted due to heat exhaustion, place cold washcloths on his neck and wrists.

4. If the physician directs, use the footstool to support the patient's legs in a raised position.
5. If the physician directs, call for emergency services.
6. Once the emergency passes, document all activities in the patient's medical record.

Patient Education

Observe the patient carefully, monitoring breathing and level of consciousness. Allow the patient to rest 10 minutes after she regains full consciousness. If the patient's vital signs are unstable or she does not respond quickly, notify the physician and be prepared to activate the emergency medical system.

Charting Example

9/18/xx 10:15 AM Patient in reception area stated that she felt faint. Patient instructed to lower her head to her knees. Instructed to and assisted with loosening of clothing. Physi-cian notified. BP 116/62, P-82 and regular, R-20. Patient remained in position for 3 minutes until symptoms subsided. Patient transferred to exam room and physician notified and evaluated patient. Maria Jimenez, NCMA (NCCT)

Emergency supplies should be easily accessible in the medical office and inventoried regularly. Staff should rotate supplies based on expiration date. In addition to items such as alcohol wipes, antimicrobial skin ointment, and cotton balls and swabs, medical offices should have elastic bandages, instant hot and cold packs, portable oxygen tanks with regulators and masks, scissors, sharps container, and Steri-Strips or suturing materials. The office should also stock such emergency pharmaceutical supplies as activated charcoal, amobarbital, apomorphine, injectable and oral antihistamine, dextrose, diazepam, furosemide, glucose tablets, syrup of ipecac, nitroglycerine tablets, injectable sodium bicarbonate, and sterile water. Every medical office should stock epinephrine, which is used for emergencies that include asthma attacks, hemorrhages, and shock.

Administering Oxygen in Emergencies

In the medical office, oxygen is often administered when a patient displays signs of respiratory distress. **Figure 16-9** ▪ highlights commons signs and symptoms of a patient in respiratory distress. When patients require oxygen in the medical office, medical assistants must be able to administer the oxygen as well as gather necessary supplies. Oxygen may be administered via nasal cannula or face mask.

Automated External Defibrillator (AED)

Every medical office must have a **defibrillator** for emergency use. This machine delivers a shock to patients with no pulse in an effort to stop ventricular fibrillation. Defibrillators work by sending an electric current into the patient's heart in order to

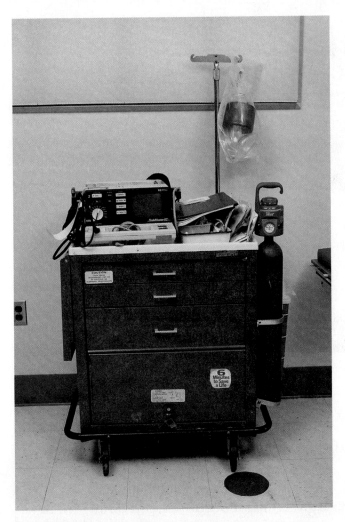

Figure 16-8 ▪ An emergency crash cart.

Source: Pearson Learning Photo Studio. Photographer: David Mager.

TABLE 16-3 Crash Cart Contents

- Cardiac monitor/defibrillator
- Conduction jelly
- EKG paper
- O₂ cylinder
- Suction catheters
- Laryngoscope
- 10 cc syringe
- O₂ face mask
- Stethoscope
- IV supplies
- 1" silk tape
- 3 cc syringes with 22 gauge needles
- Blood tubes (red tops, green tops, blue tops, and purple tops)
- Adult paddles
- Lead wires
- Suction machine
- Pocket max
- Sterile gloves
- Endotracheal tubes
- Nasogastric tube
- Nasal cannula
- Blood pressure cuff
- Tourniquets
- 4″ × 4″ sterile gauze pads
- 10 cc syringes with 20 gauge needles
- Neonatal ambu bag
- Pedi paddles
- Monitor electrodes
- Suction canister
- Oral airways
- Suction tubing
- Lidocaine jelly
- 60 cc catheter-tip syringe
- Emergency trach tray
- IV solutions
- Short arm boards
- 1 cc TB syringes
- 23 gauge butterfly needles
- Pediatric ambu bag

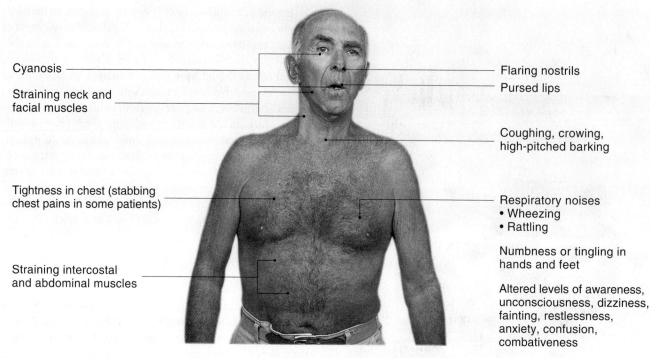

Cyanosis

Straining neck and facial muscles

Flaring nostrils

Pursed lips

Coughing, crowing, high-pitched barking

Tightness in chest (stabbing chest pains in some patients)

Respiratory noises
• Wheezing
• Rattling

Numbness or tingling in hands and feet

Straining intercostal and abdominal muscles

Altered levels of awareness, unconsciousness, dizziness, fainting, restlessness, anxiety, confusion, combativeness

Figure 16-9 ■ Signs and symptoms of respiratory distress.

 PROCEDURE 16-4 Administer Oxygen to a Patient

Theory and Rationale

A patient who is in respiratory distress might need to have oxygen administered to her in the medical office. The medical assistant should be aware of how to administer oxygen, both via nasal cannula and via oxygen mask.

Materials

- Portable oxygen tank
- Pressure regulator
- Flow meter
- Nasal cannula with connecting tubing
- Oxygen mask with connecting tubing

Competency

1. Gather all equipment.
2. Wash your hands.
3. Identify the patient and explain what you are about to do.
4. Check the pressure gauge on the oxygen tank to verify the amount of oxygen in the tank.
5. Open the cylinder on the oxygen tank one full counterclockwise turn and attach the connective tubing to the flow meter.
6. Attach either the nasal cannula or the oxygen mask to the connective tubing.

7. When using a nasal cannula, insert the cannula tips into the patient's nostrils and loop the tubing behind the patient's ears (**Figure 16-10** ■).
8. When using an oxygen mask, place the oxygen mask over the patient's nose and mouth and slip the elastic cord over their head. Adjust the cord so that the mask fits tightly yet comfortably on the patient's face.
9. Adjust the administration of the oxygen to the flow ordered by the physician.
10. Verify that oxygen is flowing through the nasal cannula or oxygen mask.

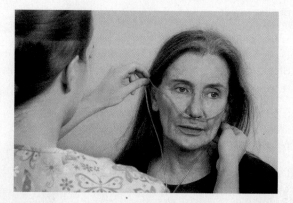

Figure 16-10 ■ Loop the tubing around the back of the patient's ears.

PROCEDURE 16-4 Administer Oxygen to a Patient (continued)

11. Wash your hands.
12. Document the procedure, including the flow rate of oxygen being given to the patient and the method of delivery (nasal cannula or oxygen mask).

Patient Education

While treating the patient with oxygen, instruct the patient to take slow deep breaths. This will allow the oxygen to

enter the blood stream at a steady and more efficient rate than with exacerbated breaths.

Charting Example

10/18/xx 3:45 PM: Patient experienced acute respiratory distress after a reaction to an injection she received in the office. Patient was given oxygen at 4 liters/minute according to physician's orders. Bryan Zindel, RMA (AMI)

---

allow the heart's natural pacemaker to return to a normal rhythm. Most ambulatory settings have automated external defibrillators that are self-contained and portable (**Figure 16-11** ■).

Every AED has a battery, a control computer, and electrodes. To use the AED, medical personnel place the electrodes on the patient, and the control computer determines the patient's rhythm or arrhythmia. The AED then sets the appropriate power levels and signals that a shock is needed. To administer a shock, the operator must press a button, but only after ensuring that no one is touching the patient. When patients do not need defibrillation, the AED allows no shock to be administered.

The Signs and Symptoms of Heart Attack

The signs and symptoms of heart attack can differ from one patient to another. Most commonly, patients complain of chest pain or pressure in the center of the chest. This pain, which patients might describe as minor, can spread to the patient's shoulder, neck, jaw, or arm. Patients experiencing heart attacks might also present with excessive sweating; nausea or indigestion; shortness of breath; or cold, clammy skin.

Women can experience different heart attack symptoms than men. Women may experience back pain or pain and

aching in the biceps or forearms, dizziness or lightheadedness, or swelling in the ankles or lower legs. Medical assistants must be familiar with all these signs and immediately bring them to the physician's attention.

In Practice

When Courtney Molino enters the medical office for her physical exam, she says she feels unwell after choosing the stairs over the elevator. In fact, she says she is having chest pain and extreme dizziness. What should the medical assistant do?

The Signs and Symptoms of Choking

Choking typically results when a foreign object becomes lodged in a patient's throat. When a choking patient can speak or make any sounds or is coughing, the medical assistant should encourage the patient to continue coughing until the object is dislodged. If the patient cannot make sounds or cough, the assistant should assume the airway is blocked and take appropriate action. The choking adult might use the universal choking sign—crossing the hands at the throat—to signal for help (**Figure 16-12** ■). Once the blockage has been removed, the patient might still be in danger of swelling in the throat, causing narrowing of the airway. For this reason, medical personnel should still be called after the blockage has been removed.

When Infants Are Choking Victims

When a choking patient is an infant up to one year of age, the medical assistant should look into the patient's mouth to see if an obstruction is visible. If so, the assistant should remove the object by swiping the finger through the child's mouth. When no object is visible or the assistant cannot remove the object, the assistant should place the infant-patient face downward with the lower portion of the patient's trunk lying across the medical assistant's forearms or thighs,. The assistant should then use the heel of the hand to administer five blows to the

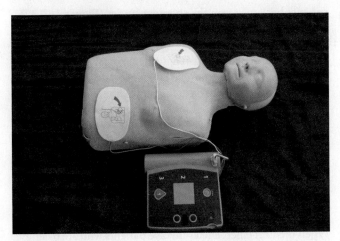

Figure 16-11 ■ An automated external defibrillator.
Source: Fotolia © Roy Pedersen.

PROCEDURE 16-5 Use an Automated External Defibrillator (AED)

Theory and Rationale

The use of AEDs as lifesaving devices is becoming more and more common. AEDs are now found in doctors' offices, malls, airplanes, and private residences. An AED works by sending an electrical current through the myocardium of the heart, briefly causing the heart to stop and allowing the heart's natural pacemaker to take over. The goal is for the heart to resume function. All AEDs function in the same manner.

The AED is brought by a second- or third-party rescuer after the initial chest compressions and rescue breathing have begun.

Materials

- Practice AED machine
- Patient chart
- Mannequin

Competency

1. Place the AED next to the victim's left ear. This position allows the rescuers clear access to the chest and airway for continued rescue measures.
2. Turn the AED on and follow the voice prompts.
3. You will be prompted to attach the electrode pads to the patient's chest, on the sternum and at the apex of the heart, following the diagram for correct placement.
4. Next, you will be directed to allow the machine to analyze the heart rhythm to determine if it is a shockable rhythm. CPR should cease while the machine is analyzing.
5. The machine will begin a charging sequence prior to shocking and warn rescuers to stand back. The voice prompt will then tell you to press the "shock" button to administer the electrical current to the patient.
6. If the machine indicates "No shock is advised," assess the patient for breathing and circulation. Continue CPR as needed until advanced medical personnel arrive.

Patient Education

If a friend or family member of the patient is present at the time of rescue, you will need to help that person remain calm and out of the way so that advanced rescue personnel can treat the victim. It is also helpful if you can explain to friends or family members what is happening and to what hospital the victim will be transported. Be careful not to make comforting statements that might not be accurate, such as "He'll be all right" or "She's going to be just fine."

Charting Example

11/25/XX 3:30 PM Patient found in stairwell, unresponsive, with absence of pulse and respirations. Emergency protocol initiated with 2 rescuer CPR and 9-1-1 services activated. Third rescuer initiated AED response and patient was analyzed for shockable rhythm. CPR and AED shocks administered a total of 8 cycles prior to advanced medical support arriving. Patient released to EMS care and transferred to Sacred Heart Medical Center. Martin Cowan, CMA (AAMA)

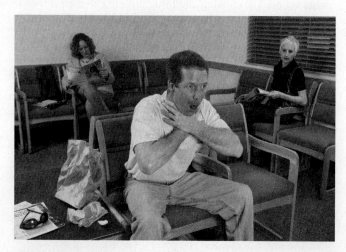

Figure 16-12 ■ The universal sign of choking.

Source: Pearson Education/PH College. Photographer: Michal Heron.

patient's back, between the shoulder blades (**Figure 16-13** ■). The medical assistant should also call for a coworker to dial for emergency personnel.

If the object fails to dislodge, the medical assistant should turn the patient over and use two fingers to administer five thrusts to the patient's chest at the nipple line (**Figure 16-14** ■). The assistant should then look in the patient's mouth again to see if an object is visible and removable. When it is not, the assistant should continue thrusting to the back and then to the front until emergency personnel arrive.

Controlling Bleeding

When medical emergencies involve patients who are bleeding, medical assistants must follow standard precautions. For bleeding patients, medical assistants should put on appropriate

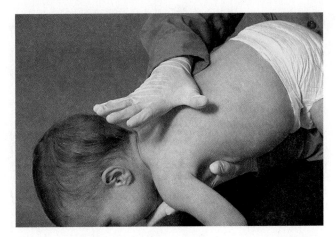

Figure 16-13 ■ Back blows for an infant.
Source: Pearson Education/PH College. Photographer: Michal Heron.

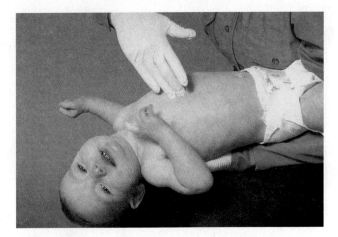

Figure 16-14 ■ Chest thrusts for an infant.
Source: Pearson Education/PH College. Photographer: Michal Heron.

 PROCEDURE 16-6 Respond to an Adult with an Airway Obstruction

Theory and Rationale

The most common object adults choke on is a bolus of food. When the food is lodged in the upper airway, the person may put his or her hands around the throat, the universal sign of choking, to let bystanders know he or she cannot breathe properly. If the person can wheeze, make a high-pitched sound, cough, or speak, do not take any action. Instead call 9-1-1 and encourage the person to continue to cough forcefully to try to dislodge the object. If the person is unable to speak or cough, he or she is in immediate danger and action must be taken.

It is important that the rescuer call 9-1-1 even if the victim's airway is not completely blocked or the Heimlich maneuver was successful. Once the object has been expelled, the throat is likely to continue to swell as a result of the irritant, so the victim should be assessed in an emergency room.

Materials

- Approved mannequin
- Gloves
- Ventilation mask with one-way valve for unconscious victim

Competency

1. Establish that the victim is choking by asking "Are you choking?" or "Can you speak?" If the victim indicates she is choking by a head shake or the universal choking sign—tell her you are going to begin emergency treatment and direct someone to call 9-1-1.

2. Stand behind the victim with your feet slightly apart, placing one foot between the victim's feet and one to the outside. This stance will give you greater stability, and if the victim should pass out, you can safely guide him or her to the ground by sliding him or her down your thigh.

3. Place the index finger of one hand at the person's navel or belt buckle. If the victim is a pregnant woman, place your finger above the enlarged uterus.

4. Make a fist with your other hand and place it, thumb side to victim, above your other hand. If the person is very pregnant, the uterus is pushing the stomach and other internal organs under the rib cage and you might have to do chest compressions.

5. Place your marking hand over your curled fist and begin to give quick inward and upward thrusts (**Figure 16-15** ■).

6. There is no set number of thrusts to give to an adult who remains conscious. Continue to give thrusts until the object is removed *or* the victim becomes unconscious.

7. If the victim becomes unconscious, gently lower him or her to the ground.

8. Activate EMS and put on gloves.

9. Immediately begin CPR with 30 chest compressions and two rescue breaths.

10. Before administering the rescue breaths, open the airway with the head tilt–chin lift and look for a foreign body in the victim's mouth and remove if visible. Blind finger sweeps are no longer recommended and should not be performed.

PROCEDURE 16-6 Respond to an Adult with an Airway Obstruction (continued)

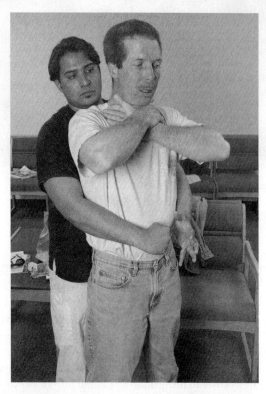

Figure 16-15 ■ Administer quick inward and upward abdominal thrusts.

Source: Pearson Education/PH College. Photographer: Michal Heron.

11. Continue with cycles of 30 compressions and two rescue breaths until the foreign body is expelled or advanced medical personal arrive to relieve you.

Patient Education

If the object has been successfully removed and the patient did not lose consciousness, the patient might feel that she no longer needs medical treatment. As a rescuer you must insist that she seek medical attention anyway. The lodged object might have caused swelling in the lining of the esophagus, constricting the throat and impairing the breathing.

Charting Example

10/25/XX 11:30 AM Jason Jones, CMA, exhibited signs of choking at lunch. Jason grabbed his throat and was unable to cough or make noise. Tina Muller, CMAA (NHA), alerted the physician and placed a call to 9-1-1. After abdominal thrusts were unsuccessful, chest compressions and rescue breaths were given until the piece of apple was expelled. EMS arrived and checked Jason for signs of throat irritation and swelling. He was transported to Sacred Heart Medical Center for assessment. Janice Walker, CMA (AAMA)

protective equipment (**Figure 16-16** ■). Personal protective equipment (**PPE**) consists of an impermeable gown, goggles that completely cover the eyes, and an impermeable mask. The medical assistant should then apply several layers of sterile dressing material directly to any wounds. Direct pressure should stop or slow bleeding until emergency personnel arrive.

Critical Thinking Question 16-3

Refer back to the case study at the beginning of the chapter. How should Adrianna respond to Mr. Whitford's emergency? Consider how she should handle the other patients waiting in the reception area who have observed his fall.

Critical Thinking Question 16-4

Referring back to the case study at the beginning of the chapter, how should the medical assistant try to control the patient's bleeding?

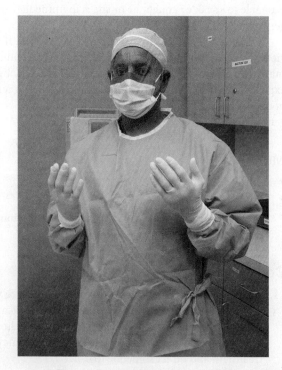

Figure 16-16 ■ A medical assistant wearing PPE gown, face shield, and gloves.

PROCEDURE 16-7 Remove an Airway Obstruction in an Infant

Theory and Rationale

When an infant has an airway obstruction, the medical assistant must be able to quickly remove the obstruction and restore the patient's airways.

Materials

- Disposable gloves
- Infant mannequin

Competency

(**Conditions**) With the necessary materials, you will be able to (**Task**) remove an airway obstruction from an infant (**Standards**) correctly within the time limit set by the instructor.

1. Call for a coworker to dial 9-1-1 for emergency services.
2. Open the infant's mouth and look to see if an object is visible. If so, use your finger to sweep the object from the infant's mouth. If the object is *not* visible, do not blindly sweep your finger through the infant's mouth, as you may push the object further back into the throat.
3. Place the baby face down over your forearm and across your thigh. The infant's head should be lower than the trunk, and you should support the infant's head and neck with one hand.
4. Using the heel of your free hand, administer five blows to the infant's back between the shoulder blades.
5. Turn the infant over, keeping the head lower than the trunk, and administer five thrusts to the midsternal area of the infant.

6. Look into the infant's mouth to see if the object is visible. If so, sweep your finger through the mouth to remove the object. If not, administer two rescue breaths into the infant by covering the infant's nose and mouth completely with your own mouth.
7. Repeat the above sequence until the object is dislodged or help arrives.
8. Once the emergency passes, document all activities in the patient's medical record.

Patient Education

Just as with an emergency involving an adult choking victim, a lodged object can cause swelling in the lining of the infant's esophagus, constricting the throat and impairing the breathing. If an infant patient chokes in the medical office, it is imperative that, after the emergency has passed, the physician provides a thorough examination and a watchful eye over the patient. The physician may request that the patient remain in the office for 30–60 minutes after the episode has occurred to ensure there are no other threats to the patient's health.

Charting Example

4/14/XX 8:45 AM. Patient (18 months old) choked on a piece of dry cereal while playing in the reception area of office. Immediate assistance was given and the object dislodged within 1 minute. Dr. Anderson assessed the pt. and pt. remained in the office for 1 hour to ensure adverse reactions were not displayed. Ryan Murphy, CMA (AAMA)

▶▶▶ Pulse Points

Controlling Nosebleeds

Sometimes patients present in medical offices with nosebleeds due to injury or the rupture of small blood vessels in the nose. Patients with mild nosebleeds should sit up, lean forward, and apply direct pressure by pinching the nose. Pressure should continue for 10 to 15 minutes until the bleeding is controlled. If the bleeding cannot be controlled, the medical assistant should notify the physician.

pupils; a weak, rapid pulse; shallow, rapid respirations; and extreme thirst. When patients exhibit signs of shock, medical assistants should ensure that those patients have an open airway and proper circulation. Assistants should encourage patients to lie down with their legs elevated to return blood to the vital organs. Next, assistants should cover patients with blankets for warmth and keep them calm until emergency personnel arrive. Most emergency treatments for shock patients will need to be administered by a physician or emergency personnel.

Assisting Patients in Shock

Patients go into shock for various reasons, including blood loss, infection, and pain. The most common signs of shock include pale gray or bluish skin; moist, cool skin; dilated

Critical Thinking Question 16-5

Referring to the case study at the beginning of the chapter, how would a medical assistant recognize the signs of shock in Mark Whitford?

PROCEDURE 16-8 Control Bleeding

Theory and Rationale

Uncontrolled bleeding can lead to further injury or even death. In a bleeding emergency, the MA should first don appropriate protective equipment and then apply several layers of sterile dressing material directly to the wound to stop or slow the bleeding until emergency personnel arrive.

Materials

- Disposable gloves
- Personal protective equipment (gown, eye protection, mask)
- Sterile dressing
- Bandage
- Biohazard waste container

Competency

1. Notify a coworker to alert the physician. If a physician is not available in the office, notify the coworker to alert emergency personnel.
2. Assemble the necessary equipment and supplies.
3. Wash your hands.
4. Don the personal protective equipment.
5. Open the sterile dressings and apply several layers directly to the wound and apply direct pressure.
6. Wrap the wound with a bandage. If the wound continues to bleed, apply more sterile dressing and bandaging material. Continue to apply direct pressure.

7. If the wound continues to bleed and if it is located on an extremity, raise the extremity to a level above the patient's heart.
8. If the bleeding continues, apply pressure to the appropriate artery.
9. Once the bleeding is under control, dispose of all contaminated materials into the biohazard waste container.
10. Wash your hands.
11. Once the emergency passes, document all activities in the patient's medical record.

Patient Education

As a medical assistant it is important to instruct the patient on proper wound care as directed by the physician. Many offices will provide patients with written instructions that document the proper steps to take in order to facilitate proper healing.

Charting Example

5/3/XX 11:15 AM Patient tripped and fell in the hallway, which resulted in a large gash on the right forearm. Sterile dressings were applied and bleeding stopped within a couple of minutes of applying pressure. Dr. Clark examined the patient and requested the patient to return in 3 days to check healing of the wound. Matilda Cruz, RMA (AMI).

Caring for Patients with Fractures

Patients with fractures most likely require emergency room care. When patients sustain fractures in or around the medical office, they must be moved only as necessary. Medical assistants should try to make these patients as comfortable as possible and notify the physician right away. The physician may ask the medical assistant to bring ice packs to the patient to reduce swelling or to apply direct pressure with sterile gauze in the event the patient is bleeding.

Assisting Patients with Burns

Medical assistants may be required to assist with emergency burn victims. First, the assistants should try to determine the cause of the burn (e.g., chemical, fire, scalding). Medical staff who know the cause of a burn can provide better care. Some burns can be treated in the ambulatory care setting; others

require hospital care. If possible, the medical assistant should immerse the burn in cool water, or soak sterile gauze in cool saline solution and apply the gauze to the burned area. In the event the burn was caused by a chemical, the medical assistant should attempt to flush the area with water. No matter what the cause of the burn, the medical assistant should seek the order of the physician in how to administer treatment to the patient.

Emergency Preparedness

The medical assistant should be knowledgeable about emergency preparedness. This includes knowing how to respond in the event of a man-made disaster, such as a terrorist event, or to a natural disaster, such as a hurricane or tornado.

Earthquake

Because earthquakes can happen at any time and without any warning, the medical assistant should know how to respond to this type of emergency. One of the first steps to preventing injury during an earthquake is to prepare before an earthquake happens. Advance preparation might save lives and prevent injuries.

According to FEMA, there are six steps involved in planning ahead for an earthquake. These steps are:

1. Check for hazards around the facility.
   - Make sure shelves are fastened securely to walls.
   - Do not place large or heavy objects on higher shelves.
   - Store any breakable items in low, closed cabinets equipped with locks.
   - Heavy items should not be hung on walls above where patients will sit or lie.
   - Overhead light fixtures should be secured.
   - Any defective electrical wiring or leaky gas connections should be repaired.
   - Water heaters should be strapped to wall studs and bolted to the floor.
   - Any deep cracks in ceilings or foundations should be repaired.
   - All flammable products should be stored in closed cabinets with locks, on the bottom shelf.
2. Identify safe places both indoors and outdoors.
   - Under sturdy furniture
   - Against an inside wall
   - Away from glass that could shatter
   - Away from bookcases or furniture that could fall over
   - In the open, away from buildings, trees, telephone or electrical lines, overpasses, or elevated expressways
3. Educate yourself and your coworkers.
   - Contact the local emergency management office or the American Red Cross chapter for information.
   - Teach all staff members how and when to turn off gas, electricity, and water.
4. Have disaster supplies on hand.
   - Flashlight and extra batteries
   - Portable battery-operated radio and extra batteries
   - First aid kit and manual
   - Emergency food and water
   - Nonelectric can opener
   - Sturdy shoes
5. Develop an emergency communication plan.
   - In case staff members are separated from one another during an earthquake, develop a plan for reuniting after the disaster.
   - Define the expectations of each staff member—who will escort patients from the building, who will check the treatment rooms?
6. Help your community get ready.
   - Provide literature for patients on how to prepare for an earthquake.

Fire

Because more than 4,000 Americans die and more than 25,000 are injured in fires each year, the medical assistant should be prepared to respond to this type of disaster. Fire spreads quickly and there is typically no time to gather belongings or make a telephone call. In just two minutes, a fire can become life-threatening and in five minutes a fire can engulf a building. Heat and smoke from fire are often more dangerous than the flames.

The medical office should be equipped with properly working smoke alarms. These should be placed on every level of the building and should be placed on the ceiling or high on the walls. Every room of the office should be equipped with a smoke detector and each should be tested and cleaned once per month. The batteries should be replaced at least twice a year and every smoke alarm should be replaced once every 10 years. In addition, ceiling-installed fire sprinkler systems are very desirable in medical offices and are usually required due to building code standards for public facilities. These systems automatically dispense water when a preinstalled heat sensitive trigger is activated.

The medical assistant should know the evacuation plans and escape routes to use in the event of a fire. Staff members should practice those escape routes. If the office is located above the first level, escape ladders may be used. It is important, and often mandated by city ordinances, that public buildings post highly visible evacuation routes that highlight emergency exits. Each room in the medical office should show a detailed evacuation route to an emergency exit. **Figure 16-17** ■ provides an example of an office evacuation route.

Fire and Electrical Safety

The medical assistant should know the location of fire exits, alarms, and fire extinguishers and should follow all emergency plans, remembering to keep all hallways and exit doors free from obstructions. *If the MA discovers a fire, he or she should pull the alarm.*

If the alarm sounds, the MA should:

- Call or direct someone to call 9-1-1 (only if it is safe to do so), or call from a safe place outside the building.
- Close all doors and windows (only if it is safe to do so).
- Check bathrooms and examination rooms to make sure all patients and staff are aware of the fire alarm.
- Evacuate with patients immediately.
- Meet at an assigned place.
- Never use the building elevator during a fire, as it can stop on the floor with the fire. Use the stairs.

Fire extinguishers should be used when the fire is between you and the exit, and for small, contained fires that are caught

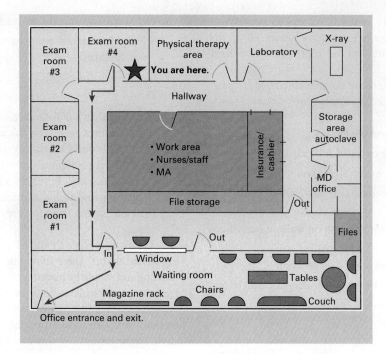

Figure 16-17 ■ Evacuation routes, that clearly mark a route to the closest exit, should be placed in every room in the medical office.

early so that they do not intensify. If it is necessary to use the extinguisher, use the PASS method: *Pull* the safety pin, *Aim* at the base of the fire, *Squeeze* the trigger to discharge the agent, and *Sweep* from side to side. It is important that you know how to use the appropriate kind of fire extinguisher before trying to use it:

- Class A Fires (ordinary combustibles) use a pressurized water or dry chemical extinguisher.
- Class B Fires (flammable liquids) use a dry chemical or carbon dioxide extinguisher.
- Class C Fires (electrical equipment) use a carbon dioxide, halon, or dry chemical extinguisher.

Local fire departments, if requested, will generally train employees regarding fire safety in the office. Electrical safety requires exercising caution. The MA must be careful with all equipment and make sure it is in good condition before using it. Tell your office manager or administrator if you see:

- Frayed wires or cords
- Overused extension cords
- Lack of ground plugs or grounded outlets
- Cracked or broken switch or receptacle plates
- Sparking when a plug is inserted into or removed from an outlet
- Broken lights

The medical assistant should be aware that if a person's clothes are on fire, that person should *stop*, *drop*, and *roll* until the fire is extinguished. Running makes the fire burn faster.

In order to escape a fire, the medical assistant should check closed doors for heat before opening. This is done by using the back of the hand to feel the top of the door, the doorknob, and the crack between the door and the door frame before opening the door. If the door is hot, it should not be opened and another route of escape should be sought. If the door is cool, it should be opened slowly.

When escaping a fire, the medical assistant should crawl low under any smoke on the way to the exit and close doors as they are passed through to delay the spread of fire. Once out of the building, the medical assistant should not attempt to reenter until or unless the fire department declares that action to be safe.

Floods

FEMA declares floods to be the most common hazard in the United States. Some floods can develop over days of rainy weather; others might be in the form of flash floods that occur very quickly. The MA should be aware of the flood dangers that exist in his or her local area.

During a flood, the medical assistant should listen to the radio for information. In the event of a flash flood, the medical assistant should move to higher ground. If there is time before evacuating, the medical assistant should be sure to disconnect any electrical equipment and shut off utilities at their main valve.

When evacuating, the medical assistant should be careful not to walk through moving water. Just six inches of moving water can make a person fall.

PROCEDURE 16-9 Develop a Safety Plan for Employees and Patients: Fire Evacuation

Theory and Rationale

A predetermined safety plan will create organization in the midst of chaos as well as a sense of security. A safety plan should be created using the input and resources of the medical office staff based on the facility where they work. However, for learning purposes the student should create a development plan that addresses general safety issues for both patients and employees. The student might also want to develop a plan utilizing the floor plan of their school building for evacuation purposes.

Materials

- Pen
- Paper
- Computer with word-processing software
- Printer
- Copy machine
- Building evacuation routes

Competency

1. Using word-processing software, create a new document that will outline the components of the safety plan.

2. Clearly identify the evacuation routes to emergency exits from every room in the building. Include copies of the evacuation routes with the final and completed safety plan. If evacuation routes do not exist, they must be created.

3. In the document, identify the safety-zones outside of the office building where everyone will gather after evacuation. If possible, include photos of the safety-zone or maps of the outside area clearly indicating the zone.

4. Create a delineation chart that outlines responsibilities of office staff members in the event of a fire. The following tasks will require an assignment of responsibility:
   a. Activate fire rescue and emergency medical services by dialing 9-1-1.
   b. Close doors and windows (if safe to do so).
   c. Secure and remove the first aid kit upon exiting the office during evacuation (only if safe to do so).

5. In the document, create a section that specifically pertains to patient safety. Include the following information:

a. Identify which office staff member will be in charge of directing and assisting the patients during evacuation. Remind patients that elevators may not be used in the event of a fire.
   b. Identify which office staff members will be in charge of checking that reception area and patient bathrooms have been evacuated.
   c. Identify which staff member will be in charge of retrieving the emergency first aid kit and transporting it to the safety zone in the event that minor injuries are sustained during evacuation.
   d. Identify the office physician who will be responsible for evaluating and treating patients at the safety-zone prior to the arrival of emergency personnel.

6. In the document, create a section that specifically pertains to employee safety. Include the following information:
   a. Identify which office staff member will be in charge of checking that employee bathrooms, break room, laboratory, and other employee-only areas have been evacuated.
   b. Identify which office staff member will be in charge of taking a roll-call at the safety-zone to ensure that all office personnel have evacuated the building.

7. The fire safety plan should also include the following information:
   a. When smoke alarm batteries should be replaced
   b. When maintenance checks on fire-extinguishers should occur
   c. A plan for ensuring that emergency first aid kits are fully stocked with products within expiration dates
   d. Contact information for the insurance company that insures the medical office building

8. Perform grammar and spell-check within the document and save the file.

9. Print the document for review by the office manager and/or office physicians. Once approved, place a copy in the medical office's policy and procedure folder.

10. Make copies of the fire-safety plan and distribute it to all employees for review and discussion.

11. Train all office staff on the fire-safety plan within the first 10 days of hire.

Hurricanes

Hurricanes can strike with little warning, though most often there is some advance warning, giving the medical office staff time to prepare. If the office is in the path of the hurricane, the windows might need to be secured. This can be done using plywood. Trees and shrubs around the office should be well trimmed.

If the medical office is to be evacuated before a hurricane, the medical assistant should listen to the radio or television for information provided by local emergency management personnel.

During the hurricane, the medical assistant should listen to the radio or television for information and prepare for high winds and possible flooding.

Tornados

While weather forecasters are able to predict and track hurricanes and give more advanced notice, tornadoes can strike with very little warning. Sometimes tornado warnings are issued within only minutes of the actual tornado strike. The effects of a tornado can be devastating and cause severe destruction to anything in its path. The best protection against a tornado is to be properly prepared. Preparation includes three key steps:

1. Know your area. Many cities and towns in the Midwest and east of the Rocky Mountains see frequent tornado activity. If your area is often threatened by tornado activity, it is important to have emergency plans in place.

2. Locate safety zones. The safest place to be during a tornado is underground. Therefore many buildings and homes use basements or storm cellars as a safety zone during a tornado. If a basement or cellar is not an option in your medical office, closets and hallways that are located away from windows on the lowest level of the building are the next best safety zone.

3. Create an emergency kit (**Figure 16-18 ■**). Emergency kits contain disaster supplies similar to those on the FEMA list discussed earlier in this section. An emergency kit may contain nonperishable food, drinking water, blankets, flashlights, batteries, battery-operated radio, a well-stocked first aid kit, plastic garbage bags, and other items that are considered to be useful in the event of an emergency situation.

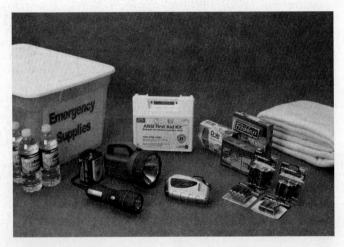

Figure 16-18 ■ Every medical office should keep emergency supplies in a waterproof container.

Source: Pearson Education/PH College. Photographer: Michal Heron.

Combine all of this information to create an emergency plan for the office. The emergency plan should also outline specific duties of key staff members and highlight when emergency drills and trainings will occur throughout the year. Procedure 16-10 expands upon this teaching through developing an environmental safety plan.

Terrorism

In the event of a terrorist attack, the medical assistant should be aware of the steps to take in an emergency such as explosions, biological threats, or a nuclear blast.

Explosions

In the event of a bomb threat, the medical assistant should try to obtain as much information from the caller as possible:

● When is the bomb going to explode?
● Where is the bomb right now?
● What does it look like?
● What kind of bomb is it?
● What will cause it to explode?

This information should be immediately provided to the police and their directions should be followed; this often includes immediate evacuation of the building.

If an explosion has occurred, the medical assistant should respond by following the steps as if an earthquake and/or fire has happened.

Biological Threats

There are four methods of delivery of a biological agent:

1. **Aerosols**—agents are dispersed into the air, forming a mist that can drift for miles.
2. **Animals**—some diseases are spread by insects or animals.
3. **Food and water contamination**—some agents are placed in the food or water supply.
4. **Person-to-person**—some spread of agents is possible via direct contact between people.

In order to prepare for a biological attack, the medical facility may have a high efficiency particulate air (**HEPA**) filter installed.

In the event of a biological attack, the medical assistant should be prepared to move away quickly, wash with soap and water, contact authorities, listen to the radio for instructions, and remove and bag clothing if contaminated.

Nuclear Blast

In the event of a nuclear attack, the medical assistant should take cover as quickly as possible, below ground if the building

PROCEDURE 16-10 Develop an Environmental Safety Plan

Theory and Rationale

Medical assistants are playing a greater role in emergency preparedness. The most important rule to follow is to always be prepared for any situation that may arise. With adequate preparation we not only help ourselves and our patients but also the community that surrounds us.

Materials

- Pen
- Paper
- Computer
- Copy machine
- Various emergency supplies
- Waterproof containers

Competency

1. Create an emergency kit that can be used by your office in the event of an environmental emergency. Supplies may include:
   - Flashlights
   - Batteries
   - Bottles of water
   - Nonperishable food
   - Bandages
   - Alcohol and hydrogen peroxide
   - Blankets
   - Vinyl or latex gloves
   - Face masks and respirator masks
   - Tweezers, scissors
   - Medication—ibuprofen, acetaminophen, antihistamines, antibiotic ointment, tetanus vaccines, etc.
   - Battery-powered radio
2. Enclose the kit in a waterproof container.
3. Place the kit in a safe area, such as a medicine closet or storage closet.
4. Create evacuation plans and make sure that every room in the medical office shows a detailed exit route.
5. Create a delineation chart that outlines responsibilities of office staff members in the event of an emergency.
6. Create a list of *safety zones* that can be used in the event of an emergency. For instance:
   - A safety zone in the event of a tornado
   - A safety zone in the event of a flood
7. Make photocopies of the safety zone list, evacuation plan, and delineation chart for everyone in the office. Laminate and hang copies in the employee break room.
8. Train all office staff on the environmental exposure plan within 10 days of hire.

has a basement. The medical assistant should remain in a safe location, listening to the radio for instructions. The medical assistant should not attempt to look at the flash or fireball, but should instead seek shelter as quickly as possible and lie flat on the ground with his head covered.

Mock Environmental Exposures

Medical assistants can play a vital role in the event of an environmental emergency. It is helpful to be prepared for such events, and to understand how to help victims and provide assistance to other health care providers.

Community organizations, colleges, and hospitals may offer mock environmental exposure events. These mock events present real-life scenarios and situations that might arise during times of disaster. Mock environmental scenarios

might include a tornado site with injured victims, exposure to a biological chemical, or treating injured victims of flash floods or hurricanes. The role of the medical assistant will vary in every situation; however, overall, MAs might be able to provide assistance by:

- Aiding in evacuation plans
- Triaging patients to determine which patients require immediate attention
- Assisting in first aid response for wounded individuals
- Administering tetanus and other vaccines under the direction of a physician
- Facilitating order and organization in the midst of chaos
- Implementing and following through on an environmental safety plan

PROCEDURE 16-11

Participate in a Mock-Environmental Exposure: Responding to an Earthquake

Theory and Rationale

Medical assistants will need to understand how to react quickly and professionally in the midst of a crisis. They will be able to assist patients by using critical thinking skills and maintaining a calm composure. Mock environmental exposure scenarios help the medical assistant student consider the appropriate actions to take in a crisis.

Materials

- Pen
- Paper

Competency

1. Evacuate the medical office or building as soon as safely possible.
   a. Make sure that staff members are following their given responsibilities during times of emergency. Someone (or a couple of staff members) must ensure the reception area, examination rooms, laboratory, physician offices, and bathrooms have all been evacuated of patients and staff members.

2. If it is reasonable and safe, gather the emergency supply kit on the way out of the building.
   a. Safety should always be your first priority. If the building is unsafe, do not bother with anything other than evacuation and finding safety.

3. After evacuation, immediately go to the predetermined safety zone.
   a. As you, the medical assistant, are exiting the building, help patients and others by providing a calm voice of reassurance. Direct patients and their family members to congregate at the specified safety zone.

4. Provide assistance to the physicians as they begin to evaluate and treat injuries.

5. Call 9-1-1 if there are injuries that are life threatening, serious, or untreatable at the scene.

6. Maintain your composure and continue to provide reassurance to those around you; addressing the needs and concerns of patients, coworkers, and physicians alike.

REVIEW

Chapter Summary

- Medical assistants have distinct and vital roles in medical emergencies.
- A number of supplies and equipment help support life-saving objectives in emergency situations.
- When an emergency arises, preparedness, training, and organization can mean the difference between measured, effective response and chaos.
- To ensure appropriate responses, members of the health care team should call emergency services to the medical office as needed.
- Rescue breathing and cardiopulmonary resuscitation (CPR) are just two means medical staff have to address emergency situations.
- A crash cart holds a number of supplies and equipment needed in emergencies.

- An automated external defibrillator is used to treat patients with no pulse.
- Medical assistants should be trained to stop bleeding, as well as to take all comfort measures for patients in varied types of emergencies.
- The medical assistant should be knowledgeable about emergency preparedness and understand how to respond in the event of a man-made disaster or a natural disaster.
- Mock environmental exposure events may be offered within the community, at colleges and hospitals. These events provide real-life scenarios and situations that may arise disasters.

Chapter Review

Multiple Choice

1. Which of the following items would be found on a crash cart?
   a. Sterile gloves
   b. Ambu bag
   c. Blood pressure cuff
   d. Tourniquet
   e. All of the above

2. The proper sequence for CPR is
   a. Circulation, airway, breathing
   b. Airway, breathing, circulation
   c. Breathing, airway, circulation
   d. Circulation, breathing, airway
   e. Airway, circulation, breathing

3. Which of the following is *not* a medical assistant's responsibility during an emergency situation?
   a. Aiding in evacuation plans
   b. Assisting in first-aid response for wounded individuals
   c. Triaging patients to determine which patients require immediate attention
   d. Providing medicine to patients from the drug supply closet
   e. Administering tetanus and other vaccines under the direction of a physician

4. The safest location during a tornado is
   a. Behind windows that have been covered in plywood.
   b. In a stairway.
   c. In closet on an exterior wall.
   d. In a basement.
   e. The highest level of the building.

True/False

T F **1.** A patient with a nosebleed should be asked to sit, lean forward, and pinch the nose.

T F **2.** One of the responsibilities of the administrative medical assistant in an office emergency is to direct patients and family members as needed.

T F **3.** When emergency personnel services must be summoned to the medical office, physicians should call because they have the greatest knowledge of the situations.

T F **4.** When administering oxygen to a patient, the medical assistant will always use a nasal cannula.

T F **5.** Standard precautions are used to prevent spread of infection.

T F **6.** Patients who are choking and have blocked airways can still speak.

T F **7.** An automated external defibrillator will not shock a patient who does not need to be shocked.

Short Answer

1. To stop bleeding, what should the medical assistant apply to the wound?
2. Describe the purpose of a CPR mouth barrier.
3. List at least five items that would be found in a medical office emergency kit.
4. What steps would make a medical office safe for small children?
5. Name three working conditions that would be considered unsafe.
6. What are two reasons a patient might be in shock?
7. What are two reasons a patient might faint?
8. How does adult choking treatment differ from child choking treatment?
9. What is the proper treatment of a patient who is in shock?

Research

1. Using the Internet as a resource, look up information on handling medical emergencies in the health care setting. What information do you find?
2. Call your local medical assisting chapter. Ask them if they offer any continuing education classes that touch on the topic of handling medical emergencies. What kind of classes do they suggest?
3. Speak with one of your instructors in the medical assisting program you are attending. Ask the instructor what kind of reading material he or she would recommend on the subject of handling medical emergencies in the medical office.

Practicum Application Experience

Willie Harrison has brought his 2-year-old daughter, Sonya, to his weekly blood draw. While Willie and his daughter are waiting in the medical office, Sonya finds an object on the floor and places it in her mouth. Seconds later, Willie begins shouting that his daughter is choking. What should the medical assistant do?

Resource Guide

American Heart Association
7272 Greenville Avenue
Dallas, TX 75231
Phone: (800) 242-8721
http://www.americanheart.org/

American Red Cross
www.redcross.org

Federal Emergency Management Agency (FEMA)
500 C Street SW
Washington, DC 20472
Disaster Assistance: (800) 621-FEMA
www.fema.gov

National Highway Traffic Safety Administration
Phone: 1 (888) 327-4236

U.S. Department of Transportation (USDOT)
400 7th St., SW
Washington, DC 20590
www.dot.gov

U.S. National Library of Medicine
8600 Rockville Pike
Bethesda, MD 20894
http://www.nlm.nih.gov/medlineplus

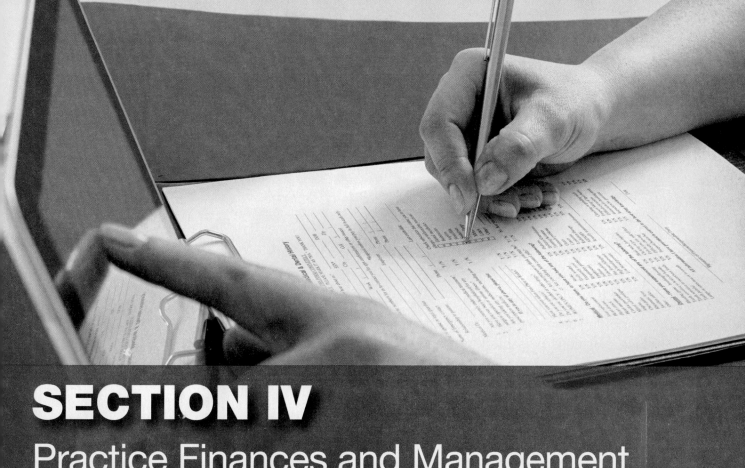

SECTION IV
Practice Finances and Management of the Medical Office

My name is William Scott, and I am an administrative medical assistant at the Middle Valley Medical Clinic. My role in the health insurance process includes working directly with patients; gathering accurate health insurance information; answering patients' questions regarding how their health insurance works; and preparing accurate insurance claim forms so that the clinic receives payment for services provided.

While a medical assistant's involvement in insurance billing may vary from one practice to the next, the MA is always considered an important team player in helping patients to access their health insurance benefits. I have found that a solid understanding of health insurance terminology and knowledge of the various types of insurance plans and types of services covered is key to my success in communicating effectively with patients.

My job is fast-paced and rewarding. I love knowing that I am able to help people by explaining insurance concepts they sometimes don't understand. When patients come to me for assistance, I do everything in my power to assist them.

17

Insurance Billing

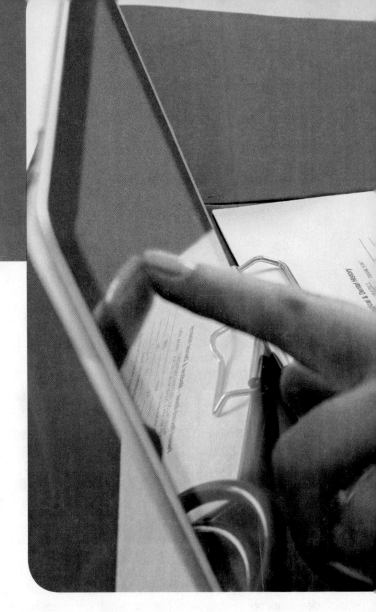

Case Study

Read the following case study and answer the critical thinking questions presented throughout the chapter.

Martin Zamora is a patient at Woodway Health Care and has PPO insurance through his employer. He recently came in with complaints of a sore throat. He was diagnosed with strep throat and was given a prescription for antibiotics. The clinic billed his insurance for $100, but the insurance did not pay anything, even though two months ago it paid $150 for his annual check-up.

Objectives

After completing this chapter, you should be able to:

17.1 Define and spell the key terminology in this chapter.

17.2 Define the medical assistant's role in insurance claim processing.

17.3 Describe the role health insurance has developed throughout history and into the future.

17.4 Define health insurance policy provisions and terminology.

17.5 Describe the types of insurance plans.

17.6 Describe the types of service coverage.

17.7 Describe the various types of private health insurance available.

17.8 Explain government insurance programs.

17.9 Describe third-party liability insurance and disability income insurance.

17.10 Explain how to gather patient information needed for filing claims.

17.11 Describe how to complete health insurance claims forms.

17.12 Explain how to work with fee schedules and reimbursement methods.

17.13 Discuss how to post payments.

17.14 Describe how to follow up on claims.

17.15 Explain how to reconcile payments and rejections.

Key Terminology

accept assignment—agreement by a physician to accept the amount approved by the insurance company as payment in full for a given service

advance beneficiary notice—a form patients sign agreeing to pay for covered Medicare services that may be denied due to medical necessity or frequency

allowed amount—the dollar amount for a service that an insurance company considers acceptable and uses to determine benefit payments

appeal—process of asking for a review of a denied service or claim

assignment of benefits—authorization by a patient for the insurance carrier to pay the health care professional directly rather than issuing monies to the patient

balance billing—billing a patient for the dollar difference between the provider's charge and the insurance approved amount; usually not permitted for participating providers

beneficiary—person who is eligible to receive benefits/services under an insurance policy

birthday rule—a coordination of benefits rule which states that, when children are covered under the policies of both parents, the insurance policy of parent with the birthday earlier in the year is the primary insurance for the children; the insurance policy of the parent with the later birthday is the secondary insurance

bundle—the act of combining multiple services under a single all-inclusive CPT code and one charge

capitation—a reimbursement method in which providers are paid set fees per month per member patients

certificate of coverage—a letter from the insurance company that provides proof of type and timeframe of coverage when a patient terminates a health insurance policy

CHAMPVA—a federal program that covers the health care expenses of the families of veterans with total, permanent, service-related, covered disabilities and the spouses and dependent children of veterans who died in the line of duty

clean claim—insurance claim with no data errors

closed-panel—an HMO in which physicians see only the patients of a specific HMO

coinsurance—percentage of medical charges patients are responsible for according to their insurance plan contracts

conversion factor—a constant dollar value multiplied by the relative value unit to determine the price of individual services

coordination of benefits—the process of determining which insurance policy should be billed first, second, or third when a patient is covered by multiple policies

copayment—the established dollar amount per visit or service that patients are responsible for according to their insurance plan contracts

covered—services potentially eligible for reimbursement

deductible—monetary amount patients must pay to the provider for health care services before their health insurance benefits begin to pay

denied—a claim processed by an insurer and determined not eligible for payment

dependent—a family member or other individual who qualifies for coverage on the insured's policy

disability income insurance—insurance that covers lost wages and certain other benefits due to a disability that prevents the individual from working; also called disability insurance

elective procedure—a medical procedure that will benefit the patient but does not need to be scheduled immediately

eligibility—the process to determine if a patient is qualified to receive coverage/paid benefits according to the insurance policy guidelines

encounter form—document on which the physician indicates procedure and diagnosis codes

exclusions—procedures or services not covered under an insurance plan

exclusive provider organization—a managed care contract with a smaller network of providers under which the employer agrees to not use any other networks in return for favorable pricing

explanation of benefits—a statement accompanying payment from the insurance company that summarizes how the payment for each billed service was calculated and gives reasons for any items not paid

fee schedule—a list of the approved fees that an insurance carrier agrees to pay to participating providers; also refers to the standard set of fees the provider charges to all insurers

fee-for-service—the payment method in which insurance companies pay providers fees for each service provided to covered patients

First Report of Illness or Injury—the initial report of a workers' compensation illness or injury that documents the circumstances of the illness, injury, treatment plan, and prognosis

geographic adjustment factor—a numeric multiplier used by Medicare to adjust fees for the varying costs of practicing medicine in different areas of the country

group health insurance—a commercial insurance policy with rates based on a group of people, usually offered by an employer

health insurance exchange—an organization created by the Patient Protection and Affordable Care Act that offers a choice of health insurance plans, certifies the plans that participate, and provides consumer information regarding options

health maintenance organization—a group of physicians or medical centers that provides comprehensive service to members under a capitated payment plan; members' care is covered only when using these designated providers

individual health insurance—a commercial health insurance policy with rates based on individual health criteria

Key Terminology (continued)

individual mandate—the requirement of the Patient Protection and Affordable Care Act that, as of 2014, requires most people to have health insurance and requires them to pay a tax penalty if they do not

insured—person who holds or owns an insurance policy; same as the member or the policyholder

Item—the name of a box to be completed on the CMS-1500 claim form

liability insurance—the type of insurance that covers injuries that occur on, in, or because of the insured's property; also called *property and casualty insurance*

lifetime maximum benefit—monetary amount allowed by an insurance carrier for a covered member's covered expenses over the member's lifetime

long-term disability—a disability income insurance policy that has a longer waiting period, usually three months to two years, and pays benefits for an extended length of time, which may be several years, to age 65, or the lifetime

managed care organization—a company that attempts to control the cost of health care while providing better outcomes by transferring financial risk to the provider

Medicaid—a joint federal and state program that helps with medical costs for some people with low incomes and limited resources

medical necessity—criteria established by payer to determine when a service is justified, based on the health care needs of a patient

Medicare—federal program that covers medical expenses for those aged 65 and over, those with end-stage renal disease, and those with long-term disabilities

Medicare Severity-Adjusted Diagnosis-Related Groups—a case-based payment method used by Medicare for inpatient hospital stays in which patients with similar conditions and care requirements are classified together and are eligible for the same amount of reimbursement

Medigap—a private insurance policy that supplements Medicare coverage, in order to fill "gaps" in Part A and Part B coverage.

member—the person who owns the insurance policy

negotiated fee schedule—a reimbursement method in which the managed care plan develops a fees schedule that participating providers agree to accept

non-covered—services not eligible for reimbursement under any circumstance

open-panel—an HMO in which providers treat both HMO patients and non-HMO patients

outliers—exceptional circumstances that cost far more or less than the average

participating provider—a health care provider who has contracted with a particular health insurance carrier

Patient Protection and Affordable Care Act—federal legislation passed in 2010 to help decrease the number of uninsured Americans and reduce the overall costs of health care through the use of mandates, subsidies, and tax credits; also referred to as the Affordable Care Act (ACA)

personal injury protection—the portion of automobile insurance that pays for injuries sustained due to an automobile accident

point of service—an insurance offering in which a patient has access to multiple plans, such as an HMO, PPO, and indemnity, and may choose to use any of them for any given service

policyholder—person who holds or owns an insurance policy; same as the *member* or the *insured*

preauthorization—approval for treatment or service obtained from an insurance company before the care is provided

pre-existing condition—condition for which a patient received treatment in a certain period before beginning coverage with a new insurance plan

preferred provider organization—organization that contracts with independent providers to perform services for members at discounted rates

premium—dollar amount paid to the insurance company to have coverage in force; usually paid monthly; employers may pay part or all of the premium as an employee benefit

preventive care—care a patient receives to maintain good health and screen for potential health risks

primary care provider—person or entity responsible for determining when and if a patient needs specific types of health care

private health insurance—health insurance not provided by the government but by an independent not-for-profit or for-profit company; also called *private insurance*, *commercial health insurance*, or *commercial insurance*

progress report—with regard to workers' compensation, a report that documents the treatment provided, the worker's current medical status, the expected plan of care, the prognosis, and the expected return-to-work date

property and casualty insurance—insurance on homes, cars, and businesses that protects the policyholder against the loss of or damage to physical property they own and against legal liability for losses caused by injury to others, including medical expenses of those injured; also called *liability insurance*

rejected—a claim that is returned without processing to the provider due to a technical error

relative value unit—unit of measure assigned to medical services based on the resources required to provide it; includes work, practice expense, and liability insurance

self-funded—type of insurance in which an employer sets aside a large reserve fund to directly reimburse employees for medical expenses, rather than purchasing a commercial insurance policy

short-term disability—a disability income insurance policy that has a short waiting period, usually 0 to 14 days, and pays benefits for a limited amount of time, usually anywhere from 3 months to 2 years

skilled nursing facility—a licensed facility that primarily provides inpatient, skilled nursing care to patients who require medical, nursing, or rehabilitative services but does not provide the level of care or treatment available in a hospital

sliding fee scale—a provider's fee schedule that charges varying fees for a service based on a patient's financial ability to pay

Social Security Disability Insurance—a federal government program that provides health care coverage to people with low income who are disabled and who do not meet the work requirements of SSI

Supplemental Security Income—a federal government program that provides Medicare coverage to disabled workers who have met Social Security requirements for quarters worked, and whose disability is not work-related

stop loss—a provision in a health insurance policy that limits the maximum amount the patient must pay out-of-pocket for deductibles, copayments, and coinsurance

subscriber—person who holds or owns an insurance policy; same as the *member* or the *insured*

third-party administrator—a company that processes paperwork for claims for a self-insured employer

third-party payer—an organization that pays for health care services on behalf of the patient

TRICARE—health insurance administered by the U.S. Department of Defense for active duty military personnel, retired service personnel, and their eligible dependents; formerly known as Civilian Health and Medical Program (CHAMPUS)

unbundling—the illegal practice of billing multiple services with separate CPT codes and separate charges that should be combined under a single CPT code and one charge

usual, customary, and reasonable—a method third-party payers use to reimburse providers based on the provider's normal or usual fee; the customary or range of fees charged by providers of the same specialty in the same geographic area; and other factors to determine appropriate or reasonable fees in unusual situations

waiting period—period after a new health insurance plan begins and during which certain services are not covered

workers' compensation—insurance coverage provided by employers for job-related illness or injury

Abbreviations

ABN—advance beneficiary notice

ACA—Affordable Care Act

ADA—American Dental Association

BC—Blue Cross

BCBSA—Blue Cross Blue Shield Association

BS—Blue Shield

CF—conversion factor

CHAMPVA—Civilian Health and Medical Program of the Veterans Administration

CHIP—Children's Health Insurance Program

CMS—Centers for Medicare and Medicaid Services

COB—coordination of benefits

CPT—Current Procedural Terminology

DEERS—Defense Enrollment Eligibility Reporting System

DI—disability income insurance

DME—durable medical equipment

EOB—explanation of benefits

EPO—exclusive provider organization

FFS—fee for service

GAF—geographic adjustment factor

GHI—group health insurance

HIE—health insurance exchange

HIPAA—Health Insurance Portability and Accountability Act

HMO—health maintenance organization

ICD-10-CM—*International Classification of Diseases,* 10th ed., *Clinical Modification*

LTD—long-term disability

MAC—Medicare administrative contractor

MCO—managed care organization

MCD—Medicaid

MCR—Medicare

MG—Medigap

MPFS—Medicare physician fee schedule

MS-DRG—Medicare Severity Adjusted Diagnosis Related Group

MSP—Medicare as secondary payer

Non-PAR—non-participating physician (Medicare)

NPI—national provider identifier

NUCC—National Uniform Claim Committee

OCR—optical character recognition

OHI—other health insurance (Medicare)

PAR—participating physician (Medicare)

P/C—property and casualty insurance

PCP—primary care provider

PIP—personal injury protection

POS—point of service

PPACA—Patient Protection and Affordable Care Act

PPO—preferred provider organization

RBRVS—resource-based relative value scale

RVU—relative value unit

STD—short-term disability

SNF—skilled nursing facility

SSDI—Social Security Disability Insurance

SSI—Supplemental Security Income

TPA—third-party administrator

UCR—usual, customary, and reasonable

WC—workers' compensation

Certification Exam Coverage

AAMA (CMA) Exam Coverage:

- Physician–patient relationship
  - Guidelines for third-party agreements
- Third-party billing
  - Types
    1) Capitated plans
    2) Commercial carriers
    3) Government plans
       a) Medicare
       b) Medicaid
       c) Tricare
       d) CHAMPVA
    4) Prepaid HMO, PPO, POS
    5) Workers' compensation
  - Processing claims
    1) Manual and electronic preparation of claims
    2) Tracing claims
    3) Sequence of filing (e.g., primary vs. secondary)
    4) Reconciling payments/rejections
    5) Inquiry and appeal process
  - Applying managed care policies and procedures
    1) Referrals
    2) Precertification
  - Fee schedules
    1) Methods for establishing fees
    2) Relative Value Studies
    3) Resource-based Relative Value Scale (RBRVS)
    4) Diagnosis Related Groups (DRGs)
    5) Contracted fees

AMT (CMAS) Exam Coverage:

- Insurance processing
  - Understand private/commercial health insurance plans (PPO, HMO, traditional indemnity)
  - Understand government health insurance plans (Medicare, Medicaid, Veteran's Administration, CHAMPUS, Tricare, use of Advance Beneficiary Notices)
  - Process patient claims using appropriate forms (including superbills) and time frames
  - Process Workers' Compensation/disability reports and forms
  - Submit claims for third-party reimbursements, including the use of electronic transmission methods
- Insurance billing and finances
  - Understand health care insurance terminology (deductible, copayment, preauthorization, capitation, coinsurance)

- Understand billing requirements for health care insurance plans
- Process insurance payments
- Track unpaid claims, and file and track appeals
- Understand fraud and abuse regulations

AMT (RMA) Exam Coverage:

- Insurance plans
  - Identify and understand the application of government, medical, disability, and accident insurance plans
  - Identify and appropriately apply plan policies and regulations for programs including:
    1) HMO, PPO, indemnity, open, etc.
    2) Short-term and long-term disability
    3) Workers' Compensation
       a) Complete first reports
       b) Complete followup reports
    4) Medicare (including Advance Beneficiary Notice [ABN])
    5) Medicaid
    6) CHAMPUS/Tricare and CHAMPVA
- Claims
  - Complete and file insurance claim forms
    1) File claims for paper and Electronic Data Interchange
    2) Understand and adhere to HIPAA Security and Uniformity Regulations
  - Evaluate claims responses
    1) Understand and evaluate explanation of benefits
    2) Evaluate claims rejection and utilize proper followup procedures
- Coding
  - Process insurance payments and contractual write-off amounts
  - Track unpaid claims
  - Generate aging reports

NCCT (NCMA) Exam Coverage:

- Insurance processing
  - Managed care models
  - Insurance plans
  - Referrals and precertification
  - Filing claims
  - Third party payers

1. Calculate deductible, coinsurance, and allowable amounts.
2. Verify a patient's insurance eligibility.
3. Obtain a managed care referral.
4. Obtain authorization from an insurance company for a procedure.
5. Handle a denied insurance claim.
6. Abstract data to complete a paper CMS-1500 form.
7. Complete a computerized insurance claim form.

Introduction

Preparing insurance claims accurately is vital to the success of any medical practice. In order to continue serving patients, medical offices must operate as a business. Their purpose is to provide needed health care services to patients. Medical offices bill insurance companies and patients to receive payment for their services. They must receive accurate payment in a timely manner in order to hire staff, pay bills, and continue serving patients. Medical assistants play a vital role in this process. Not only do they help gather information from patients, they must be able to answer patients' questions regarding how health insurance works and how amounts owed are determined for any given procedure. Medical assistants must also be able to verify patients' insurance coverage and explain that coverage to the patients. In addition, MAs must know how to prepare health insurance claims accurately, follow up on past-due claims, and pursue unpaid amounts.

Developing these skills will enable the MA to be a patient advocate, helping patients obtain the benefits they are eligible for and helping them understand the reasons when a cost is not covered. Just as in other areas of medical assisting, the medical assistant's involvement in the insurance billing area depends on the type of practice. In a large physician's office, a separate department often handles most of the insurance matters. In a smaller office, the medical assistant may have more responsibilities in this area. Regardless of the type or size of

office, in every situation the medical assistant is a vital team player in helping patients access their insurance benefits.

This chapter is presented in three sections:

- Health Insurance Policies describes the past, present, and future development of health insurance in our country, provides an overview of policy provisions and terminology, and introduces the types of health insurance plans and types of insurance coverage.
- Health Insurance Payers introduces the various types of government and private payers, as well as disability policies. The role of state insurance commissioners is also discussed.
- Health Insurance Claims and Payments walks medical assistants through the details of gathering accurate patient information, preparing the CMS-1500 claim form, and posting and reconciling payments.

Health Insurance Policies

Medical assistants are best able to help patients understand their health insurance when they have a good understanding of this complicated field. This section reviews the changing role of health insurance, introduces common health insurance terminology, describes the types of insurance plans, and summarizes the type of services covered under insurance.

The Changing Role of Health Insurance

Health insurance as it began over 150 years ago bears little resemblance to the modern array of plans and services. Recent federal legislation is expected to change the health insurance landscape further during the next decade. When medical assistants learn how the health insurance industry developed, it gives them a better appreciation of how the system operates today. Understanding where it is headed in the future helps medical assistants better adapt to the changing environment and to help patients understand the changes.

The History of Health Insurance

Health insurance in the United States began in the mid-1800s as disability income insurance, when insurance was used to replace the income of people injured in accidents or ill from certain diseases. The first group policy giving comprehensive benefits was offered by Massachusetts Health Insurance of Boston in 1847. Insurance companies issued the first individual disability and illness policies around 1890.

As medical care advanced in the early 1900s, there was a greater need for insurance that covered hospital expenses. Hospital insurance coverage began in 1929, when a group of schoolteachers in Texas formed a contract with a local hospital to guarantee up to 21 days of hospital care for a premium of $6 per year. This plan became quite popular, and other groups of employers joined the plan, which eventually became known as the Blue Cross Plan.

During the 1920s, most other industrialized countries adopted national health insurance programs which provided government-funded health care to everyone. In the 1930s, as President Franklin D. Roosevelt was developing the Social Security system, his administration looked into possibilities for creating a national health insurance program as part of that plan. The American Medical Association (AMA) opposed the concept of a national health plan, and the idea was eventually dropped.

During World War II, when wages froze, employers began offering their employees group health insurance (GHI) as a benefit. Group health insurance plans cover entire groups of individuals, usually through employers or other large associations or defined groups. These early plans were designed to protect employees from the high costs of hospitalization and eventually evolved into the health care plans common today.

Employee benefit plans became popular in the 1940s and 1950s. The unions that represented large groups of workers bargained for better benefit packages, including tax-free, employer-sponsored health insurance.

During the 1950s and 1960s government programs began to cover health care costs. Social Security coverage included disability benefits for the first time in 1954. In 1965, the federal government created Medicare, designed for the elderly, and Medicaid, targeted to low-income families. These two programs marked a substantial infusion of funding to the health care system, which became the driving force behind the expansion of health care services in the decades that followed.

The 1970s and 1980s saw a rapid rise in the cost of health care, due to advancing technology and funding from Medicare and Medicaid. In 1973, Congress passed the federal HMO Act, which allowed use of federal funds and policy to promote health maintenance organizations (HMOs). As a result, the majority of employer-sponsored group insurance plans moved to less expensive managed care plans. The Tax Equity and Fiscal Responsibility Act (TEFRA), passed in 1982, made it easier and more attractive for HMOs to contract with the Medicare program and also changed the way in which Medicare reimbursed hospitals. Medicare adopted a new hospital payment program called Diagnosis Related Groups (DRG) to help control spending.

By the mid-1990s, most Americans who had health insurance were enrolled in managed care plans. Many insurance companies had adopted hospital payment programs based on DRGs. By the end of 1995, individuals and companies paid for about one-half of the health care received in the United States, with the government paying for the other half.

Patient Education

Although most insurance plans began as safety mechanisms in the event of catastrophic health events, most plans today cover **preventive care**. Catastrophic health events are defined as chronic illnesses or serious injuries that require expensive, specialized, or long-term care. An example is a person diagnosed with cancer or a person who needs several surgeries after a serious accident. Preventive care is care a patient receives to maintain good health and screen for potential health risks. Examples include well-child checks and yearly mammograms or physicals.

Health Insurance Today

Today, Americans obtain health insurance from a variety of sources that are regulated by a multitude of state and federal laws. In addition, the landscape is changing rapidly as the result of recent federal legislation.

Sources of Health Insurance In contrast to other industrialized countries in which the government finances health care and oversees the delivery system, in the United States, Americans must find their own source of health insurance or apply for government programs, if they qualify. About 60 percent of Americans have health insurance through an employer-sponsored plan. In the past, many employees were covered by health insurance plans that covered 100 percent of all health care expenses. These plans are rare today. The vast majority of employer-provided health insurance policies require patients to share in the cost of their health care in the form of deductibles, coinsurance, and copays. These requirements can change each year when employers update their insurance offerings. In addition, when people change jobs, they also need to change their health insurance and, often, their providers. The result is a constantly evolving set of choices and requirements which can be confusing to many patients.

Despite the many options available for health insurance, it is estimated that 45 to 50 million Americans have no health insurance coverage. Often this is because individuals do not have or do not qualify for employer-based coverage, do not qualify for federal programs, and cannot afford individual policies. For these patients, many offices establish a **sliding fee scale** that charges fees based on a patient's financial ability to pay. Some cities also have free or low-cost clinics established and run by volunteers or not-for-profit agencies.

The Patient Protection and Affordable Care Act In 2010, Congress passed the **Patient Protection and Affordable Care Act** (**PPACA**), also referred to as the Affordable Care Act (**ACA**), and as Obamacare, because it was passed under the administration of President Barack Obama. PPACA represents the most significant reform of the health care system since Medicare and Medicaid were established. The goal of PPACA is to help decrease the number of uninsured Americans and reduce the overall costs of health care. It uses a number of approaches to increase the number of people covered by insurance, such as mandates, subsidies, and tax credits. Additional aspects of PPACA focus on improving health care outcomes and streamlining the delivery of health care. PPACA requires insurance companies to cover all applicants and offer the same premium rates regardless of pre-existing conditions or gender. It also prohibits insurance companies from setting a lifetime maximum amount for benefits that they pay for an individual.

PPACA established the **health insurance exchange** (**HIE**) to create a more organized and competitive market for buying health insurance. HIEs are organizations that offer a choice of health insurance plans, certify the plans that participate, and provide consumer information regarding options. They primarily serve individuals buying insurance on their own and small businesses with up to 100 employees. Each state may establish its own HIE, or opt out and allow the federal government to establish and operate it. Each state makes its information about HIEs available on the Internet.

As of 2014, PPACA requires most people to have health insurance and requires them to pay a tax penalty if they do not. This is commonly known as the **individual mandate**. Health insurance may be from employer-provided insurance, individual coverage, or Medicaid. Several groups are exempt from this requirement, due to income or employer status. Tax credits are available to U.S. citizens and legal immigrants who purchase coverage through HIEs. To be eligible for the tax credits, individuals must meet certain income requirements, not be eligible for government insurance, and not have access to health insurance through an employer.

PPACA also expanded the income criteria for who is eligible for Medicaid, the government program for low-income families. If all states implement the expansion, an additional 21.3 million individuals could gain Medicaid coverage by 2022, a 41 percent increase.

The Future of Health Insurance

With the cost of health care and health insurance coverage rising far beyond the rate of inflation in America, most experts agree that the U.S. health care system will change dramatically in the future. PPACA is expected to have a significant impact on health care delivery and health insurance in the years to come. It should decrease the number of uninsured people, improve health outcomes, and streamline health care delivery and increase overall expenditures on health care. However, the exact impact is unknown and will be experienced over the course of many years.

PPACA is expected to help two demographic groups that historically have been underserved: minorities and women.

Approximately one-third of residents of the country identify themselves as members of a specific racial or ethnic group. Minority and ethnic background is associated with poorer health status, health insurance coverage, health care access, and quality of care, which is of great concern. The federal government has made improving health care for minorities a priority, with a national goal of eliminating differences by 2020. Employers, insurers, providers, and policymakers agree with this goal, but they do not always agree on the most effective solutions.

Women are greatly impacted both by the high cost of medical care and the difficulty of obtaining health insurance. Women are major consumers of health care services, not only for themselves, especially during reproductive years, but also for their family members. One in five women (20 percent) is uninsured and often is also low-income. Women comprise the majority of beneficiaries in publicly funded programs such as Medicaid, Medicare, and welfare. For them, access to high quality, comprehensive care is even more difficult. Women are key stakeholders in public policy debates about the health care reform, but do not necessarily have the opportunity to provide adequate input.

Medical assistants play a vital role in helping patients understand their insurance benefits. By staying up to date on trends and legislation that affect health care and health insurance coverage, medical assistants become a valuable member of a patient's health care team.

Policy Provisions and Terminology

Just as medical assistants need to understand medical terminology to work in a medical office, a knowledge of insurance terminology is critical to helping patients use their health insurance policies. In many situations, multiple terms have essentially the same meaning. In other situations, terms that seem similar to the layperson have different and specific meanings in the world of health insurance. Patients are often unfamiliar with their insurance benefits and might not understand the terms they hear. Medical assistants who understand insurance terms can advocate for patients and communicate in ways that patients understand.

Members and Their Families

Health insurance, also called *medical insurance*, is a contract between an insurance carrier and the person who owns the insurance policy, known as the **member**, **subscriber**, **insured**, or **policyholder**. For those who receive insurance through their employers, the member is the employee. For those who buy individual policies, the member is the person who purchased the plan. For those covered by government policies, the term **beneficiary** is often used and refers to the individual who qualifies for the program. **Eligibility** is the process to determine if a patient is qualified to receive coverage/paid benefits according to the insurance policy guidelines.

Many commercial policies allow members to include family members on the plan. Family members are called **dependents** and may include a spouse, children, unmarried domestic partners, and stepchildren. Inclusion of family members is not automatic, and it is possible for some, but not all, family members to be covered. The member must obtain forms from the employer or the insurance company to specifically designate dependents' coverage. The medical assistant needs to ask the patient, and possibly call the insurance company, to determine who is eligible for benefits. It is also important to know exactly how each dependent is legally related to the member. Members have an opportunity to update dependent coverage each year when the policy renews and under circumstances can make changes during the year. Therefore, it is important to verify eligibility at each visit.

Premiums

In order to obtain a commercial health insurance policy, the policyholder pays a **premium** to the insurance carrier. The premium is usually paid in monthly installments for the next month's coverage. In group coverage, the employer often pays the majority of the premium and employees authorize the remainder to be deducted from paychecks. If dependent coverage is selected, the premium is higher. Some government plans require a premium as well.

Fee Schedules and Approved Amounts

Providers establish a **fee schedule** which lists their charge for each service they provide. A fee schedule is normally organized by type of service and CPT code (**Figure 17-1** ■). Providers may set their charges in any manner they desire; however, in most states they are required to charge the same fee to every patient and every insurance company. They cannot discuss their fees with other providers and use that information to set prices, a practice known as price fixing. The charge on the fee schedule is known as the provider's usual charge.

Insurance companies are not required to pay providers' usual charges. Insurers can use any method they desire to establish a payment level. Often they calculate what they determine to be an average or customary price among providers of the same specialty and in the same geographic area. This is the approved or **allowed amount**. When a provider's

New Patient Examinations		
Office Visit, Level 1	99201	$55.00
Office Visit, Level 2	99202	$110.00
Office Visit, Level 3	99203	$154.00
Office Visit, Level 4	99204	$226.00
Office Visit, Level 5	99205	$299.00
Established Patient Examinations		
Office Visit, Level 1	99211	$45.00
Office Visit, Level 2	99212	$60.00
Office Visit, Level 3	99213	$80.00
Office Visit, Level 4	99214	$123.00
Office Visit, Level 5	99215	$199.00

Figure 17-1 ■ Sample fee schedule.

actual charge is less than the allowed amount, the insurer bases payment calculations on the actual charge. Providers cannot increase their charge for a given service to selected insurance companies in order to receive higher payment. When providers' charges are more than the insurance allowable, the insurance bases payment calculations on the allowed amount. This method of determining insurance payments is **usual, customary and reasonable** (**UCR**). When calculating benefits and amounts owed, the first step is to identify the allowed charge.

Out-of-Pocket Expenses

Few health insurance plans cover 100 percent of the care patients receive, so patients experience several different kinds of out-of-pocket expenses. These are medical expenses that patients are personally responsible for paying.

Deductibles Before the insurance plan pays any benefits, patients often have a **deductible** to meet. The deductible is a monetary amount patients must pay to the provider for health care services before health insurance benefits begin to pay. Deductible amounts can be nearly any amount. For example, one patient's deductible may be as low as $100, whereas another patient's deductible could be $10,000 or more. Plans with low deductibles tend to have higher premiums than plans with high deductibles. Some government plans also have deductibles. When calculating benefits and amounts owed, the second step is to subtract the deductible from the allowed charge (**Figure 17-2** ■).

In some policies, the deductible is not be required for all services. A sick visit usually requires a deductible, but a preventive care visit usually does not. PPACA prohibits most

Scenario 1: Martina Kahlo has health insurance through her employer's plan. She has a $100 yearly deductible, and then she is covered at 100 percent. Martina sees Dr. Jacobson for an office call that includes lab work. The allowed amount for the office call is $128. How much does Martina owe for her visit?

$128 allowed for medical services

$100 for Martina's annual deductible

Martina must pay her $100 deductible. The insurance company will pay the $28 balance.

Scenario 2: Jorge Garcia has an individual health insurance plan. He has a $1,000 yearly deductible, and then he is covered at 80 percent. Jorge sees Dr. Jacobson for an office call that includes lab work and two X-rays. The allowed amount for the office call is $217. How much does Jorge owe for his visit?

$217 allowed for medical services

$1,000 for Jorge's annual deductible

Insurance company will pay $0 because Jorge has not met his $1,000 annual deductible. Jorge must pay the $217 charge.

Figure 17-2 ■ Sample scenarios: Calculating a patient's insurance deductible.

health insurance plans from charging deductibles and copayments for preventive care services. This is to encourage patients to seek preventive care. When patients include family members on the policy, there is usually an individual deductible and a family deductible. The individual deductible is the maximum deductible that any given family member must pay. The family deductible is the maximum deductible for all family members combined.

Example: Deductibles

John Jacobs is the policyholder and carries his wife, Jeanne, and his two children, Jana and James, on the policy. The individual deductible is $100 and the family deductible is $300.

- Jeanne receives medical care for which the insurance allowable is $150. She pays her deductible of $100 and insurance benefits will apply to the remaining $50.
- A short time later, Jana becomes ill and sees the doctor for an allowed charge of $50. The entire $50 is applied to her deductible and must be paid out-of-pocket. Now the family has accumulated $150 toward the family deductible.
- Next, John receives care that has an insurance allowable of $200. He has not met his individual deductible and the family deductible has not been met yet. He pays

$100 out-of-pocket for his individual deductible. Insurance benefits will apply to the remaining $100 of his bill. $250 of the family deductible has now been met.

- James becomes ill and sees the doctor for a $100 (allowable) visit. Even though he has not met his individual deductible, only $50 is owed on the family deductible, so $50 is paid out-of-pocket for James. Insurance benefits apply to the remaining $50.
- Now that the $300 family deductible has been met, no family member will be required to pay a deductible for the remainder of the year, even if the individual deductible for that dependent has not been met.
- The family deductible presents a savings for families of more than three members.

Copayments and Coinsurance After the deductible is met, most patients still have out-of-pocket expenses they are responsible for. **Copayments** are fixed dollar amounts that patients pay at the time of service, such as $5 or $10 per visit. **Coinsurance** is a fixed percentage of charges that patients pay. An 80/20 coinsurance plan means that the insurance company pays 80 percent of approved charges and the patient pays 20 percent. A 70/30 plan means that the insurance company pays 70 percent of approved charges and the patient pays 30 percent. Different types of visits or different types of providers may have different copayment or coinsurance amounts. For example, preventive care may have no copayment or coinsurance, while sick care does. A specialist visit may require a higher copayment or coinsurance than a primary care visit. The specific rules are set by the insurance company and clearly spelled out in the patient's policy. Most government programs require a copayment or coinsurance.

When calculating benefits and amounts owed, first subtract any deductible owed from the allowed amount. Then, calculate the coinsurance amount by multiplying the remaining balance times the coinsurance percentage. Finally, subtract the copayment or coinsurance amount from the remaining balance. **Figure 17-3** ■ shows how copayments and coinsurance amounts are calculated.

Generally, when medical offices bill patients' insurance, patients sign an **assignment of benefits**, which authorizes the insurance company to pay benefits directly to the provider. This helps ensure that the provider is paid in a timely manner and simplifies the billing process. If a patient refuses to sign the assignment of benefits, the insurance company should send payment to the patient and the patient pays the provider's bill. In this case, the medical office should consider requiring the patient to pay in full at the time of service or establish a regular payment plan. The concern is that the patient may forget about the provider's bill and spend the insurance payment on other expenses rather than paying the provider. In managed care plans and government programs, assignment of benefits is usually part of the provider's contract and, as a result, is automatic.

Scenario 1: Dr. Jones charges $75 for an office call. Mary Smith is insured with Premera Blue Cross Insurance and has a 20 percent coinsurance obligation. Dr. Jones is a preferred provider with Premera Blue Cross and has agreed to accept $64.25 as payment in full for his office call. Mary owes 20 percent of the $64.25 fee ($12.85).

Scenario 2: Dr. Barro charges $70 for an office call. Molly Manchero is insured with Regence Blue Shield Insurance and has a $10 copayment obligation. Dr. Barro is a preferred provider with Regence Blue Shield and has agreed to accept $62.50 as payment in full for his office call. Molly owes $10 of the $62.50 fee.

Figure 17-3 ■ Calculating copayments and coinsurance.

Balance billing is the practice of billing patients for the difference between the physician's actual charge and the amount allowed by insurance. When providers have a participating or preferred provider contract with the insurance company, they agree to accept the insurance allowed amount as payment in full and cannot balance bill patients. The insurance company calculates deductibles, coinsurance, and copayments based on the allowed amounts, which may be less than the provider's actual charge. However, when the provider is not participating or contracted with a private insurance company, the patient is responsible for the entire balance not covered by insurance and may be balance billed. Medicare patients may be billed no more than the limiting charge, an amount established by Medicare that is the maximum a nonparticipating provider can charge a patient.

Stop Loss and Lifetime Maximum

Many insurance policies have **stop loss** clauses. A stop loss is the maximum amount the patient must pay out-of-pocket for the deductible, copayments, and coinsurance. After this amount is reached in a year, the insurance pays 100 percent of the remaining expenses. The stop loss amount starts over the next year. This is helpful for patients who incur a large amount of medical expenses in a given year.

Prior to 2014, many insurance policies had **lifetime maximum benefits**. This limited the total amount the insurance company would pay for individual members over the course of the patient's life. A common lifetime maximum benefit was $1 million, but it could be as low as $100,000 in a very inexpensive policy. Sometimes patients would select a low cost policy and not be aware of provisions such as the lifetime maximum. While $1 million or even $100,000 may sound like a lot of money, medical expenses can accumulate very quickly with a serious illness such as cancer or an organ

transplant. As a result of PPACA, beginning in 2014, insurance companies can no longer have a lifetime maximum clause.

Pre-Existing Conditions

Historically, health insurance plans had **exclusions**, rules that limited when and how much the insurance plan is required to pay in benefits. Many of these restrictions have been eliminated as a result of PPACA. Starting in 2014, all health insurance companies are required to sell coverage to everyone who applies, regardless of pre-existing conditions. A **pre-existing condition** is any condition a patient was diagnosed with or treated for, including receiving prescription medications, before beginning coverage with a new insurance plan. Health insurance companies are not allowed to charge more to individuals with pre-existing conditions and they also cannot exclude coverage of the condition from the insurance policy.

HIPAA Compliance Under **HIPAA**, a pre-existing condition is covered without a **waiting period** when the patient has been continuously insured for the 24 months before joining the new plan. This allows patients to change jobs and retain pre-existing condition coverage without added waiting periods, even when they have chronic illnesses. Patients should save the HIPAA **certificate of coverage** that the previous insurance plan mails out after coverage has terminated. This letter documents the nature and length of coverage with the plan. Patients submit it to the new plan to establish proof of continuous coverage. If patients have had more than one insurance plan during the previous 24 months, they should submit certificates of coverage from each plan. Even when patients have not been insured the 24 months before joining new insurance plans, HIPAA legislation restricts insurance companies from requiring patients to wait any longer than 12 months from the dates their new insurance coverage began.

Medical Necessity

The fact that a physician determines that a patient needs a particular service or supply item does not mean that the insurance company or payer will agree. **Medical necessity** is the process of establishing the medical need for services. It is one of several criteria payers use to determine if and how much they will pay for a particular service. One of the reasons that payers establish medical necessity rules is to avoid paying unscrupulous providers who might provide a service just so they can receive payments, not because the patient actually needs the service or would benefit from it. It also helps prevent patients from demanding services they do not need, such as expensive tests or cosmetic surgery.

Each payer establishes its own definition of medical necessity and writes it into each insurance policy. Table 17-1 lists common criteria for medical necessity and examples of

PROCEDURE 17-1 Calculate Deductible, Coinsurance, and Allowable Amounts

Theory and Rationale

The medical assistant frequently explains to patients how their deductible, coinsurance, and allowable amounts are calculated. Attention to detail is very important as misquoted figures can be cause for patients to become dissatisfied with the medical staff.

Materials

- Pen
- Paper
- Insurance verification-of-benefits form
- Patient's insurance identification card
- Explanation of Benefits form
- Calculator

Competency

1. After the patient's insurance coverage has been verified, locate the information on the verification form regarding any deductible and coinsurance amount.

    Example: The patient has a $100 yearly deductible and a 20 percent coinsurance. The patient has had an examination with a charge of $95.00, an X-ray with a charge of $75.00, and laboratory work with a charge of $102.00.

2. Inform the patient of the deductible amount that needs to be paid after the beginning of the calendar or fiscal year, before insurance payments become effective.

3. Explain to the patient that the amount charged for any particular procedure in the medical office will likely be reduced to a lower amount (called the allowed amount) when processed by the insurance carrier.

4. After the insurance payment is received, use the Explanation of Benefits (**EOB**) form to identify the amount the insurance carrier allowed on the claim.

    Example: The insurance carrier allowed $72.00 for the examination, $51.00 for the X-ray, and $80.00 for the laboratory work.

5. Calculate the total allowed charges by adding together the allowed amount for each service.

    Example: $72.00 + $51.00 + $80.00 = $203.00

6. Subtract the deductible from the total of the allowed charges.

    Example: $203.00 − $100.00 = $103.00.

7. Multiply the remaining allowed amount by the coinsurance percentage to determine the patient's coinsurance amount.

    Example: $103.00 × 20% = $20.60.

8. Add the deductible to the coinsurance amount to determine the amount the patient needs to pay out-of-pocket for the visit.

    Example: $100 + $20.60 = $120.60

9. Explain the figures to the patient and collect the fees.

TABLE 17-1 Examples of Medical Necessity Criteria		
Criterion	**Appropriate Example**	**Inappropriate Example**
Improve a patient's condition	Physical therapy to treat an acute back injury	Ongoing physical therapy to maintain general back comfort
Evidence-based practice	Medications proven to benefit patients based on scientific studies	Experimental drugs or treatments
Rendered by appropriate provider	Patient going to internal medicine or family practice physician to diagnose an initial symptom stomach pain	Patient going directly to gastroenterologist and having many expensive tests performed to diagnose an initial symptom of stomach pain
Least restrictive setting	Suture removal in physician office; outpatient cataract surgery	Suture removal in the emergency department; inpatient cataract surgery without a medical reason
Not for patient or physician convenience	Liposuction for medical reasons	Liposuction for cosmetic reasons

each. By law, Medicare can pay only for services that are medically necessary, which is defined as services and supplies that:

- Are needed to diagnose or treat a medical condition or improve the functioning of a malformed body member
- Meet the standards of good medical practice in the local area
- Are not mainly for the convenience of the patient or physician

In addition to a general definition of medical necessity, payers may also establish criteria for specific conditions, such as limiting the number of physical therapy visits for back pain; requiring an X-ray before ordering a more expensive MRI; or restricting the age and frequency of preventive screening, such as a screening mammogram every 2 years for women over age 50. When providers recommend a treatment that varies from the insurance company's standard list, they may need to obtain preauthorization and provide special reports to justify the service. For some conditions, specific medical necessity criteria are not public information and patients only learn of them only after a claim is **denied** (i.e., the claim was processed and found to be ineligible for payment).

Insurance plans may limit coverage or require preapproval for **elective procedures**, those that are nonemergent, but may benefit the patient. Emergency procedures are those that must be performed immediately in order to save the patient's life, limb, or vision. Elective procedures can be scheduled at a later time and include a broad range of procedures such as back surgery, joint replacement surgery, lesion removal, vision-correction, gastric-reduction procedures, and even cosmetic surgery. Some elective procedures are considered medically necessary, based on the patient's health condition, and others might not.

Medical assistants should not manipulate codes in a way that distorts or alters the diagnoses and procedures as documented in the medical record. This is unethical and fraudulent. They need to be certain they are accurately describing everything that was done for the patient and the reasons for which the services were provided.

Types of Insurance Plans

Health insurance plans are classified either as indemnity plans or managed care plans. Indemnity plans impose few restrictions on patients while managed care plans seek to control costs by limiting patients' choices.

Indemnity Plans

Prior to the 1980s, indemnity plans were the norm. *Indemnity* means to pay for the loss experienced by another person. In health insurance, indemnity plans cover a patient's health care expenses with few restrictions. Also called **fee-for-service plans** (FFS), they allowed patients to seek care with any covered health care providers, for any covered services. Neither the list of physicians that patients may see, nor the fee schedules, were prearranged. Insurance companies reimbursed health care providers the actual fee charged for each service. This practice is believed to have contributed to the rapid rise of health care costs. Indemnity plans are rare today and, if available, are among the most expensive because they do not contain managed care or cost-control measures.

Managed Care Plans

Managed care plans, also called **managed care organizations** (**MCOs**), are companies that attempt to control the cost of health care while providing better outcomes. Managed care plans contract with physicians, hospitals, and other providers to offer services for a lower fee. Then they contract with government programs, private health insurance companies, and self-insured plans to promote an exclusive network of **participating providers**, or preferred providers. When patients use participating providers, they are responsible for lower out-of-pocket costs for deductibles, coinsurance, and copayments than if they select a nonparticipating provider, one not on the preferred list.

Medical assistants should inform patients whether providers participate with the patients' health plans. A provider may be participating with some patients' MCOs and nonparticipating with others. Most offices ask about health insurance coverage the first time patients call. When in doubt, assistants should ask patients for their insurance information and then call or research the insurance companies online.

Managed care plans are not a separate type of insurance, but rather a way of offering services to patients who are enrolled in a group health plan, self-funded plan, or individual health plan. Managed care plans also offer services to Medicare Advantage programs, Medicaid, and Workers' Compensation. Managed care companies are regulated primarily by federal laws. Well-known managed care plans include Kaiser Permanente, Group Health of Seattle, WellPoint, and Humana.

The most common types of managed care plans are health maintenance organizations (**HMOs**), preferred provider organizations (**PPOs**), and point of service (**POS**) plans.

⌐● In Practice

Georgia Collins calls the medical office to schedule an appointment as a new patient. When the medical assistant asks her about her insurance coverage, she says she is unsure of her insurance company's name and cannot locate her insurance card. How should the medical assistant respond? Is insurance information needed before patients seek care? Why or why not? If Georgia becomes angry, how should the medical assistant respond?

Health Maintenance Organizations Health maintenance organizations (HMOs) are managed care plans that cover members only when those members seek care from a list of health care providers and suppliers who have contracted

TABLE 17-2 Types of Health Maintenance Organizations

Type of HMO	Description
Exclusive provider organization (EPO)	A managed care contract with a smaller network of providers under which the employer agrees to not use any other networks in return for favorable pricing
Group model HMO	HMO in which the managed care company contracts with multi-specialty groups
Independent practice association (IPA)	An association formed by physicians with separately owned practices that contracts with managed care plans
Network model HMO	HMO that contracts with two or more group practices, or a group practice plus a combination of staff physicians and independent physicians
Staff model HMO	HMO in which the managed care company hires the physicians and owns the clinic sites and possibly the hospital

with the HMO (Table 17-2). The list of approved providers is usually somewhat limited and may be restricted to a specific clinic. An **open-panel** HMO is one in which providers treat both HMO patients and non-HMO patients. A **closed-panel** HMO is one in which physicians see only the patients of a specific HMO. Most HMOs require each patient to choose a **primary care provider** (PCP) who belongs to the network of covered providers. The primary care provider is the caretaker or gatekeeper and arranges any specialist services or hospitalizations. The specific payment rules vary among plans, but usually, copayments and coinsurance amounts are very low, often with no deductible. When members seek care from providers not on the list, they must pay for the costs out-of-pocket.

To help make health care more cost-efficient, HMOs encourage patients to take advantage of preventive health care services such as annual physicals, prostate cancer testing, and mammography. Preventive services often have no cost-sharing requirements.

HMOs are the most restrictive type of health plan because of the limited number of approved providers. However, they typically provide members with a greater range of health benefits for the lowest out-of-pocket expenses.

Preferred Provider Organizations The **preferred provider organization** (PPO) contracts with physicians and facilities to perform services for PPO members at a lower rate than for nonmembers. The PPO gives subscribers a list of network providers whom they may see for a lower cost. They usually do

not have to obtain a referral or preauthorization in order to see a specialist within the network. However, major medical procedures usually do require preauthorization. If a patient chooses to receive treatment from an out-of-network or non-preferred provider, she is responsible for higher out-of-pocket expenses and, often, higher deductibles.

Physicians may belong to several PPOs. It is also possible that not all of the physicians in a medical practice belong to the same PPOs. When this occurs, medical assistants should assist patients by scheduling them with physicians who are part of their approved network.

Point of Service Plans A **point of service (POS)** plan offers a primary HMO provider network and a secondary PPO provider network, allowing patients to choose which plan to use at the time they seek care. Out-of-pocket expenses are lowest when using HMO providers, somewhat higher when using preferred providers in the PPO, and most costly when using out-of-network providers. A POS plans provides patients with the maximum flexibility and choice when seeking services and also provides cost-effective options for those willing to use the HMO network for their care.

Critical Thinking Question 17-1

Refer back to the case study at the beginning of the chapter. What reasons can you think of as to why the insurance did not pay anything for this encounter?

Types of Service Coverage

Type of coverage refers to the specific services covered under the plan. Each insurance policy is tailored to include the benefits most desired and most affordable for each group or individual. Understanding some of the most common alternatives for coverage types enables medical assistants to clarify for patients what can be expected from their policies (Table 17-3). In addition to determining the source of patients' insurance, medical assistants need to determine what type of coverage they have.

With each type of coverage, medical assistants need to identify how patients' insurance relates to the specific services being provided in a specific situation. Research, attention to detail, careful communication, and patient advocacy are skills that successful medical assistants use in the insurance arena.

Many patients have prescription drug coverage that helps pay for the cost of prescription drugs. Plans typically have a formulary—a list of drugs they will cover. Usually the formulary is subdivided into two or more tiers with each tier having a different level of coverage (**Figure 17-4** ■). For example, tier 1 may include most generic drugs and perhaps a few brand name drugs that have no generic equivalent. Patients might have a small copayment, perhaps only a few dollars, for

TABLE 17-3 Types of Health Insurance Service Coverage

Coverage	Description
Hospital services	Inpatient hospital care such as room and board, and facility fees for special services including operating room, radiology, and laboratory
Physician services	Physicians' fees for hospital visits, office visits, and nonsurgical procedures
Surgical services	Surgeon and anesthesiologist fees for surgery performed in a hospital, in a doctor's office, or outpatient surgical center, surgical service as well as anesthesia service.
Preventive care	Annual preventive care examinations, immunizations, and screening tests
Ancillary services	Supplemental riders for prescription drugs, vision, dental, and alternative care
Disease-specific	Supplemental insurance for specific chronic or terminal illnesses, such as cancer, heart disease, stroke, Alzheimer's, Parkinson's, multiple sclerosis, kidney failure
Catastrophic care	Emergency safety net to protect against unexpected, high-cost medical services only. All routine and sick care is paid out-of-pocket.

tier 1 drugs. Tier 2 may include preferred brand name drugs, ones for which there is no generic equivalent. Patients have a slightly higher copayment for these drugs. Tier 3 may include brand name drugs that have generic equivalents or similar brand name drugs at a lower cost. Patients have the highest

Tier 1

Penicillin G Sodium

Penicillin V Potassium

Trimox

Tier 2

Avelox (Tablet)

Timentin

Tier 3

Avelox (Solution)

Penicillin G Procaine

Piperacillin Sodium

Zosyn

Figure 17-4 ■ Sample tiered drug formulary for antibiotics.

out-of-pocket expense for these drugs, perhaps as high as 50 percent coinsurance. There may be some drugs that are not on the formulary at all. Patients need to present evidence of medical necessity in order to receive coverage for non-formulary drugs. Medical assistants can advocate for patients if their plan does not cover a specific drug the provider prescribed. They can help identify potentially similar medications from the formulary or from a lower tier of the formulary that the provider could evaluate and consider prescribing for the patient. This could create financial savings for the patient while maintaining safe and high quality care.

Some plans require a referral or authorization from the PCP in order for a patient to receive benefits for alternative care services. Medical assistants often need to facilitate such requests for referrals. Other plans allow the patient to self-refer, meaning the patient receives these services without a referral or authorization. Typically, chiropractic, massage therapy, and acupuncture visits are limited in terms of how often the patient may receive them and the number of visits in a year. Anything above this cap might need a PCP referral or might not be covered at all. It is important for medical assistants to help patients understand how their policies are structured in this area.

▸▸▸ Pulse Points

Providing Coverage Information to Patients

Most patients are only vaguely aware of their insurance plan coverage. Therefore, be sure to check with patients' insurance companies before providing patients expensive treatment and to relay coverage information to patients. Remember that insurance companies only give information regarding patients' benefits. They do not guarantee what services will be covered or paid when claims are received. Make sure patients understand that you are only relaying information from their insurance carriers. Direct any questions the patient may have about coverage to those carriers.

Health Insurance Payers

In addition to the type of managed care and the type of service coverage, a patient's insurance benefits are also determined by the type of payer. **Third-party payers** are organizations that pay for health care services on behalf of the patient. In legal terms, the physician is the first party, the patient is the second party, and the payer is the third party. Third-party payers reimburse physicians and hospitals for 86 percent of all health care services in the United States. Patients pay the remaining

All data regarding national health expenditures in this chapter are from the Centers for Medicare and Medicaid Services, Office of the Actuary, National Health Statistics Group, National Health Expenditures Levels, 2009.

14 percent of services directly. Third-party payers include several government programs, over 1,300 private insurance companies, workers' compensation, and automobile "med pay" insurance. Medical assistants need to understand the various types of third-party payers because each has separate, and sometimes conflicting, rules about coding and billing.

Some employers are **self-funded**, paying directly for employees' medical bills. Individuals who do not have employer-sponsored health insurance may purchase an **individual health insurance** policy either directly from an insurance company or through a health insurance exchange (HIE). **Property and casualty insurance**, also called **liability insurance**, such as automobile and homeowner insurance, provides for medical expenses related to certain accidents.

All health care payments to hospitals, physicians, and other providers are based on coding. Procedure codes describe what services were provided to patients. Physicians and hospitals assign money charges to each procedure code. Diagnosis codes justify why the services were needed. When the diagnosis code(s) does not adequately explain why the services were provided, payment may be denied or delayed.

Private Health Insurance

Private health insurance, also called *commercial health insurance*, is coverage for health care services offered by private corporations such as Aetna, Cigna, or United Health Care, and not-for-profit organizations, such as Blue Cross and Blue Shield. Private health insurance pays for 39 percent of national health care expenses. The three major sources of private health insurance are group health plans, self-insured plans, and individual insurance. Each insurance company and each plan offered by a company can have different requirements for coding and billing. Typically, the provider's coding and billing departments maintain files on the requirements of each plan. Most laws regarding private health insurance companies are determined by each state's legislature and implemented by the state's department of insurance. Coverage amounts and premiums vary according to policy type.

Group Insurance

Group health insurance (GHI) is a policy offered to groups of people for which the risk or cost of insurance is spread across everyone equally. Approximately 60 percent of Americans are covered by a group health plan offered through their employer or union. The employer or union contracts with a private insurance company to provide a specific list of benefits to its employees. Group insurance is usually the least expensive type of insurance because statistics show that a few people in a group use a large amount of services, but many people in the group use few if any services. Everyone pays the same rate for protection, so the high costs of a few members are shared equally by everyone in the group. The most common group is the employees of a company. However, various professional organizations also offer group coverage.

Two patients, Sara and George, present Premera Blue Cross insurance identification cards. ABC Marketing, a large employer that provides its employees an extensive insurance plan, employs Sara. Lone Star Plumbing, a small employer that has purchased a plan with minimal employee coverage, employs George. Although they present similar insurance cards, Sara and George have vastly different coverage.

Figure 17-5 ■ Patient scenario: Same insurance company, different benefits.

Employers initiate negotiations with an insurance company to cover their employees. Employers determine how large their financial budget is for employee health insurance premiums and how much they want employees to contribute towards the premium. The insurance company then presents a list of benefits available for that price. The more that can be paid in premiums, the more benefits will be available. Employers select the insurance company and the benefit package that best meets the budget and the employees' anticipated needs.

It is common for an employer to allow employees to select among a variety of benefit packages from the chosen insurance company. The employer designates the amount the company will pay per month towards the premium, which is usually constant among all packages. Employees are able to select the package that best meets their needs for medical care and premium cost. Packages with high deductibles and copayments or coinsurance cost less than packages with low deductibles and out-of-pocket expenses. Employees may have the option to add dependents for an additional premium. Some employers pay part of the dependents' premiums and others require the employee to pay the full amount. Because most companies offer a variety of health insurance options for employees, two patients with the same employer and the same insurance company may have different benefits. **Figure 17-5** ■ gives such a sample scenario. To avoid giving out incorrect information, it is important for medical assistants to determine the specific benefits available to each patient. Often this information is available online through the insurer's secured Web site or by calling the insurance company.

Critical Thinking Question 17-2

Refer back to the case study at the beginning of the chapter. Assume that Martin has 100 percent coverage for preventive care, an annual deductible of $200, and coinsurance of 10 percent. How much should the insurance company pay? How should the medical assistant explain this to Martin?

Employer-based coverage typically begins with the next calendar month following 30 days of employment, but this timeframe can vary. It is important to determine when coverage begins for a patient who has recently changed jobs. It is also important to determine when coverage ends for a patient leaving a job. Coverage may end the last day of employment, the end of the month, or the end of the following month.

Blue Cross/Blue Shield Plans

Patients may have Blue Cross (**BC**) and Blue Shield (**BS**) plans through group health coverage or individual insurance. Historically BC plans provided hospital service benefits and BS plans provided physician service benefits. Each BC and BS plan was an independent not-for-profit health plan, with one or more plans in most states across the country. The national associations merged in 1977 to form the Blue Cross Blue Shield Association (**BCBSA**), with 450 member plans. Today the national association is for-profit and many of the local plans have either gone for-profit or have been purchased by for-profit insurance companies.

Patients may have a BC plan, a BS plan, or a combination BCBS plan depending on their geographic area. It is important to remember that each BCBS plan is separate and unique in terms of benefits, cost-sharing, and other requirements, just as private commercial insurance companies are unique from each other.

BCBS coverage includes fee-for-service (FFS) traditional coverage, managed care plans, a federal employee program (FEP), Medicare supplemental plans, and health care anywhere plans. The type of coverage is indicated on the member ID card. Most BCBS member ID numbers begin with three letters that are a code indicating the member's home plan. It is essential to include these letters when reporting the member ID number on a claim. Because there are many types of BCBS plans, there are many types of insurance cards. Each BCBS processes its own claims, so medical assistants need to verify the correct filing address. In the past, most local BCBS plans would forward claims to the correct home plan, but that practice has become less common in recent years as many plans have joined commercial for-profit companies.

Self-Funded Plan

Self-funded health plans, also called *self-insured*, are offered by large employers or unions who, rather than purchasing group health insurance, set aside money in a reserve fund and pay for employees' medical expenses from the fund. States regulate how much money employers must set aside in order to ensure that they will have enough money to pay catastrophic (high cost) medical expenses. For patients, health insurance through a self-insured plan is very similar to group insurance. In fact, employees often do not even recognize the difference. An employer or labor union that self-insures does not purchase a policy through a commercial insurance company. Instead, they set aside a large pool of money, or reserve, and use that fund to reimburse employees for their health care expenses. Sometimes they contract with a **third-party administrator** (**TPA**), an outside company that processes the paperwork for claims, but any payments come from the employer's or labor union's funds, not an insurance company.

Critical Thinking Question 17-3

Refer to the case study at the beginning of the chapter. Assume that upon reviewing the EOB, the medical assistant reads the explanation "Coverage terminated." In talking with Martin, the medical assistant learns that he started a new job last month. How will this affect his insurance coverage? What oversight did the medical office make when Martin came in for his most recent visit? What steps should the medical assistant take?

Other Sources of Coverage

Although employers are the primary source of private insurance coverage, patients have other options for obtaining health insurance. A patient who leaves a job with group coverage may continue the insurance under COBRA. Unemployed or self-employed individuals may also purchase individual coverage on their own or through a Health Insurance Exchange.

COBRA Coverage When employees have been covered under group insurance and leave employment, they frequently have the opportunity to continue the group coverage at their own expense. The premium is the same as that for the group, but because often the employer has been paying a large portion of the employees' premium, patients can be surprised at the cost of the premium. Nonetheless, the premium is usually less, and the benefits better, than an individual policy. This option allows employees to keep insurance in force until they obtain new insurance coverage. The federal Consolidated Omnibus Reconciliation Act (COBRA) requires employers to extend health insurance coverage at group rates, usually for up to 18 months, to any employee who is laid off, quits, or is fired, except under certain circumstances. COBRA coverage is available to employees who work for employers with 20 or more employees.

▸▸▸ Pulse Points

COBRA Overview

Congress passed COBRA health benefit provisions in 1986 to provide certain former employees, retirees, spouses, former spouses, and dependent children the right to temporarily continue health coverage at group rates. To be eligible for COBRA coverage, employees must have been enrolled in their employers' health plans when they worked and those health plans must continue to be in effect for active employees.

Individual Health Insurance Policies Another type of insurance plan is the individual plan or policy, which individuals buy directly through insurance carriers. These plans are often the most expensive, because group rates are unavailable.

The benefits are often not as good as group policies, resulting in higher deductibles and other out-of-pocket expenses. The minimum level of benefit package for individual insurance policies is regulated by each state, and in some states, only a few companies offer individual policies due to restrictive requirements. Employees who have been on a COBRA plan may be able to convert to an individual policy with the same insurance company when the COBRA benefits expire, but the group rates and benefits will no longer apply.

Health Insurance Exchanges Beginning in 2014, private health insurance may be purchased through a Health Insurance Exchange (HIE). The purpose of HIEs is to create an organized and competitive market for buying health insurance. They are aimed primarily at consumers purchasing insurance on their own and small businesses of up to 100 employees. HIEs offer consumers a choice of health insurance plans and certifies the plans that participate. They also provide information to help consumers better understand their options. States may establish their own HIEs or allow the federal government to do it. The federal government also offers technical assistance to help states with their own exchanges.

The Office of the Insurance Commissioner

Each state has an Office of the Insurance Commissioner, which is a valuable resource for both the medical office and the patient. When medical assistants or patients believe claims were incorrectly processed and appeal attempts have been fruitless, assistants may file formal written complaints with the state's insurance commissioner. It is important to involve patients in this process because they are the consumers the insurance commissioner is charged with protecting. Patients may be reluctant to appeal to the commissioner on their own initiative because they are unfamiliar with the process. One good approach is for medical assistants to write a letter on behalf of the patient and ask the patient to sign it. Sometimes, informing the insurance company that the patient intends to file a complaint with the insurance commissioner can inspire insurance carriers to review previously denied claims.

Government Insurance

The federal and state governments provide health insurance for designated groups of people such as the elderly, disabled, military personnel and retirees, and injured workers. Each of these programs has its own eligibility requirements and benefit structure. Health benefit plans funded by federal or state governments pay for 47 percent of health care services. These are *entitlement* programs for which beneficiaries (recipients of services) qualify based on specific criteria. An overview of these programs follows.

Many Americans who do not have private insurance receive health insurance benefits from the state or federal government. Government programs include **Medicare**, a federal program for persons over age 65, the disabled, and end-stage renal disease (ESRD) patients; **Medicaid**, a federal/state program primarily for low income people; **TRICARE**, for active duty and retired service personnel and their families; and **CHAMPVA** for veterans with service-related disabilities. Third-party liability plans provide coverage for injuries. These include **workers' compensation** which provides coverage for employees for job-related injuries or illnesses, and automobile **personal injury protection (PIP)** that pays for injuries sustained due to an automobile accident.

Medicare

Medicare (**MCR**), established in 1965, is a federal program that provides health insurance for approximately 43 million Americans, including people aged 65 and older, patients who have been disabled for more than 24 months, and patients with end-stage renal disease (ERSD). Medicare is the single largest payer of health care services in the United States, accounting for 24 percent of health care payments.

The program is administered by the Centers for Medicare and Medicaid Services (**CMS**) formerly known as the Health Care Financing Administration (HCFA). CMS contracts with private companies called Medicare Administrative Contractors (**MACs**) to educate and work with providers, process claims, and other functions. (Prior to 2008, the administrators for Part A were called *fiscal intermediaries* and the administrators for Part B were called *carriers*.)

Because it is so large, Medicare has a tremendous impact on health care policy and payment trends and, by extension, on coding. Other government programs and private health insurance are not required to follow Medicare rules, but it is not unusual for them to follow Medicare's lead to a considerable extent.

One of CMS's obligations is to keep providers informed about proper Medicare billing. To this end, there is vast array of information available to providers free of charge on the CMS Web site, www.cms.gov. A section called MedLearn provides free online training on many Medicare topics, free newsletters, articles, and other informative products.

The MACs also disseminate free billing information relevant to that particular region. Providers can sign up for e-mail alerts and announcements from the MAC to be sure they remain up to date. The MACs for each region are listed on the CMS Web site. Medical assistants involved in Medicare billing should learn how to access and use this vital information. Just as in many other areas of law, ignorance of Medicare rules is not an acceptable response.

All members receive Medicare identification cards that list their names, identification numbers, plans (Part A, Part B, or both), and effective dates (**Figure 17-6 ■**).

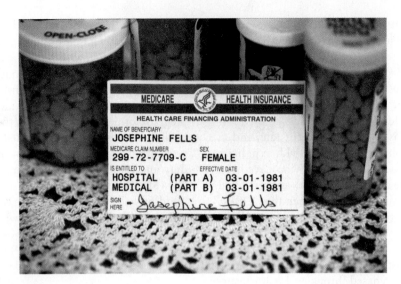

Figure 17-6 ■ A Medicare ID card.

Medicare claims should be submitted within 365 days of date of service. Those submitted later than this are not accepted, unless the provider can prove that late submission was due to factors beyond their control, such as difficulty in obtaining information from the MAC.

The Medicare program has major component parts called Part A (hospital insurance), Part B (provider coverage), Part C (Medicare Advantage), and Part D (prescription drug).

Participating Providers Medicare must accredit any health care providers who wish to participate in its program in a process very similar to the application process of any managed care plan. Because most health insurance plans follow Medicare's lead when it comes to accreditation and fee schedules, it is crucial for medical assistants or office managers to stay up-to-date by consulting Medicare's published guidelines or Web site.

As of July 2005, Medicare requires medical offices to file medical claims electronically. Some clinics may be allowed to continue to bill claims on paper. Those clinics must have no more than 10 full-time employees, or the equivalent of 10 full-time employees, such as 20 part-time employees whose combined working hours total that of 10 full-time employees.

Medicare prefers to use electronic funds transfer for payment to physicians and medical facilities. This is set up by filling out an Authorization Agreement for Electronic Funds Transfer form. This form is returned to Medicare along with a copy of a voided check or deposit ticket. After receipt of this information, Medicare begins directly depositing funds into the physician's or facility's account within three weeks.

Medicare maintains a provider directory of participating (**PAR**) providers nationwide. A search for a provider can be performed by state or specialty. This list contains the provider's name, specialty, education, residency, gender, foreign languages spoken by the physician, hospital affiliation, and practice location.

Medicare provides a variety of in-person as well as online workshops for providers to learn more about topics such as payment notices and reimbursements, the appeals process, using the Medicare Web site, and updates on changes that apply to physicians or medical facilities.

Medicare Part A Part A Medicare coverage is hospital insurance that covers most care for patients who have been hospitalized (for up to 90 days in a given period of time); patients in a **skilled nursing facility (SNF)** (facility for long-term care where patients must be monitored by nursing staff regularly) for given periods; patients who receive medical care at home, patients with life-limiting illnesses requiring hospice care (comfort care provided to patients who have six or fewer months to live); patients who require psychiatric treatment for given periods; and patients who require respite care (care provided in a skilled nursing facility on a short-term basis for patients normally treated at home). Citizens who receive Social Security benefits are automatically enrolled in Medicare Part A benefits with no premiums. Those who do not quality for Social Security may purchase Medicare Part A by paying a premium. Patients owe deductibles and coinsurance for most services in Part A.

Medicare Part B Part B Medicare coverage includes such services as physician care, therapy, and laboratory testing. Because Part B is voluntary, members must pay income-based premiums to enroll. In 2014 the standard monthly premium was $104.90 for those with individual incomes of $85,000 or less and couples with income of $170,000 or less. Patients also have out-of-pocket expenses under Part B. There is an annual deductible ($147 in 2014) which increases each year and 20 percent coinsurance on most services.

Physicians must choose whether they will participate with Medicare. A participating provider, also called PAR, must accept the Medicare fee schedule (MFS) amounts as payment in full for their services. If the MFS is higher than the physician's normal fee for a service, the normal fee is the maximum amount that can be billed. Physicians need to bill Medicare for all services, even those known not to be covered by Medicare. They also **accept assignment** on all claims, which means they accept the MFS amounts, and the payment is sent to the provider. Approximately 95 percent of all physicians are PAR.

Nonparticipating physicians (**non-PAR**) also need to bill Medicare for all services, including those not covered. However, they can decide to accept assignment on a case-by-case basis. Approximately 5 percent of all providers are non-PAR.

Example: Medicare Fee Schedule

A participating physician sees a Medicare patient for an office visit.

Normal charge: $118.00.

MFS rate: $100.00.

Reimbursement is calculated as follows.

Medicare payment: $100.00 × 80% = $80

Patient coinsurance: $100.00 × 20% = $20

Contractual allowance: $118.00 − $100.00 = $18.00

The Medicare payment is sent to the physician.

One very important aspect to billing Medicare is a form called the **Advance Beneficiary Notice (ABN)** or waiver (**Figure 17-7** ■). The ABN must be signed by patients before receiving covered services that have potential to be denied payment by Medicare. If, during the encounter, physicians recommend services that have potential to be denied, patients need to be informed and given the opportunity to accept or decline the service, knowing they are obligated to pay if Medicare does deny it. If patients do not understand that Medicare could deny the service, they are not obligated to pay for it and cannot be billed for it. Medical assistants are vital to facilitating this because they are the link between the medical care and the billing rules. Medical assistants need to review the ABN with the patient and obtain a signature before the service is provided. The ABN notifies patients that the service might not be paid by Medicare and patients agree to be responsible for payment. Medicare does not allow the ABN to be completed after the service is provided.

To understand when the ABN is needed, it is important to understand how Medicare classifies its services. **Non-covered** services are those that are not eligible for reimbursement under any circumstance and do require an ABN to be completed. **Covered** services are those potentially eligible for reimbursement; however, they are not automatically paid. Covered services must meet medical necessity and other criteria, such as frequency, in order to be paid. If services do not meet these criteria, Medicare payment may be denied. It is providers' responsibility to become familiar with what covered services may be denied under what circumstances, based on their specialty. Medicare does not allow blanket ABNs, which is the practice of having all Medicare patients sign ABNs for any service provided. The ABN must be specific to the patient's particular circumstance and service.

Example: ABN

Medicare limits how often B-12 injections are given, depending on the diagnosis. In a particular situation the physician might recommend more than the stipulated number of injections, believing the patient will receive the most benefit. The medical assistant asks the patient to sign the ABN and agree to pay for the additional injection if Medicare denies payment.

Medicare has very specific rules about what services can be billed together. For example, Medicare will not pay for an office visit and an injection on the same day, unless the office visit was clearly a distinct service, such as a physical examination. Many surgical procedures are **bundled**, meaning that multiple procedures are covered with one charge. For example, a surgeon who performs an abdominal hysterectomy with oophorectomy and salpingectomy must bill one charge only, which includes all three procedures. To bill this as three separate services is called **unbundling**, which is considered fraud.

▶▶▶ Pulse Points

Explaining Medicare Coverage

The administrative medical assistant should clearly explain to the Medicare-covered patient any services and costs that have potential to not be paid by Medicare. Medicare requires services be listed on the waiver form that the patient must sign. Be sure to give a copy of the form to the patient, and keep a copy in the patient's permanent file.

Medicare Part C: Advantage Plan   Part C Medicare is managed care, known as Medicare Advantage plans. Formerly known as Medicare + Choice, these plans are offered by private insurance companies and replace Parts A, B, and, usually, D. The benefit to the patient is potentially more comprehensive care at the same or lower cost than Medicare. The disadvantage, as with any managed care plan, is that the choice of providers is limited. Patients keep their Medicare identification

A. Notifier:

B. Patient Name: **C. Identification Number:**

Advance Beneficiary Notice of Noncoverage (ABN)

<u>NOTE:</u> If Medicare doesn't pay for **D.** _____ below, you may have to pay.
Medicare does not pay for everything, even some care that you or your health care provider have good reason to think you need. We expect Medicare may not pay for the **D.** _____ below.

D.	E. Reason Medicare May Not Pay:	F. Estimated Cost

WHAT YOU NEED TO DO NOW:
- Read this notice, so you can make an informed decision about your care.
- Ask us any questions that you may have after you finish reading.
- Choose an option below about whether to receive the **D.** _____ listed above.
  Note: If you choose Option 1 or 2, we may help you to use any other insurance that you might have, but Medicare cannot require us to do this.

G. OPTIONS: Check only one box. We cannot choose a box for you.

☐ **OPTION 1.** I want the **D.** _____ listed above. You may ask to be paid now, but I also want Medicare billed for an official decision on payment, which is sent to me on a Medicare Summary Notice (MSN). I understand that if Medicare doesn't pay, I am responsible for payment, but **I can appeal to Medicare** by following the directions on the MSN. If Medicare does pay, you will refund any payments I made to you, less co-pays or deductibles.

☐ **OPTION 2.** I want the **D.** _____ listed above, but do not bill Medicare. You may ask to be paid now as I am responsible for payment. **I cannot appeal if Medicare is not billed**.

☐ **OPTION 3.** I don't want the **D.** _____ listed above. I understand with this choice I am **not** responsible for payment, and **I cannot appeal to see if Medicare would pay**.

H. Additional Information:

This notice gives our opinion, not an official Medicare decision. If you have other questions on this notice or Medicare billing, call **1-800-MEDICARE** (1-800-633-4227/**TTY:** 1-877-486-2048).
Signing below means that you have received and understand this notice. You also receive a copy.

I. Signature:	J. Date:

According to the Paperwork Reduction Act of 1995, no persons are required to respond to a collection of information unless it displays a valid OMB control number. The valid OMB control number for this information collection is 0938-0566. The time required to complete this information collection is estimated to average 7 minutes per response, including the time to review instructions, search existing data resources, gather the data needed, and complete and review the information collection. If you have comments concerning the accuracy of the time estimate or suggestions for improving this form, please write to: CMS, 7500 Security Boulevard, Attn: PRA Reports Clearance Officer, Baltimore, Maryland 21244-1850.

Form CMS-R-131 (03/11)   Form Approved OMB No. 0938-0566

Figure 17-7 ■ Advance Beneficiary Notice Form (ABN).

card and receive an additional card from the Advantage plan. Because patients might not understand the difference between the two cards, it is a good practice for medical assistants to ask patients if they belong to an Advantage plan or have another identification card. When billing, the Medicare Advantage plan is billed, not Medicare. When patients have secondary coverage, medical assistants bill the secondary plans after the Medicare Advantage plan has made a payment or decision.

Medicare Part D Part D Medicare coverage, also called prescription drug coverage, is offered by private insurance companies through contracts with Medicare and provides limited benefits for prescription drugs. Patients choose from a variety of private plans, each of which may cover different medications, and select the one that covers the majority of their most costly prescriptions. Patients pay premiums, deductibles, and coinsurance. Members covered by Medicare may opt to purchase Part D coverage, which covers both name-brand and generic prescription drugs at participating pharmacies. Not all drugs are covered under every plan, so patients need to determine which plans cover their most common or most expensive medications.

Medical assistants can assist patients by providing them with complete medication lists. The Medicare Web site for patients, www.medicare.gov, has a prescription drug plan finder tool to assist patients in evaluating their options. Medicare Part D has an annual deductible, copayments or coinsurance, a maximum benefit level, and a stop loss for patients who have out-of-pocket costs over a certain level. The deductible and stop loss levels are updated annually.

Medigap Plans Medigap (**MG**) is a private insurance policy that supplements Medicare coverage, in order to fill "gaps" in Part A and Part B coverage. In most states, patients choose from ten standardized plans labeled Plan A through Plan J. Medigap policies are used only with Original Medicare, not Part C. All Medigap plans cover the patient's coinsurance. Each type of Medigap plan (A–J) covers different expenses, such as coverage of deductibles for Parts A and B, skilled nursing facility coinsurance, foreign travel, and other specific expenses. Patients need to select the policy that best meets their personal needs. Medigap is billed after Medicare has determined its portion of the payment. Most Medigap plans have an agreement with CMS so that the MACs electronically send the claims information to the Medigap carrier, relieving the provider of the need to directly bill the Medigap policy.

Medical assistants should ask patients if they have a Medigap policy so that information can be included on the billing to Medicare.

Medicare and Other Health Insurance (OHI) Patients may have other health insurance (**OHI**) in addition to Medicare. CMS requires providers to be very vigilant in determining when Medicare is obligated to pay first and when they are the secondary payer. These are known as Medicare Secondary Payer (**MSP**) rules. When Medicare is the secondary payer they pay a lower portion of the bill than when they are primary. Medicare provides a detailed questionnaire on the CMS Web site that medical assistants should review with patients to determine MSP. In general, Medicare is primary to Medicaid and secondary to most other insurance, including workers' compensation, liability, TRICARE, or when covered by a spouse's group health policy. Medicare is usually secondary when patients over age 65 are still working and covered by an employer's group health plan. There are exceptions to this, which the MSP questionnaire aids in determining.

Medicaid

Medicaid (**MCD**) coverage is a health benefit program for low-income patients that accounts for 18 percent of national health care payments. CMS establishes the general plan requirements, but states have considerable latitude in determining eligibility and coverage rules. Billing and coding requirements are also determined and administered by each state. The federal government provides funds to every state, and every state adds its own funds to cover qualified enrollees. As of 2011, the last year for which Medicaid has compiled extensive data, approximately 53 million persons received health care services through the Medicaid program, making it the largest health care program in the country.

Because Medicaid reimbursement is extremely low in most states, most health care providers cannot afford to treat a large number of Medicaid patients. The low reimbursement rate has caused many health care providers to stop accepting Medicaid patients altogether, or to limit the number of patients. As a result, Medicaid-covered patients might wait longer for care or be required to travel to find accepting providers. This situation is likely to become more pronounced with the implementation of the PPACA and the expected large increase in the number of Medicaid-covered patients.

If they wish to accept Medicaid patients, health care providers must apply to become Medicaid accredited in their state. As part of this process, which is very similar to any other managed care application process, Medicaid provides physicians fee schedules of covered expenses. Medicaid programs offer coverage on a month-to-month basis in most states, which means that just because Medicaid covered the patient in a previous month, does not guarantee that the patient is covered this month. Medical assistants must verify Medicaid eligibility each month the patient comes in. Many states provide patients with identification cards that medical offices can swipe through a card reader to verify a patient's current eligibility. If the patient is new to Medicaid or the state does not provide for electronic verification, a paper coupon may be presented at the time of service. Because every state runs its own Medicaid program, identification cards or coupons differ.

Low-income elderly or disabled patients often have both Medicare and Medicaid coverage. Medicare is always primary in these cases, and Medicaid is secondary. Often, Medicare's reimbursement rate is higher than what Medicaid allows, resulting in no Medicaid payment. The CMS estimates that there are approximately 6.5 million people receiving benefits from both Medicare and Medicaid. When physicians accept assignment from both Medicare and Medicaid, or participate in both programs, those physicians must accept what the two agencies together pay as payment in full for covered services. In these cases, billing patients for any portion of covered services is illegal. To do so can result in fines and/or removal from the Medicare and/or Medicaid programs as a participating provider.

It is important to note that Medicaid coverage is not simply based upon a person's income level. An individual may be considered low income yet not qualify for Medicaid benefits within their state. Medicaid coverage is based upon a list of qualifications, including the person's age, whether the patient is pregnant, disabled, or blind, whether or not the person is a U.S. citizen or a lawfully admitted immigrant, as well as on income level. Medicaid also includes special rules for persons who live in nursing homes or disabled children who live at home.

Medicaid is always the "payer of last resort," meaning that all other insurances should be billed before Medicaid. If the payment from the other insurance is higher than Medicaid's approved rate, Medicaid pays nothing.

Medicaid has introduced cost-sharing in recent years, which means that some patients might be responsible for copayments, deductibles, or premiums based on income level, family size, and other factors. If working for Medicaid providers, medical assistants should become familiar with their state's Medicaid identification card and eligibility verification system, as these tools provide much information about patients' coverage, eligibility, and financial responsibility.

Children's Health Insurance Program (CHIP)
The Children's Health Insurance Program (**CHIP**), complements Medicaid by providing coverage to low-income children who are uninsured but not eligible for Medicaid. Congress originally created the State Children's Health Insurance Program (SCHIP) in 1997. The program was extended, expanded, and renamed in 2009. CHIP is funded by the states (30 percent), with federal matching funds (70 percent) up to a predetermined capped allotment per state. Every state has a CHIP program, which has created coverage for 7 million children, in addition to the 29 million covered under Medicaid.

TRICARE

TRICARE, formerly called CHAMPUS, is a federal program that provides health care benefits to families of current and retired military personnel. The active duty service member is called a *sponsor*. Eligible family members are called *beneficiaries*. To be eligible for TRICARE, sponsors and beneficiaries must be enrolled in the Defense Enrollment Eligibility Reporting System (**DEERS**).

TRICARE offers three plans, each with different types of benefits:

1. TRICARE Standard, a fee-for-service plan
2. TRICARE Extra, a PPO
3. TRICARE Prime, an HMO

All TRICARE enrollees are automatically enrolled in TRICARE Standard and TRICARE Extra. Most patients on TRICARE Standard and TRICARE Extra owe copayments and deductibles. TRICARE Prime is an optional plan which enrollees must specifically enroll in and requires no copayments or deductibles. Medical assistants should be alert to the fact that TRICARE's deductible year begins October 1.

Some patients have TRICARE for Life, a plan that acts as secondary insurance coverage for patients over age 65. For primary insurance, these patients have Medicare. TRICARE requires preauthorization for medical services, and patients must use in-network providers.

TRICARE requires participating providers to submit claims within 60 days of the date care was provided. Non-network providers have up to one year from the date the care was provided to submit claims.

CHAMPVA The Civilian Health and Medical Program of the Veterans Administration (**CHAMPVA**) is a federal program that covers the health care expenses of the families of veterans with total, permanent, service-related, covered disabilities, and the spouses and dependent children of veterans who died in the line of duty. Patients with CHAMPVA coverage may use any civilian health care provider, without preauthorization.

If a patient has other coverage besides CHAMPVA, the other coverage should be billed first. By law, CHAMPVA is always the secondary payer, with the following exceptions: Medicaid, State Victims of Crime Compensation, and supplemental CHAMPVA policies. After the primary insurance carrier has made payment, a CMS-1500 claim form is sent to CHAMPVA along with a copy of the primary carrier's explanation of benefits.

CHAMPVA requires preauthorization only in the following areas:

● Organ and bone marrow transplants
● Hospice care
● Dental care
● Durable medical equipment (**DME**) worth more than $300
● Most mental health or substance abuse services

Third-Party Liability Insurance

Third-party liability insurance is insurance in which someone other than the patient is ultimately responsible for the medical bills, usually due to injury or negligence. The most common of these are workers' compensation insurance and property and casualty insurance.

Workers' Compensation Insurance

Workers' compensation (**WC**) insurance covers employees injured in the workplace or suffering from a workplace-related illness. Occupational injuries are those that occur during the course of employment, but do not have to be on company property or while performing work duties. WC covers accidents that occur off-site, such as while driving on company business or at a remote work site, and those that occur during a paid break. Occupational illnesses are conditions that arise from short- or long-term exposure to a workplace hazard or condition, such as dust, chemical allergens, radiation, repetitive motion, and loud noises. The challenge with occupational illnesses is identifying, diagnosing, and reporting them, because some, such as repetitive stress injuries (RSI), hearing loss, and various respiratory disorders, may take years to manifest themselves.

All employers must offer WC. Each state establishes its own requirements for WC insurance, but must comply with federal minimums. Insurance may be obtained from a state-managed fund, private insurers, or self-funded by the employer. Some states do not allow private insurers to offer workers' compensation policies, so coverage must be obtained from the state or through self-funding. Federal laws cover workers in Washington, D.C, coal miners, federal employees, and maritime workers.

A workers' compensation claim is initiated by filing the **First Report of Illness or Injury**. The First Report describes the circumstances of the illness or injury, the expected plan of care, and expected prognosis. Most states have a specific form that must be used for the First Report. State laws vary widely on the time frame required for filing and the responsible party. In some states, the employer may be required to file this report and in other states the first provider who treats the injured worker is responsible. Medical assistants need to be familiar with how the filing process works in their state. Most states also require that reports be filed periodically throughout the duration of treatment. **Progress reports**, also called *followup reports*, document the treatment provided, the patient's current medical status, the expected plan of care, the prognosis, and the expected return-to-work date.

Benefits to the injured worker include coverage of the cost of medical care related to the illness or injury, wages for time lost from work due to illness or injury, death benefits for survivors when the accident is the cause of the worker's death, and rehabilitation or retraining benefits that enable the worker to return to work or learn a different line of work if necessary.

WC has three types of claims:

- **Non-disability (ND) claim**—one in which the worker was injured and treated by a physician, but no time was lost from work

- **Temporary disability (TD) claim**—one in which the worker is able to return to previous or modified work at a later time
- **Permanent disability (PD) claim**—one in which no further improvement is expected and the worker is unable to return to work

Health care providers must enroll with their state's workers' compensation programs before accepting workers' compensation cases. Providers receive identification numbers for billing purposes. Workers' compensation programs reimburse physicians based on an established schedule. If physician charges are higher than the reimbursement amount, patients cannot be balance billed. In some states, workers' compensation operates under a managed care model.

To ensure the program runs properly, health care providers must keep good records on workers' compensation cases. This includes verifying patients' injuries with employers and contacting insurance companies to obtain claim numbers and verify the date of injury on file. Medical assistants must become familiar with their state requirements for preauthorization. They should also create new medical records and financial records for patients with work-related injuries in order to maintain confidentiality and keep reporting and claim filing accurate. Most states' labor departments provide free physician reporting forms and claim information for injured workers.

WC programs are not subject to HIPAA regulations because they do not qualify as a health insurance plan. However, states have separate privacy and security rules that govern WC. WC plans may have unique coding and billing requirements, such as their own private code sets.

Property and Casualty Insurance

Property and casualty insurance is insurance on homes, cars, and businesses. The *property* portion protects the policyholder (person or business) against the loss of or damage to physical property they own. The *casualty* portion protects the policyholder against legal liability for losses caused by injury to others, including medical expenses of those injured. When patients are injured in an accident involving automobiles, watercraft, private or public property, they may file a claim with a property and casualty (**P/C**) insurance company.

The most common form of P/C insurance that medical assistants encounter is automobile insurance. Automobile insurance policies often include medical payments (*med pay*) coverage or personal injury protection (**PIP**), which pays for medical expenses incurred as the result of an automobile accident. However, medical assistants might also encounter P/C insurance for boating and personal watercraft accidents and any type of injury caused by the negligence of another person or entity.

P/C insurance is regulated by each state's department of insurance, not by federal or HIPAA laws that govern health insurance companies. P/C companies tend to have specialized requirements and their own forms for submitting claims. They often contract with external bill review companies to review medical claims and recommend payment amounts. Medical assistants should keep a file of these requirements for each P/C company it deals with.

 ## Pulse Points

Medical Claims for Injuries

Any patient who has a medical claim for an injury, whether through workers' compensation or other liability insurance, is assigned a claim number and a claims manager or department to handle the claim. At the beginning of the patient's care in the medical office, locate the name and phone number of the claims manager. Readily available contact information allows the office easily to contact the claims manager in the event the physician orders tests or procedures that require preauthorization.

HIPAA Compliance

Workers' compensation programs and automobile injury policies are not HIPAA covered entities. Separate rules established by each state govern these types of claims. By filing a WC claim, the patient automatically authorizes the release of medical information related to the injury to be released in order to process the claim. However, be careful not to release information about any other illnesses or injuries. A separate file for injury claims makes it easier to determine the information that is to be copied and sent.

Disability Income Insurance

Disability income (DI) insurance reimburses a patient for lost wages due to a non-work-related disability that prevents the individual from working. Disability income insurance is offered by federal, state, and private sources. Benefits are based on a percentage of employees' wages, often 66 percent, because benefits are not subject to income tax. Lost wages due to a work-related disability are covered by workers' compensation insurance; lost wages due to a disability related to an automobile or other liability accident are covered by liability insurance.

DI policies may be short-term or long-term. The policies differ in the waiting period and the length of benefits. **Short-term disability (STD)** DI policies have a short waiting period, usually 0 to 14 days, and pay benefits for a limited amount of time, usually anywhere from three months to two years. **Long-term disability (LTD)** DI policies have a longer waiting period, usually three months to two years, and pay benefits for an extended length of time, which may be several years, to age 65, or the lifetime.

The federal government provides two long-term DI programs under Social Security:

- **Supplemental Security Income (SSI)**—Provides coverage to disabled workers who have met Social Security requirements for quarters worked, and whose disability is not work-related.
- **Social Security Disability Insurance (SSDI)**—Provides coverage to people who are disabled and have low incomes and who do not meet the work requirements of SSI.

With only a few exceptions, disability insurance does not pay for medical treatment; therefore, medical assistants do not often bill a disability plan for medical services. However, medical assistants might need to assist patients who are applying for disability coverage or benefits by providing information from the medical record regarding a patient's past health history or current disability. Even though patients have disability insurance, they might not have medical coverage because they are not employed and cannot afford or are not eligible for individual health insurance policies.

No standard definition of a disability exists; rather, the conditions of a disability are defined by each individual plan. The Social Security definition of a disability is the strictest and own-occupation disability offered by some private companies is the most liberal. Under the Social Security definition, patients are considered disabled if they cannot do work that they did before, they cannot adjust to other work because of their medical condition(s), and their disability has lasted or is expected to last for at least one year or to result in death. Social Security pays no benefits for temporary or partial disability. Own-occupation disability means that, because of sickness or injury, patients are not able to perform the substantial duties of their occupation which they were performing at the time of disability.

The Medical Assistant's Role with Disability Insurance

Medical assistants' role with disability insurance varies, depending on the role of the physicians in the office. Medical assistants should be familiar with the various ways physicians may be involved with the disability determination process, for both government and private insurers.

Treating Physician Physicians may treat disability applicants and need to provide medical records or testimony regarding patients' functioning. Information provided may include facts such as the date the disability occurred, a description of how the disability occurred, description of how the disability prevents the patient from working, examination and test results that document the extent of disability, and the level and time frame of expected recovery. The wording of information provided by physicians can affect the determination, based on the disability definition being used by the insurer.

Consultative Examiner Physicians may also work as paid consultative examiners who provide an outside medical or psychological examination of applicants. In this case, patients who are disability applicants, and not part of the physician's established patient base, may come to the office.

Medical Review Officer Physicians also may be paid medical review officers who review claims from a medical perspective for the insurer. Part of the physician's regular schedule may be set aside for this activity.

Billing Most disability policies do not provide coverage for medical services, but veterans' disability benefits do include certain medical services. For these patients, medical assistants submit bills and must accept the insurance payment as payment in full.

Health Insurance Claims

There are many steps involved in converting a patient encounter into a paid insurance claim. Each step needs to be completed in a timely and accurate manner in order for providers to receive correct payment for their services. The exact procedures are not the same in every office, but the general process is similar. The process begins with the medical assistant gathering accurate patient information. Next, the claims must be prepared and submitted, either electronically or on paper. Finally, payments must be posted and medical assistants must follow up on unpaid claims to be sure that all monies are received.

Gathering Patient Information

The first step in receiving proper reimbursement for insurance claims is obtaining accurate patient information. The life cycle of an insurance claim begins when the patient calls the physician to make an appointment, a patient arrives at the emergency department, or a physician admits a patient to the hospital. Although providers do not code or bill for scheduling an appointment, the insurance process begins when providers begin collecting insurance information. When time allows, patients pre-register by completing paperwork regarding their health condition and insurance prior to the appointment. The provider verifies eligibility with the insurance company through a telephone call or secure Web site in order to determine if the patient is covered by insurance and what services are covered and/or require preauthorization.

Each new patient in the medical office should complete a registration form (**Figure 17-8 ■**) that is verified at each visit and updated annually. When time allows, patients pre-register by completing paperwork regarding their health condition and insurance prior to the appointment. Many medical offices ask patients for their health insurance information over the phone, before their first visits. Other offices simply ask patients for their insurance type over the phone and then ask those patients to bring their insurance card to their visit. Yet others mail or e-mail the paperwork to new patients, so they can complete the forms at home, without pressure, and bring them to the first visit. The provider verifies eligibility with the insurance company through a telephone call or secure Web site in order to determine if the patient is covered by insurance and what services are covered and/or require preauthorization.

Patient registration forms include a place for patients to authorize the release of their medical information in order to process insurance claims. This is required by the CMS-1500 billing form. HIPAA allows medical offices to share patient information with insurance companies that is necessary to process the claim because such information is part of the treatment, payment, and operations provision. Patients consent to this when they receive the medical office's notice of privacy practices. Insurance claim forms give patients' names, addresses, birth dates, diagnoses, and types of treatment.

After obtaining pertinent patient information, medical assistants must identify the name and birth date of the insured. When the patient is the spouse or child of the insured, the medical assistant must ask the patient for the additional information. The assistant needs to know if the patient is covered by more than one plan. If so, the assistant then must determine which plan is primary and which is secondary.

Medical assistants must photocopy both sides of patients' insurance identification cards when patients arrive for their first visits. The front of an insurance card typically contains the name and identification number of the insured or member. Each patient is uniquely identified by a member identification number assigned by the insurance company. Patients have a different number with each separate insurance plan they have. HIPAA originally made provision for a unique patient identification number that would be the same for all insurance companies, but concerns about privacy and identity theft have put this on hold indefinitely.

In today's world of identity theft, most insurance plans no longer use Social Security numbers for identification. Instead, many identification numbers now have alphabetic prefixes followed by numbers. Some have alphabetic characters only. Plans may have their own group or plan numbers, as well. A *payer number*, a unique number that identifies an insurance company, allows medical offices to submit claims electronically. The back of the card typically has the claims mailing addresses. Insurance telephone numbers appear on the front or back of cards. Typically, one number is for "customer or member service" and another is for "providers." Medical assistants call the latter for information on patients' coverage or claims.

Verification of Benefits

After obtaining insurance information from patients, medical assistants should verify coverage with the insurance company. To verify coverage, medical assistants contact the insurance company to determine what services are covered. They should confirm the following information and record the answers on a verification of benefits (VOB) worksheet (**Figure 17-9 ■**).

- What is the effective date of the policy?
- Who is the insured?

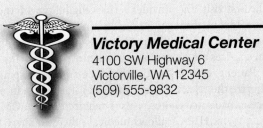

Victory Medical Center
4100 SW Highway 6
Victorville, WA 12345
(509) 555-9832

Patient Name: _____
            Last Name   First Name   Middle Initial

Address: _____
            Street   City   State   Zip

Home Phone: _____ Work Phone: _____

Mobile Phone: _____ Birthdate: _____

Social Security Number: _____ Age: _____

Sex: _____ Marital Status: S M D W Children: _____

How do you prefer to be addressed? _____

Spouse's Name: _____

Primary Care Physician: _____ Phone No: _____

Name of Person Responsible for Bill: _____

Relationship to Patient: _____ Phone No: _____

Address of Person Responsible for Bill: _____

Patient's Employer: _____ Phone No: _____

Occupation: _____

Spouse's Employer: _____ Phone No: _____

Occupation: _____

INSURANCE INFORMATION

Primary Insurance: _____ Policy No: _____

Name of Policyholder: _____ Birthdate: _____

SS#: _____ Relationship to Insured: _____

Secondary Insurance: _____ Policy No: _____

Name of Policyholder: _____ Birthdate: _____

If Injured: Date: _____ Place: _____

Claim Number: _____ Nature or Cause of Injury: _____

Employer at Time of Injury: _____ Phone No: _____

EMERGENCY INFORMATION

In case of emergency, local friend or relative to be notified (not living at same address)

Name: _____ Relationship to Patient: _____

Address: _____ Phone No: _____

I hereby authorize the health care professionals in this clinic to diagnose and treat my condition. I clearly understand and agree that all services rendered me are charged directly to me and that I am personally responsible for payment. I agree that I am responsible for all bills incurred at this clinic. I hereby authorize assignment of my insurance rights and benefits directly to the provider for services rendered. I also authorize the health care professionals to discuss my care with other health care providers who I am currently treating with.

_____   _____   _____   _____
Patient's Signature   Date   Parent or Guardian Signature   Date

Figure 17-8 ■ Sample new patient registration form.

```
Patient's Name: _____ Chart #: _____ Appt. Date: _____
D.O.B._____ Policy ID # _____ Gr# _____
Policyholder: _____ DOB: _____
Insurance Co. Name: _____ Referral# Required: ☐ No ☐ Yes
Telephone #_____ Referral #: _____
Mailing Address: _____
Employer's Name: _____
Employer's Phone #: _____
Effective Date: _____ Lifetime maximum: _____
Pre-Cert Required: ☐ Yes ☐ No

Deductible Met:
Copay _____ Deductible_____ ☐ No ☐ Yes
Pays @_____%
Exclusion/Preexisting: _____
Chief Complaint/Diagnosis: _____
Insurance Rep's Name: _____
Insurance Company Phone #: _____ Date: _____ Time: _____
Verified by _____
```

Figure 17-9 ■ Verification of benefits worksheet.

- Is the type of service the patient is seeking (office visit, laboratory test, X-ray, etc.) covered?
- What are the deductible, copayment, and/or coinsurance amounts for this service?
- Is a referral or preauthorization required for this service?
- Where should a paper claim be submitted? For electronic claims, what is the payer number?
- What is the full name and phone number of the person you spoke to?

Insurance companies may have a separate phone number for verification. The process may be completely automated or may include personally speaking with a representative. It is becoming more common for insurance companies to offer the option of verifying benefits online through a secure Web site, especially if the physician is a preferred provider. It is worthwhile to make arrangements to perform verification online because it is usually faster and more convenient for medical assistants.

Verifying benefits with the insurance company is not a 100 percent guarantee of payment because there might have been recent changes in the patient's status, such as adding or dropping coverage, that have not been input into the computer system at the time of verification.

Determining Coordination of Benefits

Patients may be covered by more than one insurance plan. Most often this is because spouses each have a group health plan and each has purchased coverage for the other. Also, both spouses may elect to cover their children under both policies. Insurance companies, in cooperation with state insurance commissioners, have established specific rules that determine which coverage is primary (the one billed first) and which is secondary (the one billed second). This process of determining which company is primary and which is secondary is **coordination of benefits** (**COB**). Patients do not have the option of specifying which insurance should be primary or secondary.

When spouses or partners are covered by each other's policy, the patient's own policy is always primary, and the spouse's or partner's policy is secondary. Likewise, when spouses are patients, their own policy is primary. Medical assistants should not assume that spouses are covered by each other's policy because such coverage is entirely patients' choice, based on their insurance needs and costs associated with covering other family members. It is possible, for example, for the husband's insurance to cover himself and his wife, but the wife's insurance to cover only her. In this case, the husband would have only one insurance, his own. The wife would have two policies; hers would be primary and her husband's would be secondary.

When both parents carry coverage for the children, most health insurance plans decide which insurance plan is primary and which is secondary based on the **birthday rule** (**Figure 17-10** ■). According to this rule, the parent with the birthday earlier in the calendar year is the primary carrier for the children; the parent with the later birthday is the secondary carrier for the children.

The birthday rule relies only on the month and day of the parent's birthday. The year is not used. The insurance commissioners of most states have agreed to use the birthday rule. If a state does not use the birthday rule, the COB rules of plan in the non-birthday rule state apply. Medical assistants need to ask about this when verifying benefits.

PROCEDURE 17-2 Verify a Patient's Insurance Eligibility

Theory and Rationale

Many patients who seek medical care are covered by some form of medical insurance. Verifying a patient's eligibility is an important part of the medical assistant's job. Verifying benefits with the insurance company ensures that the medical assistant has the most current and accurate information possible.

Materials

- Insurance identification card
- Patient's registration form
- Insurance verification of benefits worksheet
- Telephone or computer
- Paper
- Pen

Competency

1. Look at the patient's registration form and locate the patient's birthdate and the patient's relationship to the insured.
2. Look at the patient's insurance identification card and locate the name of the insured, the insured's member

identification number, and the telephone number of the insurance company.

3. Call the insurance company at the provider customer service telephone number listed on the insurance identification card, or access the insurance company's secure Web site, if available.
4. When the customer service representative answers the call, write down the name of the customer service representative, and the date and time of the call.
5. Verify spelling of policyholder's name and birthdate.
6. Verify patient's name and birthdate.
7. Verify coverage for type of service to be rendered, including frequency or number of visits.
8. Verify when preauthorization is needed.
9. Verify patient's financial responsibility for deductible, copayment, or coinsurance amounts.
10. Verify coordination of benefits rules if more than one policy covers the patient.
11. Verify provider's participating or non-participating status.
12. Verify the address where insurance claims are to be mailed or the payer number needed for electronic billing.

Complicated issues can arise with child patients covered by three companies, perhaps through both biological parents and one stepparent. In these cases, typically the custo-

dial parent's plan is primary, the spouse of the custodial parent's plan is secondary, and the noncustodial parent's plan is tertiary. The easiest way to get patients' claims paid on time is to ask the insurance carriers to identify the order in which to bill.

Mary and Josiah Banks have a son, Ian. Mary has an insurance policy through Aetna U.S. Health Care that provides family coverage. Josiah has an insurance policy through Premera Blue Cross that also provides family coverage. Mary's birthday is January 10, 1977, and Josiah's birthday is April 15, 1968. According to the birthday rule, the primary and secondary coverage for this family would be as follows:

	Primary Coverage	Secondary Coverage
Mary	Aetna U.S. Healthcare	Premera Blue Cross
Josiah	Premera Blue Cross	Aetna U.S. Healthcare
Ian	Aetna U.S. Healthcare	Premera Blue Cross

Because Mary's birthday falls earlier in the year than Josiah's, her policy is primary for her and Ian. Because Josiah's birthday falls later, his plan is secondary for Ian. Policyholders are primary on their own policies, so Josiah's primary carrier is his own policy through Premera Blue Cross.

Figure 17-10 ■ Patient scenario: Using the birthday rule.

Critical Thinking Question 17-4

Refer back to the case study at the beginning of the chapter. Assume that Martin's insurance policy has a $150 deductible, which he has already met this year, and a $15 copayment. How much should the insurance company pay? What does Martin owe? What should the medical assistant do next?

Obtaining Authorizations and Referrals

Authorizations and *referrals* refer to approvals patients must receive, to comply with insurance company rules, before receiving certain services or procedures. Before scheduling any nonemergency procedures or costly tests, medical assistants should call insurance carriers both to verify patients' eligibility for those services and to complete any needed **preauthorizations**. Preauthorization, called *precertification* by some third-party payers, is the process of contacting the patient's insurance carrier to obtain permission for patients to receive prescribed procedures. This generally involves submitting a form to the insurance company that explains the service, the reasons the patient needs it, and the anticipated cost. The insurance company reviews the request and, if approved, provides a preauthorization number that should be reported when the service is billed. Insurance companies are required by law to have an appeals process for patients to use when a preauthorization request is denied. The medical office and patient need to communicate and work together to file an appeal and work through the progressive steps of the appeal process. Preauthorizations may be valid for a limited period of time, such as 60 or 90 days. Medical assistants should make the physician and patient aware of any such time limit, so the procedure can be scheduled in a timely manner. If patients do not receive the procedure within that time frame, a new request must be submitted.

▸▸ Pulse Points

Insurance Terminology

Insurance companies use a variety of terms to refer to the approval process. One insurance company may use the term *preauthorization* and another may use *precertification*. Yet another company may use the terms *preauthorization*, *precertification*, and *predetermination* to describe three different types of approval. Medical assistants should be aware of this variation and verify with each insurance company how they use these terms and what their specific requirements are.

When patients require specialist care, managed care plans often require referrals from patients' PCPs. Medical assistants who work for PCPs may be asked to arrange those specialist referrals, which entails verifying which specialists are covered under patients' managed care plans. To accomplish this task, assistants can phone insurance carriers' customer service departments or look online, understanding that online information may not be completely up-to-date. When a specialist is selected, it is a good idea to verify current participation with the specialist's office. Medical assistants in specialist offices must ensure that patients' PCPs have arranged referrals before those patients visit the specialists' offices.

HMOs may penalize physicians who fail to obtain an authorization or referral before rendering service. Many insurance carriers deny claims that are not properly preauthorized. In managed care, physicians are prohibited from billing patients for services denied due to lack of authorization. In effect, the physicians perform the procedures for free. With penalties this severe, it is imperative that health care providers verify the need for referrals and authorizations before providing service.

Documenting Insurance Company Calls

While comprehensive, in-depth knowledge of all insurance plans is unrealistic, administrative medical assistants should know where to find answers and information. Many insurance companies provide coverage information online. Insurance companies' Web site addresses typically appear on patients' identification cards. These resources are recommended for general information, not procedure authorization. When assistants have questions about patients' insurance coverage, the provider customer service department of the patients' insurance carrier is the best place to call.

 PROCEDURE 17-3 Obtain a Managed Care Referral

Theory and Rationale

Medical assistants in primary care or family practice physicians' offices are often required to obtain managed care referrals for patients who need to see specialists or other health care providers. Whenever needed, medical assistants in specialists' office should ensure that managed care referrals are obtained for patients covered by managed care policies.

Materials

- Telephone
- Patient's medical chart
- Name and telephone number of patient's primary care provider

Competency

1. Call the patient's primary care provider's office, and ask for the person in charge of referrals.

2. Give the referral assistant the patient's information, including name and birthdate.

3. Inform the referral assistant of the need for a referral to the physician, including the reason for the patient's visit in the medical office.

4. Ask the referral assistant if any information from the patient's file is needed to process the referral.

5. Ask the referral assistant when to expect the referral. If needed, provide the office fax number for information transmittal.

6. Document in the patient's file the content of the telephone call.

7. Notify the physician and the patient of the content of the telephone call.

PROCEDURE 17-4 Obtain Authorization from an Insurance Company for a Procedure

Theory and Rationale

Most insurance companies require preauthorization before physicians perform any nonemergency services. Without insurance carrier authorization, physicians are usually not paid for their services.

Materials

- Patient insurance information (i.e., ID number, birthdate of the insured, name and telephone number for provider customer service at the insurance company)
- Paper and pen
- Description of the procedure the doctor has prescribed, including Current Procedural Terminology (**CPT**) code
- Patient's diagnosis pertaining to the needed procedure
- Location where procedure is to be performed (e.g., office, outpatient surgery, inpatient hospitalization)
- Date by which the procedure must be performed

Competency

1. Write down the date and time of the call, the name of the insurance company, and the name of the insurance company representative on the phone.

2. Give the insurance company representative your name and your office's/physician's name.

3. Give the insurance company representative the name of the patient, the name of the insured, and the insured's ID number.

4. Let the representative know what procedure your doctor has prescribed for the patient and the date by which the procedure must be performed.

5. Provide the representative any other requested information (e.g., procedure code, diagnosis code, and place where the procedure is to be performed).

6. Write down the authorization number the representative provides.

7. Ask the representative if any supporting documentation (e.g., chart notes, operative report, laboratory report, or pathology report) is needed with the CMS-1500 billing form. If so, write down the required documentation.

8. Keep all preceding information in the patient's file for reference in case the claim is not paid by the insurance carrier.

Medical assistants should document any calls made to an insurance carrier, including date and time, number used, party on the phone, and information obtained. Such data becomes part of patients' permanent financial record and can be referenced should there ever be a discrepancy between what the medical assistant was told by the insurance carrier and how the insurance carrier processed the claim.

Preparing Health Insurance Claims

After the proper patient information has been gathered and the service has been provided, medical assistants prepare the claim to submit to the insurance company. Whether submitting claims electronically or on paper, specific guidelines must be followed.

The National Provider Identifier (NPI)

The national provider identifier (**NPI**) is a unique, ten-digit number assigned to health care providers by the CMS. NPI use was mandated as part of HIPAA administrative simplifications language as of May 2007. Before that date, each health insurance company issued its own identification number. The Medicare number was the unique provider identification number (UPIN).

NPI numbers must be used by all covered entities for submitting health insurance claims. A covered entity is any provider who submits electronic claims to Medicare. Specialists who receive referrals from other physicians must report their NPI number on the CMS-1500 claim form, as well as the referring physician's name and NPI number. Not only does each individual provider have an NPI, but the facility or medical group that bills for individual providers has a facility or group NPI. Both the rendering provider NPI and group NPI are reported on the CMS-1500 in specific locations.

The CMS-1500 Claim Form

Although most physicians submit insurance claims electronically, some smaller offices still use paper forms. Regardless of which submission method is used, the same information is required. Medical assistants must submit all paper claims using the CMS-1500 form, a uniform billing format used for medical claims (**Figure 17-11** ■). Dental claims are prepared using the American Dental Association (**ADA**) standard form. The ADA form and the CMS-1500 are the only two insurance claim forms medical assistants use to submit paper claims. Effective April 2014, a new version of the CMS-1500 is required, due to the implementation of the **ICD-10-CM** coding system.

HEALTH INSURANCE CLAIM FORM

APPROVED BY NATIONAL UNIFORM CLAIM COMMITTEE (NUCC) 02/12

CARRIER

| | PICA | | | | | | | | PICA | |

1. MEDICARE ☐ (Medicare#)   MEDICAID ☐ (Medicaid#)   TRICARE ☐ (ID#/DoD#)   CHAMPVA ☐ (Member ID#)   GROUP HEALTH PLAN ☐ (ID#)   FECA BLK LUNG ☐ (ID#)   OTHER ☐ (ID#)

1a. INSURED'S I.D. NUMBER   (For Program in Item 1)

2. PATIENT'S NAME (Last Name, First Name, Middle Initial)

3. PATIENT'S BIRTH DATE   MM | DD | YY   SEX   M ☐   F ☐

4. INSURED'S NAME (Last Name, First Name, Middle Initial)

5. PATIENT'S ADDRESS (No., Street)

6. PATIENT RELATIONSHIP TO INSURED   Self ☐ Spouse ☐ Child ☐ Other ☐

7. INSURED'S ADDRESS (No., Street)

CITY   STATE

8. RESERVED FOR NUCC USE

CITY   STATE

ZIP CODE   TELEPHONE (Include Area Code) (   )

ZIP CODE   TELEPHONE (Include Area Code) (   )

9. OTHER INSURED'S NAME (Last Name, First Name, Middle Initial)

10. IS PATIENT'S CONDITION RELATED TO:

11. INSURED'S POLICY GROUP OR FECA NUMBER

a. OTHER INSURED'S POLICY OR GROUP NUMBER

a. EMPLOYMENT? (Current or Previous) ☐ YES ☐ NO

a. INSURED'S DATE OF BIRTH   MM | DD | YY   SEX   M ☐   F ☐

b. RESERVED FOR NUCC USE

b. AUTO ACCIDENT? ☐ YES ☐ NO   PLACE (State)

b. OTHER CLAIM ID (Designated by NUCC)

c. RESERVED FOR NUCC USE

c. OTHER ACCIDENT? ☐ YES ☐ NO

c. INSURANCE PLAN NAME OR PROGRAM NAME

d. INSURANCE PLAN NAME OR PROGRAM NAME

10d. CLAIM CODES (Designated by NUCC)

d. IS THERE ANOTHER HEALTH BENEFIT PLAN? ☐ YES ☐ NO   *If yes*, complete items 9, 9a, and 9d.

READ BACK OF FORM BEFORE COMPLETING & SIGNING THIS FORM.

12. PATIENT'S OR AUTHORIZED PERSON'S SIGNATURE I authorize the release of any medical or other information necessary to process this claim. I also request payment of government benefits either to myself or to the party who accepts assignment below.

SIGNED _____   DATE _____

13. INSURED'S OR AUTHORIZED PERSON'S SIGNATURE I authorize payment of medical benefits to the undersigned physician or supplier for services described below.

SIGNED _____

PATIENT AND INSURED INFORMATION

14. DATE OF CURRENT ILLNESS, INJURY, or PREGNANCY (LMP)   MM | DD | YY   QUAL.

15. OTHER DATE   QUAL.   MM | DD | YY

16. DATES PATIENT UNABLE TO WORK IN CURRENT OCCUPATION   MM | DD | YY FROM   MM | DD | YY TO

17. NAME OF REFERRING PROVIDER OR OTHER SOURCE   17a.   17b. NPI

18. HOSPITALIZATION DATES RELATED TO CURRENT SERVICES   MM | DD | YY FROM   MM | DD | YY TO

19. ADDITIONAL CLAIM INFORMATION (Designated by NUCC)

20. OUTSIDE LAB? ☐ YES ☐ NO $ CHARGES

21. DIAGNOSIS OR NATURE OF ILLNESS OR INJURY Relate A-L to service line below (24E)   ICD Ind.

A. _____ B. _____ C. _____ D. _____
E. _____ F. _____ G. _____ H. _____
I. _____ J. _____ K. _____ L. _____

22. RESUBMISSION CODE   ORIGINAL REF. NO.

23. PRIOR AUTHORIZATION NUMBER

24. A. DATE(S) OF SERVICE					B. PLACE OF SERVICE	C. EMG	D. PROCEDURES, SERVICES, OR SUPPLIES (Explain Unusual Circumstances)		E. DIAGNOSIS POINTER	F. $ CHARGES	G. DAYS OR UNITS	H. EPSDT Family Plan	I. ID. QUAL.	J. RENDERING PROVIDER ID. #
From MM	DD	YY	To MM	DD	YY			CPT/HCPCS	MODIFIER						
1														NPI
2														NPI
3														NPI
4														NPI
5														NPI
6														NPI

PHYSICIAN OR SUPPLIER INFORMATION

25. FEDERAL TAX I.D. NUMBER   SSN ☐ EIN ☐

26. PATIENT'S ACCOUNT NO.

27. ACCEPT ASSIGNMENT? (For govt. claims, see back) ☐ YES ☐ NO

28. TOTAL CHARGE $

29. AMOUNT PAID $

30. Rsvd for NUCC Use

31. SIGNATURE OF PHYSICIAN OR SUPPLIER INCLUDING DEGREES OR CREDENTIALS (I certify that the statements on the reverse apply to this bill and are made a part thereof.)

SIGNED _____   DATE _____

32. SERVICE FACILITY LOCATION INFORMATION

a.   b.

33. BILLING PROVIDER INFO & PH # (   )

a.   b.

Figure 17-11 ■ CMS-1500 claim form.

HEALTH INSURANCE CLAIM FORM

APPROVED BY NATIONAL UNIFORM CLAIM COMMITTEE (NUCC) 02/12

ABC INSURANCE CO
999 MAIN STREET
NEW YORK NY 12345

CARRIER

| | PICA | | | | | | | | PICA | |

1. MEDICARE	MEDICAID	TRICARE	CHAMPVA	GROUP HEALTH PLAN	FECA BLK LUNG	OTHER	1a. INSURED'S I.D. NUMBER (For Program in Item 1)
☐ (Medicare#)	☐ (Medicaid#)	☐ (ID#/DoD#)	☐ (Member ID#)	☐ (ID#)	☐ (ID#)	☒ (ID#)	9874653

2. PATIENT'S NAME (Last Name, First Name, Middle Initial)	3. PATIENT'S BIRTH DATE MM DD YY — SEX	4. INSURED'S NAME (Last Name, First Name, Middle Initial)
ABNER AARON	01 28 1976 M ☒ F ☐	ABNER MELISSA

5. PATIENT'S ADDRESS (No., Street)	6. PATIENT RELATIONSHIP TO INSURED	7. INSURED'S ADDRESS (No., Street)
	Self ☐ Spouse ☒ Child ☐ Other ☐	98 N ROSEWOOD DR

CITY	STATE	8. RESERVED FOR NUCC USE	CITY	STATE
			TOWNSHIP	NY

ZIP CODE	TELEPHONE (Include Area Code)		ZIP CODE	TELEPHONE (Include Area Code)
	( )		12345	( )

PATIENT AND INSURED INFORMATION

9. OTHER INSURED'S NAME (Last Name, First Name, Middle Initial)	10. IS PATIENT'S CONDITION RELATED TO:	11. INSURED'S POLICY GROUP OR FECA NUMBER
		01536

a. OTHER INSURED'S POLICY OR GROUP NUMBER	a. EMPLOYMENT? (Current or Previous) ☐ YES ☒ NO	a. INSURED'S DATE OF BIRTH MM DD YY — SEX
		08 04 1974 M ☐ F ☒

b. RESERVED FOR NUCC USE	b. AUTO ACCIDENT? PLACE (State) ☐ YES ☒ NO	b. OTHER CLAIM ID (Designated by NUCC)

c. RESERVED FOR NUCC USE	c. OTHER ACCIDENT? ☐ YES ☒ NO	c. INSURANCE PLAN NAME OR PROGRAM NAME
		ABC INSURANCE CO

d. INSURANCE PLAN NAME OR PROGRAM NAME	10d. CLAIM CODES (Designated by NUCC)	d. IS THERE ANOTHER HEALTH BENEFIT PLAN? ☐ YES ☒ NO If yes, complete items 9, 9a, and 9d.

READ BACK OF FORM BEFORE COMPLETING & SIGNING THIS FORM.

12. PATIENT'S OR AUTHORIZED PERSON'S SIGNATURE I authorize the release of any medical or other information necessary to process this claim. I also request payment of government benefits either to myself or to the party who accepts assignment below.

SIGNED **SOF** DATE _____

13. INSURED'S OR AUTHORIZED PERSON'S SIGNATURE I authorize payment of medical benefits to the undersigned physician or supplier for services described below.

SIGNED **SOF**

14. DATE OF CURRENT ILLNESS, INJURY, or PREGNANCY (LMP) MM DD YY QUAL.	15. OTHER DATE QUAL. MM DD YY	16. DATES PATIENT UNABLE TO WORK IN CURRENT OCCUPATION FROM MM DD YY TO MM DD YY

17. NAME OF REFERRING PROVIDER OR OTHER SOURCE	17a.	18. HOSPITALIZATION DATES RELATED TO CURRENT SERVICES FROM MM DD YY TO MM DD YY
	17b. NPI	

19. ADDITIONAL CLAIM INFORMATION (Designated by NUCC)	20. OUTSIDE LAB? ☐ YES ☒ NO $ CHARGES

21. DIAGNOSIS OR NATURE OF ILLNESS OR INJURY Relate A-L to service line below (24E) ICD Ind. **0**

A. F41.0	B. F17.210	C. Z82.49	D. Z82.5
E.	F.	G.	H.
I.	J.	K.	L.

22. RESUBMISSION CODE ___ ORIGINAL REF. NO. ___

23. PRIOR AUTHORIZATION NUMBER

PHYSICIAN OR SUPPLIER INFORMATION

24. A. DATE(S) OF SERVICE From MM DD YY To MM DD YY	B. PLACE OF SERVICE	C. EMG	D. PROCEDURES, SERVICES, OR SUPPLIES (Explain Unusual Circumstances) CPT/HCPCS MODIFIER	E. DIAGNOSIS POINTER	F. $ CHARGES	G. DAYS OR UNITS	H. EPSDT Family Plan	I. ID. QUAL.	J. RENDERING PROVIDER ID. #
1	12 01 YY 12 01 YY	11		99203	ABCD	85 00	1		NPI	1234567890
2	12 01 YY 12 01 YY	11		85025	ABC	95 00	1		NPI	1234567890
3	12 01 YY 12 01 YY	11		93000	ABC	75 00	1		NPI	1234567890
4	12 01 YY 12 01 YY	11		80053	ABC	75 00	1		NPI	1234567890
5	12 01 YY 12 01 YY	11		36415	ABC	15 00	1		NPI	1234567890
6									NPI	

25. FEDERAL TAX I.D. NUMBER SSN EIN	26. PATIENT'S ACCOUNT NO.	27. ACCEPT ASSIGNMENT? (For govt. claims, see back)	28. TOTAL CHARGE	29. AMOUNT PAID	30. Rsvd for NUCC Use
750246810 ☐ ☒	B2	☒ YES ☐ NO	$ 345 00	$	

31. SIGNATURE OF PHYSICIAN OR SUPPLIER INCLUDING DEGREES OR CREDENTIALS (I certify that the statements on the reverse apply to this bill and are made a part thereof.)	32. SERVICE FACILITY LOCATION INFORMATION	33. BILLING PROVIDER INFO & PH # (555) 555 1234
SIGNED PHIL WELLS MD DATE 12/01/20YY	a. NPI b.	CAPITAL CITY MEDICAL 123 UNKNOWN BLVD CAPITAL CITY NY 12345 a. 151317216 b.

NUCC Instruction Manual available at: www.nucc.org **PLEASE PRINT OR TYPE** APPROVED OMB-0938-1197 FORM 1500 (02-12)

Figure 17-12 ■ A completed CMS-1500 claim form.

The boxes to be completed on the CMS-1500 form are referred to as **Items**, *blocks*, or *form locators*. The form is divided into two major sections: Patient and Insured Information (Items 1–13) and Physician or Supplier Information (Items 14–33). The top right margin is the Carrier's Area and is used to print the insurance company's address on the form.

The National Uniform Claim Committee (**NUCC**), chaired by the American Medical Association (AMA), maintains and updates the CMS-1500 form. NUCC also provides specific guidelines for completing a CMS-1500 claim form that are consistent with those for preparing electronic claims. NUCC guidelines are published in the *1500 Health Insurance Claim Form Reference Instruction Manual* which is updated each year in July.

TRICARE, CHAMPVA, Medicare, Medicaid, and workers' compensation carriers each have their own rules for completing the CMS-1500 form. Private insurance companies also have their own variations. Because guidelines for completing the CMS-1500 vary at the state and local levels, the medical assistant should check with the local intermediaries and private carriers. For Blue Cross Blue Shield claims, the medical assistant should refer to the provider manual for their state's Blue Cross Blue Shield plans for guidelines.

When completing the form, medical assistants *abstract data*, meaning they use several source documents to find the required information. It is the medical assistant's responsibility to locate all needed data on established documents and accurately transfer it to the CMS-1500 form. Medical assistants obtain most information for completing the CMS-1500 from the patient registration form, the insurance card, the encounter form, and the medical record:

- The patient registration form provides information about the patient's and insured's name, address, birthdate, and related data.

- The insurance card provides information on the insurance policy, identification number, group number, mailing address for claims, as well as basic coverage and copayment information.

- The **encounter form** provides the date of service, services rendered, and treating provider. The encounter form may contain fees; if it does not, the medical assistant may need to refer to the clinic's fee schedule for charges. The encounter form or patient registration form may contain the clinic's address, tax identification number, and NPI numbers, or the medical assistant may need to refer to other office records for this information. Many names are used for encounter form, including *charge slip*, *routing slip*, *superbill*, or *multi-purpose billing form*.

- The medical record provides additional details that do not always appear on the encounter form, such as the date the illness, injury, or hospitalization began, supporting documentation for the diagnosis, and procedure reports.

Medical assistants may also need to refer to the EOB of a denied claim, referral forms, or other documents to complete some claims.

Table 17-4 provides general guidelines for completing the form and identifies the most common source documents needed for each item. Accuracy in identifying and transferring the data is essential. A single transposition mistake in a critical field such as name, identification number, birthdate, or CPT code could cause the claim to be rejected. A few extra minutes spent proofreading data helps prevent the need to rework claims later. An example of a completed CMS-1500 form appears in **Figure 17-12** ■.

▶▶ Pulse Points

Documenting the Medical Record

Any service billed by the medical office must be documented in the patient's medical record. Billing for services that have not been documented is considered fraud and is illegal. Therefore, it is crucial that all billed-for services are documented as services performed by members of the health care team. All diagnoses reported on claims should be documented by the physician as patient complaints or as outcomes of the examination.

▶▶ Pulse Points

Patient Account Numbers

While not required, it is a good idea to include the medical office's patient account number on the CMS-1500 claim form. This helps identify the patient when payment is received. Most insurance companies list offices' patient account numbers on the explanation of benefits, making patient accounts easier to find and payments easier to post in computer systems.

Optical Character Recognition The CMS-1500 form was developed so insurance carriers could process claims efficiently by optical character recognition (**OCR**). OCR devices (scanners) read printed or typed text and bar codes and convert it to data that the insurance company's computer can process. Scanners reduce the cost of data entry and decrease the processing time. OCR improves accuracy, thus reducing coding errors, because the claim is entered exactly as coded by the medical assistant.

The CMS-1500 form is printed in a specific color of red ink so that it is recognizable by OCR scanners. The red portion drops out, or becomes invisible to the scanner, so the scanner can read only the data entered. The office should not attempt to reprint or copy the form on a color device because the dropout red does not reproduce accurately. Original approved forms must be used.

Successful OCR begins with the proper submission of claims data. Keying a form for OCR scanning requires specific

TABLE 17-4 Instructions for Completing the CMS-1500 Claim Form

Item Number, Name, and Use (R = required; C = conditional, depending on claim)	Source Document
Carrier Area (top right hand margin) The carrier block is located in the upper center and right margin of the form. In order to distinguish this version of the form from previous versions, the Quick Response (QR) code symbol and the date approved by the NUCC have been added to the top, left hand margin. Enter the insurance plan's mailing address for claims from this policy. Be sure to verify. Some insurance companies have different addresses and different P.O. boxes for different types of plans, such as group, individual, or government. When printing page numbers on multiple page claims, print the page numbers in the Carrier Block on Line 8 beginning at column 32. Page numbers are to be printed as: Page XX of YY. This is generally done by clearinghouses when printing an electronic submission on the paper CMS-1500 claim form.	Insurance ID card
Items 1–13: PATIENT AND INSURED INFORMATION	
Item 1: Type of Insurance (R) Item 1 identifies what type of insurance the patient carries. The form lists five government plans: Medicare, Medicaid, TRICARE/CHAMPUS, CHAMPVA, and FECA/Black Lung. There are two other options: Group Health Plan and Other. Other indicates health insurance including HMOs, commercial insurance, automobile accident, liability, workers' compensation, and, usually, BCBS.	Insurance ID card
Item 1a: Insured's ID Number (R) In Item 1a, enter the insured's insurance ID number as given on the insurance card. The insured could be the patient or it could be someone else such as spouse, mother, or father. If the patient can be identified by a unique member identification number, the patient is considered to be the "insured." Report the patient as the insured in the insured data fields (Items 1a, 4, 5, and 7) and not in the patient fields (Items 2 and 5). For Workers Compensation Claims: Enter Employee ID For Other Property and Casualty Claims: Enter the Federal Tax ID or SSN of the insured person or entity.	Insurance ID card
Item 2: Patient's Name (C) In Item 2, enter the name of the patient who received services. This information is input last name, first name, and middle name or initial. The spelling should match the insurance card exactly. If the name on the card is misspelled, then the name in the computer should be misspelled until the patient provides a new card with the correct spelling. *When the patient is the insured, then it is not necessary to report the patient's name in Item 2.*	Patient registration form Encounter form
Item 3: Patient's Date of Birth/Sex (R) In Item 3, enter the patient's date of birth and sex/gender. Enter the date of birth using the eight-digit format: MMDDCCYY. Enter an X in the correct box for male or female. If gender is unknown, leave blank. Do not try to guess the gender based on the patient's name.	Patient registration form Encounter form
Item 4: Insured's Name (R) Item 4 is the name of the person who is the insured. This may or may not be the patient. The insured's name should be entered last name, first name, middle name or initial. If the patient can be identified by a unique Member Identification Number, the patient is considered to be the "insured." Report the patient as the insured in the insured data fields (Items 1a, 4, 5, and 7) and not in the patient fields (Items 2 and 5). For Workers Compensation Claims: Enter the name of the employer. For Other Property and Casualty Claims: Enter the name of the insured person or entity.	Insurance ID card
Item 5: Patient's Address (R) Enter the patient's home address and telephone number in Item 5, *if different from the insured's* address and telephone number. This information is taken from the patient information form when the patient registers in the office. The address includes the street name and number, city, state (two-letter abbreviation), and zip code. Do not use commas, periods, or other punctuation in the address. Do not use the # sign for apartment numbers. When entering a nine-digit zip code, include the hyphen. "Patient's Telephone" does not exist in the electronic claims standard, so NUCC recommends that the phone number *not* be reported. For Workers' Compensation and Other Property and Casualty Claims: If required by a payer to report a telephone number, do not use a hyphen or space as a separator within the telephone number.	Patient registration form

TABLE 17-4 Instructions for Completing the CMS-1500 Claim Form (*continued*)	
Item Number, Name, and Use (R = required; C = conditional, depending on claim)	**Source Document**
Item 6: Patient's Relationship to the Insured (R) After Item 4 has been completed, in Item 6 enter an X in the correct box to indicate the patient's relationship to the insured. Options include Self, Spouse, Child, or Other. If the patient is the insured person, the "Self" entry is marked here. Only one box can be marked. *If the patient is a dependent but has a unique member identification number* and the payer requires the identification number be reported on the claim, then report "Self," because the patient is reported as the insured.	Patient registration form
Item 7: Insured's Address (R) In Item 7, enter the insured's address. This information should include the street name and number, city, state (two-letter abbreviation), and zip code. "Insured's Telephone" does not exist in the electronic claims standard, so NUCC recommends that the phone number not be reported. For Workers Compensation Claims: Enter the address of the Employer.	Patient registration form
Item 8: Reserved for NUCC Use This field was previously used to report "Patient Status." "Patient Status" does not exist in the electronic claims standard, so this field has been eliminated. This field is reserved for NUCC use. The NUCC will provide instructions for any use of this field.	Patient registration form
Item 9: Other Insured's Name (C) If Item 11d is marked YES, also complete Items 9 and 9a–d; otherwise, leave them blank. Item 9 indicates that there is another policy that covers the patient. When there is additional group health coverage, enter the other insured's full last name, first name, and middle initial of the enrollee in another health plan if it is different from that shown in Item 2. If there is no secondary policy, leave this field blank.	Insurance ID card
Item 9a: Other Insured's Policy or Group Number (C) Enter the policy number or group number of the secondary insurance policy in Item 9a. Enter the number exactly as it appears on the insurance card.	Insurance ID card
Item 9b: Reserved for NUCC Use (C) Item 9b was previously used to report date of birth of the insured of the secondary policy. This data does not exist in the electronic claims standard, so this field has been eliminated. This field is reserved for NUCC use. The NUCC will provide instructions for any use of this field.	
Item 9c: Reserved for NUCC Use (C) Item 9c was previously used to report insured's employer or school. This data does not exist in the electronic claims standard, so this field has been eliminated. This field is reserved for NUCC use. The NUCC will provide instructions for any use of this field.	
Item 9d: Insurance Plan Name or Program Name (C) In Item 9d, enter the name of the secondary insurance plan, if any. This information is taken directly from the secondary insurance card. Enter the name exactly as it appears on the card.	Insurance ID card
Item 10a–c: Is Patient's Condition Related To? (R) Item 10 identifies whether the patient's visit was related to an employment accident, auto accident, or other accident. Enter an X in the correct box. Mark YES when filing workers' compensation claims, auto accident claims, or claims for other types of injuries. Mark NO when the patient's visit does not pertain to an accident. If this box is not marked, or is marked incorrectly, the claim could be delayed.	Encounter form Medical record
Item 10d: Claim Codes (C) Claim codes or condition codes, originally used on institutional claims, identify additional information about the patient's condition or the claim. A limited number of these codes are reported on the CMS-1500. The Condition Codes approved for use on the CMS-1500 Claim Form are available at www.nucc.org under Code Sets. For Medicaid Claims: Condition Codes are required to report the reason for an abortion. For Workers Compensation Claims: Condition Codes are required when submitting a bill that is a duplicate or an appeal. (Original Reference Number must be entered in Box 22 for these conditions). Do not use Condition Codes when submitting a revised or corrected bill.	
Item 11: Insured's Policy Group or FECA Number (C) If Item 4 is completed, then also complete Item 11. Item 11 identifies the insured's policy group number listed on the insurance card. This number should be entered exactly as it appears on the insurance card. For Workers' Compensation claims for Federal employees: Enter the FECA number (nine-digit alphanumeric identifier).	Insurance ID card

(continued)

TABLE 17-4 Instructions for Completing the CMS-1500 Claim Form (*continued*)	
Item Number, Name, and Use (R = required; C = conditional, depending on claim)	**Source Document**
Item 11a: Insured's Date of Birth/Sex (C) In Item 11a, list the date of birth of the insured that appears in Item 1a. Use the eight-digit format MMDDCCYY. Mark an X in either male or female accordingly. If gender is unknown, leave blank.	Insurance ID card Patient registration form
Item 11b: Other Claim ID (C) Item 11b is used only for Workers Compensation or Property and Casualty claims. Enter the qualifier Y4 (Property Casualty Claim Number) to the left of the vertical, dotted line. Enter the identifier number to the right of the vertical, dotted line.	Insurance ID card Patient registration form
Item 11c: Insurance Plan Name or Program Name (C) Item 11c identifies the insurance plan name. The information should be taken directly from the insurance card and spelled exactly as it appears on the card. Some payers require an identification number of the primary insurer rather than the name in this field.	Insurance ID card
Item 11d: Is There Another Health Benefit Plan? (R) In Item 11d, indicate whether there is another health benefit plan, in addition to the one shown in Item 1a. If there is another plan, mark YES with an X and enter the information into Items 9a–d. If there is no additional insurance plan, mark NO.	Patient registration form
Item 12: Patient's or Authorized Person's Signature (R) Item 12 is where the patient or guarantor signs, allowing the release of any medical information to the insurance company for billing purposes. This release is only valid for billing information. Any other request for records will require a formal release of information form to be signed by the patient or guarantor. This signature is good for one year from the date it is signed and should be updated annually. The words "Signature on File" or "SOF" may be printed here in place of a signature if a current signature is on file in the patient's chart. In this case, do not enter a date. If the patient signs the form, enter the date in the six-digit format (MM/DD/YY) or eight-digit format (MM/DD/CCYY). If there is no signature on file, leave blank or enter "No Signature on File."	Patient registration form
Item 13: Insured's or Authorized Person's Signature (C) Item 13 is where the patient or insured signs, authorizing the insurance company to reimburse the physician or supplier directly. The words "Signature on File" or "SOF" may be printed here in place of a signature if a current signature is on file in the patient's chart. In this case, do not enter a date. If the patient signs the form, enter the date in the six-digit format (MM/DD/YY) or eight-digit format (MM/DD/CCYY). If there is no signature on file, leave blank or enter "No Signature on File." Not required for government claims such as Medicare, Medicaid, or Workers' Compensation because those programs automatically send payment directly to participating providers.	Patient registration form
Items 14–33 PHYSICIAN OR SUPPLIER INFORMATION	
Item 14: Date of Current: Illness, Injury, Pregnancy (C) Report the first date of the current illness, injury, or pregnancy in Item 14. Use the six-digit (MMDDYY) or eight-digit format (MMDDCCYY). For a pregnancy, report the first day of the woman's last menstrual period (LMP). Enter one of the following qualifiers to the right of the vertical dotted line to identify which date is being reported. 431 Onset of Current Symptoms or Illness 484 Last Menstrual Period If this information is not known, leave blank.	Encounter form Medical record
Item 15: Other Date (C) Item 15 reports other dates related to the patient's condition or treatment. Use the six-digit (MMDDYY) or eight-digit (MMDDYYYY) format. Enter the applicable qualifier between the vertical, dotted lines after the word "Qualifier" to identify which date is being reported. 454 Initial Treatment 304 Latest Visit or Consultation 453 Acute Manifestation of a Chronic Condition 439 Accident 455 Last X-ray 471 Prescription 444 First Visit or Consultation Previous pregnancies are not a similar illness. Leave this field blank if unknown.	Encounter form Medical record

TABLE 17-4 Instructions for Completing the CMS-1500 Claim Form *(continued)*	
Item Number, Name, and Use (R = required; C = conditional, depending on claim)	**Source Document**
Item 16: Dates Patient Unable to Work in Current Occupation (C) In Item 16, list the dates the patient is unable to work due to his illness or injury. These dates are required when filing workers' compensation or disability claims. Use the six-digit (MMDDYY) or eight-digit format (MMDDCCYY). If the information is not required, leave blank.	Encounter form Medical record
Item 17: Name of Referring Physician or Other Source (C) Item 17 requests the name of the provider who referred, ordered, or supervised the services on the claim. Some insurance companies, such as health maintenance organizations (HMOs) or exclusive provider organizations (EPOs), require the referring provider to be reported here. Enter the provider's last name, first name, and credentials. Enter the applicable qualifier code to the left of the vertical, dotted line. If multiple providers are involved, enter one provider using the following priority order and Qualifier: **1.** DN Referring provider **2.** DK Ordering provider **3.** DQ Supervising provider	Encounter form Referral form
Item 17a: Other ID # (C) Enter the non-NPI identification number of the referring, ordering, or supervising provider in Item 17a, if required by the plan. In the Qualifier field, enter the two-character designation of what type of ID number is being reported: 0B State License Number 1G Provider UPIN Number G2 Provider Commercial Number LU Location Number (This qualifier is used for Supervising Provider only.)	Referral form
Item 17b: NPI Number (C) Enter the NPI number of the referring, ordering, or supervising provider in Item 17b.	Referral form
Item 18: Hospitalization Dates Related to Current Services (C) In Item 18, enter the hospital admission and discharge dates the patient was hospitalized as an inpatient. Use the six-digit (MMDDYY) or eight-digit format (MMDDCCYY).	Encounter form or medical record
Item 19: Additional Claim Information (C) Item 19 is required by some payers to report certain identifiers such as alternate provider numbers and provider taxonomy codes. Each identifier requires a two-character Qualifier. Refer to the most current instructions from the applicable public or private payer regarding the use of this field. NUCC provides a list of qualifiers to be used. For Workers' Compensation: Enter the type of attachment or supplemental claim information if required. Enter PWK followed by the NUCC approved code(s) for report type and transmission type.	
Item 20: Outside Lab (C) Item 20 is used only if lab tests appear in section 24. If the physician's office is billing on behalf of an outside lab, mark YES. This indicates that an entity other than the entity billing for the service performed the purchased services. Enter the purchased price under Charges and complete Item 32. If the lab tests were performed by the provider's office mark NO. If no lab tests were ordered, leave this Item blank.	Encounter form Medical record
Item 21: Diagnosis or Nature of Illness or Injury (R) In Item 21, enter the patient's ICD diagnosis code(s) for this claim. In the upper right corner, enter the number to identify which version of codes is being reported: 9 ICD-9-CM 0 ICD-10-CM Enter between one and 12 codes, in order of priority. Line 1 is the primary diagnosis. Enter the decimal point as part of the code number. Do not enter narrative descriptions. Ensure that the diagnosis codes support the medical necessity of the services (CPT codes) listed in Item 24D. Relate each diagnosis (A-I) to the lines of service in 24E by letter (A, B, C, etc.).	Encounter form Medical record
Item 22: Resubmission Code and Original Reference Number (C) If required, use Item 22 on **resubmitted** claims to report the payer's reference number for the original claim. Enter the appropriate bill frequency code left justified in the left hand side of the field. 7 Replacement of prior claim 8 Void/cancel of prior claim Consult with the payer for specific instructions on the use of this Item.	EOB Phone call to insurance company

(continued)

TABLE 17-4 Instructions for Completing the CMS-1500 Claim Form (*continued*)	
Item Number, Name, and Use (R = required; C = conditional, depending on claim)	**Source Document**
Item 23: Prior Authorization Number (C) Some insurance plans, such as those of HMOs and PPOs, require a prior authorization number. If required, when preauthorization is obtained from an insurance company for services, enter the number assigned in Item 23. HMOs may require that referral numbers be entered here. If this field is left blank when the payer requires prior authorization or referral, the claim will be denied. If no prior authorization is required, leave blank.	Referral form
Section 24 The six service lines in Section 24 are divided horizontally to accommodate submission of supplemental information. Enter the service information in the *white* portion of each line. Each CPT code must be entered on a separate line. When the same CPT code is provided multiple times, on non-sequential dates, use a separate line for each date and repeat the CPT code. When the same CPT code is provided multiple times on a single date, enter the date once in Item 24A and enter the number of procedures in Item 24G. Enter the appropriate NUCC qualifier and code for supplemental information in the *shaded* portion. Providers must verify requirements for supplemental information with the payer. Supplemental information that may be entered includes: • Narrative description of unspecified codes • National Drug Codes (NDC) for drugs • Vendor Product Number—Health Industry Business Communications Council (HIBCC) • Product Number Health Care Uniform Code Council—Global Trade Item Number (GTIN), formerly Universal Product Code (UPC) for products • Contract rate • Tooth numbers and areas of the oral cavity	
Item 24A: Dates of Service (R) In Item 24A, enter the dates of service for the service provided as listed in the CPT code. Use the six-digit format (MM/DD/YY). Use a separate line for each CPT code. When the same CPT code is provided on multiple, sequential dates, enter both the "From" date and the "To" date. When there is only one date of service for a CPT code, as is frequently the case in physician offices, payers require varying formats for this Item. Some payers require that the both the "To" and "From" dates to be entered. Some require that only the "From" date be listed.	Encounter form Medical record
Item 24B: Place of Service (R) Place of service in Item 24B is a mandatory field because it describes the place where the procedure or service was performed. The most common places of service are the physician's office, hospital, emergency department, or skilled nursing facility. Enter the Place of Service Code (see following list) in the white portion of this field. Note that the CMS has stated that if the place of service is other than the provider's normal location in FL32, the place of service must be fully written out in Item 32. Consider this example: The patient was an inpatient (at the hospital) and the physician saw the patient in the hospital for an evaluation and management service. Therefore, the code 21 (see following list) would be entered in Item 24B and the name and address of the hospital entered in Item 32: Common place-of-service codes include the following: 11 Physician's office 20 Urgent care facility 21 Inpatient hospital 22 Outpatient hospital 23 Hospital emergency department 31 Skilled nursing facility	Encounter form Medical record
Item 24C: EMG (Emergency) (C) Item 24C is used only with Medicaid to indicate whether the service was provided on an emergency basis. Enter Y for YES. Leave blank for NO or not applicable. The definition of an emergency is defined differently by each payer.	Encounter form Medical record
Item 24D: Procedures, Services, or Supplies (R) In Item 24D, enter the CPT or HCPCS code to identify the procedures, services, or supplies provided. Also enter up to four modifiers in Item 24D. Do not enter the narrative description of the code. Enter each unique CPT or HCPCS code on a separate line. Use only the white portion of the line for CPT and HCPCS codes. If more than six codes are required, continue the claim to a second page. Do not use the gray portion of the line to accommodate more than six codes.	Encounter form Medical record

TABLE 17-4 Instructions for Completing the CMS-1500 Claim Form (*continued*)	
Item Number, Name, and Use (R = required; C = conditional, depending on claim)	**Source Document**
Item 24E: Diagnosis Pointer (R) Item 24E indicates the reference letter (A–L) of the diagnosis code in Item 21 as it relates to each service or procedure. If more than one diagnosis is attached to a single procedure or service, enter the primary diagnosis first, followed by the additional diagnoses. Up to four letters may be entered, with no spaces or commas between them. Do not enter the actual code number, only the reference letter. Be certain that each CPT code has a corresponding diagnosis code to justify the need. Some payers, such as Medicare, require only one diagnosis reference number per service.	Encounter form Medical record
Item 24F: Charges (R) Item 24F lists the charges for each CPT or HCPCS code listed. The amount should be entered without a decimal point or dollar sign. Enter 00 in the cents area if the charge is an even dollar amount. If multiple units are entered in Item 24G, the charges should reflect the total charges for amount of the procedure *times* the number of units. It is not a per unit charge. The charge entered should be the provider's established fee schedule, not the discounted or contracted rate. Medicare claims should contain the Medicare fee schedule charge.	Encounter form Physician fee schedule
Item 24G: Days or Units (R) Enter the number of units per procedure or service provided to a patient in Item 24G. If multiple units are entered in 24G, the charges should reflect the amount of the procedure multiplied by the number of units. This field is most commonly used for multiple visits, units of supplies, anesthesia units or minutes, or oxygen volume. If only one service is performed, enter "1." For anesthesia, report the number of *minutes*. Report units for anesthesia services only when the code description includes a time period (such as "daily management"). When required by payers to provide supplemental information such as the National Drug Code (NDC) units in addition to the HCPCS units, enter the applicable NDC units' qualifier and related units in the shaded line. The following qualifiers are to be used when reporting NDC units: F2 International Unit, ML Milliliter, GR Gram, UN Unit.	Encounter form Medical record
Item 24H: EPSDT Family Plan (C) Item 24H is used on Medicaid claims only, to identify whether the patient is receiving her services through Medicaid's Early and Periodic Screening, Diagnosis, and Treatment (EPSDT) program. Enter "Y" for yes or "N" for no or follow state-specific guidelines.	Insurance (Medicaid) ID card
Item 24I: ID Qualifier (C) If the insurance plan requires use of a plan specific provider ID number for the provider who delivered the service, enter the code for type of plan in the shaded portion of 24I. Otherwise, leave blank.	Office records
Item 24J: Rendering Provider (R) The provider rendering the service is reported in Item 24J. Enter the NPI number in the unshaded area of the field. If the insurance plan also requires use of a plan-specific provider ID number for the provider who delivered the service, or if the provider does not have an NPI, enter Qualifier in 24I and the other ID number in the shaded portion of 24J. Otherwise, leave the shaded portion blank.	Encounter form Medical record
Item 25: Federal Tax ID Number (R) In Item 25 enter the provider's federal tax ID number or the employer identification number (EIN) of the billing entity. This number should be consistent with the billing provider listed in Item 33. Do not enter hyphens with numbers. The appropriate box (SSN or EIN) should be marked with an X.	Encounter form Office records
Item 26: Patient's Account Number (C) In Item 26, enter the patient's account number assigned by the medical office. The computer system used in the office will generate the number and it should be entered on the claim. This in turn will allow for the account number to appear on the Explanation of Benefits (EOB) form, which makes it easier to locate the correct patient to post insurance payments.	Encounter form Medical record
Item 27: Accept Assignment? (C) Item 27 is used with Medicare claims to indicate whether or not the physician accepts assignment on this claim. PAR physicians must always mark YES. Non-PAR physicians must select YES or NO on each claim.	Encounter form Office records
Item 28: Total Charge (R) Item 28 lists the total charges, added together from those listed in Item 24F. The charges should be checked for accuracy to ensure proper reimbursement. Do not use decimal points or dollar signs in this entry. Enter 00 in the cents field if the amount is a whole number.	Calculator

(*continued*)

TABLE 17-4 Instructions for Completing the CMS-1500 Claim Form *(continued)*	
Item Number, Name, and Use (R = required; C = conditional, depending on claim)	**Source Document**
Item 29: Amount Paid (C) Item 29 indicates the amount paid by primary insurance when submitting secondary claims. This amount is added after the primary EOB is received and payment is posted. A secondary claim is printed to be sent to the secondary insurance carrier along with a copy of the primary insurance carrier's EOB. Do not use decimal points or dollar signs in this entry. Do not enter any patient payments unless instructed to do so by the insurance plan. Some managed care plans require copayments to be reported here.	Encounter form
Item 30: Reserved for NUCC Use (C) Item 30 was previously used to report "Balance Due." This data does not exist in the electronic claims standard, so the field has been eliminated. This field is reserved for NUCC use. The NUCC will provide instructions for any use of this field.	
Item 31: Signature of Physician or Supplier Including Degrees or Credentials (R) In Item 31, enter the legal signature of the physician or supplier who has provided the services to the patient along with professional credentials (M.D., PA-C, or NP). "Signature on File" or "SOF" is also acceptable in this Item. Enter a six-digit date (MM/DD/YY), eight-digit date (MM/DD/CCYY), or alphanumeric date (Month 30, 20YY). A signature stamp may be used instead of a written signature. The stamp must leave a clear, non-smeared image on the claim.	Typed Signature stamp
Item 32: Name and Address of Facility Where Services Were Rendered (C) Item 32 identifies the name of the facility where services were provided. Enter the name, address, zip code, and NPI number. When more than one supplier is used, use a separate CMS-1500 form for each supplier.	Encounter form Medical record
Item 32a: NPI Number (C) Enter the NPI number of the service facility location in Item 32a.	Encounter form Office records
Item 32b: Other ID Number (C) If required by the insurance plan, enter the Qualifier and plan-specific ID number in the shaded portion.	Encounter form Office records
Item 33: Billing Provider Information and Phone Number (R) Enter the provider's or supplier's billing name, address, zip code, and phone number in Item 33. This should be the same entity as the Tax ID in Item 25. Enter the phone number in the area to the right of the field title. Electronic claims require a physical location, not a P.O. Box, and NUCC recommends that the physical address be entered in on the CMS-1500 form as well. Enter the name and address information in the following format: First line: Name Second line: Address Third line: City, state, and zip code.	Encounter form Office records
Item 33a: NPI Number (R) Enter the NPI number of the billing provider in Item 33a.	Encounter form Office records
Item 33b: Other ID Number (C) If required by the insurance plan, enter the Qualifier and plan-specific ID number in the shaded portion.	Encounter form Office records

techniques. Printed characters must conform to the preprogrammed specifications relative to character size and alignment on the CMS-1500 form. OCR guidelines include:

- Use original approved forms only.
- Use all capital letters.
- Use a standard mono-spaced serif font (one that has little lines on the ends of the letters such as Courier).
- Do not use any punctuation such as . , / # -.
- Keep all text within the boundaries of the red box for each Item.
- Use eight digit dates for birthdates. Other dates can be either six or eight digits, but should be consistent.
- Do not erase, strike out, overtype, or white out. If you make a mistake, start over.

- Do not use highlighters or pen to make any extra markings on the form.
- Do not tape or staple anything to the form.

HIPAA Compliance

Once completed, CMS-1500 claim forms contain confidential patient information. As a result, these forms must be protected from view by anyone who is unauthorized to see patient information. Keep these forms in a secure area, never in a nonsecure area, even when in envelopes. When errors are made on CMS-1500 claim forms and new ones must be printed, shred the forms with errors to protect patient privacy.

Electronic Transactions

One of the purposes of HIPAA is to standardize how electronic transmissions are handled. Electronic transactions, also called electronic data interchange (EDI), are exchanges involving the computerized transfer of health care information between two parties for specific purposes, such as a health care provider submitting medical claims to a health plan for payment. Version 5010 is the set of standards used for all health care transactions.

Each process that was once handled on paper has a corresponding electronic format. Just as the CMS-1500 form is the standard for paper claims, the 837P is the standard format for electronic claims. Each data element in the 837P corresponds to a field on the CMS-1500. In addition to submitting claims, medical assistants may use electronic transactions for tracking claim status, receiving EOBs, coordination of benefits, eligibility inquiries, referrals, and authorization requests.

Electronic claims, also called electronic media claims (EMC), are the leading method of claims submission by providers. Electronic claims are never printed on paper and may be submitted to the insurance carrier via direct data entry, direct wire, telephone line via modem, or disc. When claims are sent electronically to the insurance carriers for processing, an electronic signature is used to verify that the information received is true and correct. Medicare requires electronic transmission of claims for providers with 10 or more employees or facilities with 25 or more employees. Paper claims will not be processed for these submitters.

Electronic claims have a number of advantages:

- Administrative costs are lower because fewer personnel hours are needed to prepare forms, and supply and postage costs are lower.
- Fewer claims are rejected because technical errors are detected and corrected before the claim arrives at the payer.
- Processing is faster with fewer errors. An electronic claim is received by the payer in minutes. The payer does not have to perform data entry, so there is less opportunity for errors to be introduced. In addition, most claims can be automatically adjudicated by the computer, rather than being processed by a claims analyst.
- Errors can be corrected faster. If errors are found on claims by carriers or the claim is denied, the office is notified immediately and medical assistants can begin work on resolving the issue.
- Payment is faster. Payment can be transferred electronically to the provider's bank, eliminating delays in cash flow. These payments are referred to as electronic remittances. Medicare is required by law to process electronic claims in 14 days, and is prohibited from processing paper claims for at least 28 days after receipt.

Electronic claims also have disadvantages:

- Claims transmission can be disrupted occasionally due to power failures, or computer hardware or software problems that might require claims to be resubmitted.

- Many patient billing programs cannot create an electronic attachment, so when a claim attachment is required, the electronic claim must be sent separately from mailed attachments, which sometimes causes problems for the payer in matching up the two. In some cases, the claim must instead be submitted on paper when it must be accompanied by a claim attachment.

Medical assistants enter patient, insurance, and service information into practice management software, which then converts the data into the standard format required by HIPAA. Claims may be submitted daily, weekly, or on any schedule the office determines is best.

Electronic claims are submitted through a clearinghouse, a billing service, or directly to the carrier. A physician who plans to use electronic billing must contact all major insurers and carriers for a list of the vendors approved to handle electronic claims, and must have a signed agreement with each. Each carrier has special electronic billing requirements and is knowledgeable in which systems meet their criteria and which are compatible in format. Insurance carriers also provide information about how to submit an electronic bill for patients who have secondary coverage.

Medicare, Medicaid, TRICARE, and many private insurance carriers allow providers to submit insurance claims directly to them with no "middle man." In this type of system, the medical practice must have special software or the physician must lease a terminal from the carrier to key in claims data. The data is transmitted via modem (dedicated telephone line) directly to the carrier's computer for processing. Medicare provides software and training for electronic submissions of Medicare claims.

If the physician is not sending the data directly to the carrier, he or she may use a clearinghouse. A clearinghouse is a company that receives claims from providers, processes them through a series of audits to check for errors, and then forwards them to the appropriate insurance carrier in the required data format. Clearinghouses may charge a flat fee per claim or charge a percentage of the claim's dollar value. It is very important for physicians' practices to negotiate the best possible fee for using a clearinghouse's services.

The clearinghouse conducts an audit to determine if any data on the claim is incorrect or missing. A claim with incorrect or missing information is a dirty claim, and is not transmitted to the carrier. The results of the audit are sent back to the provider from the clearinghouse in the form of an audit/edit report. The medical assistant needs to correct any claims with incorrect data (as indicated on the audit/edit report) and resubmit them to the clearinghouse. When the claims are corrected and resubmitted to the clearinghouse, they are **clean claims**, which are then formatted and forwarded to the carrier. Each time the claim is returned there is an additional charge, so the medical assistant should ensure that clean claims are transmitted initially.

Filing Timelines

Most insurance carriers accept claims up to 1 year from the date of service, although some have much shorter timelines, such as

90 days. After filing timelines pass, claims are considered past timely filing limits and will likely be rejected. With most managed care plans, claims rejected due to timely filing limits cannot be billed to the patient. To avoid rejection, it is best to submit claims soon after service is rendered.

Sending Supporting Documentation

Many insurance plans require supporting documentation, such as chart notes, surgical/operative reports, laboratory reports, or pathology reports, before they agree to pay for certain, usually high-cost services, such as surgeries (**Figure 17-13** ■). When

---

OPERATION DATE: 10/17/xx

SURGEON: GREGORY PROVENCE, MD

PREOPERATIVE DIAGNOSIS:

Right parotid mass.

POSTOPERATIVE DIAGNOSIS:

Same.

PROCEDURE:

Right deep lobe parotid resection, removal of right parotid tumor with facial nerve preservation and with facial nerve monitoring.

DESCRIPTION OF PROCEDURE:

The patient is a 54-year old female who noted a growing mass in the right parotid area. Fine needle biopsy reported benign cells and CT scan confirmed a large bilobed cystic lesion. Risks, expectations, complications, procedure and alternative treatment measures were discussed prior to consent.

FINDINGS:

A bilobed tumor extending medial to the facial nerve branches into the "turquoise" space superior to the thyroid process and most of the deep lobe parotid were absent. Facial nerve was preserved with the facial nerve monitoring.

General endotracheal anesthesia was given. 1% Xylocaine was used for facial skin infiltration. Incision was drawn with an ink pen and incision was carried along the preauricular crease around the "yellow" lobule to the upper neck along the skin crease. Incision carried through the platysmas and the sternomastoid muscle and the external ear canal. The posterior facial vein was identified and dissected laterally, lifting the gland away from the facial vein for the purpose of identifying the lower branch of the facial nerve. Superiorly, the facial branch was identified. It was then carefully preserved and as the parotid gland was lifted, the superficial lobe of the parotid gland was lifted laterally and anteriorly. The lower division of the facial nerve was found and medial to the nerve was the tumor. The tumor was then gently grasped with forceps and the lower division was carefully lifted and shifted superiorly as the tumor was shifted inferiorly for excision. Blunt and sharp dissection was made to free the nerve from surrounding tissue. The deep lobe of the parotid was generally absent because of the size of the mass. The mass was cylindrical bilobed-shaped, and extending beyond the styloid process, placed superior to the styloid process into the "turquoise" space.

Finally the entire tumor was isolated and removed. Bleeding was controlled with bipolar cautery. An Avitene sheet was used for hemostasis. A 15 Blake drain was inserted, secured with 3-0 nylon. The skin incision was closed with 4-0 chromic and 5-0 nylon. Blood loss was about 25 cc. Dressing applied. Antibiotic ointment was placed on the incision.

The patient was then extubated and sent to the recovery room in good condition. Postop facial nerve function was intact. She was given Keflex for prophylaxis and Lortab 7.5 mg for pain. She will be seen as needed and drain will be removed in the next 48 hours.

GREGORY PROVENCE, MD

Figure 17-13 ■ Sample operative report.

calling insurance carriers to obtain preauthorization for services, medical assistants should ask customer service representatives if they need supporting documentation with the insurance claim forms. Sending proper documentation with the initial billing, when required, helps avoid delayed payment. Most claims that require attachments must be prepared on paper, although insurance companies increasingly have the ability to accept electronic attachments.

The insurance company may ask for additional documentation while reviewing the claim. The request usually comes in the form of a letter. When replying to such requests, medical assistants should be certain to identify exactly what information is being requested and respond specifically. It is not necessary to send a voluminous amount of records when only one or two specific items are requested.

With workers' compensation and other third-party liability claims, carriers may request a progress report. A written progress report clearly describes the extent of the patient's recovery since the injury, what further treatment is needed, and the expected result. Include any test results such as X-rays, lab tests, or physical function tests, such as range of motion or lifting capacity, to document the patient's status. Medical assistants should respond to such requests immediately because no further payment will be made on the claim until the report is received. Medical assistants may have the responsibility of abstracting the pertinent information from the medical record, drafting the report, and presenting it to the provider for review and signature.

Working with Reimbursement Schedules

As a result of the growth of managed care and ongoing concerns about controlling health care costs, insurance companies use a variety of methods to determine how much to pay providers. Medical assistants need to understand how the payment method impacts the practice.

Physician Fee Schedules

Providers may use a variety of methods in determining their fee structure (the amount charged for each procedure performed). Physicians are free to set their fees at any level they believe fairly reflects the cost of providing a service and the value of their professional judgment and skill. The most common methods used to establish fees are charge-based fees and resources-based fees.

Charge-Based Fee Schedules A charge-based fee schedule is determined by comparing the fees that other providers charge for similar services. To determine how their fees for specific services compare with other providers of the same specialty, they may purchase information from a nationwide fee database. For each procedure code, the database reports the average fee amounts, as well as the highest and lowest amount, charged by similar providers within a zip code region.

It shows what percentage of providers charge above or below that amount. Based on this research, providers can decide if their fees should be on the high, low, or midpoint of the range.

Resource-Based Fee Structures Resource-based fee structures, also called relative value systems (RVS) are determined objectively, based on the factors that contribute to a provider's costs. Three types of costs are considered:

1. **Work**—the difficulty level for the provider to perform the procedure
2. **Practice expense**—the amount of office overhead involved in the procedure
3. **Malpractice**—the relative risk that the procedure presents to the patient and the provider

These cost elements, also referred to as the **relative value unit (RVU)**, are added together to determine the fee for a particular procedure.

Medicare's Resource-Based Relative Value Scale The Medicare physician fee schedule (**MPFS**) is a list of approved Medicare fees for each procedure. The resource-based relative value scale (**RBRVS**) is Medicare's relative value system formula. Medical offices receive a comprehensive MPFS from Medicare each year that is usually programmed into the computer system, so medical assistants do not normally need to calculate individual fees. However, it can be helpful to have a basic understanding of how Medicare determines its fees.

The RBRVS formula has three components:

1. National relative value unit (RVU)
2. **Geographic adjustment factor (GAF)**
3. National uniform **conversion factor (CF)**

The RVU reflects the type of work a physician does, office overhead expense, and the cost of the provider's medical malpractice insurance. An RVU of 1.0 represents the average procedure. A more complicated procedure has a higher RVU and a less complicated service has a lower RVU. The second component of RBRVS, the GAF, considers the area of the country in which a physician practices, adjusting higher or lower based on that area's cost of living. The third component of RBRVS, the CF, is a dollar amount used to convert the RVU and GAF for each service into the price that Medicare allows. Each year, Medicare adjusts the CF according to the cost-of-living index.

The RBRVS formula helps ensure that different Medicare providers are reimbursed equally for the same service, with appropriate adjustments for costs in various parts of the country.

Insurance Plan Reimbursement Schedules

Insurance companies are not obligated to pay the amount the physician charges and usually establish their own reimbursement schedules. Before agreeing to participate with any insurance plan, health care providers should carefully review the reimbursement schedules the managed care companies provide. After contracts are in place, physicians have little leverage to adjust payment amounts and may find some, or all, fees are lower than they can afford to accept. Insurance companies may adopt a reimbursement schedule based on provider fees or they may use a risk-based approach.

Fee-Based Reimbursement

Fee-based reimbursement determines the payment amount in relationship to the provider's published fee schedule. This is usually determined by a usual, customary, and reasonable (UCR) fee or a negotiated discount.

Usual, Customary, and Reasonable (UCR) Reimbursement   The most traditional reimbursement method is a usual, customary, and reasonable (UCR) schedule maintained by each insurance company. The insurer establishes an acceptable fee, referred to as *customary*, based on the range of what other providers of the same specialty in the same geographic area charge. The insurer pays the lesser of either this amount or the provider's normal fee, referred to as *usual*. In unusual circumstances, they negotiate a specific fee, referred to as *reasonable*, for a given bill. The insurer is not required to publicize their UCR, so the practice learns by experience the amount each company approves.

Negotiated or Discounted Fee Schedule   A common reimbursement method of PPOs is a **negotiated fee schedule**. The managed care plan develops of list of fees for providers that they agree to accept. Fees may be determined based on a percentage of the provider's usual fee (for example, 80 percent) or may be arrived at through negotiation.

Risk-Based Reimbursement

Risk-based reimbursement methods are those in which the provider shares responsibility for minimizing the cost of care. Insurance companies believe this type of reimbursement discourages physicians from ordering unnecessary or costly procedures. The disadvantage is that it may also discourage physicians from providing medically necessary services, due to potential financial penalties.

Capitation   The most common risk-based reimbursement for physicians is **capitation**. Capitation, which literally means "per head" pays providers a flat amount per member per month, regardless of what services the patient uses. If a patient comes in many times, or not at all, the provider receives the same payment. This method is most often used by HMOs. The objective of capitation is to put the responsibility and risk on the provider to manage the patient's care in a cost effective, yet medically appropriate, manner.

Per Diem   For inpatient care, a *per diem* or *per day* payment method may be used. The insurance company pays the facility a flat amount per day the patient is in the hospital, regardless of what services are provided. This method places much cost management on the facility to provide the services that are medically appropriate because they will not be paid more if they provide unnecessary services. The risk is partially shared

with the insurer, who pays more for a longer stay than a shorter one. However, there may be a maximum number days that the insurance company pays for any given condition.

Per Case   *Per case* payment is also used for hospitals. Under this method, the insurance company pays the hospital a pre-established amount per patient for the entire stay, based on the patient's diagnosis, regardless of how long they are in or what services are provided. Medicare uses a form of per-case reimbursement, which is called **Medicare Severity-Adjusted Diagnosis-Related Groups (MS-DRG)**, because patients with similar conditions and care requirements are classified or grouped together and all are eligible for the same amount of reimbursement.

Under all risk-based reimbursement methods, insurance companies usually make additional payments for **outliers**, or exceptional circumstances that cost far more or far less than the average. Most contracts also include *carve outs*, services that are reimbursed in addition to the base rate for the patient. The details of each MCO contract are different; there are no general rules. The medical assistant needs to become familiar with the details of each contract the provider has to be sure the billing and payment are appropriate.

Receiving Payments

To post insurance payments, medical assistants must read and interpret the explanation of benefits, enter data into the computer, and follow up on unpaid claims. After the payer has processed the claim, the provider receives a check or electronic deposit and an explanation of benefits (EOB). Depending on the sophistication of the provider's computer system, the payment can be automatically posted to the patient's account or the medical assistant might need to manually enter it into the computer or manual bookkeeping system. If the medical assistant is responsible for posting payments, she also reconciles the EOB by comparing the EOB to the original bill to verify that each service billed was paid in the amount expected.

Explanation of Benefits (EOB)

After an insurance carrier has processed a claim, a check is sent to the health care provider with an **Explanation of Benefits** (EOB) statement. With large insurance carriers, providers may receive one EOB and check as payment for several patients. The EOB lists the name of the patient, the name of the insured, the date of service, the amount billed, the amount allowed, the amount paid, and the amount the provider may bill the patient. Medical assistants must check EOBs to ensure all services that were billed are accurately listed and that service payment matches the amount in the insurance company contract.

An EOB is not always accompanied by payment, but it does state the status of unpaid claims, such as *pending*. A pending claim is one that is received but not processed by the carrier because additional information is needed or because it contains an error. When claims are submitted electronically, the electronic EOB is referred to as the *Electronic Remittance Advice* (ERA). The EOB lists the patient, dates of services, types of service, and the charges filed on the insurance claim form. The EOB also describes how the amount of the benefit payment was determined. If claim forms were filed for more than one patient with the same insurance carrier at the same time, the provider's EOB can include information on more than one patient.

The format and contents of each EOB vary based on the benefit plan and the services provided. No universal form for explaining benefits is available. Terminology is also different on various EOBs. For example, some EOBs show the "Allowed Amount or Charge" and some EOBs read "Deducted Amount." The medical assistant eventually becomes accustomed to the carriers with whom the provider contracts, but should always review all EOBs carefully prior to entering data.

Insurance carriers often use reason codes or remark codes on the EOB to identify reasons for payment adjustments and denials. These are usually three or four character alphanumeric codes, for which a key appears on the face or back of the EOB. Reason codes provide important information about how the insurance company processed the claim. Although the format of EOBs varies among insurance companies, policy information, service information, and payment information is always provided (**Figure 17-14** ■).

Policy information

1. Insurance company name
2. Name of employer or group
3. Date the EOB statement was finalized
4. Member's or insured's name and ID number
5. Patient's identification number as it appears on his ID card
6. Control number assigned to the claim

Service information:

7. Name of the person who received the service (the patient)
8. Provider's name
9. Dates of the services provided (DOS)
10. Procedures performed (CPT codes)
11. Total charge for each procedure

Coverage determination:

12. The contractual allowed amount
13. Patient's copayment or coinsurance amount
14. Patient's deductible
15. Non-covered procedures or amounts
16. Total payment to the provider
17. The total amount that is the patient's responsibility

After medical assistants post the patient's payment to the specific date and procedure, they often need to make an adjustment. An adjustment is a positive or negative change to a patient's account balance. Corrections, changes, and write-offs to patients' accounts are made by means of adjustments to the

existing transactions. The medical assistant also adjusts a patient's bill as a result of any discounts given. If the provider is participating in the plan, the medical assistant adjusts off (subtracts) the difference between the billed amount and the allowed amount so the patient is not billed. When providers contract with insurance carriers, they must accept the allowed amount of the claim as payment in full. Billing the patient for the difference between the billed amount and the allowed amount, a practice called balance billing, violates the health care provider's contract with the insurance carrier. **Figure 17-15** ■ shows how this works. If providers are not contracted with the carriers, they should balance bill.

When patients have defined copayment amounts, those copays should be collected at the time of service. When patients owe coinsurance or deductible amounts, medical assistants bill patients after receiving the EOB and payment.

Secondary Insurance

When patients have a secondary insurance policy, it is billed after the primary policy has paid. This is because the secondary company needs to know how much the primary company paid in order to determine benefits. In some cases the secondary insurance pays 100 percent of the balance remaining and in other cases, it does not. The calculations depend on the provisions of each policy.

To bill secondary insurance, medical assistants create a CMS-1500 form, attach a copy of EOB from the primary insurance, and send the entire package to the secondary company.

The secondary CMS-1500 is identical to the one sent to the primary with two changes:

1. Enter the name and address of the secondary insurance company in the Carrier Area.
2. Enter the amount paid by the primary insurance company in Item 29.

When an office uses computer software to create CMS-1500 forms, the software normally generates a form for the secondary company with the required changes. When submitting electronic claims, some insurance companies automatically forward the EOB information to the secondary company, eliminating the need for a second billing by the medical office.

Claims Followup

Claims followup is an important part of the insurance billing process, because medical assistants must ensure that all claims are processed and paid correctly by the insurance company. Some claims can be delayed, meaning it takes longer than usual to receive payment. Other claims might contain services that are denied and some claims can be denied in their entirety.

Most medical office software can print a variety of reports that list past due claims, making it easy to identify the claims that require further investigation. An aging report lists all outstanding insurance claims and identifies how long it has been since the claim was submitted, using date ranges, such as less than 30 days, 31–60 days, 61–90 days, 91–120 days, and over 130 days.

Explanation of Benefits

¹ Ultimate Medical Plan

CHRIS PATIENT
999 MAIN STREET
ANYTOWN WA 99999

This is not a bill.
³ 06/08/20YY

⁵ Your ID Number: W125370058
⁴ Subscriber Name: CHRIS R LONEMA
⁷ Patient Name CHRIS R LONEMA
⁶ Claim Number: K100925-0038
² Group Name: XYZ Company

Provider Information

⁸ CATHERINE S JONES MD
2525 NE 44TH ST
ANYTOWN WA 99999

If you have questions, contact us:

By Mail:
Ultimate Medical Plan
PO Box 0000
New York, NY 10000

By Phone/E-mail:
Local: 425-555-3000
Toll Free: 1-800-555-6004
E-mail: abc@ump.xxx

Provider Name: ⁹	Date(s) of Service	¹⁰ Service(s) Provided	¹¹ Amount Charged	¹² Allowed	PPO Savings	¹⁵ Non-Cov'd Amount	Deductible	¹³ Copay	Co-Ins. %	¹⁶ Paid	¹⁷ Patient's Responsibility	See Notes Section
CATHERINE S JONES MD	05 07 20YY– 05 07 20YY	87621 90 PATHOLOGY-PHYS CHGS	125.00	66.94	58.06			6.69	90	60.25	6.69	PPU
CATHERINE S JONES MD	05 07 20YY– 05 07 20YY	88142 90 PATHOLOGY-PHYS CHGS	72.00	28.31	43.69			2.83	90	25.48	2.83	PPU
		TOTAL\S	197.00	95.25	101.75	0.00	0.00	9.52		85.73	9.52	

Other Insurance Paid Amount 0.00
(*) See Notes Adjustment 0.00
Final Paid Amount/Check .... 85.73 # 43984431

Total Payment to Provider: *******85.73   **Total Payment to Enrollee:** *********0.00

NOTES:

THANK YOU FOR USING A PARTICIPATING PROVIDER

PPU   THIS IS YOUR PLANS PARTICIPATING PROVIDERS CONTRACTUAL ALLOWANCE FOR THIS SERVICE. PROVIDER AGREES TO REDUCE THE FEE TO THE AMOUNT ALLOWED.

DEDUCTIBLE

YOU HAVE MET 200.00 OF YOUR 200.00 DEDUCTIBLE FOR 01/01/20YY - 12/31/20YY

Figure 17-14 ■ Explanation of Benefits (EOB).

How much should the patient be billed?

❑ Corey Johansen is insured with Medicare.

❑ His service with Dr. Anholm was billed at $100.00.

❑ Dr. Anholm is a participating provider with Medicare.

❑ Medicare allows $78.45 for this service.

❑ Medicare paid $62.76.

How much does Corey owe?

$100 for the service

$78.45 is allowed

Provider must write off the difference between the amount charged ($100.00) and the amount allowed ($78.45). This means the provider must write off $21.55.

Corey owes the difference between the allowed amount ($78.45) and the amount paid by Medicare ($62.76). Corey owes $15.69 for his service with Dr. Anholm.

Figure 17-15 ■ Patient scenario: Sample billing when provider is contracted with the insurance carrier.

Each state has its own guidelines that outline the time frame within which an insurance carrier must pay or deny a claim. In Washington State, for example, the time frame is 30 days. Any claims that have not been processed within that time frame are subject to interest in the amount allowed by state law. As a general rule, any claim that has not been paid or denied within 45 days of submission on paper, or within 20 days of submission electronically, may be considered past due and warrants a telephone call to the insurance carrier.

When a claim is past due, the medical assistant should call the insurance carrier to follow up on or trace the claim. During this call, the medical assistant may be told that the insurance carrier does not have the claim on file. If this is the case, the medical assistant can request a fax number to send the claim to the customer service representative for processing personally. The medical assistant might also be told that there was an error on the claim. Sometimes, the medical assistant can clarify the error over the phone; other times, the claim must be resubmitted. The medical assistant should always document any phone call made to an insurance carrier, noting the date and time of the call, the name of the person spoken to, and the results of the call.

When payment is denied for one service or for the entire claim, the medical assistant needs to *trace the claim*, or investigate the reason. Usually the reason is stated on the EOB, but the medical assistant might need to call the insurance company for clarification. Solutions might involve obtaining additional information from the patient, asking the coding department to review the documentation and the codes assigned, or providing copies of documentation. The provider needs to respond to insurance company inquiries quickly because any delay by the provider adds to the time it takes to receive payment.

Rejections, Denials, and Appeals

Claims are sometimes denied or rejected, many times for errors made in the medical office. Incorrect identification numbers, incorrect birthdates, missing diagnosis codes, and missing supporting documentation all delay payment of insurance claims (Table 17-5). Attention to detail in the claim submission process saves time and effort in the end.

TABLE 17-5 Reasons for Denied Claims and Solutions	
Reason for denial	**Solution**
Need supporting documentation	When calling for preauthorization of any procedure, ask the insurance company customer service representative if supporting documentation will be required. If so, copy the chart notes, operative report, laboratory report, or other documentation and send it in with the CMS-1500 billing form.
Diagnosis code does not match procedure performed	Before sending the claim, look at the diagnosis codes the physician assigns to the patient in the *ICD-10-CM* coding manual to verify that the code matches the diagnosis.
Patient is no longer eligible for coverage	Before scheduling any procedure, call to verify coverage with the insurance carrier.
Missing information on the CMS-1500 claim form	Quickly scan all CMS-1500 claim forms prior to sending to determine any missing information or blank boxes.
Preauthorization was not obtained	Before scheduling any procedure, call to verify coverage with the insurance carrier.
Patient age or gender does not match the procedure	Proofread all data entry to ensure accuracy.
Past timely filing limits	Submit all insurance claim forms in a timely manner, usually within 30 days of the date of the procedure.

PROCEDURE 17-5 Handle a Denied Insurance Claim

Theory and Rationale

Even after all information has been carefully entered into the computer system management software program, insurance claims are occasionally returned to the medical office. To determine the cause of the denial and the proper action to take, denied claims must be acted on in a timely fashion.

Materials

- Patient insurance information (i.e., ID number, birthdate of the insured, name and provider customer service telephone number of insurance company)
- Paper and pen
- Copy of the explanation of benefits (EOB) received
- Description of the procedure the doctor has performed, including CPT code
- Patient's diagnosis pertaining to the procedure performed
- Location where procedure was performed (e.g., office, outpatient surgery, inpatient hospitalization)
- Date the procedure was performed
- Any documentation of the service having been preauthorized by the office

Competency

1. Organize all materials.
2. Call the insurance company's provider customer service phone number as listed on the patient's insurance identification card.

3. Write down the date and time of the telephone call, the number called, and the name of the customer service representative on the phone.
4. Self-identify to the customer service representative, and provide the patient's identification number and date of service.
5. If the service was preauthorized, give that information to the customer service representative.
6. Ask the customer service representative why the procedure was not paid as anticipated.
7. If there was an error in processing the service for payment, ask the customer service representative if any other information is needed to process the claim correctly. Ask the customer service representative when the office can expect payment for the procedure.
8. If the customer service representative says the claim was correctly processed, request the reason for the denial.
9. If the reason for the denial was lack of supporting documentation, ask the customer service representative if faxing the information is a solution. If the answer is yes, get the customer service representative's direct fax line and fax the needed documentation.
10. If the reason for the denial requires that an appeal be filed, ask the customer service representative to explain the insurance company's process for appeals.
11. Write down any pertinent information, such as where to mail the appeal and what information the appeal should contain.
12. Call the patient with the findings and get the patient involved as needed.

A **rejected** claim is one that never entered the carrier's system due to an incorrect identification number or similar technical problem. These are often returned to the provider during the EMC process. Rejected claims should be corrected and resubmitted as a new claim.

Be careful to differentiate between denied claims and disallowances:

- A denied claim is one the carrier received and processed but did not pay due to benefits or coverage issues. The reason for denial is usually listed on the EOB.
- Disallowances represent partial payment on claims because they are above the maximum allowable fee.

If the reason for payment reduction cannot be determined, or the medical assistant or patient disagrees with the reason, the medical assistant should place a telephone call to the insurance company. If a corrected claim needs to be resubmitted, the carrier should provide specific directions on how to do this so it will not be automatically rejected by the system. Denied claims

that are resubmitted as new claims, rather than corrected claims, are usually rejected due to a duplicate date of service.

Submitting a formal **appeal** is very different from submitting a new claim because an appeal involves extra time and research. Additional information and paperwork must be supplied, and detailed clinical information from the physician might also be requested by the carrier. Because the appeals process is time consuming, it is often not done properly or consistently.

When deciding to submit an appeal, the first step is to know and follow the appeals policy of the payer. For example, medical assistants must submit the appeal in a timely manner because there is often a cutoff date for doing so. Most practices learn about the appeals policies of the major plans they work with by referring to physician administrative manuals, contracts, and newsletters. Medical assistants may also call the insurance plan to learn about specific policies.

In general, an appeal includes writing a letter that clearly states why the provider believes the denial was not justified. It is best to be clear and factual rather than emotional, angry, or threatening when writing appeal letters. Attach the EOB and any supporting documentation to the letter. Be aware that some plans are instituting paperless review procedures, which decreases the time spent gathering and documenting detailed information.

Medical assistants should also send a copy of the appeal to the patient. Because health care coverage is an agreement between the patient and the insurance carrier, the patient often gets better results when requesting an appeal. For this reason, the medical assistant should always ask the patient to become involved in any appeal process.

After all insurance payments are received and followup is complete, the office sends the patient a bill for any deductible, coinsurance, or patient responsibility amounts that have not been paid.

PROCEDURE 17-6 Abstract Data to Complete a Paper CMS-1500 Claim Form

Theory and Rationale

Even though few offices still complete CMS-1500 forms manually and without the aid of a computer, some small offices do. Proper completion of a paper CMS-1500 claim acquaints medical assistants with the Item fields and data requirements, all of which are required when using a computer program. This procedure allows medical assistants to focus on how to abstract or locate required information from the source documents without learning a computer software program at the same time.

Materials

- Klaus Davies patient registration form (**Figure 17-16** ■)
- Insurance ID card (**Figure 17-17** ■)
- Encounter form (**Figure 17-18** ■)
- Capital City Medical fee schedule (**Figure 17-19** ■)
- Table 17-4: Instructions on Completing the CMS-1500 Claim Form
- Blank CMS-1500 form (photocopy Figure 17-11 or obtain from instructor)
- Black ink pen
- Calculator

Competency

Refer to Table 17-4 to identify how each field is to be completed and where to find the information. Print all information neatly, in capital letters, with a pen. Erasing, cross-outs, write-overs and white-out may not be used. You may wish to fill in a draft form in pencil, then recopy it in ink when finished.

1. Enter the insurance company name and mailing address in the Carrier Area.
2. Check the correct box in Item 1.
3. Enter the insured's ID number in Item 1a.
4. Enter the patient's name in Item 2, if different from the insured.
5. Complete Item 3, using MMDDCCYY date format.
6. Complete Item 4.
7. Leave Item 5 blank because it is the same as Item 7.
8. Complete Item 6.
9. Complete Item 7. Note there are 3 lines of information to complete.
10. Leave Item 8 blank.
11. Leave Item 9a to 9d blank because there is no secondary insurance.
12. Complete Item 10a, 10b, and 10c.
13. Leave Item 10d blank.
14. Enter the group number in Item 11.
15. Complete Item 11a, using MMDDCCYY date format.
16. Leave Item 11b blank.
17. Enter the insurance plan name in Item 11c.
18. Mark NO in Item 11d.
19. Enter "SOF" in Item 12.
20. Enter "SOF" in Item 13.
21. Leave Item 14 to Item 19 blank.
22. Mark NO in Item 20.
23. Enter the first diagnosis code in Item 21, line A.
24. Enter the second diagnosis code in Item 21, line B.
25. Leave Item 22 to Item 23 blank.
26. In Item 24A, line 1, enter the date of service in both the FROM and TO fields.
27. Enter the code number for place of service in Item 24B.
28. Leave Item 24C blank.
29. Enter the first CPT code in Item 24D.
30. In Item 24E enter "A B" to designate that both diagnoses 1 and 2 relate to this service.
31. Look on the encounter form to find the description for CPT code 99231. Then look on the fee schedule to find the fee for this service and enter it in Item 24F.
32. Enter 1 for units in Item 24G.
33. Leave blank Item 24H and Item 24I.
34. Enter the physician's NPI number on the unshaded portion of 24J. You will find the number on the encounter form.

(continued)

PROCEDURE 17-6 Abstract Data to Complete a Paper
CMS-1500 Claim Form (continued)

Capital City Medical—123 Unknown Boulevard, Capital City, NY 12345-2222 (555)555-1234	Patient Information Form
Phil Wells, MD, Mannie Mends, MD, Bette R. Soone, MD	Tax ID: 75-0246810
	Group NPI: 1513171216

Date of Visit: _____

Patient Information:

Name: (Last, First) Davies, Klaus_____ ☒ Male ☐ Female Birth Date: 10/24/1965

Address: 19 Willow Rd. Capital City, NY 12345_____ Phone: (555) 555-1276_____

Social Security Number: 631-03-4305_____ Full-Time Student: ☐ Yes ☒ No

Marital Status: ☐ Single ☒ Married ☐ Divorced ☐ Other

Employment:

Employer: ___Organic Food Mart_____ Phone: ( ) (555) 555-5619_____

Address: ___13 Mile Blvd, Township, NY 12345_____

Condition Related to: ☐ Auto Accident ☐ Employment ☐ Other Accident

Date of Accident: _____ State _____

Emergency Contact: _____ **Phone: ( )** _____

Primary Insurance: Capital Health Insurance Company_____ Phone: ( ) _____

Address: 111 Main St, Capital City, NY 12345_____

Insurance Policyholder's Name: Same_____ ☐ M ☐ F DOB: _____

Address: _____

Phone: _____ Relationship to Insured: ☒ Self ☐ Spouse ☐ Child ☐ Other

Employer: _____ Phone: _____

Employer's Address: _____

Policy/ID No: YY28436489_____ Group No: 32643_ Percent Covered: ___%, Copay Amt: $ 35.00

Secondary Insurance: _____ Phone: ( ) _____

Address: _____

Insurance Policyholder's Name: _____ ☐ M ☐ F DOB: _____

Address: _____

Phone: _____ Relationship to Insured: ☐ Self ☐ Spouse ☐ Child ☐ Other

Employer: _____ Phone: ( ) _____

Employer's Address: _____

Policy/ID No: _____ Group No: _____ Percent Covered: ___%, Copay Amt: $_____

Reason for Visit: Need my blood pressure and cholesterol checked today_____

Known Allergies: _____

Were you referred here? If so, by whom?: _____

Figure 17-16 ■ Klaus Davies patient registration form.

PROCEDURE 17-6 Abstract Data to Complete a Paper — CMS-1500 Claim Form (continued)

CAPITAL HEALTH INSURANCE COMPANY

Group Name   **ORGANIC FOOD MART**

ID **YY28436489**   Group **32643**

Subscriber/Dependents	M RX
01: KLAUS DAVIES	Y Y
02: SARA DAVIES	Y Y

Card Issue Date   10/09/XX

Provider: Please submit medical and/or vision claims to 111 MAIN STREET CAPITAL CITY NY 12345

Member: To locate a preferred or participating Provider outside your service area please call 1 (555) 810-9999. For all other questions, please call 1-555-9978
This card is not an authorization for services or a guarantee of payment.

PPP Network   DED $300: COMP CARE $35 COPAY
                                    IN-NTWK 20%/OUT-NTWK 40%

RX BIN **09870**   PCN **246800**

OV $35   ER $100 $10 GEN
SP $50 $35 FORM
                         $50 NON-FORM

Figure 17-17 ■ Klaus Davies sample insurance ID card.

---

35. Repeat these steps for lines 2 through 6. In Item 24E be certain you designate the correct diagnoses reference for each service, as some lines will be only "A" or only "B."

36. When all services are completed, enter the EIN in Item 25 and mark X in the appropriate box. You will find this information on the patient registration form.

37. Enter the patient's account number in Item 26. You will find this number on the patient registration form.

38. Mark YES in Item 27.

39. Add up the total charges in column 24F. Write the total in Item 28.

40. Leave Item 29 and Item 30 blank.

41. Enter the physician's signature, credentials, and the date in Item 31. Be certain to stay within the lines of the box.

42. In Item 33, enter the clinic's phone number in the top right corner.

43. Enter the clinic's name and address in Item 33.

44. Enter the clinic's NPI number in Item 33a.

45. Leave Item 33b blank.

46. Proofread your work. Check all spelling and numbers against your source documents.

47. Check your claim against the sample CMS-1500 form in **Figure 17-20** ■.

(continued)

Patient Name Klaus Davies

Capital City Medical
123 Unknown Boulevard, Capital City, NY 12345-2222

Physician: Phil Wells, MD NPI 9876543210

Date of Service
10-26-20YY

New Patient			Other Invasive/Noninvasive / Injections			Laboratory		
Problem Focused	99201		Arthrocentesis/Aspiration/Injection			Amylase	82150	
Expanded Problem, Focused	99202		Small Joint	20600		B12	82607	
Detailed	99203		Interm Joint	20605		CBC & Diff	85025	X
Comprehensive	99204		Major Joint	20610		Comp Metabolic Panel	80053	
Comprehensive/High Complex	99205		Other Invasive/Noninvasive			Chlamydia Screen	87110	
Well Exam Infant (up to 12 mos.)	99381		Audiometry	92552		Cholesterol	82465	
Well Exam 1–4 yrs.	99382		Cast Application			Digoxin	80162	
Well Exam 5–11 yrs.	99383		Location Long Short			Electrolytes	80051	
Well Exam 12–17 yrs.	99384		Catheterization	51701		Ferritin	82728	
Well Exam 18–39 yrs.	99385		Circumcision	54150		Folate	82746	
Well Exam 40–64 yrs.	99386		Colposcopy	57452		GC Screen	87070	
			Colposcopy w/Biopsy	57454		Glucose	82947	
			Cryosurgery Premalignant Lesion			Glucose 1 HR	82950	
			Location (s):			Glycosylated HGB A1C	83036	
Established Patient			Cryosurgery Warts			HCT	85014	
Post-Op Follow Up Visit	99024		Location (s):			HDL	83718	
Minimum	99211		Curettement Lesion			Hep BSAG	87340	
Problem Focused	99212		Single	11055		Hepatitis panel, acute	80074	
Expanded Problem Focused	99213	X	2–4	11056		HGB	85018	
Detailed	99214		>4	11057		HIV	86703	
Comprehensive/High Complex	99215		Diaphragm Fitting	57170		Iron & TIBC	83550	
Well Exam Infant (up to 12 mos.)	99391		Ear Irrigation	69210		Kidney Profile	80069	
Well exam 1–4 yrs.	99392		ECG	93000		Lead	83655	
Well Exam 5–11 yrs.	99393		Endometrial Biopsy	58100		Liver Profile	80076	X
Well Exam 12–17 yrs.	99394		Exc. Lesion Malignant			Mono Test	86308	
Well Exam 18–39 yrs.	99395		Benign			Pap Smear	88155	
Well Exam 40–64 yrs.	99396		Location			Pregnancy Test	84703	
Obstetrics			Exc. Skin Tags (1–15)	11200		Obstetric Panel	80055	
Total OB Care	59400		Each Additional 10	11201		Pro Time	85610	
Injections			Fracture Treatment			PSA	84153	
			Loc			RPR	86592	
Drug			w/Reduc w/o Reduc			Sed. Rate	85651	
Dosage			I & D Abscess Single/Simple	10060		Stool Culture	87045	
Allergy	95115		Multiple or Comp	10061		Stool O & P	87177	
Cocci Skin Test	86490		I & D Pilonidal Cyst Simple	10080		Strep Screen	87880	
DTaP<7yr	90700		Pilonidal Cyst Complex	10081		Theophylline	80198	
Hemophilus	90646		IV Therapy—To One Hour	96365		Thyroid Uptake	84479	
Influenza	90658		Each Additional Hour	96366		TSH	84443	
MMR	90707		Laceration Repair			Urinalysis	81000	
OPV	90712		Location Size Simp/Comp			Urine Culture	87088	
Pneumovax	90732		Laryngoscopy	31505		Drawing Fee	36415	X
TB Skin Test	86580		Oximetry	94760		Specimen Collection	99000	
Tdap>=7yr	90715		Punch Biopsy			Other:		
Unlisted Immun	90749		Rhythm Strip	93040				
Tetanus Toxoid	90703		Treadmill	93015				
Vaccine/Toxoid Admin <=18 Yr Old w/Counseling	90460		Trigger Point or Tendon Sheath Inj.	20550				
Vaccine/Toxoid Administration for Adult	90471		Tympanometry	92567				

Diagnosis/ICD-9: **401.9, 272.0**
Diagnosis/ICD-10: **I10, E78.0**

		Lipid Panel	80061	X

I acknowledge receipt of medical services and authorize the release of any medical information necessary to process this claim for health care payment only. I do authorize payment to the provider.

Patient Signature *Klaus Davies*

Total Estimated Charges: _____

Payment Amount: _____

Next Appointment: _____

Figure 17-18 ■ Klaus Davies encounter form.

Capital City Medical
Fee Schedule

New Patient OV		Laceration Repair various codes	$60
Problem Focused 99201	$45	Punch Biopsy various codes	$80
Expanded Problem Focused 99202	$65	Nebulizer various codes	$45
Detailed 99203	$85	Cast Application various codes	$85
Comprehensive 99204	$105	Laryngoscopy 31505	$255
Comprehensive/High Complex 99205	$115	Audiometry 92552	$85
Well Exam infant (less than 1 year) 99381	$45	Tympanometry 92567	$85
Well Exam 1–4 yrs. 99382	$50	Ear Irrigation 69210	$25
Well Exam 5–11 yrs. 99383	$55	Diaphragm Fitting 57170	$30
Well Exam 12–17 yrs. 99384	$65	IV Therapy (up to one hour) 96365	$65
Well Exam 18–39 yrs. 99385	$85	Each additional hour 96366	$50
Well Exam 40–64 yrs. 99386	$105	Oximetry 94760	$10
Established Patient OV		ECG 93000	$75
Post Op Follow Up Visit 99024	$0	Holter Monitor various codes	$170
Minimum 99211	$35	Rhythm Strip 93040	$60
Problem Focused 99212	$45	Treadmill 93015	$375
Expanded Problem Focused 99213	$55	Cocci Skin Test 86490	$20
Detailed 99214	$65	X-ray, spine, chest, bone—any area various codes	$275
Comprehensive/High Complex 99215	$75	Avulsion Nail 11730	$200
Well exam infant (less than 1 year) 99391	$35	**Laboratory**	
Well Exam 1–4 yrs. 99392	$40	Amylase 82150	$40
Well Exam 5–11 yrs. 99393	$45	B12 82607	$30
Well Exam 12–17 yrs. 99394	$55	CBC & Diff 85025	$95
Well Exam 18–39 yrs. 99395	$65	Comp Metabolic Panel 80053	$75
Well Exam 40–64 yrs. 99396	$75	Chlamydia Screen 87110	$70
Obstetrics		Cholestrerol 82465	$75
Total OB Care 59400	$1700	Digoxin 80162	$40
Injections		Electrolytes 80051	$70
Allergy 95115	$35	Estrogen, Total 82672	$50
DTaP<7yr 90700	$50	Ferritin 82728	$40
Drug various codes	$35	Folate 82746	$30
Influenza 90658	$25	GC Screen 87070	$60
MMR 90707	$50	Glucose 82947	$35
OPV 90712	$40	Glycosylated HGB A1C 83036	$45
Pneumovax 90732	$35	HCT 85014	$30
TB Skin Test 86580	$15	HDL 83718	$35
Tdap>=7yr 90715	$40	HGB 85018	$30
Tetanus Toxoid 90703	$40	Hep BSAG 83740	$40
Vaccine/Toxoid Administration for Younger		Hepatitis panel, acute 80074	$95
Than <=18 Years Old w/ counseling 90460	$10	HIV 86703	$100
Vaccine/Toxoid Administration for Adult 90471	$10	Iron & TIBC 83550	$45
Arthrocentesis/Aspiration/Injection		Kidney Profile 80069	$95
Small Joint 20600	$50	Lead 83665	$55
Interm Joint 20605	$60	Lipase 83690	$40
Major Joint 20610	$70	Lipid Panel 80061	$95
Trigger Point/Tendon Sheath Inj. 20550	$90	Liver Profile 80076	$95
Other Invasive/Noninvasive Procedures		Mono Test 86308	$30
Catheterization 51701	$55	Pap Smear 88155	$90
Circumcision 54150	$150	Pap Collection/Supervision 88142	$95
Colposcopy 57452	$225	Pregnancy Test 84703	$90
Colposcopy w/Biopsy 57454	$250	Obstetric Panel 80055	$85
Cryosurgery Premalignant Lesion various codes	$160	Pro Time 85610	$50
Endometrial Biopsy 58100	$190	PSA 84153	$50
Excision Lesion Malignant various codes	$145	RPR 86592	$55
Excision Lesion Benign various codes	$125	Sed. Rate 85651	$50
Curettement Lesion		Stool Culture 87045	$80
Single 11055	$70	Stool O & P 87177	$105
2–4 11056	$80	Strep Screen 87880	$35
>4 11057	$90	Theophylline 80198	$40
Excision Skin Tags (1–15) 11200	$55	Thyroid Uptake 84479	$75
Each Additional 10 11201	$30	TSH 84443	$50
I & D Abscess Single/Simple 10060	$75	Urinalysis 81000	$35
Multiple/Complex 10061	$95	Urine Culture 87088	$80
I & D Pilonidal Cyst Simple 10080	$105	Drawing Fee 36415	$15
I & D Pilonidal Cyst Complex 10081	$130	Specimen Collection 99000	$10

Figure 17-19 ■ Capital city fee schedule.

(continued)

PROCEDURE 17-6 Abstract Data to Complete a Paper — CMS-1500 Claim Form (continued)

HEALTH INSURANCE CLAIM FORM

APPROVED BY NATIONAL UNIFORM CLAIM COMMITTEE (NUCC) 02/12

CAPITAL HEALTH INSURANCE CO
111 MAIN STREET
CAPITAL CITY NY 12345

↑ CARRIER

PICA | PICA

1. MEDICARE MEDICAID TRICARE CHAMPVA GROUP HEALTH PLAN FECA BLK LUNG OTHER	1a. INSURED'S I.D. NUMBER (For Program in Item 1)
(Medicare#) (Medicaid#) (ID#/DoD#) (Member ID#) (ID#) (ID#) [X] (ID#)	YY28436489

2. PATIENT'S NAME (Last Name, First Name, Middle Initial)	3. PATIENT'S BIRTH DATE SEX	4. INSURED'S NAME (Last Name, First Name, Middle Initial)
DAVIES KLAUS	MM 10 DD 24 YY 1965 M [X] F [ ]	DAVIES KLAUS

5. PATIENT'S ADDRESS (No., Street)	6. PATIENT RELATIONSHIP TO INSURED	7. INSURED'S ADDRESS (No., Street)
19 WILLOW RD	Self [X] Spouse [ ] Child [ ] Other [ ]	19 WILLOW RD

CITY	STATE	8. RESERVED FOR NUCC USE	CITY	STATE
CAPITAL CITY	NY		CAPITAL CITY	NY

ZIP CODE	TELEPHONE (Include Area Code)	ZIP CODE	TELEPHONE (Include Area Code)
12345	( )	12345	( )

9. OTHER INSURED'S NAME (Last Name, First Name, Middle Initial)	10. IS PATIENT'S CONDITION RELATED TO:	11. INSURED'S POLICY GROUP OR FECA NUMBER
		32643

a. OTHER INSURED'S POLICY OR GROUP NUMBER	a. EMPLOYMENT? (Current or Previous) [ ] YES [X] NO	a. INSURED'S DATE OF BIRTH SEX MM 10 DD 24 YY 1965 M [X] F [ ]

b. RESERVED FOR NUCC USE	b. AUTO ACCIDENT? [ ] YES [X] NO PLACE (State)	b. OTHER CLAIM ID (Designated by NUCC)

c. RESERVED FOR NUCC USE	c. OTHER ACCIDENT? [ ] YES [X] NO	c. INSURANCE PLAN NAME OR PROGRAM NAME CAPITAL CITY HEALTH INS

d. INSURANCE PLAN NAME OR PROGRAM NAME	10d. CLAIM CODES (Designated by NUCC)	d. IS THERE ANOTHER HEALTH BENEFIT PLAN? [ ] YES [X] NO *If yes*, complete items 9, 9a, and 9d.

READ BACK OF FORM BEFORE COMPLETING & SIGNING THIS FORM.

12. PATIENT'S OR AUTHORIZED PERSON'S SIGNATURE I authorize the release of any medical or other information necessary to process this claim. I also request payment of government benefits either to myself or to the party who accepts assignment below.

SIGNED **SOF**   DATE

13. INSURED'S OR AUTHORIZED PERSON'S SIGNATURE I authorize payment of medical benefits to the undersigned physician or supplier for services described below.

SIGNED **SOF**

→ PATIENT AND INSURED INFORMATION

14. DATE OF CURRENT ILLNESS, INJURY, or PREGNANCY (LMP) MM DD YY QUAL.	15. OTHER DATE QUAL. MM DD YY	16. DATES PATIENT UNABLE TO WORK IN CURRENT OCCUPATION FROM MM DD YY TO MM DD YY

17. NAME OF REFERRING PROVIDER OR OTHER SOURCE	17a. 17b. NPI	18. HOSPITALIZATION DATES RELATED TO CURRENT SERVICES FROM MM DD YY TO MM DD YY

19. ADDITIONAL CLAIM INFORMATION (Designated by NUCC)	20. OUTSIDE LAB? $ CHARGES [ ] YES [X] NO

21. DIAGNOSIS OR NATURE OF ILLNESS OR INJURY Relate A-L to service line below (24E)   ICD Ind. **0**

A. **I10**   B. **E78.0**   C. _____   D. _____
E. _____   F. _____   G. _____   H. _____
I. _____   J. _____   K. _____   L. _____

22. RESUBMISSION CODE   ORIGINAL REF. NO.
23. PRIOR AUTHORIZATION NUMBER

24. A. DATE(S) OF SERVICE						B. PLACE OF SERVICE	C. EMG	D. PROCEDURES, SERVICES, OR SUPPLIES (Explain Unusual Circumstances)		E. DIAGNOSIS POINTER	F. $ CHARGES		G. DAYS OR UNITS	H. EPSDT Family Plan	I. ID. QUAL.	J. RENDERING PROVIDER ID. #
From MM	DD	YY	To MM	DD	YY			CPT/HCPCS	MODIFIER							
1	10 26	YY	10 26	YY	11		99213		AB	55	00	1		NPI	9876543210
2	10 26	YY	10 26	YY	11		85025		A	95	00	1		NPI	9876543210
3	10 26	YY	10 26	YY	11		80061		B	95	00	1		NPI	9876543210
4	10 26	YY	10 26	YY	11		80076		B	95	00	1		NPI	9876543210
5	10 26	YY	10 26	YY	11		36415		AB	15	00	1		NPI	9876543210
6													NPI	

↓ PHYSICIAN OR SUPPLIER INFORMATION

25. FEDERAL TAX I.D. NUMBER SSN EIN	26. PATIENT'S ACCOUNT NO.	27. ACCEPT ASSIGNMENT? (For govt. claims, see back)	28. TOTAL CHARGE	29. AMOUNT PAID	30. Rsvd for NUCC Use
750246810 [ ] [X]	A8	[X] YES [ ] NO	$ 355 00	$	

31. SIGNATURE OF PHYSICIAN OR SUPPLIER INCLUDING DEGREES OR CREDENTIALS (I certify that the statements on the reverse apply to this bill and are made a part thereof.)

PHIL WELLS MD   10/26/20YY
SIGNED   DATE

32. SERVICE FACILITY LOCATION INFORMATION	33. BILLING PROVIDER INFO & PH # (555) 555 1234
a. NPI b.	CAPITAL CITY MEDICAL 123 UNKNOWN BLVD CAPITAL CITY NY 12345 a. 151317216 b.

Figure 17-20 ■ Klaus Davies completed CMS-1500 form.

PROCEDURE 17-7 Complete a Computerized Insurance Claim Form

Theory and Rationale

Proper completion of the CMS-1500 insurance claim form is vital to prompt payment of claims in the medical office. So that forms print properly, medical assistants must accurately enter necessary patient data in the computer system.

Materials

* Computer with medical billing software
* Patient medical chart
* Fee slip for patient's visit

Competency

1. Choose the patient's account ledger in the computer billing software.
2. Verify that the fee slip is for the patient with the account opened on the computer.
3. Enter the charges and coding as appropriate.
4. Complete the patient insurance information field.
5. Enter the patient's information, including address, telephone number, and birthdate.
6. Enter the insured's information, including address, telephone number, and birthdate.
7. Enter the patient's relationship to the insured.
8. Enter the insured's identification and group number.
9. Check the appropriate box to indicate the patient has authorized the release of information to the insurance company.
10. Check the appropriate box to indicate the patient has assigned the benefits (payment) to the provider.
11. Check the appropriate boxes to indicate if the visit was related to an accident.
12. If the visit was due to an accident, enter the date of the accident.
13. Enter any information regarding a referring physician, if applicable.
14. Enter any information regarding the patient's need for hospitalization for these charges, if applicable.
15. Enter the treating provider's name, address, telephone number, national provider identification (NPI) number, and Internal Revenue Service (IRS) tax identification number.
16. Enter information regarding the facility where the services were performed if not performed in the provider's office.
17. Check the appropriate box to indicate the provider accepts assignment.
18. Print the patient's insurance claim form.
19. Review the form for accuracy and completeness.
20. Send the claim to the insurance company.

REVIEW

Chapter Summary

* Medical assistants play a vital role in the health insurance process by gathering accurate information from patients, answering patients' questions regarding how health insurance works, and preparing accurate insurance claims so the office receives payment for services provided.

* As medical care advanced in the early 1900s, there was a greater need for insurance that covered hospital expenses.

* In 1965, the federal government created Medicare, designed for the elderly, and Medicaid, targeted to low-income families. These two programs marked a substantial infusion of funding to the health care system.

* Today, Americans obtain health insurance from a variety of sources that are regulated by a multitude of state and federal laws.

* The goal of Patient Protection and Affordable Care Act of 2010 is to help decrease the number of uninsured Americans and reduce the overall costs of health care.

* A knowledge of insurance terminology related to health insurance policy provisions is critical to helping patients utilize their health insurance policies.

* Health insurance plans are classified either as indemnity plans, which impose few restrictions on patients, or managed care plans, which seek to control costs by limiting patients' choices.

- Understanding the types of services covered by health insurance enables medical assistants to clarify for patients what can be expected from their policies.
- Third-party payers are entities other than the patient or physician who pay for health care services, accounting for 86 percent of all health care payments in the United States.
- The three major sources of private health insurance are group health plans, self-insured plans, and individual insurance.
- The federal and state governments provide health insurance for designated groups of people, such as the elderly, disabled, military personnel and retirees, and injured workers.
- The first step in receiving proper reimbursement for insurance claims is obtaining accurate patient information.
- Whether submitting health insurance claims electronically or on the paper CMS-1500 form, specific guidelines must be followed.
- With the growth of managed care and ongoing concerns about controlling health care costs, insurance companies use a variety of methods to determine how much to pay providers.
- Physicians may establish their fees by comparing their charges to other providers or by using a resource-based formula.
- Insurance companies may determine payment based on physician fees or by using risk-based reimbursement methods.
- RBRVS is Medicare's method of determining the Medicare physician schedule that calculates fees based on the relative value of each service, a geographic adjustment factor, and an annual conversion factor.
- MS-DRGs are a risk-based reimbursement method for hospitals, in which Medicare pays hospitals a predetermined amount for each patient stay, rather than actual costs.
- To post insurance payments, medical assistants must read and interpret the explanation of benefits, enter data into the computer, and follow up on unpaid claims.

Chapter Review

Multiple Choice

1. Under PPACA, people who need to purchase health insurance may do so using:
   a. Medicare
   b. Medicaid
   c. Health insurance exchanges
   d. TEFRA
   e. CHIP

2. With most insurance carriers, timely filing limits refer to submitting claims within _____ days from the date of service.
   a. 365
   b. 120
   c. 45
   d. 30
   e. 20

3. What is the best way to follow up on an overdue insurance claim?
   a. Send another copy of the original claim
   b. Send a bill to the patient
   c. Call the insurance company regarding the claim
   d. Call the state's Office of the Insurance Commissioner
   e. Send the claim to a collection agency

4. Which of the following is a risk-based reimbursement method?
   a. RVS
   b. RBRVS
   c. UCR
   d. MS-DRG
   e. FFS

5. When the patient is also the insured, where on the CMS-1500 form should the name be entered?
   a. Item 2 Patient's Name
   b. Item 4 Insured's Name
   c. Both Item 2 and Item 4
   d. Item 6 Patient's Relationship to Insured
   e. Item 9c Insurance Plan or Program Name

6. Balance billing occurs when the physician:
   a. Bills the secondary insurance company after receiving payment from the primary insurance company
   b. Bills the primary insurance company
   c. Bills Medicare
   d. Bills the patient for their deductible
   e. Bills the patient an amount that should be written off under the preferred provider contract

7. Using the birthday rule, the parent who is usually primary when billing for a child's services is the parent who:
   a. Has a birthday earlier in the year
   b. Has birthday later in the year
   c. Is older
   d. Is younger
   e. Is randomly selected by the insurance company

8. Which type of service may require an authorization from the insurance company?
   a. Emergency room visit
   b. Elective joint replacement surgery
   c. Removal of foreign body from the eye in order to save an injured worker's vision
   d. Annual preventive care visit
   e. Treatment for strep throat

9. HIPAA requires medical offices to give patients:
   a. Copies of the office's privacy practices
   b. Access to their medical records on request
   c. Accounts of any disclosures of their medical records on request
   d. Access to other patients' medical records
   e. All of the above

True/False

T F **1.** Many managed care plans require the medical office to obtain preauthorization before rendering certain services to patients.

T F **2.** When insurance companies deny payment for services, the only recourse is to bill the patient for the fee directly.

T F **3.** Medicare fee schedules are the same wherever physicians practice.

T F **4.** Medicaid is funded entirely by each state.

T F **5.** Sending any information to an insurance company without the patient's permission violates HIPAA.

Short Answer

1. Explain the term *pre-existing condition* as it applies to health care.
2. Why is it a good idea to start a new file for an existing patient who has just recently been involved in a workers' compensation claim?
3. Which other terms mean the same as *subscriber* with regard to health insurance coverage?
4. What is another term for the Medicare advance beneficiary notice?
5. List two reasons a claim might be denied by an insurance company, and suggest how to avoid those denials.
6. What does CMS stand for, and what is its role?

Research

1. Interview a person who works in a medical office. How does that office handle insurance authorizations for patients with managed care?
2. Look at the Medicare Web site. Where is the office for providers in your state to call for help with claims processing or questions?
3. Look at your state's Medicaid Web site. What telephone number do providers in your state call in order to obtain authorization for procedures on a Medicaid-covered patient?

Practicum Application Experience

Phyllis Allen is a patient of Dr. King's. The physician would like to have Phyllis scheduled for a biopsy procedure to be performed in the office. What information should the medical assistant gather before calling the insurance carrier? What information should the assistant write down during the telephone call?

Resource Guide

Centers for Medicare and Medicaid Services
7500 Security Boulevard
Baltimore, MD 21244
Phone: (877) 267-2323
www.cms.gov/

Kaiser Family Foundation
2400 Sand Hill Road
Menlo Park, CA 94025
Phone: (650) 854-9400
http://www.kff.org/

National Uniform Claim Committee
c/o American Medical Association
515 N. State St.
Chicago, IL 60654
www.nucc.org

Patient Protection and Affordable Care Act/Health Insurance Exchange
c/o Centers for Medicare and Medicaid
7500 Security Boulevard
Baltimore, MD 21244
Phone: (800) 318-2596
www.healthcare.gov

U.S. Department of Defense Military Health System
Skyline 5, Suite 810
5111 Leesburg Pike
Falls Church, VA 22041-3206
http://www.tricare.org/

U.S. Department of Health and Human Services
200 Independence Avenue, SW
Room 509F, HHH Building
Washington, DC 20201
Phone: (800) 368-1019
http://www.hhs.gov/ocr/hipaa/

U.S. Department of Labor
Frances Perkins Building, 200 Constitution Ave., NW
Washington, DC 20210
Phone: (866) 4-USA-DOL
www.dol.gov

18

Diagnostic Coding

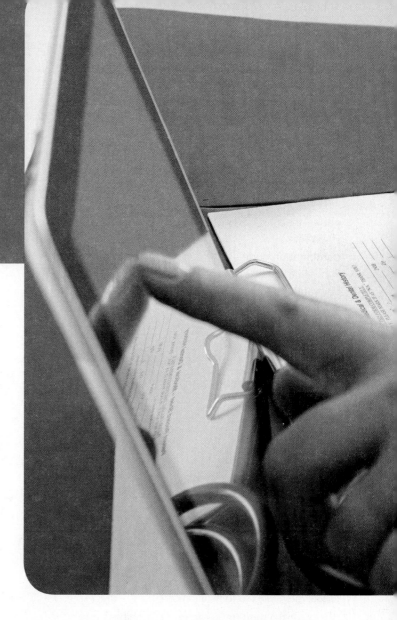

Case Study

Read the following case study and answer the critical thinking questions presented throughout the chapter.

Recently hired in the billing department of Dr. Johnson's medical office, Mary is asked to assign a diagnostic code to a patient's visit and bill for the charges. Unfortunately, Mary has a difficult time deciphering Dr. Johnson's handwriting. After deciding she cannot read the writing in the patient's chart, she says, "Well, it looks like the visit has something to do with the patient's ear, so I'll just code the visit as an earache."

Objectives

After completing this chapter, you should be able to:

18.1 Define and spell the key terminology in this chapter.

18.2 Explain the history and recent changes in diagnostic coding.

18.3 Define the purpose of diagnostic coding.

18.4 Define the medical assistant's role in diagnostic coding.

18.5 Describe the function and layout of the ICD-10-CM coding manual.

18.6 List the steps to correctly assign diagnosis codes.

18.7 Accurately assign diagnosis codes for basic patient situations.

18.8 Discuss examples for coding special diagnostic situations.

18.9 Describe how the medical assistant might pursue coding certification.

Competency Skills Performance

1. Perform diagnostic coding using ICD-10-CM.

Key Terminology

category—a three-digit code in ICD-10-CM Tabular List

chapter—one of 21 major sections of the ICD-10-CM Tabular List, organized by body system and etiology

chief complaint—statement in the patient's own words of the reason for seeking medical care

code—the most specific entry that requires no additional characters

combination code—a single code that describes two or more conditions that frequently occur together

conventions—coding rules, abbreviations, symbols, or formatting intended to ensure consistency in coding

etiology—cause of a disease or an illness

first listed—the diagnosis that is chiefly responsible for the outpatient services provided; formerly called *primary diagnosis*

Index to Diseases and Injuries—the portion of the ICD-10-CM manual that lists conditions and diseases in alphabetical order by Main Term

Main Term (ICD-10-CM)—words by which conditions and diseases are alphabetized in the ICD-10-CM Index; may be name of condition, eponym, acronym, or synonym, but not an anatomical site

morbidity—cause of illness or injury

mortality—cause of death

multiple coding—a diagnosis that requires more than one code to completely describe it; often indicated by a second code in slanted brackets

neoplasm—the medical term for an abnormal growth of new tissue; often referred to as a tumor

nonessential modifiers—words in parentheses after a Main Term in the ICD-10-CM that clarify the Main Term but that need not be present in the medical record

primary diagnosis—patient's chief complaint or reason for visit

qualified—diagnosis statement accompanied by terms such as *possible*, *probable*, *suspected*, *rule out* (R/O), or *working*

diagnosis, indicating that the physician has not determined the root cause; also called an *uncertain* diagnosis

secondary diagnoses—conditions, diseases, or reasons for seeking care in addition to the first-listed diagnosis; they may or may not be related to the first-listed diagnosis

section—an organizational division of a chapter that groups together multiple categories

sequela—an abnormal condition resulting from a previous injury, condition, or disease

sign—a physical sign of a condition that can be observed or measured by a physician

subcategory—a four- or five-character entry in ICD-10-CM Tabular List that is not a final code

subterm—a word indented two spaces under the boldfaced Main Term in the ICD-10-CM which further describes the Main Term in terms of etiology, co-existing conditions, anatomic site, episode, or similar descriptor

symptom—indication of a condition reported by the patient that the physician cannot observe or measure

Tabular List (ICD-10-CM)—the portion of the ICD-10-CM manual that lists diagnostic codes in alphanumeric order

verify—the process of consulting the Tabular List to read detailed code descriptions, conventions, and instructional notes, and to assign additional specificity

Abbreviations

AAPC—formerly known as the American Academy of Professional Coders

AHIMA—American Health Information Management Association

APHA—American Public Health Association

CCS-P—Certified Coding Specialist–Physician based

CPC—Certified Professional Coder

ICD-9-CM—*International Classification of Diseases,* 9th Rev., *Clinical Modification*

ICD-10-CM—*International Classification of Diseases,* 10th Rev., *Clinical Modification*

Certification Exam Coverage

AAMA (CMA) Exam Coverage:
- Coding systems
  - International Classification of Diseases, Clinical Modifications (ICD-CM) (*current schedule*)
  - Relationship between procedure and diagnosis codes

AMT (CMAS) Exam Coverage:
- Coding
  - Understand diagnosis coding

Introduction

Diagnostic coding is the process of assigning a number to a description of the patient's condition, illness, disease, or other reason for the encounter as it appears in the health care provider's documentation in the patient's medical record. Diagnostic codes identify the reasons that health care services were provided. Procedure codes describe services performed for patients. Diagnostic codes must be accurate because they inform insurance companies of the severity of patients' conditions and therefore the need for services, procedures, or tests. The combination of diagnostic codes and related procedure codes provide the basis for health care reimbursement. On a broader scale, diagnostic codes are used within the United States and worldwide to group and identify diseases and illnesses in order to track causes of **morbidity** and **mortality**.

Diagnostic coding requires a great deal of learning and attention to detail. This chapter provides an introduction to diagnostic coding for services provided in the medical office. It does not cover diagnostic coding for services physicians provide to hospital inpatients or for outpatient services provided outside of the medical office. Medical assistants who enjoy this topic may wish to pursue further training and practice.

Overview and History of Diagnostic Coding

ICD-10-CM is a listing of alphanumeric codes, three to seven characters long, and descriptions used to report causes of mortality and morbidity. ICD-10-CM codes identify the reason that health care services were provided to patients. As a result, ICD-10-CM is the standard for efficient and effective communication among health care providers, regulators, and payers.

The History of Diagnostic Coding

Diagnostic coding has existed for more than a century, beginning in 1893 with French physician Jacques Bertillon. Dr. Bertillon created the Bertillon Classification of Causes of Death, which the American Public Health Association (**APHA**) adopted in 1898. At the time, the classification contained an alphabetic Index and a Tabular List, and was quite small compared to coding references used today.

In 1901, the APHA published a coding manual called the *International Classification of Diseases (ICD), Volume I.* The *ICD-1* was used until 1910 when revisions were published about every 10 years. In 1948, with ICD-6, the World Health Organization (WHO) took responsibility for maintaining and publishing updates. When ICD-8 was published in 1965, the United States decided to develop an adaptation tailored to the needs of clinicians in this country. The adaptation, *International Classification of Diseases, Adapted* (ICDA-8), was published by the United States Public Health Service in 1968. By 1979, when ICD-9 was published, the United States again issued an adapted version, *International Classification of Diseases, Volume 9, Clinical Modification* (**ICD-9-CM**). At that time, WHO recommended waiting 10 or more years to publish major ICD updates. However, the United States issued annual updates to ICD-9-CM to refine the code set and keep pace with changes in medicine. ICD-9-CM is discussed in Appendix A.

Diagnostic Coding Today

WHO began work on ICD-10 in 1983, with adoption in 1990. Most countries were using ICD-10 by 2000. The United States used ICD-10 for worldwide mortality reporting beginning in 1999, but continued to use ICD-9-CM for morbidity reporting and health care claims. The United States also began work on an adaptation to ICD-10. In 2008, the U.S. Department of Health and Human Services (HHS) approved ICD-10-CM for use in the United States. A series of delays has repeatedly postponed the ICD-10-CM implementation date. As this text went to press, the October 1, 2014, implementation date had been again delayed, and the new implementation date had not yet been established. Refer to www.cms.gov for information on the current status of ICD-10-CM. ICD-10-CM provides a revised and expanded code structure that incorporates updated terminology and greater specificity and consistency.

Work has already begun on the international version of ICD-11, with a beta version released in 2012. ICD-11 is being developed with an Internet-based platform and will be fully integrated into electronic health records (EHR).

The Transition to ICD-10-CM

The transition from ICD-9-CM to ICD-10-CM is one of health care's top priorities and expenditures for the next several years because it will take several years after the implementation date for providers and payers to fully adjust to the new system. Coding changes impact every aspect of health care organizations. Everyone who is part of the health care system or uses its data has been impacted, including providers, payers, regulators, vendors, claims clearinghouses, medical billing services, researchers, educational institutions, and support staff in each of these settings. All computer systems that collect, transmit, receive, or store diagnostic data require updating due to the expanded length, format, and structure of codes. These changes further impact the budgets of organizations and the productivity of workers.

With the implementation of ICD-10-CM, ICD-9-CM will no longer be used in the daily operations of clinics. ICD-9-CM will become a legacy system, one that has historical value and is used when comparing statistics gathered under the previous system to statistics gathered under the ICD-10-CM system. It may also be used by organizations that are not HIPAA-covered entities, such as worker's compensation and property and casualty claims. Table 18-1 compares the ICD-9-CM and ICD-10-CM code sets.

The ICD-10-CM code set is updated annually. Code definitions are revised, new codes are added, and outdated codes are deleted. Updates are effective each year on October 1, to coincide with the beginning of the federal fiscal year. Each HIPAA-covered entity must update its systems and paperwork to incorporate the changes.

The Purpose of Diagnostic Coding

Diagnostic codes describe the medical need for health care encounters. Medical offices report diagnosis codes on CMS-1500 forms and electronic claims to justify the reasons that services were provided. Without proper diagnosis codes, a claim may not be paid.

Example: Justifying services

A patient presents in the office complaining of a headache and sore throat. The physician orders a throat culture to check for strep throat. The medical assistant must ensure the claim form carries a diagnostic code that relates to a sore throat in order to justify the throat culture. If the medical assistant codes only for a headache, the insurance company will likely not pay for the throat culture.

Incorrect diagnostic coding not only is likely to impede the office's ability to get paid by the insurance carrier, it also can adversely affect the patient's ability to obtain health insurance coverage in the future. An insurance company might see a past diagnosis and, not knowing it was coded incorrectly, believe the patient has a condition when, in fact, the information is not accurate. The patient could then be denied coverage, or charged more, due to a false pre-existing condition. However, this problem is becoming less common under PPACA because limitations have been placed on the ability of insurance companies to discriminate based on pre-existing conditions. It is also improper to code for a more complex condition than what the patient actually has, in the hope of receiving higher reimbursement. Doing so is considered fraud and carries severe penalties, including fines and possible imprisonment. Medical assistants must also be attentive to entering codes correctly into the computer or onto the CMS-1500 billing form. A typographic error in a code number can result in a rejected insurance claim, which must be corrected and rebilled, thus delaying the payment the office receives.

Example: Improper diagnosis coding

A patient presents to the office complaining of chest pain. The physician believes the pain is symptomatic of heartburn and treats the patient for heartburn. The medical assistant sees they symptom of chest pain and incorrectly assigns a diagnostic code for acute myocardial infarction (AMI). The patient's insurance company flags the patient as having AMI, which could create coverage issues in the

TABLE 18-1 Comparison of Codes in ICD-9-CM and ICD-10-CM

Feature	ICD-9-CM	ICD-10-CM
Number of codes	16,000	70,000 +
Code length	3 to 5 digits	3 to 7 characters
Code structure	3-digit category	3 character category
	4th and 5th digits for etiology, anatomic site, manifestation	4th, 5th, 6th characters for etiology, anatomic site, severity
		7th character used for additional information
First character	Always numeric, except E codes and V codes	1st character is always alphabetic
Subsequent characters	All numeric	2nd character is always numeric; all other characters may be alphabetic or numeric
Decimal point	Mandatory after 3rd character, except E codes where decimal point is after 4th character	Mandatory after 3rd character on all codes
7th character	None	Some codes use a 7th character to provide additional information
Placeholders	None	Character "X" is a placeholder in certain 5- and 6-character codes

future, such as denial of coverage or increased premiums. Although this coverage situation is becoming less common under PPACA, the correct codes should always be used.

Critical Thinking Question 18-1

Referring to the case study at the beginning of the chapter, what is the preliminary harm in Mary's guessing at the patient's diagnostic code?

The Role of Medical Assistants in Diagnostic Coding

Medical assistants usually do not perform medical coding as a regular part of their job because most offices hire or contract with professional certified coders who are trained in the details of assigning medical codes. However, the need occasionally arises for medical assistants to research a code. In addition, medical assistants hold one of the few staff positions within a medical office that is trained in both the administrative and clinical aspects of health care. Therefore, medical assistants play an important role in communication and understanding of medical codes in the following ways:

- Assist in communication between coders and physicians when a question arises.
- Provide appropriate diagnosis codes when an insurance pre-authorization is required for a procedure, or a patient is referred to another provider for a procedure or consultation.
- Facilitate communication with attorneys when they need information about medical codes related to injured patients they represent. (Specific written authorization by patients is required for the release of protected health information (PHI) to attorneys.)
- Answer patient questions about the meaning of codes on their insurance claims or other paperwork.
- Review or facilitate medical documentation to help ensure it provides adequate specificity (detail) for coding.

Medical coding requires knowledge of anatomy and physiology, clinical procedures, local, state, and federal regulations, and attention to detail. Medical assistants should understand the scope and limitations of their training in medical coding, should provide assistance whenever possible, and should consult with a certified coder whenever they are not completely confident regarding the coding information requested.

Organization of the ICD-10-CM Manual

ICD-10-CM provides the codes that identify all diagnoses physicians give patients. ICD-10-CM lists over 68,000 diagnostic codes in one volume. ICD-10-CM codes are updated annually and take effect October 1 of each year. Code changes are published by the National Center for Health Statistics (NCHS) and the Centers for Medicare and Medicaid Services

(CMS), in conjunction with the WHO. Medical assistants should use the edition of the ICD-10-CM that was in effect on the date of service.

EXAMPLE: The correct edition (year) of the ICD-10 manual

On October 3, a medical assistant is coding services for patients seen during the past week and needs to decide which ICD-10-CM manual to use. For patients seen on September 30, she uses the previous ICD-10-CM manual. For patients seen on October 1, she uses the new ICD-10-CM manual.

The ICD-10-CM manual is a single volume and is not separated into three volumes as the ICD-9-CM was. Several companies publish the ICD-10-CM manual, so the exact order of information may vary, based on which publisher's book is used. A table of contents page near the front of the manual outlines the contents, organization, and page numbers of the ICD-10-CM (Table 18-2). The Centers for Medicare and Medicaid Services (CMS) provides electronic files for ICD-10-CM, which can be downloaded (www.cms.gov).

Introductory Material

The introductory material that appears at the beginning of the ICD-10-CM manual provides important information for medical assistants. Not only does it provide instructions on how to use ICD-10-CM, it also outlines the Official Guidelines for Coding and Reporting (OGCR), official (universal) conventions, and publisher-specific conventions.

HIPAA requires that coders adhere to the ICD-10-CM Official Guidelines for Coding and Reporting (OGCR) when assigning diagnosis codes. The OGCR serves several purposes. It provides directions for how to code selected conditions. It establishes the rules for how to identify which diagnoses should be reported on a claim for any given patient (**Figure 18-1** ■). The OGCR also explains the official coding conventions.

Conventions

Conventions are specialized rules, abbreviations, formatting, and symbols that alert users to important information. The official conventions are described at the beginning of the manual. A key to selected symbols usually appears at the bottom of each page. Certain conventions are universal to all ICD-10-CM manuals. Here, the term "Official" should appear before the term "manuals." While others are specific to each publisher. Conventions are described at the beginning of the manual. A key to selected symbols usually appears at the bottom of each page. The official conventions are universal to all ICD-10-CM manuals. In addition, individual publishers provide enhanced conventions such as color coding and special symbols to further assist the coder. These are called publisher-specific conventions.

Official ICD-10-CM Conventions Conventions that are an official part of the ICD-10-CM code set are explained in

TABLE 18-2 Organization of the ICD-10-CM Manual		
Type of Information	**Name of Section**	**Purpose**
Introductory Material	Preface Introduction How to Use the ICD-10-CM ICD-10-CM Conventions ICD-10-CM Official Guidelines for Coding and Reporting	Useful information and rules on how to use the manual
Index	ICD-10-CM Index to Diseases and Injuries (Index) ICD-10-CM Table of Neoplasms ICD-10-CM Table of Drugs and Chemicals ICD-10-CM Index to External Causes	Alphabetical list of diseases and injuries, reasons for encounters, and external causes. Two tables provide quick look-ups, one for neoplasms and one for drugs and chemicals causing injury. Coders must always reference one of these indices or tables when searching for a code. All codes found in the index must be verified in the Tabular List.
Tabular List	ICD-10-CM Tabular List of Diseases and Injuries	Alphanumeric list of diseases and injuries, reasons for encounters, and external causes. Provides additional instruction on how to use, assign, and sequence codes. Coders must always reference the Tabular List to verify a code, after consulting the Index, and before assigning the final code.

4. **Chapter 4: Endocrine, Nutritional, and Metabolic Diseases (E00-E89)**

   a. **Diabetes mellitus**

   The diabetes mellitus codes are combination codes that include the type of diabetes mellitus, the body system affected, and the complications affecting that body system. As many codes within a particular category as are necessary to describe all of the complications of the disease may be used. They should be sequenced based on the reason for a particular encounter. Assign as many codes from categories E08—E13 as needed to identify all of the associated conditions that the patient has.

   1) **Type of diabetes**

   The age of a patient is not the sole determining factor, though most type 1 diabetics develop the condition before reaching puberty. For this reason type 1 diabetes mellitus is also referred to as juvenile diabetes.

   2) **Type of diabetes mellitus not documented**

   If the type of diabetes mellitus is not documented in the medical record the default is E11.-, Type 2 diabetes mellitus.

   3) **Diabetes mellitus and the use of insulin**

   If the documentation in a medical record does not indicate the type of diabetes but does indicate that the patient uses insulin, code E11, Type 2 diabetes mellitus, should be assigned. Code Z79.4, Long-term (current) use of insulin, should also be assigned to indicate that the patient uses insulin. Code Z79.4 should not be assigned if insulin is

   ICD-10-CM Official Guidelines for Coding and Reporting **2014**
   Page 32 of 117

Figure 18-1 ■ Example of the Official Guidelines for Coding and Reporting.

the OGCR and appear in Table 18-3. The most important of these for medical assistants are Excludes1 and Excludes2. These notations explain which codes cannot be used together.

Excludes1 Excludes1 notes appear immediately under a code or heading in the Tabular List. The note is followed by a list of other conditions and codes. Excludes1 means that the condition represented by the code and the condition listed as excluded are mutually exclusive and should not be coded together. When an Excludes1 note appears under a code, none of the codes that appear after it should be used with the code where the note appears. This occurs frequently with conditions that may be either congenital or acquired.

Example: Excludes1

K55 Vascular disorder of intestine

Excludes1: necrotizing enterocolitis of newborn (P77.-)

The second condition, necrotizing enterocolitis of newborn, is not included in codes that begin with K55 Vascular disorder of intestine, and the codes are mutually exclusive. A patient cannot have both conditions. When coding for necrotizing enterocolitis of newborn, the correct code begins with P77, not K55.

Excludes2 Excludes2 notes also appear immediately under a code or heading in the Tabular List. The note is followed by a list of other conditions and codes. Excludes2 means that the condition excluded is not part of the condition represented by the code, but the patient may have both conditions at the same time. These conditions are not mutually exclusive. When an Excludes2 note appears under a code, it is acceptable to use the main code and the excluded code if the patient is documented to have both conditions.

TABLE 18-3 ICD-10-CM Conventions

Convention	Meaning/Use
- Short dash	**Index and Tabular:** Additional characters should be assigned in place of the - . The additional characters may be number or letters.
( ) Parentheses	**Index and Tabular:** Nonessential modifiers which describe the default variations of a term. These words are not required to appear in the documentation in order to use the code.
: Colon	**Tabular:** Appears after an incomplete term that requires one or more modifiers following the colon to be classified to that code or category
[ ] Square brackets	**Tabular:** Synonyms, alternative wording, explanatory phrases **Index:** Indicates sequencing on etiology/manifestation codes or other paired codes. The code in square brackets [ ] should be sequenced second.
And	**Tabular:** Means "and/or"
Boldface **(Heavy type)**	**Index:** Main Terms **Tabular:** Code titles
Code Also	**Tabular:** More than one code may be required to fully describe the condition.
Code First/Use Additional Code	**Tabular:** Provides sequencing instructions for conditions that have both an underlying etiology and multiple body system manifestations and certain other codes that have sequencing requirements
Excludes1	**Tabular:** Mutually exclusive codes. None of the codes that appear after it should be used with the original code itself.
Excludes2	**Tabular:** The condition excluded is not part of the condition represented by the code, but both conditions may be reported together if documented.
Includes notes	**Tabular:** Begin with the word "Includes" and further define, clarify, or give examples
Inclusion terms	**Tabular:** A list of synonyms or conditions included within a classification
Italics *(Slanted type)*	**Tabular:** Exclusion notes, manifestation codes
NEC	**Index and Tabular:** Not Elsewhere Classifiable. The medical record contains additional details about the condition, but there is not a more specific code available to use.
NOS	**Tabular:** Not Otherwise Specified. Information to assign a more specific code is not available in the medical record.
See	**Index:** It is necessary to reference another Main Term or condition to locate the correct code.
See Also	**Index:** Coder may refer to an alternative or additional Main Term if the desired entry is not found under the original Main Term.
With	**Tabular:** In a code title, means "both" or "together"
With/Without	**Tabular:** Within a set of alternative codes, describes options for final character
X	**Tabular:** A placeholder in codes with less than six characters that require a 7th character extension. The X itself has no meaning and is not replaced with an actual number or letter. In some codes, the X is used to reserve room for future expansion.

Example: Excludes2

K86.0 Alcohol induced chronic pancreatitis

Excludes2: alcohol induced acute pancreatitis (K85.2)

The second condition, alcohol induced acute pancreatitis, is not included in code K86.0, but may be reported together with it if the documentation states that the patient has both the acute and chronic forms of the condition.

Placeholders A placeholder is a filler character that has no meaning by itself. Some codes that are five or six characters long use the X to reserve a position for future use. In the examples that follow, X is used to hold the fourth position of the code open for future use and has no meaning. The fifth and sixth characters are part of the core code.

- J09.X1 Influenza due to identified novel influenza A virus with pneumonia

- M01.X21 Direct infection of right elbow in infectious and parasitic diseases classified elsewhere

Seventh Character The seventh character of an ICD-10-CM code is reserved for special use, most commonly the episode of care for injuries (Table 18-4). The seventh character must be assigned from the Tabular List. When a seventh character is required on a code of five or fewer characters, add the placeholder X to fill out the empty characters in the code. In the example that follows, the core code is S69.80. The seventh characters A and D identify the initial and subsequent encounter for the injury and must appear in the seventh position, so X is used to expand the length of the code.

- S69.80XA Other specified injuries to the wrist, initial encounter

- S69.80XD Other specified injuries to the wrist, subsequent encounter

TABLE 18-4 Definition of Common Episode of Care Characters

Value	Description	Definition
A	Initial encounter	The patient is receiving active treatment for the condition. Examples of active treatment are: surgical treatment, emergency department encounter, and evaluation and treatment by a new physician.
D	Subsequent encounter	The patient has completed active treatment of the condition and is receiving routine care for the condition during the healing or recovery phase. Examples of subsequent care are: cast change or removal, removal of external or internal fixation device, medication adjustment, other aftercare and follow up visits following treatment of the injury or condition.
S	Sequela	The patient presents with complications or conditions that arise as a direct result of a condition. An example is scar formation after a burn. The scars are sequelae of the burn. The 7th character "S" identifies the injury responsible for the **sequela**. The "S" is added only to the injury code, not the sequela code. The specific type of sequela (e.g. scar) is sequenced first, followed by the injury code.

Publisher-Specific Conventions Publishers of the ICD-10-CM manual may use color-coding and special symbols to alert users to important information. Conventions that vary among publishers are publisher-specific conventions. Medical assistants can read the introductory material to learn about these conventions. A key that explains the conventions often appears at the bottom of the page in the Tabular List. Conventions are commonly used to indicate the following:

- New Code
- Revised Code
- Additional character(s) required
- Placeholder required
- 7th character required
- Age-specific requirement
- Gender-specific requirement

Index to Diseases and Injuries

The **Index to Diseases and Injuries** (Index) lists conditions, diseases, and reasons for seeking medical care alphabetically by **Main Term** and **subterms** that aid in locating the most appropriate code. After identifying preliminary codes in the Index, verify them in the Tabular List. Final codes should never be based only on the Index.

Specialized Index Locations

Although most conditions and reasons for the encounter are located in the Index to Diseases and Injuries, ICD-10-CM has three additional references for specialized purposes.

- **Table of Neoplasms**—Neoplasms are indexed on the Table of Neoplasms, located under "N" in the alphabetic Index. Some publishers may place this table at the end of the Index.
- **Table of Drugs and Chemicals**—Poisonings, adverse effects, and underdosing are indexed on the ICD-10-CM Table of Drugs and Chemicals, which is located at the end of Index in most manuals.

- **Index to External Causes**—External causes of illness and injury are located in a separate index, the ICD-10-CM Index to External Causes, which follows the Table of Drugs and Chemicals in most manuals.

Tabular List

The Tabular List is an alphanumerically sequenced list of all diagnosis codes, divided into 21 chapters based on cause, or **etiology**, and body system (Table 18-5). After locating the diagnosis in the Index, medical assistants need to **verify** the code by referencing the Tabular List. Verifying a code means consulting the Tabular List to read detailed code descriptions, conventions, and instructional notes, and to assign additional specificity. Medical assistants need to know where to find the beginning of each chapter, because the beginning of the chapter provides global instructions that apply to all codes within the chapter.

Assigning ICD-10-CM Diagnosis Codes

Coding begins and ends with the patient's medical record. Medical assistants abstract information from the medical record in order to code for services and the reasons they were provided. Coding is to be performed to the highest level of certainty. All relevant information in the chart should be coded, but missing information should not be assumed or coded. Only conditions, diseases, and symptoms documented in the medical record can be coded and billed. If the medical record is incomplete or inaccurate, it should be corrected or amended before attempting to code (**Figure 18-2** ■). In some cases, you need to query the provider for more information. Any changes to the medical record should be made by the original author and should be signed and dated. Information that is not relevant to the current encounter, such as resolved conditions, should not be coded.

TABLE 18-5 ICD-10-CM Tabular List

Chapter	Title	Code Range
Chapter 1	Certain infectious and parasitic diseases	A00-B99
Chapter 2	Neoplasms	C00-D49
Chapter 3	Diseases of the blood and blood-forming organs and certain disorders involving the immune mechanism	D50-D89
Chapter 4	Endocrine, nutritional, and metabolic diseases	E00-E89
Chapter 5	Mental, behavioral, and neurodevelopmental disorders	F01-F99
Chapter 6	Diseases of the nervous system	G00-G99
Chapter 7	Diseases of the eye and adnexa	H00-H59
Chapter 8	Diseases of the ear and mastoid process	H60-H95
Chapter 9	Diseases of the circulatory system	I00-I99
Chapter 10	Diseases of the respiratory system	J00-J99
Chapter 11	Diseases of the digestive system	K00-K95
Chapter 12	Diseases of the skin and subcutaneous tissue	L00-L99
Chapter 13	Diseases of the musculoskeletal system and connective tissue	M00-M99
Chapter 14	Diseases of the genitourinary system	N00-N99
Chapter 15	Pregnancy, childbirth, and the puerperium	O00-O9A
Chapter 16	Certain conditions originating in the perinatal period	P00-P96
Chapter 17	Congenital malformations, deformations, and chromosomal abnormalities	Q00-Q99
Chapter 18	Symptoms, signs, and abnormal clinical and laboratory findings, not elsewhere classified	R00-R99
Chapter 19	Injury, poisoning, and certain other consequences of external causes	S00-T88
Chapter 20	External causes of morbidity	V01-Y99
Chapter 21	Factors influencing health status and contact with health services	Z00-Z99

Diagnosis coding involves three basic steps:

1. Identify the first-listed diagnosis.
2. Research the diagnosis in the Index.
3. Verify the code(s) in the Tabular List.

In Practice

Sharon is the administrative medical assistant who completes billing work in the office. One day when she receives a patient file for billing, Sharon notices that the fee slip the physician completed indicates that he drained a cyst on the patient's wrist. When Sharon reviews the chart notes to assign a diagnosis code, she finds that the physician has written nothing in the chart about the cyst or the procedure. In situations like these, Sharon usually just "jots something" in the chart. What might be wrong with this scenario?

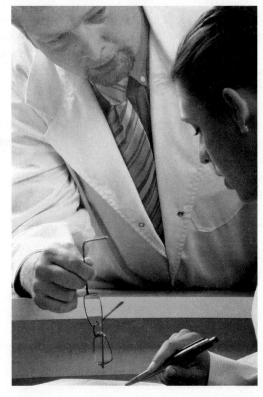

Figure 18-2 ■ The medical assistant may need to consult the physician to obtain additional information required to assign the correct code.

Source: Fotolia © endostock.

Critical Thinking Question 18-2

Referring back to the case study presented at the beginning of the chapter, what should Mary do when she cannot decipher the physician's handwriting?

HIPAA Compliance

Some physicians outsource their billing services. Because the information needed to process insurance claims is confidential, offices using outside billing services must obtain a Business Associates Agreement, which verifies that the services are HIPAA compliant, and the billing service will keep patient information confidential.

Several documents within the medical record may contain information needed for coding. When coding for office-based or other outpatient services, medical assistants refer to the patient registration form, the encounter form, visit notes, lab and radiology reports, and to operative reports for outpatient procedures. When coding for services physicians provide to inpatients, medical assistants refer to the admitting history and physical (H&P), daily progress notes, operative reports, lab and radiology reports, and the discharge summary.

It is important to keep in mind that the diagnosis must describe 1) the reasons that the specific service was provided, and 2) related medical conditions that may affect the specific service. Diagnosis codes should not repeat patients' entire problem list. The problem list is a comprehensive list of all active conditions that often appears in the front of the medical record, but it does not document the reason(s) for a specific encounter.

Example: Code actively managed conditions.

The physician sees a patient for a sinus infection, who also has chronic gastric reflux. The physician prescribes an antibiotic for the sinus infection and inquires how the gastric reflux is doing. The physician does not document that he further evaluates, treats, or manages the gastric reflux. The medical assistant should code only the sinus infection.

Example: Code all relevant medical conditions.

A diabetic patient comes into the office for a burn on the hand. The physician treats the burn and indicates that the diabetes may slow the healing process and requires more frequent followup visits as a result. The medical assistant codes both the burn and the diabetes. The first listed diagnosis is the burn. The secondary diagnosis is diabetes.

The following coding steps provide the practical details medical assistants need in order to patiently and accurately execute the process. This discussion is oriented toward office-based coding.

Step 1: Identify the First-listed Diagnosis in the Medical Record

Medical assistants abstract information from the medical record in order to code for services and the reasons they were provided. Often the physician indicates a diagnosis code on the encounter form, but medical assistants may need to verify it against the medical record. Look for a definitive diagnostic statement by the physician regarding the reason for the visit. The diagnosis may be indicated with the word *Impression* or, in SOAP notes, under

A (Assessment). This is the **first-listed** or **primary diagnosis**, the reason chiefly responsible for the services provided.

Uncertain or **qualified** diagnoses are those accompanied by terms such as *possible, probable, suspected, rule out (R/O),* or *working diagnosis,* indicating the physician has not determined the root cause. For outpatient coding, do not use uncertain diagnoses. Instead, look for the **signs** and **symptoms** that are part of the patient's **chief complaint**. The chief complaint is a statement in the patient's own words of the reason for the visit. Signs are indications of a condition that the physician can observe or measure, such as a rash. Symptoms are indications reported by the patient that the physician cannot observe or measure, such as a headache.

Additional conditions or complaints are **secondary diagnoses**, which are coded in the same way as the primary, but listed after them on the CMS-1500 billing form. Signs and symptoms that are routinely associated with the first-listed diagnosis are not coded as secondary diagnoses.

The following sample patient scenarios illustrate the difference between a definitive diagnosis and signs and symptoms. These same scenarios are further developed throughout this chapter as each step in the coding process is discussed.

Sample Patient Scenario

Identify the First-Listed Diagnosis

Scenario 1—A patient presents with difficulty breathing and fever. The physician takes a sputum culture and diagnoses acute pneumonia. The first-listed diagnosis is pneumonia, acute. Difficulty breathing and fever are commonly associated symptoms of pneumonia, so they are not coded.

Scenario 2—A patient presents with difficulty breathing and fever. The physician orders a chest X-ray for "suspected pneumonia." Because the pneumonia has not been confirmed, it is not coded. The first-listed diagnosis is difficulty breathing. The secondary diagnosis is fever.

Step 2: Research the Diagnosis in the Index

After determining the diagnosis in the patient's medical record, use the ICD-10-CM coding manual to assign the actual code number. The first step in using the coding manual is to identify the diagnosis in the Index. Using the Index involves three steps:

1. Locate the Main Term.
2. Read the subterms and modifiers.
3. Identify the preliminary code(s).

Step 2.1 Locate the Main Term

Identify the word(s) from the first-listed diagnosis to be looked up as the Main Term in the Index (**Figure 18-3 ■**). The

fracture of left tibia

chest <u>pain</u>

<u>sore</u> throat

congestive heart <u>failure</u>

benign <u>hypertension</u>

Figure 18-3 ■ Examples of diagnostic statements with Main Term underlined.

Main Term is always boldfaced with an initial capital letter. The Main Term may be any of the following:

- A condition, such as *Fracture*
- A disease, such as *Pneumonia*
- Reason for a visit, such as *Screening*
- Eponym (a disease or condition named after an individual), such as *Colles' fracture*
- Abbreviation or acronym, such as *AIDS*
- Nontechnical synonym (a word similar in meaning), such as *Broken* instead of fracture
- An adjective, such as *Twisted*.

Some Main Terms are rather generic with pages of subterms, such as *Disease*, while others are quite specific with only a single code, such as *Duroziez's disease*.

Main Terms usually do not include anatomic sites. To locate a condition that affects a specific site, look up the condition itself as the Main Term. Then read the subterms to locate the anatomic site (**Figure 18-4** ■).

Example: Anatomic sites

A medical assistant needs to code for an ankle sprain. She looks in the Index under *A* for the Main Term *Ankle*, and finds an entry with the cross reference *Ankle—see condition*. The condition is a sprain. She looks under *S* for the Main Term *Sprain* in the Index. Under *Sprain*, she locates the subterm, *ankle*. The subterm entry *ankle* provides additional subterms for the exact site and type of sprain.

Anisocytosis R71.8

Anisometropia (congenital) H52.31

Ankle—*see* condition

Ankyloblepharon (eyelid) (acquired)—*see also* Blepharophimosis
  filiforme (adnatum) (congential) Q10.3
  total Q10.3

Figure 18-4 ■ Example of Index entry for an anatomic site with a cross reference.

Source: Papazian-Boyce, L. M. ICD-10-CM/PCS Coding: A Map for Success. © 2013. Reprinted by permission of Pearson Education, Inc. Upper Saddle River, NJ.

Sample Patient Scenario
Locate the Main Term

Continue with the examples about a patient with pneumonia and a patient with difficulty breathing and fever.

Scenario 1—Diagnosis: Acute pneumonia. Main Term: *Pneumonia*.

Scenario 2—Diagnosis: Difficulty breathing. Fever. Suspected pneumonia. Main Term: *Breathing* is the Main Term for the first-listed diagnosis. In the Index, the subterm *labored* cross-references us to *Hyperventilation*. Fever is the Main Term for a secondary diagnosis. "Suspected" pneumonia is a qualified or uncertain diagnosis and should not be coded.

▶▶ Pulse Points

Main Terms

In the beginning, you may experience a process of trial and errors while learning how to identify Main Terms. Do not let this frustrate you and do not be disturbed by cross-reference notes in the Index. This is ICD-10-CM's way of pointing you in the right direction and is a normal part of coding.

Exercise 18-1
Getting Acquainted with the Index

Matching: Look up the following Main Terms (underlined word) in the Index. Match the letter of the choice that describes the type of Main Term with each Main Term.

Example: <u>C.</u> Colles' fracture

Choices:

a. condition

b. disease

c. eponym

d. acronym

e. synonym

Main Terms:

1. ___ <u>Crocq's</u> disease

2. ___ <u>HELLP</u> syndrome

3. ___ <u>Infertility</u>

4. ___ <u>Melanoma</u>

5. ___ <u>Sore</u> throat

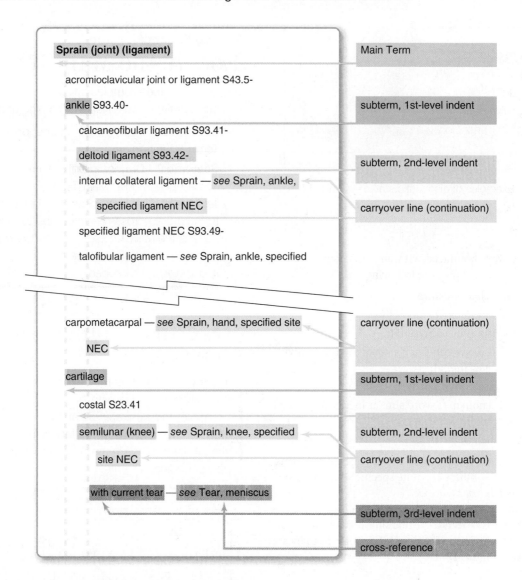

Figure 18-5 ◼ Example of Main Term, subterms, and carryover lines in the Index.

Source: Papazian-Boyce, L. M. ICD-10-CM/PCS Coding: A Map for Success. © 2013. Reprinted by permission of Pearson Education, Inc. Upper Saddle River, NJ.

Step 2.2: Read the Subterms and Modifiers

Modifiers and subterms provide additional information and variations on the condition described in the Main Term (**Figure 18-5** ◼).

Nonessential modifiers are words that appear in parentheses immediately after the Main Term. These words do not have to be present in the medical record in order to use the code, but if they are present, they confirm that the user has located the appropriate code. For example, the Main Term *Pneumonia* has many nonessential modifiers including *(acute), (double), (migratory),* and others (**Figure 18-6** ◼). Terms that are essential modifiers for one Main Term can be nonessential modifiers for a different Main Term.

Subterms are words indented two spaces under the bold-faced Main Term that further describe variations of the condition. Examples of types of subterms (shown in *italics*) are:

- Etiology: Pneumonia, *allergic*

- Coexisting condition: Pneumonia, *with influenza*
- Anatomic site: Pneumonia, *interstitial*
- Episode: Pneumonia, *chronic,* or similar descriptors

Subterms often have additional levels of one or more of their own subterms, each of which are indented another two spaces.

Carry-over lines are indented more than two spaces from the level of the preceding line. If the Main Term or subterm is too long to fit on one line, a carryover line is used. It is important to read carefully to distinguish between carry over lines and subterms.

Main terms or subterms may contain instructional notes, such as *see* or *see also,* which direct the user to other entries.

Pneumonia (acute) (double) (migratory) (purulent) (septic) (unresolved)

Figure 18-6 ◼ Example of Main Term with nonessential modifiers in the Index.

Dementia (degenerative (primary)) (old age) (persisting) F03.90
    Lewey body G31.83 *[F02.80]*

Figure 18-7 ■ Example of the multiple coding convention in the Index.

For example, *Pneumonia, alveolar—see Pneumonia, other.* This instructs the user where to look for the code needed.

Entries under the Main Term may contain special formatting, such as slanted brackets, indicating that **multiple coding** may be required (**Figure 18-7** ■). The second code in slanted brackets is required in addition to the first code to completely describe the condition. Multiple coding also is frequently indicated by instructional notes in the Tabular List to *Code first* a specific condition or to *Use additional code* to report an additional condition.

Exercise 18-2
Index Conventions

Matching: Look up the Main Term *Pneumonia* in the Index. Match the choices below with the type of convention used.

Example: B adenoviral

Choices:

a. nonessential modifier

b. subterm

c. main term

d. instructional note

e. multiple coding

Conventions used with the Main Term *Pneumonia*.

1. ____ basal, basic, basilar see Pneumonia, by type

2. ____ (acute) (double)

3. ____ atypical

4. ____ schistosomiasis B65.9 *[J17]*

5. ____ Pneumonia

Sample Patient Scenario
Identify Conventions in the Index

Continue with the examples about a patient with pneumonia and a patient with difficulty breathing and fever.

Scenario 1—Main Term: *Pneumonia.* Nonessential modifier: *(acute)* Subterm: No further description is provided, so there are no additional subterms to identify.

Scenario 2—Main Term: *Breathing.* Nonessential modifier: None. Subterm: The word "difficulty" is not listed as a subterm, but the synonym *labored* appears and is an appropriate choice. The entry cross-references to the

Main Term *Hyperventilation.* Turn to the entry for *Hyperventilation.* Main Term: *Hyperventilation.* Nonessential modifier: *(tetany).* Subterm: No subterms apply.

Step 2.3: Identify the Preliminary Code(s)

When the appropriate subterms are located, the preliminary code(s) appears immediately to the right. It is helpful to jot down the appropriate codes before verifying in the Tabular List. Never use the Index to make the final code selection.

Sample Patient Scenario
Identify the preliminary code(s)

Continue with the examples about a patient with pneumonia and a patient with difficulty breathing and fever.

Scenario 1—*Pneumonia (acute) J18.9*

Scenario 2—*Breathing, labored, see Hyperventilation R06.4*

Step 3: Verify the Code in the Tabular List

The final step in coding is to verify the code in the Tabular List. To verify the code, read the detailed code description, interpret conventions and instructional notes, read and apply the OGCR, and assign the highest level of specificity. Verification requires five steps:

1. Locate the preliminary code(s) in the Tabular List.
2. Interpret the conventions, instructional notes, and OGCR.
3. Assign the highest level of specificity.
4. Compare the final code to the documentation.
5. Assign the code.

Step 3.1: Locate the Preliminary Code(s) in the Tabular List

Look for the preliminary code number in the Tabular List which lists the code in alphanumeric order. The Tabular List contains 21 **chapters** based on etiology or the body system. The chapter numbers do not correlate directly with the code numbers. Refer back to Table 18-2. Chapters are divided into **sections** with boldfaced or highlighted headings. Within the sections, the actual code numbers are tabulated in three levels: **category** (three-character entries), **subcategory** (four- and five-character entries), and **code** (the most specific entry that requires no additional characters) (**Figure 18-8** ■). It is helpful to learn the specific meanings of these designations, because the terms are used frequently in coding instructions.

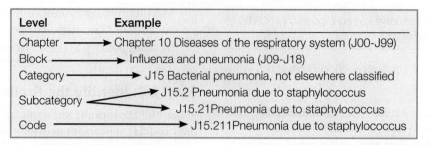

Level	Example
Chapter ⟶	Chapter 10 Diseases of the respiratory system (J00–J99)
Block ⟶	Influenza and pneumonia (J09–J18)
Category ⟶	J15 Bacterial pneumonia, not elsewhere classified
Subcategory ⟶	J15.2 Pneumonia due to staphylococcus
⟶	J15.21 Pneumonia due to staphylococcus
Code ⟶	J15.211 Pneumonia due to staphylococcus

Figure 18-8 ■ Organizational structure of ICD-10-CM chapters.

Step 3.2: Interpret the Conventions, Instructional Notes, and OGCR

Before verifying and finalizing the code, medical assistants must interpret the conventions presented with the code and its category. Tabular List conventions include punctuation, instructional notes, and symbols. Conventions may appear on the same line with the code, above it, below it, or at the beginning of a subcategory, category, section, or chapter. Look carefully for any information that may be relevant to the code selection. Additional information may direct you when to use a different code or an additional code, depending on your original diagnostic statement. In the Tabular List, the way in which punctuation is used has meaning (see Table 18-3). Medical assistants should become familiar with these meanings. Coders should always review the information at the beginning of the chapter, category, and subcategory as part of the verification process. In addition, they should read the general and chapter-specific OGCR for additional instructions.

▶▶▶ Pulse Points

Easily Confused Characters

Be on the watch for letters that can be easily confused with numbers. The letter capital I can be confused with the number 1. The letter S can be confused with the number 5. The letter capital O can be confused with the number 0. The number zero is sometimes written as Ø to help distinguish it from the capital letter O.

Sample Patient Scenario

Interpret Conventions and Instructional Notes

Continue with the examples about a patient with pneumonia and a patient with difficulty breathing and fever.

Scenario 1—Preliminary code *J18.9* is designated as an "Unspecified Code" in the Tabular List of most coding manuals. This is a publisher-specific convention that may appear as a special symbol or color coding. (Look for a key at the bottom of the page in the Tabular List.) Review the documentation for any additional specific information. None appears.

Because the Index directed us to this code for acute pneumonia, this choice is acceptable. Also note that the category contains an *Excludes1* statement; *Excludes1* is an official convention that, in this occurrence, indicates that specific types of pneumonia should be coded from other categories. None of these apply to this patient scenario because the type of pneumonia is not documented.

Scenario 2—Preliminary code *R06.4* is a subcategory. First locate the category (*R06 Abnormalities of breathing*) headings for conventions. An official convention, *Excludes1*, appears indicating certain types of respiratory problems that should not be coded here. A publisher-specific convention might appear, indicating that additional digits must be used. Under code *R06.4 Hyperventilation* there is another *Excludes1* note indicating that psychogenic hyperventilation should not be coded here. This does not apply to our patient because the hyperventilation is not psychogenic.

Step 3.3: Assign the Highest Level of Specificity

ICD-10-CM codes are between 3 and 7 characters in length. There is no general rule regarding how many characters any given code will have. The number of characters is determined only after reading the instructional notes and conventions available in the category, section, and chapter. Use the most specific code available in the Tabular List for the condition. Most coding manuals display a symbol or color-coding with entries that provide a more specific code (Table 18-6).

Codes of the highest level of specificity may provide options for anatomic site, laterality, with or without manifestations, and other details.

The seventh character of an ICD-10-CM code is reserved for special use, most commonly the episode of care. Episode of care characters do not appear sequentially within the Tabular List. They appear at the beginning of a subcategory or category and apply to all codes within that division. Be certain to review the subcategory and category headings thoroughly to locate the correct seventh characters when required. It sometimes requires a little detective work and reviewing several pages of codes to locate the appropriate listing (**Figure 18-9** ■).

TABLE 18-6 Examples of ICD-10-CM Codes with Varying Number of Characters

Code Length	Example
3-character code	I10
4-character code	F52.8
5-character code	K70.30
6-character code	L89.511
7-character code	T22.761A
7-character code with placeholder X	T51.0X1D V52.0XXS O33.4XX0

Source: Papazian-Boyce, L. M. ICD-10-CM/PCS Coding: A Map for Success. ©2013. Reprinted by permission of Pearson Education, Inc. Upper Saddle River, NJ.

Sample Patient Scenario
Assign the Highest Level of Specificity

Continue with the examples about a patient with pneumonia and a patient with difficulty breathing and fever.

Scenario 1—*Pneumonia, unspecified organism, J18.9.* This code matches the physician's diagnostic statement, and there are no subcategories available.

Scenario 2—*Hyperventilation R06.4.* This code matches the physician's diagnostic statement and there are no subcategories available.

Exercise 18-3
Assign the Highest Level of Specificity

Completion: Look up each entry in the Tabular List. Locate the code with greatest specificity for the condition listed

and write the remaining characters of the code in the space provided

Example: M05.01*2* Felty's syndrome, left shoulder

1. H60.0___ Abscess of the left external ear

2. J86.___ Pyothorax without fistula

3. H66.0____ Acute suppurative otitis media, without spontaneous rupture of ear drum, recurrent, right ear

4. L03.11 ___ Cellulitis of right upper limb

5. H02.41__ Mechanical ptosis of bilateral eyelids

Exercise 18-4
Episode of Care

Completion: Look up each entry in the Tabular List. Assign the episode of care for each entry. If the code is less than 6 characters, add the placeholder X to fill up the empty positions so the episode of care character always appears in the seventh position.

Example: S09.22*XA* Traumatic fracture of left ear drum, initial encounter

1. S21.011_____ Laceration without foreign body of right breast, initial encounter

2. S32.012_____Unstable burst fracture of first lumbar vertebra, initial encounter for open fracture

3. S46.012_____Strain of muscle and tendon of rotator cuff of left shoulder, sequela

4. T20.17_____Burn of first degree of neck, subsequent encounter

5. S14.4____ Injury of peripheral nerves of neck, initial encounter

---

S94 Injury of nerves at ankle and foot level

The appropriate 7th character is to be added to each code from category S94

A - initial encounter

D - subsequent encounter

S - sequela

   S94.0 Injury of lateral plantar nerve

      S94.02 Injury of lateral plantar nerve, right leg

Final codes with placeholder X and episode of care characters:

S94.02 X A Injury of lateral plantar nerve, right leg, initial encounter

S94.02 X D Injury of lateral plantar nerve, right leg, subsequent encounter

S94.02 X S Injury of lateral plantar nerve, right leg, sequela

Figure 18-9 ■ Example use of a placeholder (X) and episode of care characters.

PROCEDURE 18-1 Perform Diagnostic Coding Using ICD-10-CM

Theory and Rationale

Accurate diagnostic coding is critical to proper reimbursement from third-party payers. The medical assistant must know precisely where to look in the ICD-10-CM coding manual in order to obtain proper codes, as well as which steps to take when unsure of the correct code.

Materials

- Patient's medical chart
- Current ICD-10-CM coding manual
- Superbill with doctor's written diagnosis

Competency

1. Locate the patient's diagnostic code(s) or description on the superbill or in the chart notes.

2. Verify that the diagnostic code(s) or description on the superbill is documented in the patient's chart.

3. Look in the Index of the ICD-10-CM coding manual to find the Main Term, subterm, and preliminary diagnosis code.

4. Look up the preliminary code(s) in the Tabular List. Confirm that the written description matches the chart notes. If in doubt, check with the physician.

5. Read and apply the conventions in the Tabular List.

6. Assign the code for each diagnosis, beginning with the appropriate first-listed diagnosis.

Step 3.4: Compare the Final Code to the Documentation

As a final check, with coding manual instructions fresh in your mind, refer back to the original documentation and verify that all conditions of the code agree with the medical record. If a discrepancy arises, work through the process again from the beginning.

Sample Patient Scenario

Compare the Final Code to the Documentation

Continue with the examples about a patient with pneumonia and a patient with difficulty breathing and fever.

Scenario 1—*Pneumonia, unspecified organism, J18.9.* The final code matches the documentation.

Scenario 2—*Hyperventilation R06.4.* The final code matches the documentation.

Repeat this entire process to code for the other symptom, fever.

Step 3.5: Assign the Code

Write down the final code where indicated on your worksheet or documentation. Be certain to proofread the number as you wrote or keyboarded it, to avoid transcription errors that are easy to make.

Repeat this process for any additional codes required by the medical record.

Selecting a diagnosis code might seem like a long and tedious process at first. As medical assistants become familiar with the services and codes used by their medical office, coding becomes faster and easier, but accuracy and attention to detail is always paramount. Taking time and care to learn the fundamentals correctly helps create long-term success in the medical assistant's coding role.

▶▶ Pulse Points

Medical Billing Software Updates

Medical billing software typically provides the ability to access ICD-10-CM codes. To keep current and insert accurate diagnosis code information in insurance claims, it is crucial that such software be updated regularly. Claims with outdated or expired codes usually result in delays or denials by insurance carriers.

Exercise 18-5

ICD-10-CM Coding Practice

Underline the Main Term. Look up each condition in the Index, then verify it in the Tabular List. Write the code on the line provided.

1. _____ Benign hypertension

2. _____ Alcohol addiction

3. _____ Chondromalacia, right ankle

4. _____ Nausea with vomiting

5. _____ Lower back strain, initial encounter

6. _____ Tuberculosis of the lung

7. _____ Central corneal ulcer, left eye

8. _____ Beta thalassemia

9. _____ Supervision of pregnancy, young primigravida (less than 16 years of age at expected date of delivery) third trimester

10. _____ Hereditary hemochromatosis

Coding for Special Diagnostic Situations

As with any activity, there are always special situations that require additional information and knowledge. Diagnosis coding is the same. There are a number of conditions and circumstances that have unique tables, codes, and guidelines. An overview of the OGCR for these situations is provided in the remainder of the chapter. We will discuss hypertension, neoplasms, Z-codes, fractures, external cause codes, poisonings and adverse effects, burns, HIV, influenza, obstetrics, and diabetes.

Some conditions that frequently occur together may be described with a **combination code**. Careful reading of subterms in the Index and instructional notes in the Tabular list category, such as *Includes* and *Excludes*, guide the medical assistant as to when a combination code is available. Combination code descriptions frequently contain specific words that indicate more than one condition is covered, such as *associated with, due to, secondary to, without, with, complicated by*, and *following*.

Medical assistants often work in offices that hire certified coders to assign and audit diagnosis codes. Whenever medical assistants are unsure of how to select a code, they should reach out to their supervisor or a certified coder. Reporting incorrect diagnosis codes on an insurance claim can create problems such as denial, improper reimbursement, inaccurate patient medical history, and fraud. Awareness of special coding situations enables medical assistants to show their professionalism by recognizing when additional expertise is required.

Hypertension

Hypertension is a condition of elevated blood pressure over an extended period of time. It has been called "the silent killer" because it damages organs and causes numerous health issues without manifesting any symptoms until severe damage has occurred. This is the reason that all patients should have their blood pressure taken on a regular basis.

To code for hypertension, locate the Main Term *Hypertension* in the Index. When manifestations exist, locate the subterm that identifies each manifestation or complication. Verify the code in the Tabular List.

Neoplasms

Neoplasm is the medical term for an abnormal growth of new tissue, often referred to as a *tumor*. Neoplasms can occur in any type of tissue anywhere in the body, and they can be either malignant or benign. Tumors that have cellular characteristics that cause them to invade adjacent healthy tissue or spread to distant sites are malignant, or life threatening. The spreading of malignant neoplasm is called metastasis. Tumors that do not have these characteristics are benign. The Table of Neoplasms provides the index to the behaviors and anatomic sites of neoplasms (**Figure 18-10** ■).

	Malignant Primary	Malignant Secondary	Ca in situ	Benign	Uncertain Behavior	Unspecified Behavior
Neoplasm, neoplastic	C80.1	C79.9	D09.9	D36.9	D48.9	D49.9
abdomen, abdominal	C76.2	C79.8-	D09.8	D36.7	D48.7	D49.89
cavity	C76.2	C79.8-	D09.8	D36.7	D48.7	D49.89
organ	C76.2	C79.8-	D09.8	D36.7	D48.7	D49.89
viscera	C76.2	C79.8-	D09.8	D36.7	D48.7	D49.89
wall	C44.59	C79.2-	D04.5	D23.5	D48.5	D49.2
connective tissue	C49.4	C79.8-	-	D21.4	D48.1	D49.2
abdominopelvic	C76.8	C79.8-	-	D36.7	D48.7	D49.89

Figure 18-10 ■ Example of the Table of Neoplasms.

Source: Papazian-Boyce, L. M. ICD-10-CM/PCS Coding: A Map for Success. © 2013. Reprinted by permission of Pearson Education, Inc. Upper Saddle River, NJ.

The Table of Neoplasms lists the anatomical sites alphabetically. For each site, there are up to six possible codes, based on the type of neoplasm behavior.

Primary—site of origin. Malignant neoplasms are coded as primary unless otherwise stated in the medical record.

Secondary—site of metastasis, so stated in the medical record.

Ca in situ—cells that have begun to change but have not yet invaded normal tissue, so stated in the medical record.

Benign—non-invasive.

Uncertain behavior—the pathologist clearly indicates that further study is needed before determining the benign or malignant behavior.

Unspecified—the medical record does not contain adequate description of the neoplasm, which may happen with a patient who has relocated and whose previous medical records are not yet available.

After determining the anatomic site and the type of behavior, select the code from the appropriate column, then verify it in the Tabular List.

Example: Coding for Neoplasms

Patient presents with primary carcinoma of the abdominal cavity. Carcinoma iscoded from the Table of Neoplasms. Locate the term *Abdomen*. Locate the column *Primary*. Select the code where the row and column intersect. Verify the code in the Tabular List.

ICD-10-CM Code: C76.2 Malignant neoplasm of abdomen

Z-Codes (Factors Influencing Health Status and Contact with Health Services)

Not all patients who seek health care services have a specific disease or condition. They may receive services such as preventive care, therapy, followup, suture removal, or pregnancy supervision. They might have problems that require screening, carry certain risk factors, or have a health status that affects treatment and requires coding. All of these are examples of situations that require codes from the chapter entitled "Factors Influencing Health Status and Contact with Health Services." Because these codes begin with the letter Z, they are commonly referred to as Z-codes.

Z-codes fall into three general categories: problems, services, or factual.

1. **Health Status Problems:** Z-codes identify a problem that could affect a patient's overall health status but is not itself a current illness or injury. The Z-code in this example is supplemental.

Example: Z-code for a health status problem

A patient with strep throat needs an antibiotic, but is allergic to penicillin.

ICD-10-CM Codes: J02.0 Streptococcal pharyngitis
Z88.0 Allergy status to penicillin

2. **Reason for the Encounter:** As mentioned, a Z-code can be used to describe circumstances other than an illness or injury that prompted the patient's visit. This is an exception to the general rule for coding Z-codes because the sequencing is dictated in the OGCR. Although there is a disease, the Z-code is coded primary because it is the main reason for the encounter. The disease is coded supplemental to the Z-code.

Example: Z-code to identify the reason for the encounter

Patient is seen for chemotherapy to treat her colon cancer.
ICD-10-CM Codes: Z51.11 Encounter for antineoplastic chemotherapy
C18.8 Malignant neoplasm of overlapping sites of colon
For cases such as this, the Z-code describes the reason for the encounter. A CPT® procedure code that identifies the nature of the treatment must also be assigned.

3. **Factual:** Z-codes are used to describe certain facts that do not fall into the "problem" or "service" categories.

Example: Z-code for family history

A patient who has a family history of colon cancer presents with rectal bleeding.
ICD-10-CM Codes: K62.5 Hemorrhage of anus and rectum
Z80.0 Family history of malignant neoplasm of digestive organs

Example: Z-code to identify exposure to a contagious disease

A patient presents to a health care facility for care after having unprotected sex with a partner who has tested positive for human immunodeficiency virus (HIV).
ICD-10-CM Code: Z20.6 Contact with and (suspected) exposure to human immunodeficiency virus [HIV]

Fractures

Fractures may be traumatic (due to injury) or pathological (due to disease). When coding fractures, the following information is required:

- Anatomic site and laterality
- Type of fracture (transverse, spiral, comminuted, etc.)
- Open or closed
- Displaced or nondisplaced
- Episode of care (initial, subsequent, sequela, per ICD-10 definitions)

Search the Index for the Main Term *Fracture, traumatic* or *Fracture, pathological*. Locate subterms for the anatomic site and type of fracture. Verify the code in the Tabular List to confirm all details of the fracture, assign laterality, and assign a seventh character for the episode of care.

Example: Coding for fractures

A patient is treated for a nondisplaced Type II transverse fracture of the shaft of the left ulna.
> *ICD-10-CM Codes:* S52.225B Nondisplaced transverse fracture of shaft of left ulna, initial encounter for open fracture type I or II

External Cause Codes

External cause codes, classified with codes V00 to Y99.9, describe the external cause of illness or injury. They are never the first-listed diagnosis and are never used alone. They must be preceded by a diagnostic code that describes the injury or condition. Multiple external cause codes are used to fully identify the causal event, the activity, the place of occurrence, and the employment status of the person injured at the time the injury occurred. External cause codes are located using the Index to External Causes (Table 18-7).

Examples of when external cause codes are used include:

- A patient was involved in a motor vehicle accident.
- A patient was a pedestrian who was struck by a car while crossing the street.
- A patient fell off a ladder at home.
- A patient was injured as a result of a medical mistake, such as the physician operating on the wrong limb.
- A patient was bitten by a poisonous spider.

- A patient was knocked down at a sporting event.
- A patient was assaulted by another person.

Example: Coding for external causes

A patient is treated for a nondisplaced Type II transverse fracture of the shaft of the left ulna because he fell off a ladder in the yard of his single-family home while painting the house.
> *ICD-10-CM Codes:* (*Diagnosis*) S52.225B Nondisplaced transverse fracture of shaft of left ulna, initial encounter for open fracture type I or II
>
> (*Causal event*) W11.XXXA Fall on and from ladder, initial encounter
>
> (*Activity*) Y93.H9 Activity, other involving exterior property and land maintenance, building and construction
>
> (*Place of occurrence*) Y92.017 Garden or yard in single-family (private) house as the place of occurrence of the external cause
>
> (*Status, for leisure*) Y99.8 Other external cause status

Poisonings and Adverse Effects

When coding for injuries that have resulted from the use of drugs, chemicals, or biologicals, the medical assistant will need to determine the type of drug or chemical involved, if the event was accidental or purposeful, and whether the substance was prescribed by a health care provider. Table 18-8 provides the definitions and examples of injuries from drugs, chemicals, and biologicals.

TABLE 18-7 Commonly Used Main Terms in the Index to External Causes	
• Accident	• Incident
• Activity	• Jump
• Assault	• Legal
• Bite	• Military operations
• Burn	• Misadventure
• Complication	• Place
• Contact	• Radiation
• Drowning	• Status
• Explosion	• Striking against
• Exposure to	• Struck by
• Failure	• Suicide
• Fall	• War operations
• Forces of nature	

TABLE 18-8 Definitions for the Table of Drugs and Chemicals	
External Cause	**Description**
Poisoning, Accidental	Accidental overdose, wrong substance given or taken, drug or substance used or ingested by mistake, accidental use of a drug or chemical during a procedure.
Poisoning, Intentional Self-harm	Ingesting or using a substance, or taking a planned overdose, with the intent of harming oneself.
Poisoning, Assault	Substance contact or ingestion inflicted by another person with the intent to harm or kill.
Poisoning, Undetermined	The medical record states that the intent of the poisoning is unknown.
Adverse Effect	The correct substance(s), used or taken in the correct manner, caused an undesired reaction.
Underdosing	Injury due to using or taking less of a substance than directed.

Substance	Poisoning, Accidental (unintentional)	Poisoning, Intentional self-harm	Poisoning, Assault	Poisoning, Undetermined	Adverse effect	Underdosing
Trimethobenzamide	T45.0X1	T45.0X2	T45.0X3	T45.0X4	T45.0X5	T45.0X6
Trimethoprim	T37.8X1	T37.8X2	T37.8X3	T37.8X4	T37.8X5	T37.8X6
with sulfamethoxazole	T36.8X1	T36.8X2	T36.8X3	T36.8X4	T36.8X5	T36.8X6
Trimethylcarbinol	T51.3X1	T51.3X2	T51.3X3	T51.3X4	-	-
Trimethylpsoralen	T49.3X1	T49.3X2	T49.3X3	T49.3X4	T49.3X5	T49.3X6
Trimeton	T45.0X1	T45.0X2	T45.0X3	T45.0X4	T45.0X5	T45.0X6
Trimetrexate	T45.1X1	T45.1X2	T45.1X3	T45.1X4	T45.1X5	T45.1X6

Figure 18-11 ■ Example of the Table of Drugs and Chemicals.

Source: Papazian-Boyce, L. M. ICD-10-CM/PCS Coding: A Map for Success. © 2013. Reprinted by permission of Pearson Education, Inc. Upper Saddle River, NJ.

ICD-10-CM provides the Table of Drugs and Chemicals (**Figure 18-11** ■) to assist in coding these circumstances. It is a cross-tabulated index to poisoning and adverse effects of drugs and other chemical substances. Codes identify the substance used and the intent. Use this table as follows:

1. Locate the row in the Substance column that contains the name of the substance, listed alphabetically on the left side of the table.
2. Identify the column (second to sixth column), that corresponds to the intent.
3. Locate the preliminary code where the substance row and intent column intersect.
4. Verify the preliminary code in the Tabular List to identify the full code and assign the appropriate extension for the episode of care.
5. When more than one substance is involved, assign separate codes for each substance.

Assign additional codes to identify the condition that resulted from the use of the substance. When coding a poisoning, the poisoning code from the table is sequenced first, followed by the code(s) for the condition that resulted. When coding therapeutic use or underdosing, sequence the condition (effect) code first, followed by the code from the table.

Burns

Burns caused by a source of heat or radiation are classified under the Main Term *Burn* in the Index. Burns caused by contact with a chemical are classified under the Main Term *Corrosion* in the Index. When coding for burns, identify the anatomic site and degree (first, second, third).

Assign a code for the highest degree of burn at each site and an additional code for the extent of the total body surface

area (TBSA) affected by third-degree burns. Codes are based on the "rule of nines" in estimating the body surfaces involved, as illustrated in **Figure 18-12** ■. Assign external cause codes where applicable.

Example: Coding for burns

A patient suffered third-degree burns to the back and the back of the left arm, and second-degree burns to the back of the right arm when she fell into a campfire.

> *ICD-10-CM Codes:* T21.33XA Burn of third degree of upper back, initial encounter
> T22.392A Burn of third degree of multiple sites of left shoulder and upper limb, except wrist and hand, initial encounter
> T22.291A Burn of second degree of multiple sites of right shoulder and upper limb, except wrist and hand, initial encounter
> T31.32 Burns involving 30–39% of body surface with 20–29% third degree burns
> X03.0XXA Other exposure to controlled fire, not in building or structure, initial encounter
> W18.30XA Fall on same level, unspecified, initial encounter

HIV

Codes for HIV and AIDS differ based on the stage in the disease cycle, as summarized in Table 18-9. In addition, assign codes for all AIDS-related illnesses.

Influenza

Influenza is a condition that medical assistants encounter frequently. Influenza is caused by one of several types of viruses,

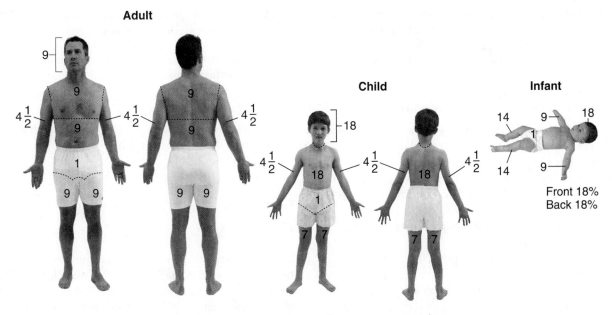

Note: Each arm totals 9% (front of arm $4\frac{1}{2}$ %, back of arm $4\frac{1}{2}$ %)

Figure 18-12 ■ Rule of nines.
Source: Pearson Education/PH College. Photographer: Michal Heron.

such as avian, novel A, H1N1, and swine. Influenza may have manifestations that affect the respiratory system, digestive system, or heart. To code for influenza, locate the Main Term *Influenza*; then locate the subterm for the specific virus or *unidentified (J11.-)*; then locate the next level of subterm to identify the manifestations. Verify the code in the Tabular List.

Example: Coding for Influenza

A patient presents with laryngitis that the physician diagnoses as an unidentified influenza virus.

ICD-10-CM Code: J11.1 Influenza due to unidentified influenza virus with other respiratory manifestations

Obstetrics

Obstetric coding is one of the more complex areas of coding because multiple codes are nearly always required. Coding guidelines for obstetrics are summarized in Table 18-10. Prenatal visits require a code for supervision of the pregnancy, codes for any complications that exist, and a code from category

TABLE 18-9 Coding for Stages of HIV/AIDS

Stage of Disease	ICD-10-CM Code
Exposure to HIV virus	Z20.6 Contact with and (suspected) exposure to human immunodeficiency virus [HIV]
HIV testing	Z11.4 Encounter for screening for human immunodeficiency virus [HIV]
Inconclusive test results	R75 Inconclusive laboratory evidence of human immunodeficiency virus [HIV]
Confirmed HIV (seropositive)	Z21 Asymptomatic human immunodeficiency virus [HIV] infection status
HIV counseling	Z71.7 Human immunodeficiency virus [HIV] counseling
AIDS manifestations or illnesses	B20 Human immunodeficiency virus [HIV] disease

TABLE 18-10 Obstetrics Coding

Type of Encounter	Index Main Term and Subterms
Routine prenatal visit	*Pregnancy, supervision* *Weeks of gestation (Z3A.-)*
Complications of pregnancy	*Pregnancy, complicated by*
Normal delivery	Tabular List: O80 Encounter for full-term uncomplicated delivery Z37.0 Single live birth
Delivery with complications	*Delivery, complicated by* *Outcome of delivery (Z37.-)*
Cesarean delivery	*Delivery, cesarean* *Outcome of delivery (Z37.-)*
Birth encounter for the newborn	Tabular List: Z38.- Liveborn infants according to place of birth and type of delivery *Newborn, born in hospital, born outside hospital, twin, triplet, quadruplet, quintuplet*

Z3A for the weeks of gestation. Most complications of pregnancy have a unique code from ICD-10-CM Chapter 15 Pregnancy, Childbirth, and the Puerperium (O00-O9A) that is to be used in place of, or in addition to, a code for the same condition in a nonpregnant person.

Example: Pregnancy-related condition

A pregnant woman, age 29, presents for a prenatal visit at 30 weeks of gestation. She has gestational diabetes (diabetes caused by pregnancy) that has been successfully controlled with diet. This is her first pregnancy.
>   *ICD-10-CM Codes:* Z34.03 Encounter for supervision of normal first pregnancy, third trimester
>   O24.410 Gestational diabetes mellitus in pregnancy, diet controlled
>   Z3A.30 30 weeks gestation of pregnancy

Example: Pre-existing condition affecting pregnancy

A pregnant woman, age 32, presents for monitoring of pre-existing Type 1 diabetes. This is her second pregnancy and she has completed 14 weeks of gestation.
>   *ICD-10-CM Codes:* O24.012 Pre-existing diabetes mellitus, type 1, in pregnancy, second trimester
>   E10.9 Type 1 diabetes mellitus without complications

The birth episode requires codes for the delivery, any complications, and the outcome of delivery. A normal delivery is defined as a vaginal delivery needing minimal or no assistance, resulting in a single liveborn infant. Multiple births, caesarean sections, and complicated deliveries require multiple codes that describe all the circumstances. All delivery encounters require an additional code to identify the number of live births and still births. These codes appear in category Z37 and are indexed under the Main Term entry *Outcome of delivery*.

A separate medical record is opened for all liveborn infants. The newborn record requires a code from category Z38 as the first diagnosis code to describe the location of birth, type of delivery, and number of liveborn mates. Any complications affecting the infant are also coded.

Diabetes

Not only is diabetes mellitus (DM) a common condition, it causes and impacts many other conditions, so medical assistants will frequently encounter the need to code for it. Diabetes requires the use of combination codes that identify the type of diabetes and any complications or manifestations when they exist. To code for diabetes, locate the Main Term *Diabetes* in the Index. Select the appropriate subterm for the type of diabetes: *type 1, type 2, due to drug or chemical,* or *due to underlying condition*. Follow the indented subterms under the type of diabetes to locate combination codes for the complications or manifestations. Assign codes for all conditions that coexist. Verify the combination code in the Tabular List to verify the type of diabetes and the complication.

When a type 2 diabetic requires long-term insulin use, assign the additional code Z79.4 to report this information.

Example: Combination code for diabetes and manifestation

A patient is seen for type 2 diabetes with diabetic nephropathy. The diabetes is managed with insulin.
>   *ICD-10-CM Codes:* E11.21 Type 2 diabetes mellitus with diabetic nephropathy
>   Z79.4 Long term (current) use of insulin

Pursuing Professional Certification

Medical assistants who enjoy the problem-solving and detective work involved in diagnostic coding may choose to pursue certification as a professional coder. This career path allows them to use their clinical knowledge to enhance their coding skills. Although many organizations offer certifications, the most widely recognized are the Certified Professional Coder (**CPC**), offered by the **AAPC** (formerly the American Academy of Professional Coders), and the Certified Coding Specialist-Physician based (**CCS-P**), offered by the American Health Information Management Association (**AHIMA**). Both certifications require an in-depth knowledge of both diagnostic and procedural coding, as well as reimbursement basics. Certification is obtained by passing a written examination that takes most people several hours to complete. Both organizations offer entry-level apprentice options for graduating students, as well as certification for hospital-based coders and advanced certification for a variety of physician and administrative specialties. Local chapter meetings provide opportunities for professional networking, education, and employment searches. AAPC and AHIMA Web sites, listed at the end of the chapter, provide more detailed information and requirements.

▸▸▸ Pulse Points

If It Wasn't Charted, It Wasn't Done

The saying in the medical office, "If it wasn't charted, it wasn't done," holds true for coding. A provider can only charge for items documented in patients' charts.

Whether medical assistants decide to become certified professional coders or remain in a general purpose administrative role, diagnostic coding skills are important to their career. Some medical assistants may perform hands-on coding, while others review encounter forms or serve as an interpreter or communication link for other coders. Medical assistants play a vital role in supporting both patients and their medical office when they understand how to abstract diagnostic information from the medical record and accurately translate it into codes that justify reimbursement.

REVIEW

Chapter Summary

- Diagnostic coding is the process of assigning a number to a description of the patient's condition, illness, disease, or other reason for the encounter as it appears in the health care provider's documentation in the patient's medical record.

- ICD-10-CM is a listing of alphanumeric codes, three to seven characters long, and descriptions used to report causes of mortality and morbidity.

- Diagnostic coding has existed for more than a century, beginning in 1893 with French physician Jacques Bertillon who created the Bertillon Classification of Causes of Death

- ICD-10-CM provides an expanded code structure that incorporates updated terminology and greater specificity and consistency. The implementation date was unknown at the time this text went to press.

- The implementation of ICD-10-CM is one of health care's top priorities and expenditures for the next several years as providers adjust to the new system.

- Medical offices report diagnosis on CMS-1500 forms and electronic claims to justify the reasons that services were provided, for reimbursement purposes.

- ICD-10-CM lists over 70,000 diagnostic codes in one volume, consisting of an Index and a Tabular List, which is updated annually and takes effect October 1 of each year.

- There are a number of documents within the medical record that may contain information needed for coding.

- The introductory material at the beginning of the ICD-10-CM provides instructions on how to use ICD-10-CM and outlines the Official Guidelines for Coding and Reporting (OGCR), official conventions, and publisher-specific conventions.

- The Index to Diseases and Injuries (Index) lists conditions, diseases, and reasons for seeking medical care alphabetically by Main Term and subterms that aid in locating the most appropriate code.

- The Tabular List presents codes in alphanumeric order by body system and/or etiology.

- The first step in diagnostic coding is to identify the first-listed diagnosis.

- The second step in diagnostic coding is to research the diagnosis in the Index.

- The third step in diagnostic coding is to verify the code(s) in the Tabular List.

- Reporting incorrect diagnosis codes on an insurance claim can create problems such as improper reimbursement, inaccurate patient medical history, and fraud, so medical assistants should show their professionalism by recognizing when additional expertise is required.

- A number of conditions and circumstances have unique tables, codes, and guidelines, including hypertension, neoplasms, Z-codes, fractures, external causes of injury, poisonings and adverse effects, burns, HIV, influenza, obstetrics, and diabetes.

- Medical assistants who enjoy the problem-solving and detective work involved in diagnostic coding may choose to pursue certification as a professional coder.

Chapter Review

Multiple Choice

1. On what date do updated ICD-10-CM codes go into effect each year?
   a. January 1
   b. March 1
   c. July 1
   d. October 1
   e. December 1

2. How are nonessential modifiers indicated in the Index?
   a. * asterisk
   b. + plus sign
   c. ( ) parentheses
   d. [ ] square brackets
   e. < > pointed brackets

3. ICD-10-CM codes have a maximum of how many characters?
   a. 3
   b. 4
   c. 5
   d. 6
   e. 7

4. Which coding situation does the following statement describe? A single code may describe multiple conditions, which requires careful attention to Index subterms and Tabular List conventions.
   a. Multiple coding
   b. Combination coding
   c. Uncertain diagnoses
   d. External cause
   e. Single coding

5. What character is a placeholder in codes with less than six characters that require a seventh character?
   a. X
   b. Z
   c. 0
   d. 9
   e. #

True/False

T F **1.** Diagnosis coding begins with the Tabular List.

T F **2.** Simple conditions can be coded directly from the Index.

T F **3.** Physician offices are the providers required to use ICD-10-CM.

T F **4.** Medical assistants should consult the Index before the Tabular List.

T F **5.** Medical assistants can show their professionalism by not asking for assistance in coding.

T F **6.** Diagnosis codes describe the need for medical care.

T F **7.** Each visit a patient has with a health care provider can only have one diagnosis code.

Short Answer

1. How do you determine the first-listed diagnosis assigned to a patient?
2. What is the Index and how should it be used?
3. What are the three steps in diagnosis coding?
4. Why would a physician code a condition as *suspected*?
5. What does the saying, "If it wasn't charted, it wasn't done" mean?
6. What is the Tabular List and how should it be used?
7. What are publisher-specific conventions? Give three examples.

Coding Exercises

Underline the Main Term. Look up each condition in the Index, then verify it in the Tabular List. Write the code on the line provided.

1. _____ Bronchial croup
2. _____ Allergic enteritis
3. _____ Furuncle, back
4. _____ Diabetes with cataract
5. _____ Rectocele with uterine prolapse (female)

Research

1. Interview a person who works in the billing department of a local medical office. How does that office handle the process of coding? Do the physicians assign the codes? What is the role of medical assistants in coding?
2. Look at the Medicare Web site. What are some of the rules Medicare applies regarding the use of diagnostic codes?
3. Look at your state's Medicaid Web site. What are some of the rules Medicaid applies regarding the use of diagnostic codes?

Practicum Application Experience

Mabel Donchez, a patient of Dr. Bridges, is being seen today for a painful elbow after falling. Dr. Bridges is uncertain whether the elbow is fractured or sprained, so she orders an X-ray. What diagnosis should be listed for the office visit encounter?

Resource Guide

AAPC
2480 South 3850 West
Suite B
Salt Lake City, UT 84120
Toll Free Phone: (800) 626-CODE (2633)

Phone: (801) 236-2200
Fax: (801) 236-2258
Email: info@aapc.com
http://www.aapc.com

American Health Information Management Association
233 N. Michigan Avenue, 21st Floor
Chicago, IL 60601-5800
Toll Free Phone: (800) 335-5535
Phone: (312) 233-1100
Fax: (312) 233-1090
Email: info@ahima.org
http://www.ahima.org

American Medical Association
515 N State Street
Chicago, IL 60610
Phone: (800) 621-8335
http://www.ama-assn.org/

Centers for Disease Control and Prevention
1600 Clifton Road
Atlanta, GA 30333
Phone: (800) 311-3435
http://www.cdc.gov

Flash Code (provides information on proper coding)
Phone: (800) 711-7873
http://flashcode.com/

OptumInsight
13625 Technology Drive
Eden Prairie, MN 55344
Phone: (888) 445-8745
Fax: (952) 833-7201
http://www.optuminsight.com/

19

Procedural Coding

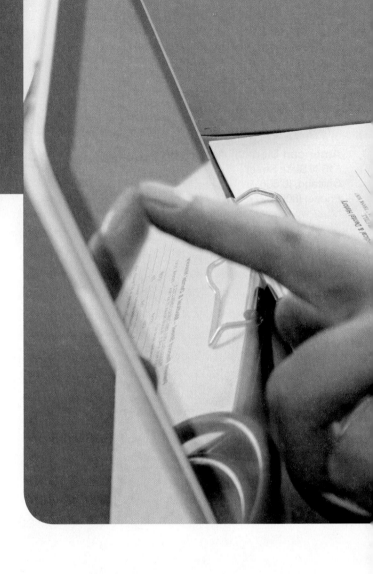

Case Study

Read the following case study and answer the critical thinking questions presented throughout the chapter.

At Monday morning's staff meeting, Dr. Anderson mentions she is unhappy with the amount she is being reimbursed for her Medicare patients' office visits. To boost reimbursement, Dr. Anderson asks her medical assistant, Lydia, to use higher codes for those patients.

Objectives

After completing this chapter, you should be able to:

19.1 Define and spell the key terminology in this chapter.

19.2 Understand the history of procedural coding.

19.3 Describe the organization of the CPT® coding manual.

19.4 List the steps to accurate CPT coding.

19.5 Discuss how modifiers are used in procedural coding.

19.6 List the steps to Evaluation and Management coding.

19.7 Explain the coding guidelines for surgery, radiology, pathology, laboratory, and medicine.

19.8 Explain the use of the Healthcare Common Procedure Coding System (HCPCS).

19.9 Explain the relationship between accurate documentation and reimbursement.

19.10 Assign CPT and HCPCS codes to patient encounters.

Competency Skills Performance

1. Code for a procedure.

CPT is a registered trademark of the American Medical Association.

Key Terminology

abuse—improper behavior and billing practices that result in improper financial gain but are not fraudulent

add-on code—a CPT code designated by the plus sign (+) that cannot be used alone; must be used with another CPT code

audit—a review process that verifies that every detail of a CPT code is clearly documented in the medical record

bilateral—on both sides of the body

bundling—the act of combining multiple services under a single, all-inclusive CPT code and one charge

category (CPT)—a division of a subheading within the CPT Tabular List

Category I codes—CPT codes numbered 00100 to 99999 representing widely used services and procedures approved by the FDA

Category II codes—optional codes used to collect and track data for performance measurement; four numbers followed by the letter F, such as 1002F

Category III codes—temporary codes for data collection and tracking the use of emerging technology, services, and procedures; four numbers followed by the letter T, such as 0162T

common descriptor—the portion of a standalone code before the semicolon that is shared with the indented codes that follow

contributing factors—three secondary criteria, in addition to the key components, that may influence the selection of an E&M code; include presenting problem, counseling/coordination of care, and physicians' face-to-face time with patients and families

coordination of care—a contributory factor in E&M coding that describes physicians' work in arranging care with other providers

counseling—a contributory factor in E&M coding that describes physicians' discussion with patients and family members regarding diagnosis, treatment options, instructions, and followup

Current Procedural Terminology—Level I of the HCPCS code set used to code procedures and services in outpatient health care settings

downcode—to assign a code for a lower level of service than was actually performed; done by some insurance companies to save money; done by some physicians to avoid fraud or abuse charges

edit—a specific coding or billing criterion that is checked for accuracy based on predetermined rules

established patient—a patient who has seen the same provider, or another provider of the same specialty or subspecialty, in the same practice within the past three years

Evaluation and Management—CPT codes used for billing physician services to evaluate and manage patient care, such as office visits

examination—a key component of E&M coding that describes the complexity of the physical assessment of the patient

face-to-face time—a contributory factor in E&M coding that measures the amount of time the provider spent in the presence of the patient and/or family, as opposed to time spent documenting the visit or arranging referrals

fraud—the act of intentionally billing for services that were never given, including billing for a service that has a higher reimbursement than the service provided

global period—the number of days surrounding a surgical procedure during which all services relating to that procedure—preoperative, during the surgery, and postoperative—are considered part of the surgical package

guidelines—specific instructions at the beginning of each section of the CPT manual that define terms and describe specific information about how to use codes in that section

Healthcare Common Procedure Coding System—the code set used to code procedures and services in the outpatient health care setting

history—a key component of E&M coding that describes the background, onset, and progression of the patient's current condition

indented code—a CPT code whose description is indented 3 spaces under another (standalone) code and whose definition includes the portion before the semicolon (;) in the standalone code

Index (CPT)—the alphabetical listing of CPT codes by procedure name, condition, eponym, and acronym

inpatient—a patient who has been formally admitted to a facility with written admission orders from a physician

instructional notes—directions in the Tabular List, which appear in parentheses before or after a code entry, to point the user to alternative codes for closely-related procedures or to codes that must or must not be used together

key component—three primary determining criteria in selecting an E&M code; include history, examination, and medical decision making

Level I codes—same as Current Procedural Terminology

Level II codes—HCPCS alphanumeric codes created by CMS to bill supplies, drugs, and certain services

Main Term (CPT)—words by which procedures and services are alphabetized in the CPT Index; may be a procedure, service, anatomic site, condition, synonym, eponym, or abbreviation

medical decision making—a key component of E&M coding that describes the complexity of establishing a diagnosis and/or selecting a management option

modifier—a two-character alphanumeric code appended to CPT (Level I) or Level II codes to further describe circumstances

modifying term—descriptive words in the Index that appear indented under the Main Term to further describe the service or procedure

new patient—a patient who has not seen the same provider, or another provider of the same specialty and subspecialty in the same practice, for more than three years

Key Terminology (continued)

outpatient—a patient who has not been formally admitted to a facility, such as one seen for office visits, emergency department visits, and observation status

panel—a group of laboratory tests ordered together to detect particular diseases or malfunctioning organs

parent code—see *standalone code*

patient status—the classification of patients as new or established

presenting problem—a contributory factor in E&M coding that consists of a disease, condition, illness, injury, symptom, sign, finding, complaint, or other reason for the encounter, as stated by the patient

procedural coding—the process of assigning codes to health care services and procedures

procedures—services health care providers perform or for patients

professional component—the portion of a test or procedure in which a qualified physician interprets the results and writes a report

relative value unit—unit of measure assigned to medical services based on the resources required to provide it; includes work, practice expense, and liability insurance

resequenced code—a CPT code that appears out of numerical sequence within a subsection in order to group it with similar codes

section—one of six major divisions of the CPT manual: evaluation and management; anesthesia; surgery; radiology; pathology and laboratory; and medicine

semicolon (;)—a punctuation mark in a standalone code; the part of the definition before the semicolon is used by the indented codes that follow

special instructions—directions within each section describing specific rules and definitions for use of codes within a particular category or subcategory

standalone code—a CPT code that contains a full description and is not dependent on another code for complete meaning

standardized—uniform practice

subcategory—a division of a category within the CPT Tabular List

subheading—a division of a subsection within the CPT Tabular List

subsection—subdivisions within a section of the CPT Tabular List

surgical package—the group of services included in the CPT code for a surgical procedure, as defined in the CPT Surgery Section guidelines

Tabular List—the numerical listing of all CPT codes, accompanied by guidelines and notes

technical component—the portion of a test or procedure that involves administering the procedure and providing the necessary personnel and equipment

unbundling—the illegal act of billing multiple services with separate CPT codes and separate charges that should be combined under a single CPT code and one charge

upcode—to illegally code and bill for a higher level of service than was actually provided

Abbreviations

AMA—American Medical Association

CMS—Centers for Medicare and Medicaid Services

CPT—Current Procedural Terminology

DME—durable medical equipment

E&M—Evaluation and Management

E/EX—examination

FDA—Food and Drug Administration

H/HX—history

HCPCS—Healthcare Common Procedure Coding System

MDM—medical decision making

POS—place of service

RVU—relative value unit

Certification Exam Coverage

AAMA (CMA) Exam Coverage:

- Coding systems
  - Current Procedural Terminology (CPT)
  - Healthcare Common Procedure Coding System (HCPCS)
  - Relationship between procedure and diagnosis codes

AAMA (CMA) certification exam topics are reprinted with permission of the American Association of Medical Assistants.

AMT (CMAS) Exam Coverage:

- Coding
  - Understand procedure coding
  - Employ Current Procedural Terminology (CPT) and Evaluation and Management codes appropriately
  - Employ Healthcare Common Procedure Coding System (HCPCS) codes appropriately

AMT (CMAS) certification exam topics are reprinted with permission of American Medical Technologists.

Introduction

Procedural coding is the act of assigning a code to a patient's procedure or service. Since 1966, procedure codes have been **standardized**, which has rendered coding both more efficient and more accurate. Accuracy in procedural coding is essential, because incorrect or inadequate coding may lead to denial or delay of insurance claims.

Overview and History of Procedural Coding

Current Procedural Terminology (CPT®), Fourth Edition, (CPT-4) is a listing of five-character alphanumeric codes and descriptions used to report outpatient medical services and **procedures**. The Health Insurance Portability and Accountability Act (HIPAA) mandates the use of CPT for all covered entities that handle electronic claims related to outpatient health care services. As a result, CPT is the standard for efficient and effective communication among health care providers, regulators, and payers.

The History of CPT Coding

Before the mid-1960s, most patients paid for their services out-of-pocket. When they had health insurance, they submitted their own claims to insurance companies and were reimbursed directly. There were no standard medical billing forms or procedure codes. Reimbursement was cost-based, meaning that the insurance companies paid whatever fees providers charged.

With the passage of Medicare and Medicaid in 1965, industry recognized the need to standardize the description of health care services. The Health Care Financing Administration (HCFA), now known as the Centers for Medicare and Medicaid Services (**CMS**), assigned the task of developing codes to the American Medical Association (**AMA**). The AMA developed and published the first edition of CPT in 1966, the year that the Medicare and Medicaid programs were implemented, and has been responsible for CPT codes ever since. The first edition of CPT primarily contained surgical procedures, with limited sections on medicine, radiology, and laboratory. Codes were four numbers in length.

In 1970, the second edition of CPT was published, which expanded surgical procedures and identified them as diagnostic or therapeutic. It also added procedures relating to internal medicine and expanded the other sections of the manual. The third edition was published within a few years and, in 1977, the fourth edition, still in use today, was adopted. At that time, a process was established to update the code set on a regular basis.

In 1983, the federal government adopted CPT as part of its Healthcare Common Procedure Coding System (HCPCS). This action mandated the use of HCPCS/CPT to report services billed to Medicare Part B. In October 1986, state Medicaid agencies were required to use HCPCS. In 1987, as part of the Omnibus Budget Reconciliation Act, HCFA mandated that CPT be used to report outpatient hospital surgical procedures.

The passage of HIPAA in 1996 required that uniform standards be established for electronic transactions. Effective October 16, 2003, CPT was designated a mandated procedure code set for covered entities for physician services and most other types of outpatient claims.

CPT codes must be used on the CMS-1500 claim form and its electronic equivalent, the 837P. To standardize medical fees and increase the accuracy of the coding process, in 1992 the U.S. Congress developed a system that assigned a **relative value unit** (**RVU**) to every health care procedure or treatment. The RVU is the basis used to determine Medicare fees.

CPT Coding Today

Today, the CPT manual covers all procedures approved by the Food and Drug Administration (**FDA**). The CPT lists over 8,800 procedural codes. The CPT manual is updated every year, with changes taking effect January 1 when a new manual is published. Code changes are published by the AMA in conjunction with CMS. CPT updates are made in order to clarify code descriptions and incorporate new technologies and equipment. Medical assistants should use the edition of the CPT that was in effect on the date of service.

Example: CPT Dates

On January 3, a medical assistant is coding services for patients seen during the past week and needs to decide which CPT manual to use. For patients seen on December 31, she uses the CPT manual for the old year. For patients seen on January 2, she uses the CPT manual for the new year.

▶▶▶ Pulse Points

Effective Date

Medical assistants should note that the transition date for CPT manuals is January 1. This differs from the transition date for ICD-10-CM diagnosis coding manuals, which is October 1.

The Role of the Medical Assistant in Procedure Coding

Medical assistants are most often involved with assigning procedure codes to basic procedures and services provided in the medical office or clinic. These services are the focus of this chapter.

In addition to providing services in the medical office, physicians also provide services in other settings such as an ambulatory surgery center; outpatient hospital departments such as radiology or cardiac catheterization lab; and inpatient hospitals. Although the services are provided in a location other than the medical office, physicians are still responsible for coding and billing the services they provide in those settings. These services usually require more complex coding than basic office services, and are coded by a certified coder who has advanced training. Medical assistants should understand the scope of their training and recognize when they need to reach out to a certified coder for assistance.

The Purpose of Procedure Coding

Procedure codes identify billable services provided to patients. Medical offices report CPT procedure codes on CMS-1500 forms and electronic claims to identify the services provided and the cost of those services. Physicians are paid for CPT codes, but diagnosis codes are required to explain the reason(s) for the encounter and/or the reason services were provided.

Example: Billable Services

An established patient presents in the office complaining of a sore throat. The physician performs a problem-focused history, a problem-focused examination, and straightforward medical decision making. The physician then takes a throat culture that will be processed in the office, to check for strep throat. The medical assistant reports an evaluation and management procedure code, 99212, that identifies the complexity of the encounter. An additional procedure code, 87880, is reported for the strep test. The diagnosis code, J02.9, identifies the sore throat, which was the reason for the visit and for the lab test.

On the CMS-1500 form, each CPT code must be cross-referenced to one or more diagnosis codes that identify the medical reason each service was provided. Diagnosis codes are entered in Item 21. Date(s) of service, CPT codes, charges and related information are entered on lines 1 through 6 of Item 24. In column 24E, enter the letter from Item 21 (A through L) that corresponds to the diagnosis that supports each service (**Figure 19-1** ■). Each service must be linked to one or more diagnosis codes. A diagnosis code can be linked to as many services as appropriate.

Medical assistants may find it challenging to find the most appropriate and accurate code for each patient encounter. For example, a patient encounter for what is commonly referred to as an "office visit" may be reported with any of 30-plus codes, depending on a number of circumstances surrounding the visit. However, only one code is correct in any given situation, so medical assistants must become familiar with the nuances among codes that might appear to be similar. Likewise, more than 50 codes exist for a patient who receives sutures for a wound. The correct code is based on the location, length, and depth of the wound. Medical assistants need to be familiar with all of the criteria for coding services offered by their office to be certain they select the accurate code.

It is improper to code for a more complex service than what was actually provided, in the hope of receiving higher reimbursement. Doing so is considered fraud and carries severe penalties, including fines and possible imprisonment. Medical assistants must also be attentive to entering codes correctly into the computer or onto the CMS-1500 billing form. A typographic error in a code number can result in a denied or rejected insurance claim, which must be corrected and rebilled, thus delaying the payment the office receives.

Figure 19-1 ■ CMS-1500 form showing linkage of CPT and diagnosis codes.

Compliance, Fraud, and Abuse

Compliance means following the rules. Accuracy in coding is important in order to prevent fraud or abuse. **Fraud** is the act of intentionally billing for services that were never given, which includes upcoding. **Abuse** is improper behavior and billing practices that result in improper financial gain but are not fraudulent.

When uncertain of the best code, it might be tempting to "guesstimate" and assign an approximate code. This practice might result in **upcoding**, which is coding for a higher level of service than was actually provided in order to gain higher reimbursement. Guessing could also result in **downcoding**, which is coding for a lower level of service than was actually provided, in order to avoid potential fraud or abuse. Downcoding may seem prudent to avoid fraud, but it deprives the medical office of reimbursement to which it is legally entitled.

Examples of fraud include knowingly doing any of the following:

- Billing for services not provided
- Billing for services not documented
- Misrepresenting the diagnosis to justify payment
- Billing for appointments that the patient failed to keep
- Altering documentation to receive a higher payment amount
- Soliciting, offering, or receiving a kickback (a financial incentive provided by another physician, laboratory, hospital, or pharmaceutical representative for using their services)
- Unbundling (billing separately for services that are included in a single procedure code)
- Falsifying certificates of medical necessity, plans of treatment, and medical records to justify payment
- Upcoding (billing for a service at a higher level than was actually provided)

Examples of Medicare abuse include:

- Charging excessively high fees for services or supplies
- Billing for services that were provided but not medically necessary
- Routinely filing duplicate claims for the same encounter, even if they do not result in duplicate payments
- Billing for supplies that were given to the patient but not medically necessary

Investigation of Medicare fraud and abuse is primarily the responsibility of the Department of Health and Human Services (HHS) Office of the Inspector General (OIG). The purpose of the OIG is to fight waste, fraud, and abuse in Medicare, Medicaid, and more than 300 other HHS programs. The CMS Web site offers consumers and patients information to encourage them to identify and report fraud.

The OIG has provided guidance to assist health care entities to develop effective internal controls to help them be aware of and follow the requirements of federal, state, and private health plans. The OIG believes that health care institutions that adopt and implement compliance programs significantly reduce fraud, abuse, and waste. Compliance programs identify internal controls to help providers be aware of and follow the requirements of federal, state, and private health plans. The OIG has issued sample compliance programs that include seven major characteristics:

- Develop and distribute written standards of conduct, policies, and procedures that address specific areas of potential fraud
- Designate a high level manager to be the chief compliance officer who oversees compliance activities
- Develop and implement education and training for employees
- Establish a process for reporting exceptions
- Develop an internal system to respond to accusations or reports of improper activities, and implement disciplinary measures when appropriate
- Develop an auditing and monitoring system
- Investigate and correct system-wide problems and develop policies regarding employment or retention of sanctioned individuals

The Patient Protection and Affordable Care Act (PPACA), passed in 2010, mandates compliance programs for providers who contract with Medicare and Medicaid. The timeline for defining and implementing compliance programs has not yet been established.

As in all areas of health care, ignorance is no excuse. Medical assistants need to be aware of the legal issues surrounding coding, but do not need to feel fearful. Many resources are available to help you be informed and confident. The CMS Web site provides several resources, including newsletters, Web pages, conference calls, and online training, to help keep providers and their staff informed. When you are unsure regarding a coding issue, talk to your supervisor, a certified coder, the physician, or a professional organization.

Organization of the CPT Manual

Medical assistants need to become familiar with the organization of the CPT manual (Table 19-1) so that they can find needed information quickly. Various editions or publishers sometimes organize the features differently and might not include some features. The content and labeling of specific topics sometimes changes from year to year when the manual is updated. For this reason, it is important to become familiar with the specific edition of the manual you use.

Introductory Matter

Introductory matter provides valuable reference material for medical assistants. This information appears within the first several pages of the CPT manual, before the code listing begins, and, in some editions, inside the front and back covers.

TABLE 19-1   Typical Organization of the CPT Manual

Location	Name	Description
Introductory Matter	Symbols, Modifiers, Anesthesia Physical Status Modifiers, Modifiers Approved for Hospital Outpatient Use, Place of Service Codes for Professional Claims, Contents, Introduction, Illustrated Anatomical and Procedural Review, Molecular Pathology, Evaluation and Management Tables	Provides a quick reference guide for commonly used information, including: CPT symbols Commonly used modifiers Place of service (**POS**) codes used on the CMS-1500 form Provides instructions on how to use the CPT manual. Lists common medical terms. Lists all illustrations contained within the manual. Provides basic anatomical diagrams. Provides overview of molecular pathology codes. Provides tables summarizing key components of evaluation and management codes.
Tabular List	N/A	Provides a numerical listing of all CPT codes, descriptions, and guidelines: Category I (Evaluation and management, anesthesia, surgery, radiology, pathology, medicine) Category II (Performance measures) Category III (Emerging technology, services, procedures).
Appendix A	Modifiers	Presents a complete description of all modifiers applicable to the current year codes.
Appendix B	Summary of Additions, Deletions and Revisions	A valuable reference at the beginning of the year when the new CPT codes are released.
Appendix C	Clinical Examples	Provides examples of E&M code scenarios for many medical specialties.
Appendix D	Summary of CPT Add-on Codes	Lists the code numbers for those codes than cannot be used alone.
Appendix E	Summary of CPT Codes Exempt from Modifier 51	A summary (not exhaustive) list of code numbers that do not require modifier 51, multiple procedures.
Appendix F	Summary of CPT Codes Exempt from Modifier 63	Lists code numbers that do not require modifier 63 procedure performed on infants less than 4 kg.
Appendix G	Summary of CPT Codes That Include Moderate (Conscious) Sedation	A list of codes in which moderate sedation by the surgeon is an inherent part of the procedure.
Appendix H	Alphabetical Clinical Topics Listing	A cross reference between Category II codes and situations in which they might be used.
Appendix I	Genetic Testing Code Modifiers	Lists modifiers for reporting molecular laboratory procedures related to genetic testing.
Appendix J	Electrodiagnostic Medicine Listing of Sensory, Motor, and Mixed Nerves	Used in accurately coding nerve conduction studies with CPT codes 95900, 95903, and 95904.
Appendix K	Product Pending FDA Approval	Lists CPT Category I codes for vaccines expected to be approved by the FDA at some point after the CPT manual is published, often in July.
Appendix L	Vascular Families	Depicts the structure of first, second, and third order vascular branches.
Appendix M	Deleted CPT Codes	Provides a cross reference to deleted and renumbered codes from 2007 to 2009. CPT no longer deletes and renumbers codes. Instead, they are **resequenced**.
Appendix N	Summary of Resequenced CPT Codes	Lists CPT codes that do not appear in numeric sequence in the Tabular Listing of CPT codes.

(continued)

TABLE 19-1 Typical Organization of the CPT Manual (*continued*)

Location	Name	Description
Appendix O	Multianalyte Assays with Algorithmic Analyses	A list of administrative codes for Multianalyte Assays with Algorithmic Analyses (MAAA) procedures that tend to be unique to a single clinical laboratory or manufacturer with cross references to Category I codes.
Index	CPT Index	Cross references conditions, anatomical sites, procedures, eponyms, and acronyms with the most likely codes or code ranges in the Tabular List.

The introductory matter provides a table of contents by page number, instructions for use of the codebook, and other valuable information, depending on the version of the manual used. Possible inclusions are a review of medical terminology and anatomical plates.

Inside the front cover or within the first few pages of most CPT manuals is a list of commonly used symbols, **modifiers**, and place-of-service codes. These are provided for quick reference for users who fully understand the correct use of these items. Inside the back cover of most CPT manuals are commonly used medical abbreviations. Publishers other than the AMA may place these features in different locations, or may not include them at all.

Tabular List

The **Tabular List** is a numerical listing of all CPT codes, divided into **Category I, Category II** and **Category III**. The Tabular List provides the official descriptions of CPT codes and the guidelines for using them. When coding, medical assistants first search for a code in the Index, then verify it in the Tabular List.

Category I

Category I codes, which comprise the bulk of the CPT, are numbered 00100 to 99999. They describe widely used services and procedures approved by the FDA. The CPT manual does not specifically label codes as Category I. Rather, Category I codes carry the names of the six **sections** (see Table 19-2).

TABLE 19-2 Sections of CPT Category I Codes

Section	Code Range(s)
Evaluation and Management (E&M)	99201–99499
Anesthesiology	00100–01999
	99100–99140
Surgery	10021–69990
Radiology	70010–79999
Pathology/Laboratory	80047–89398
Medicine	90281–99199
	99500–99607

While most of the codes are in numeric order, the codes 99201 through 99499 appear in the first section, Evaluation and Management (**E&M**). E&M codes are the most frequently used and are used by all medical specialties, so they are placed first for convenience. Other codes are used more selectively, based on the specific services provided by each office. The majority of this chapter discusses Category I codes.

Category II

Category II codes are optional codes used to collect and track data for performance measurement. They consist of four numbers followed by the letter F, such as 1002F. They identify certain services or test results that contribute to quality patient care and are usually included in a routine examination or other service. Examples include documentation of:

- Disease-specific assessments (heart failure, osteoarthritis)
- Certain types of care plans (prenatal flow sheet, pain management)
- Select patient history elements (fall history, tobacco use history)
- Components of physical assessment (blood pressure, weight, mental status)
- Test results (mammogram, oxygen saturation)

By using Category II codes, the medical office reduces the amount of time spent auditing charts to collect this information. The codes themselves are not billable and carry a charge of $0.00, but Medicare pays physicians a separate financial incentive for reporting Category II codes for data collection purposes.

Category III

Category III codes are temporary codes for data collection and for tracking the use of emerging technology, services, and procedures. The codes are four numbers followed by the letter T; for example, 0163T. If a Category III code is available, medical assistants should use it in place of a Category I code. Category III technology and procedures generally are in the FDA approval process. Services generally are items that the AMA is considering adding to Category I. For example, online medical evaluation was a temporary code, 0074T, from 2005 to 2007. In 2008, it was assigned to Category I with the code number 99444.

Appendices

The CPT manual has appendices that provide reference information. Several appendices summarize codes designated with special symbols throughout the CPT manual. Other appendices provide technical information used by medical practices that perform specialized procedures, such as nerve conduction studies, cardiac catheterization, or genetic testing. Table 19-1 lists appendices in the 2014 CPT manual; these may be updated in subsequent years. The appendices used most often by medical assistants in the medical office setting include the following:

> **Appendix A**—*Modifiers* presents a complete description of all modifiers applicable to the current year codes. Modifiers are two-character alphanumeric codes appended to CPT (Level I) or Level II codes to further describe circumstances. An abbreviated list of commonly used modifiers appears inside the front cover, but medical assistants should develop the habit of referring to Appendix A until they are familiar with the details of how a specific modifier is to be used. Use of modifiers is introduced later in the chapter.

> **Appendix B**—*Summary of Additions, Deletions and Revisions* is useful at the beginning of the year when the new CPT codes are released. Medical assistants can quickly cross reference the CPT codes on encounter forms to Appendix B in order to determine what commonly used codes in their office might be affected by the annual revision.

> **Appendix C**—*Clinical Examples* provides examples of E&M code scenarios for many medical specialties. These should not be used for coding, but for learning and understanding how various patient encounters might be coded. The most commonly used E&M codes each have at least one example.

Index

The Index lists procedures and services in the CPT manual alphabetically by **Main Term** and **modifying terms** that aid in locating the most appropriate code or range of codes. The CPT coding process begins with the **Index**. After identifying potential codes in the Index, users should verify them in the Tabular List. Never make the final code selection made based only on the Index, even if only one code appears.

How to Assign CPT Procedure Codes

Procedure coding consists of three basic steps:

1. Abstract procedures from the patient's medical record
2. Look up the procedure(s) in the Index.
3. Select and verify the code in the Tabular List.

Each of these steps is discussed below and the additional sub-steps are demonstrated in detail. Medical assistants need to patiently and accurately execute the process of procedural coding.

Step 1. Abstract Procedures from the Patient's Medical Record

Procedure coding is based on the patient's medical record. Medical assistants abstract clinical information from the medical record in order to code for services and the reasons they were provided. Coding must be performed to the highest level of certainty, meaning that all relevant information in the chart should be coded, but missing information should not be assumed or coded. In some cases, you need to query the provider for more information. If the medical record is incomplete or inaccurate, it should be corrected or amended following proper protocols before attempting to code. Any changes to the medical record should be made by the original author and must be signed and dated.

A number of documents within the medical record contain information needed for coding. When coding for office-based or other outpatient services, medical assistants refer to the encounter form, visit notes, in-house lab and radiology reports, and operative reports for outpatient procedures. When coding for services that physicians provide to inpatients, medical assistants refer to the daily rounds sheet, which lists the patients seen in the hospital; daily progress notes; and operative reports for inpatient procedures.

Keep in mind that when performing procedure coding, medical assistants must code and bill only for the services actually delivered on a specific date by a specific provider. Do not bill for services previously completed, performed by a different provider, or ordered to be completed in the future.

Example: Identifying Services to Code

A patient, Henry, makes a followup visit to Dr. Jessop related to back pain. Dr. Jessop discusses Henry's progress and current condition, performs a physical examination, reviews X-rays taken by the hospital outpatient department, adjusts Henry's medication, provides therapeutic ultrasound, and orders a magnetic resonance imaging (MRI) study. The medical assistant, Heather, codes for the two services that Dr. Jessop performed today:

- E&M visit, such as code 99214
- therapeutic ultrasound, 97035

Heather does NOT code for the following services, because Dr. Jessop did not perform them today:

- The X-ray was performed previously at another location and is billed by that facility.
- The E&M medical decision making includes Dr. Jessop reviewing the X-ray, adjusting the medication, writing the prescription, and ordering the MRI, so he does not bill separately for performing these tasks.
- The patient fills the prescription at the pharmacy, so the pharmacy bills for these services.
- The MRI will be performed in the future at another location and will be billed by the facility that performs the procedure.

Abstracting procedures from the patient's medical record involves three steps:

1. Identify the primary service or procedure.
2. Identify secondary services or procedures.
3. Identify the quantity of each procedure.

Identify the Primary Service or Procedure

Often the physician indicates procedure codes on the encounter form, but it is necessary to verify the codes on the encounter form against the medical record. When abstracting from the medical record, be certain not to write in the record. Make a photocopy of the pertinent pages that you wish to annotate or highlight, or keep a separate paper for notes. Remember to shred copies of medical records when you are done with them.

First, look for the chief complaint or reason for the visit. The primary service or procedure is the one most closely related to the reason for the encounter. Services or procedures may be indicated in SOAP notes, under O (Observation). Then, identify the primary procedure or the main service provided during the encounter. Often, this may simply be the E&M encounter—the history, examination, and medical decision making. It is common for the E&M to be the only service provided.

Identify Secondary Services or Procedures

Medical assistants should identify the secondary procedures, which are any additional services documented in the medical record in addition to the primary procedure. Secondary procedures are coded in the same way as primary procedures and prioritized from highest cost to lowest cost on the CMS-1500 form. This is because many insurance companies pay the first procedure in full, but discount additional procedures performed at the same time. Generally, the E&M is identified first, with additional procedures to follow. However, some insurers request that all services be listed in descending cost order.

Identify the Quantity of Each Procedure

For many procedures, such as E&M, the quantity is one. For services such as removal of lesions, identify the type and number of lesions removed. For services based on time, identify the number of minutes spent providing the service, then convert to the unit of time required by the code description. For example, therapeutic ultrasound is reported in 15-minute increments, so when 30 minutes of treatment are provided, report a quantity of 2 units on the CMS-1500 form.

The following sample patient scenario illustrates how to identify procedures. The same scenario is developed throughout the chapter for each step in the coding process.

Sample Patient Scenario

Select the Primary and Secondary Procedures

Patient presents with a lesion on the back. The physician prepares the area, administers local anesthetic, and removes a 0.7 cm benign lesion from the back. The site is closed with simple sutures.

The primary procedure is removal of a lesion on the back. The quantity is 1.

Step 2. Look Up the Procedure(s) in the Index

For each procedure, use the Index to locate the preliminary code(s). This involves determining the Main Term, modifying terms, and codes or code ranges. Never code directly from the Index. After completing this step, then you must verify the code(s) in the Tabular List. Using the Index involves three steps:

1. Identify the Main Term.
2. Review the modifying terms and/or instructional notes.
3. Identify the preliminary code(s).

Identify the Main Term

The Main Term is the word you look up in the Index to find the code(s). The CPT Index classifies Main Terms in four ways. Medical assistants may use any of these methods to locate a code in the Index. If one method does not provide adequate information, then another method may be used (**Figure 19-2** ■).

1. Look up the name of the *procedure* or *service,* such as *Endoscopy* or *Splint.*

Eponym/ Acronym	Procedure	Anatomic Site	Condition	Synonym
(Eponym) Colles fracture	Repair	Wrist	Fracture	
(Acronym) EKG	Electrocardiogram	Heart		Monitoring
	Excision	Eye	Cataract	Removal

Figure 19-2 ■ Alternative methods for locating the CPT Main Term.

2. Look up the name of the *organ* or *anatomic* site, such as *Colon* or *Tibia*.

3. Look up the name of a *condition* or *disease*, such as *Fracture* or *Polyp*.

4. Look up the *eponym* (a disease or condition named after an individual) such as *Colles fracture*; an abbreviation or *acronym*, such as *AIDS*; a nontechnical *synonym* (a word similar in meaning) such as *Removal* instead of *Excision*.

Medical assistants should be aware that in the CPT Index, Main Terms include organs and anatomic sites, whereas in ICD-10-CM, anatomic site is not an option in the Index. Because there are many choices of how to locate a Main Term, a good guideline is to search in this order: eponym or abbreviation; procedure or service name; organ or anatomic site; disease or condition; synonym.

The Main Term is always boldfaced with each word beginning with a capital letter. Some Main Terms are broad, with several pages of modifying terms, such as *Excision*, while others are quite specific with only a single code, such as *Color Vision Examination*.

Exercise 19-1

Getting Acquainted with the Index

Instructions: Below is a list of Main Terms that appear in the Index and a list of the types of Main Terms that the CPT manual uses. Next to each Main Term, write the name of the type of term. If possible, look up the Main Terms in the CPT Index.

Example: EKG *procedure*

Main Term	Type of Term
1. Abdomen _____	eponym
2. Ablation _____	acronym
3. Abscess _____	procedure
4. ADH _____	organ
5. Dana Operation _____	condition
6. Femur _____	synonym
7. Fibroadenoma _____	
8. Iridotomy _____	
9. Release _____	
10. Uterus _____	

Sample Patient Scenario

Identify the Main Term

Continue with the example of a patient who presents with a lesion on the back. There are four ways to look up the procedure. Using the acronym or eponym does not apply

to this case because there is no acronym or eponym for removal of lesions. You may look up the name of the procedure, *Excision*. You may also look up the organ system or anatomic site, *Skin*. Remember that the skin is an organ. These lesions are located on the "skin," not on the back or other body area. In the CPT manual, entries for back procedures reference the internal musculoskeletal structure of the back, not the skin of the back. Finally, you may look up a Main Term for the condition under *Lesion*.

Review the Modifying Terms and Instructional Notes

Main Terms rarely provide the exact code needed. Frequently, Main Terms function as major headings that have up to three levels of modifying terms. *Modifying terms* are descriptive words in the Index that appear indented under the Main Term to further describe the service or procedure. When modifying terms appear, it is important to review the entire list of options before selecting the most specific term (**Figure 19-3** ■). Medical assistants should be aware that *modifying terms* are different than two-digit *modifiers* that are appended to Category I codes.

The first level of modifying terms is aligned on the same margin as the Main Term, but in smaller, non-boldfaced type. The second and third levels of modifying terms are each indented several spaces beyond the previous level. They further describe the Main Term in reference to anatomical site (e.g., *Endoscopy, Anus*); extent (e.g., *Excision, Clavicle, Partial*); procedure—(e.g., *Electrocardiography, 24-Hour Monitoring*); or by similar descriptors.

When the Main Term or modifying term is too long to fit on one line, a carry-over line is used. Carry-over lines are indented the same number of spaces as the beginning of the line. It is important to read carefully to distinguish between carry-over lines and modifying terms.

Main Terms and modifying terms contain instructional notes, such as *see* or *see also*, which direct the user to synonyms for the code. For example, the entry *Pneumonotomy— see Incision, Lung* instructs the user to look under the Main Term *Incision* and the modifying term *Lung* in order to locate the codes for removal of the lung. In **Figure 19-3**, the instructional note under the Main Term *Endoscopy* states *See Arthroscopy; Thoracoscopy*. This instructional note directs the user to other Main Terms related to endoscopy.

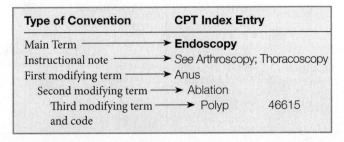

Type of Convention	CPT Index Entry
Main Term ⟶	**Endoscopy**
Instructional note ⟶	*See* Arthroscopy; Thoracoscopy
First modifying term ⟶	Anus
Second modifying term ⟶	Ablation
Third modifying term ⟶ and code	Polyp 46615

Figure 19-3 ■ Example of CPT conventions in the Index.

Codes next to a Main Term may be single codes, a range of codes, or a nonsequential list, as follows:

- A single code is one code that is presented for a specific modifying term. In Figure 19-3, *Polyp 46615* is an example of a single code.
- A range of codes is presented with a hyphen "-", such as *Bone Graft, Harvesting 20900–20902*. This indicates that all codes beginning with 20900 and ending with and including 20902 should be reviewed.
- Nonsequential codes are presented with a comma ",," such as *Biopsy, Urethra 52204, 52250, 52354, 53200*. This indicates that three codes should be reviewed, but the intervening code numbers are often not applicable.

Exercise 19-2
Identifying Conventions in the CPT Index

Instructions: Look up the Main Term *Blood* in the Index and read through the indented entries under it. Write the name of the type of convention next to each entry in the list below. Options for the type of convention appear in the right-hand column. All of the entries below appear under the Main Term *Blood*.

Example: Assay   *First-level modifying term*

Index Entry under *Blood*	Type of Convention
1. Blood _____	Main term
2. *See* Blood Cell Count; Compete Blood Count _____	Instructional note
3. Concentration 85046 _____	First-level modifying term
4. Hemoglobin _____	
5. Plasma Depletion 38214 _____	Second-level modifying term
6. 85306–85307, 85335, 85337 _____	Third-level modifying term
7. Transfusion 36430 _____	
8. Exchange 36455 _____	
9. Newborn 36450 _____	Carry-over line
10. *See* Blood Banking _____	

Sample Patient Scenario
Interpret CPT Index Conventions

Main Term: **Excision**

First modifying term: Lesion

Second modifying term: Skin

Third modifying term: Benign.

Continue with the example of a patient who presents with a lesion on the back. The medical assistant turns to the Index and looks for the Main Term *Excision*. She then locates the first modifying term, *Lesion*, because a lesion was excised. The second modifying term, *Skin*, identifies the body system and the third modifying term, *Benign*, describes the type of lesion. There is no modifying term for the location of the lesion. The anatomic site is identified in the Tabular List.

Identify the Preliminary Code(s)

When the appropriate modifying terms are located, the preliminary code(s) is printed immediately to the right. It is helpful to jot down the potential appropriate codes before verifying in the Tabular List, being careful not to transpose any digits. Never use the Index to make the final code selection. Even when only one code appears, it must be verified in the Tabular List to be certain the code selection is accurate, and any instructional notes must be read.

Sample Patient Scenario
Select the Preliminary Code(s)

Excision
  Lesion
    Benign 11400–11404, 11406, 11420–11424, 1426, 11440–11444, 11446, 11450, 11451, 11462, 11463, 11470, 11471

Continue with the example of a patient who presents with a lesion on the back. The entry for excision of a benign lesion lists multiple codes and code ranges that must be reviewed to select the appropriate code.

Step 3. Verify the Code in the Tabular List

All codes must be verified in the Tabular List to ensure that the description accurately represents the service provided. Medical assistants also need to read the guidelines, special instructions, and instructional notes printed in the Tabular List. Verifying the code in the Tabular List involves the following steps:

1. Locate the preliminary code(s) in the Tabular List.
2. Interpret Tabular List conventions.
3. Select the code with the highest level of specificity.
4. Review the code for bundling, add-on codes, and quantity.
5. Append modifiers, if needed.

Level	Description					
Section	Anesthesia		Surgery			
Subsection	HEAD	NECK	CARDIOVASCULAR SYSTEM			
Subheading	*none*	*none*	Heart and Pericardium			Arteries & Vessels
Category	*none*	*none*	*Pericardium*	*Cardiac Valves*	*Arterial Grafting*	*multiple*
Subcategory	*none*	*none*	*none*	**Aortic** **Mitral** **Tricuspid** **Pulmonary**	*none*	*multiple*

Figure 19-4 ■ Example of Tabular List organization levels and formatting.

6. Compare the final code with the documentation.
7. Assign the code.

Locate the Preliminary Code(s) in the Tabular List

Look for the preliminary code number in the Tabular List, where codes are arranged in numerical order. The Tabular List contains six sections, each of which is divided into **subsections**, **subheadings**, **categories**, and **subcategories** based on anatomy, procedure, condition, or descriptor **Figure 19-4** ■. Medical assistants should be aware that due to the expanding nature of the code set, some codes are not in strict numerical order. These are resequenced codes and are highlighted with the symbol "#" for easy identification.

Interpret Tabular List Conventions

Before medical assistants verify and finalize the code, they first need to interpret the conventions presented with the code. CPT codes are five-digit numbers with no decimal point, and a description to the right. Tabular List conventions include formatting, punctuation, narrative instructions, and symbols. Conventions may appear on the same line with the code, above it, below it, or at the beginning of a **subcategory**, category, subheading, subsection, or section. Look carefully for any information that may be relevant to the preliminary code selection, because this additional information can direct you to use a different code or an additional code. The Tabular List conventions of the semicolon, narrative instructions, and symbols are discussed next.

Semicolon In the Tabular List, an important convention is the use of the **semicolon** (;) and indented code descriptions. To conserve space and avoid having to repeat common terminology, some of the procedure descriptors in the Tabular List are not printed in their entirety, but rather refer back to a common portion of the procedure descriptor listed in a preceding entry. The **standalone** or **parent code** is the one whose description is left-justified and begins with a capital letter. The shared portion of the code before the semicolon is the common descriptor, which is shared with indented codes. The portion after the semicolon is the unique descriptor that applies to only one code number. The **indented code** description is indented three spaces and begins with a small letter. This description is the unique descriptor for that code number. The unique descriptor must be combined with the shared descriptor from the standalone code in order to obtain a full description of the code. Within a series of indented codes, medical assistants *must* refer back to the preceding standalone code to determine the common descriptor of the indented code(s). Indented codes describe variations on the standalone code, such as an alternative anatomic site, alternative procedure, or extent of services.

Figure 19-5 ■ illustrates this formatting convention. The standalone code is 27134. The words before the semicolon (*Revision of total hip arthroplasty*) are the common part of its description. This **common descriptor** should be considered part of each of the following indented codes in that series. For example, the full procedure descriptor represented by code 27137 is as follows:

27137 Revision of total hip arthroplasty; acetabular component only, with or without autograft or allograft

An indented code should not be billed together with the parent code, unless both services were provided. These are considered two distinct procedures or services. The common descriptor is simply a space-saving convention in the printed book.

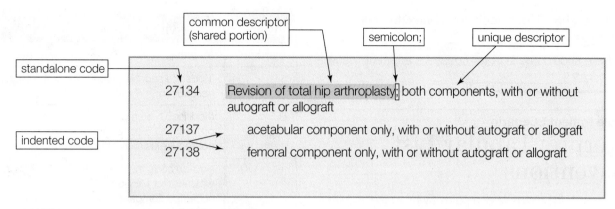

Figure 19-5 ■ Example of standalone and indented codes.

Exercise 19-3
Interpreting the Semicolon

Instructions: Look up the following codes in the CPT manual and circle whether each is a parent code or an indented code.

1. 11420	Parent	Indented
2. 62010	Parent	Indented
3. 81000	Parent	Indented
4. 31622	Parent	Indented
5. 27517	Parent	Indented

Instructions: Look up the following indented codes. Write the code number of its parent code.

6. 31578	Parent code _____
7. 11307	Parent code _____
8. 78315	Parent code _____
9. 98942	Parent code _____
10. 11422	Parent code _____

Narrative Instructions The CPT manual provides several types of narrative instructions which guide medical assistants in proper coding:

● **Guidelines** are instructions that appear at the beginning of each of the six sections and apply to all codes in that section. Guidelines also list commonly used modifiers and provide subsection information.

● **Special instructions** are directions within each section describing specific rules and definitions for use of codes within a particular category or subcategory. Read and interpret the special instructions before assigning a code, even if it means going back to the top of the page or a previous page to find them.

● **Instructional notes**, which appear in parentheses, direct the user to alternative codes for closely-related procedures or to codes that must or must not be used together (**Figure 19-6** ■).

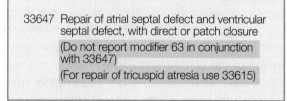

Figure 19-6 ■ Example of instructional notes.

Symbols Symbols in the Tabular List alert the user to certain circumstances that can affect use or interpretation of codes. A key appears at the bottom of each page. Medical assistants should become familiar with these meanings (Table 19-3).

Exercise 19-4
Interpreting Special Instructions

Look up CPT code 11400 in the Tabular List. Locate the special instructions under the subheading *Excision—Benign Lesions*. Read the instructions, then write down answers to the questions below:

1. Is local anesthesia included? _____

2. Where should one look for codes for shave removal?
_____

3. Where should one look for codes for electrosurgical and other methods of removal? _____

4. What is the definition of *Excision*? _____

5. What is the margin? _____

6. What is included in the size of the excised lesion?
_____

7. What type of closure is included? _____

8. Where should one look for codes for intermediate closures? _____

9. Where should one look for codes for complex closures? _____

10. Where should one look for codes for adjacent tissue transfer? _____

Sample Patient Scenario

Interpret Tabular List Conventions

Continue with the example of a patient who presents with a lesion on the back. The Index directed us to *Excision*, *Lesion*, *Skin*, *Benign*, and a list of several codes and code ranges. The task now is to look up these codes in the Tabular List to select the one that best describes the procedure (0.7 cm lesion from the back, closed with simple sutures, benign). First, read the special instructions at the beginning of the subheading *Excision—Benign Lesions* and complete exercise 19-4 on interpreting special instructions to help understand what is being said.

Upon looking at the Tabular List, you see that all of the codes listed appear under the heading *Excision—Benign Lesions*. Scan all the codes in this heading. The last six codes, 11450 to 11471, describe *Excision of skin and subcutaneous tissue for hidradenitis*, which is not appropriate for this case.

You quickly see among codes 11400 to 11446 that there are many indented codes that appear to be the same. For example, 11401, 11421, 11441 all state *excised diameter 0.6 to 1.0 cm*.

To understand the differences between these codes, it is necessary to compare the common portion of the accompanying standalone codes, 11400, 11420, 11440. The first part of the common portion of the standalone codes is also the same *Excision, benign lesion including margins, except skin tag (unless listed elsewhere)*. The last half line of the common portion that describes the body area is what varies among the standalone codes, as follows:

- Codes 11400 through 11406 identify lesions of the trunk, arms, or legs.
- Codes 11420 through 11426 identify lesions of the scalp, neck, hands, feet, and genitalia.
- Codes 11440 through 11446 identify lesions of the face, ears, eyelids, nose, lips, and mucous membrane.

Select the Code with the Highest Level of Specificity

There is no universal rule that describes how many codes need to be reviewed to identify the one with the highest specificity.

TABLE 19-3 CPT Symbols

Symbol	Meaning
⊙	Moderate sedation is bundled in the code description.
⊘	Modifier 51 exempt. When billing multiple procedures, a code with this symbol does not require using modifier 51.
+	Add-on code must be used in conjunction with another CPT code. Frequently, the accepted companion codes are provided in an instructional note. (When an add-on code is also an indented code, then report both the parent code and indented code.)
⁄	FDA approval pending. FDA approval of the vaccine described is expected to come during the current year.
( )	Parentheses enclose synonyms, eponyms, or supplementary descriptors for clarity. These terms do not have to appear in a physician's statement of condition in order to use the code.
●	New code in this edition of the CPT manual.
▲	Revised code. The code number is the same, but the descriptor has been updated. The descriptor should be reviewed to determine if it is still appropriate.
►◄	Contains new or revised text. Alerts users to the fact that guidelines or instructions have been updated and should be reviewed.
#	Resequenced code. Some codes do not appear in strict numerical sequence within a section of the Tabular Listing. Rather than deleting and renumbering codes, which was done prior to 2010, resequencing allows existing codes to be relocated to an appropriate place within the CPT subsection, based on the code concept, regardless of the numerical order. This symbol is used in front of the resequenced code to help the medical assistant locate it.

Sometimes, the best code is the first one listed; other times, there can be a dozen or more codes to review and additional ones to cross-reference. There also is no universal rule that describes how precise the correct code will be in its description. For example, many codes on the integumentary system include the size of the area treated, but the size is usually a range, such as 1.1 cm to 2.0 cm. If a treatment covers 1.5 cm exactly, there is not a more specific code or modifier to describe the exact size. The medical record often contains more detail than what is coded. Only by carefully interpreting the conventions associated with each code, category, and section can one be certain. As medical assistants become experienced in a particular office, they become very familiar with the most frequently used codes.

Sample Patient Scenario
Select the Code with the Highest Level of Specificity

Continue in the Tabular Listing with the example of a patient who presents with a lesion on the back. First, select the standalone code that contains the description for this patient. The term *back* does not appear, but using knowledge of anatomy, you know that *trunk* includes the back. Code 11400, *trunk, arms, or legs* is the appropriate standalone code.

Now select the indented code that describes the diameter of 0.7 cm. Code 11401 is *excised diameter 0.6 to 1.0 cm*, so this is the best code.

Review the Code for Appropriate Edits

Carefully review code descriptions, instructional notes, and special instructions one more time to be certain that the code selected is accurate. **Edits** are specific coding and billing criteria that are checked for accuracy based on predetermined rules. Payers' computer systems reject claims that violate edit rules. Edits that should be reviewed are bundling, add-on codes, and quantity definitions.

Bundling Edits Pay special attention to **bundling** edits, frequently triggered by the words *includes* and *not separately reportable*. These phrases indicate that multiple services are included in a single code. The words *report separately* or *use in conjunction with* indicate that additional codes should be used.

For example, the special instructions for codes *33510* to *33516 Coronary artery bypass, vein only* include both bundling and multiple coding situations.

- Regarding bundling, the instructions state *Procurement of the saphenous vein graft is included in the description of the work for 33510–33516 and should not be reported as a separate service or co-surgery.*
- Regarding multiple coding, an additional code is needed in some situations: *to report harvesting of an upper extremity vein, use 35500 in addition to the bypass procedure.*

Add-On Codes **Add-on codes** should be verified. Use of add-on codes might be limited to only a few codes that are listed in instructional notes. For example, when coding for discectomy of multiple disks, the code for each additional interspace is reported in addition to a specific primary procedure code. CPT add-on code 63078 should be used in conjunction with 60377.

Quantity Edits CPT codes differ regarding how the quantity of procedures is to be reported. This information is provided in the code description or special instructions. For example:

- To report removal of skin tags, a single code, 11200, describes *up to and including 15 lesions*. While the code is reported with a quantity of *1* on the CMS-1500 form, Item 24G, it describes any quantity from 1 to 15 lesions.
- To report shaving of epidermal or dermal lesions (11300–11313), each code describes a single lesion; multiple lesions of the same size and body area are reported by designating the number of lesions in Item 24G on the CMS-1500 form.
- To report end-stage renal disease services, use a single code for the entire month (90960–90961); the special instructions describe the scope of services included.

Codes that include a time-based element also vary in how quantity is reported. For example, codes for certain physical therapy treatments (97032–97039) describe 15 minutes of treatment with a quantity of *1* on the CMS-1500 form, Item 24G. Thirty minutes of treatment is reported with a quantity of *2* on the CMS-1500 form, Item 24G.

Sample Patient Scenario
Review Bundling, Add-on Codes, and Quantity Edits

Continue with the example of a patient who presents with a lesion on the back. The special instructions describe that local anesthesia and simple closure are included (bundled) with the codes in this subheading. No add-on codes apply. No additional coding is required for these services. Only a single lesion was excised, so there are no quantity edits.

Append Modifiers, If Needed Modifiers affect the complete description of a service and frequently have a significant impact on reimbursement and coding compliance. Use of modifiers may be described in the instructional notes, special instructions, or guidelines. The experience of the medical assistant is an important factor when determining if the situation calls for any modifiers.

Modifiers are two-digit suffixes used with CPT codes to report a service or procedure that has been modified by some specific circumstance without altering or modifying the basic definition or CPT code. The proper use of modifiers can speed up claims processing and increase reimbursement. Improper use of CPT modifiers may result in claim delays or denials. A complete list of modifiers, with their full definitions, appears in the CPT manual in Appendix A. Modifiers are used for a variety of reasons:

- To report only the professional component of a procedure or service
- To report a service mandated by a third-party payer
- To indicate that a procedure was performed **bilaterally**
- To report multiple procedures performed at the same session by the same provider
- To report a portion of a service or procedure that was reduced or eliminated at the physician's discretion

Modifier	Name	Application
24	Unrelated Evaluation and Management Service by the Same Physician during a Postoperative Period	Indicates that an evaluation and management service was performed during a postoperative period for a reason(s) unrelated to the original procedure. Append modifier 24 to the E&M code.
25	Significant, Separately Identifiable Evaluation and Management Service by the Same Physician on the Same Day of the Procedure or Other Service	Indicates that, on the day a procedure or service identified by a CPT code was performed, the patient's condition required a significant, separate E&M service above and beyond the usual preoperative and postoperative care associated with the procedure that was performed. Append modifier 25 to the E&M code.
26	Professional Component	Certain procedures are a combination of a physician or other qualified health care professional component and a technical component. When the physician or other qualified health care professional component is reported separate from the technical component, append modifier 26 to the procedure code.
32	Mandated Services	Identifies that a service was mandated by a third-party payer, governmental, legislative or regulatory requirement. Append modifier 32 to the basic procedure code.
50	Bilateral Procedure	When a procedure is performed on paired organs or anatomic sites at the same operative session, append modifier 50 to the procedure code. When a code description includes bilateral, then do not use modifier 50.
51	Multiple Procedures	When multiple procedures other than evaluation and management (E&M) services are performed at the same session by the same provider, the primary procedure should be listed first. The additional procedures are identified by appending modifier 51 to the additional procedure code. Modifier 51 should not be appended to add-on codes or those with the symbol ⊘, which means *exempt from modifier 51*.
57	Decision for Surgery	An evaluation and management service that resulted in the initial decision to perform the surgery may be identified by adding modifier 57 to the appropriate level of E&M service. This indicates that the encounter involved more than the typical preoperative assessment that is bundled with the surgical procedure and should be paid in addition to the surgical procedure.

TABLE 19-4 CPT Modifiers Used for Medical Office Services

- To report a portion of the surgical package provided by other than the primary surgeon.
- To report assistant surgeon services

The modifiers most commonly used in an office-based setting appear in Table 19-4. For more information on all modifiers, refer to Appendix A in the CPT manual.

Sample Patient Scenario

Append Modifiers, If Needed

Continue with the example of a patient who presents with a lesion on the back. No modifiers are required for this case. If more than one lesion had been excised, of a different size range or body area, modifier –51, multiple procedures, would be used on the subsequent procedures.

Compare the Final Code with the Documentation

As a final check, with coding manual instructions fresh in your mind, refer back to the original documentation and verify that all conditions of the code agree with the medical record. If a discrepancy arises, work through the process again from the beginning.

Sample Patient Scenario

Compare the Final Code with the Documentation

Continue with the example of a patient who presents with a lesion on the back. Code *11401 Excision, benign lesion including margins, except skin tag, trunk, arms or legs, excised diameter 0.6 cm to 1.0 cm* accurately matches the documented description of excision of

0.7 cm lesion from the back, closed with simple sutures, benign.

Assign the Code

Write down the final code where indicated on your worksheet or documentation. Be certain to proofread the number as you wrote or keyed it to catch transcription errors that are easy to make.

Repeat this process for any additional codes required by the medical record.

Selecting a procedure code might seem like a long and tedious process at first. As medical assistants become familiar with the services and codes used by their medical office, coding becomes faster and easier, but accuracy and attention to detail is always important. Taking time and care to correctly learn the fundamentals helps create long-term success in your coding role.

Coding for Evaluation and Management Services

Evaluation and Management (E&M) codes describe patient encounters with a physician for the evaluation and management of a health problem. Although these codes begin with the numbers 99, they are located out of numerical sequence in the CPT manual. The E&M section is the first section in the manual. This placement is for convenience, because these are the most commonly used group of CPT codes.

In some offices, the physician marks the E&M code on the encounter form. Medical assistants need to ensure that documentation in the medical record is consistent with the codes checked off. Offices should **audit** bills on a regular basis. Auditing is a detailed process that verifies that every detail of the E&M code is clearly documented. E&M coding possesses some differences from the rest of CPT coding. The key steps for E&M coding are summarized next. This provides a general overview of the criteria for E&M coding. Additional details can be found in the E&M section guidelines in the CPT manual and professional reference resources. The general process for coding E&M services includes the following steps:

1. Identify the type of service.
2. Determine the key components and contributing factors.
3. Verify the final code with the documentation.
4. Identify bundled and separately billable services.
5. Append modifiers, if needed.

Step 1. Identify the Type of Service

The first step in coding E&M services is to identify the category and subcategory of service, before trying to determine the specific code. The category and subcategory identify the general location, type of service, and type of patient. These elements must be selected correctly before a code can be assigned. Identifying the type of service involves three steps:

1. Identify the category.

TABLE 19-5 Categories of E&M Codes Used for Medical Office Services

E&M Category	Code Range
Office (and Other Outpatient) Services	99201–99215
Consultations (Office and Inpatient)	99241–99245
Emergency Department Services	99281–99288
Preventive Medicine Services	99381–99429

Source: CPT only Copyright 2013 American Medical Association. All rights reserved.

2. Identify the subcategory.
3. Read the reporting instructions.

Identify the Category

E&M codes are selected based on the category of service, which is the location or the type of service provided. A category may describe the location of service, such as office visit or hospital inpatient visit, or the type of service, such as consultation, critical care, or preventive care. This can be confusing because the *Office Visit* category does not list all services provided in the medical office. Office-based services also appear in other categories, such as *Consultation* and *Preventive Care*. It is important to be familiar with CPT definitions of these services, which are described in special instructions at the beginning of each subsection. Table 19-5 lists the most commonly used categories of E&M service with a brief description of each. To locate codes, look first in the Index, under the Main Term *Evaluation and Management*, then select the appropriate category.

Identify the Subcategory

Most of the E&M categories are further subdivided based on patient status (new vs. established), location (office vs. inpatient), frequency (initial vs. subsequent), or other relevant characteristic. Special instructions in the subsections describe these criteria. Commonly used terms are discussed next.

Medical assistants frequently need to determine **patient status**; that is, to distinguish between **new patients** and **established patients**. This criterion is used for office visits and preventive care. For coding purposes, a new patient is one who has not received any professional services from the physician, or another physician of the same specialty or subspecialty who belongs to the same group practice, within the past three years. An established patient is one who has received professional services from the physician, or another physician of the same specialty or subspecialty who belongs to the same group practice, within the past three years. Although the medical office may use other definitions for classifying new and established patient files, for coding purposes these definitions, which are presented in the CPT manual, must be used.

Codes that describe the frequency of the encounter, such as codes 99221 through 99223 for *Initial hospital care*, and codes

99231 through 99232 for *Subsequent hospital care*, identify whether this is the first encounter with a particular physician (or substitute from the same specialty and subspecialty) for the current hospital admission. The first, or initial, encounter requires a more extensive history and examination than subsequent visits during the same admission. Be aware that the meanings of initial and subsequent for CPT codes are different from the ICD-10-CM definitions for the initial and subsequent episodes of care.

Some codes are determined based on whether the patient is an **outpatient** or an **inpatient**. An inpatient is someone who has been formally admitted to a facility with written admission orders from a physician. All others are considered outpatients, even though they may occupy a hospital bed. For example, observation status and emergency department patients are outpatients. Observation status is a designated type of care in which a patient is hospitalized for monitoring, but not formally admitted.

Read the Reporting Instructions

Each category and subcategory within the E&M section contains definitions and instructions that describe key terms, how the codes are to be reported, and what may be bundled into the code description. Even though the instructions can sometimes be lengthy, take time to read and understand what is being said. For example, when reporting critical care services, special instructions provide examples of what comprises critical care, where it can be provided, and the age of the patient appropriate for the codes. In addition, the instructions list the CPT codes that are bundled into critical care and cannot be reported separately.

Step 2. Determine the Key Components and Contributing Factors

Within each subcategory, there are three to five levels of codes, in increasing order of complexity. It is necessary to determine the **key components** or other criteria used for code selection within each subcategory of E&M codes. Many codes are based on the extent of the history (H), the examination (E), and the medical decision making (MDM). Other codes are based on time or age. A summary of the three key components (H, E, MDM) follows. More detailed guidelines can be found in the CPT guidelines and advanced coding texts.

History

History (H, HX) describes the background, onset, and progression of the patient's current condition. The complexity of the history may be classified as follows:

- **Problem focused**—patient's problem is small; he has only one chief complaint and gives a brief history of his present illness or problem.
- **Expanded problem focused**—patient's problem is mild to moderate; he has more than one chief complaint and/or a more extensive history of his present illness or problem.

- **Detailed**—patient's problem is moderate to severe and he has pertinent past, family, and/or social history that is directly related to his current problem.

Each of these levels of history has specific definitions in the CPT manual and official documentation guidelines.

Examination

Examination (E/EX) describes the complexity of the physical assessment of the patient. The complexity of the examination may be classified as follows:

- **Problem focused**—A limited examination of the affected body area is done.
- **Expanded problem focused**—A limited examination of the affected body area and other related organ systems is done.
- **Detailed**—An extended examination of the affected body area and other related organ systems is performed.
- **Comprehensive**—A general multisystem examination is performed.

Each of these levels of examination has specific definitions in the CPT manual and official documentation guidelines.

Medical Decision Making

Medical decision making (MDM) describes the complexity of establishing a diagnosis and/or selecting a management option. The four types of medical decision making are:

- **Straightforward**—minimal diagnoses, minimal complexity, and minimal risk of complications
- **Low complexity**—limited diagnoses, limited complexity, and low-risk of complications
- **Moderate complexity**—multiple diagnoses, moderate complexity, and moderate risk of complications
- **High complexity**—extensive diagnoses, extensive complexity, and high risk of complications

Each of these levels of medical decision making has specific definitions in the CPT manual and official documentation guidelines.

The specific E&M code is selected based on how it meets the criteria of the key components. The criteria for each component are described in the code definition in the CPT manual. Some categories of E&M codes require that all three key components be at the level specified in the code description or a higher level in order to assign the code. Other categories require that only two of the key components be at the level specified in the code description or a higher level in order to assign the code. The number of components required is stated in the code description.

Contributing Factors

Contributing factors are **counseling, coordination of care**, and nature of the **presenting problem**. These factors rarely determine the E&M code, but should be consistent with the code selected.

- **Counseling**—provider's discussion with the patient and/ or a family concerning the patient's diagnosis, test results, impressions, prognosis, risks and benefits of treatment options, and instructions for management of the condition
- **Coordination of care**—working with other providers or agencies to provide the patient with needed care, such as referral to home health care
- **The presenting problem**—the primary reason the patient is seeing the provider

E&M codes take the following into consideration in determining the nature of the presenting problem:

- **Minimal**—The problem may not require the presence of the physician, but service is provided under the physician's supervision.
- **Self-limited or minor**—The problem runs a definite and prescribed course, is temporary, and is not likely to permanently alter the patient's health status.
- **Low severity**—The problem has a low risk of causing the patient's death without treatment, and full recovery is expected.
- **Moderate severity**—The problem has a risk of death without treatment, there is an uncertain prognosis or an increased likelihood the problem will cause permanent health problems for the patient.
- **High severity**—The problem has a high risk of causing the patient's death without treatment, or there may be a high probability of prolonged functional impairment to the patient as a result of this condition.

Time is also a consideration in E&M coding. Codes with the three key components also include an indication of the amount of time the physician typically spends **face-to-face** with the patient and/or family. Although these E&M codes should never be selected based on time, there are situations in which a code level can be increased due to time. When the time spent in counseling and coordination of care is more than 50 percent of total visit time, it may be considered a *controlling factor* to qualify for a higher level E&M code. Documentation needs to indicate the total amount of time spent with the patient and/or family, the amount of time spent in counseling and coordination of care, and a description of why the additional time was required.

Example: Coding for Evaluation and Management Services

The physician sees an established patient with type 2 diabetes mellitus for a six-month follow up visit. She performs an expanded problem focused history, a detailed examination, and medical decision making of moderate complexity. The physician marks CPT code 99213 on the encounter form. The medical assistant needs to verify that the code is correct.

1. The medical assistant identifies the category of service as office visit. In the CPT Index, she looks up the Main Term *Evaluation and Management*, then the modifying term *Office Visit*. The Index leads her to the code range 99201–99215.
2. The medical assistant reviews the subcategories of service in the Tabular List, which are *New Patient* and *Established Patient*. She identifies the patient status as established, because the patient has been seen within the past three years. This leads her to the subcategory *Established Patient*, codes 99211–99215.
3. She reads the subcategory instructions and code descriptions. She identifies that two of the three key components must be at the same level or higher in order to assign a code.
4. The history is expanded problem focused, which qualifies for code 99213.
5. The examination is detailed, which qualifies for code 99214 or lower.
6. The medical decision making is of moderate complexity, which qualifies for code 99214 or lower.
7. Two of the three components qualify for code 99214, so she determines that 99214 is the correct code. This is a higher level code than 99213 that the physician circled on the encounter form. Because the code requires only two of the three key components, she can assign 99214 even though one key component, history, does not qualify for this level.
8. The medical assistant double checks the key components in the medical record against the requirements of code 99214 in the CPT Tabular List, to ensure she did not overlook anything. She assigns code 99214 to the encounter. Code 99214 has a higher reimbursement rate than 99213.

Step 3. Compare the Final Code with the Documentation

As a final check, with coding manual instructions fresh in your mind, refer back to the original documentation and verify that all conditions of the code agree with the medical record. If a discrepancy arises, work through the process again from the beginning.

After verifying documentation against CPT guidelines, special instructions, and code descriptions, finalize the appropriate code and write it on your coding worksheet or enter it into the computer system. Be certain to double-check the accuracy of the code number, as transposition errors easily occur.

Step 4. Identify Bundled and Separately Billable Services

Medical assistants must determine which services are bundled in the E&M code and which should be billed separately. This ensures that coding is accurate, no fraud is committed, and the office receives reimbursements for all services provided.

An E&M code includes the following services, which cannot be billed separately:

- Discussions with patients and their families about the current problem
- Physical examination
- Reviewing test results, reports from other providers, and records of outside services
- Ordering tests and services
- Writing prescriptions
- Scheduling procedures
- Obtaining preapproval and precertifications
- Providing instructions and education to patients and their families

Certain codes, such as critical care, include a more specific list of bundled services. Surgical codes include postoperative followup. When an office or emergency department encounter develops into another E&M service on the same date, such as inpatient admission, the services may be combined into one code. For example, when a physician sees a patient in the emergency department and then admits the patient, the emergency department services are bundled into an E&M code for the hospital admission (*Initial Hospital Care 99221–99226*).

Identify any other services provided in the office that may be billed in addition to the E&M code, such as:

- Venipuncture
- Immunizations
- EKGs
- X-rays
- Lab tests performed in the office

Step 5. Append Modifiers, If Needed

Certain modifiers are used specifically for E&M coding and tell payers that an E&M service should be reimbursed and not bundled into another service. Refer to Table 19-4 or the CPT manual for more information about modifiers.

Example: E&M Modifiers

During a postoperative period for surgical repair of a fractured femur, the patient sprains a wrist and sees the same physician for treatment. The physician performs a detailed history, detailed exam, and medical decision making of moderate complexity. The physician bills the office visit E&M with modifier –24 to indicate that this visit is not part of the postoperative followup for the fracture.

> 99214-24 Evaluation and management of an established patient; unrelated evaluation and management service by the same physician during a postoperative period

What should Lydia tell Dr. Anderson about the relationship between appropriate codes and medical chart documentation?

Exercise 19-5
Coding for Evaluation and Management Services

Underline the Main Term. Use the CPT manual to look up each condition in the Index, then verify it in the Tabular List. Write the code on the line provided.

1. _____The physician sees a 16-year-old patient for followup after acute bacterial tonsillitis. He performed a problem focused examination and straightforward medical decision making.

2. _____The physician sees a new patient who is 63 years old. The patient has congestive heart failure, hypertension, and type 2 diabetes. She performed a comprehensive history, a comprehensive examination, and medical decision making of high complexity.

3. _____The physician admits a 16-year-old patient to the hospital due to acute bacterial tonsillitis so that IV antibiotics could be administered. The initial visit consists of a comprehensive history, a comprehensive examination, and medical decision making of moderate complexity.

4. _____The physician sees a 35-year-old patient for an annual comprehensive medical examination.

5. _____The emergency department physician sees a patient with acute eye pain due to an embedded glass fragment. He performs an expanded problem focused history, an expanded problem focused examination, and medical decision making of moderate complexity.

Coding for Special Situations
Coding for Surgery

The surgical section of CPT is the largest section and is divided into 14 subsections by body system (**Figure 19-7** ■). CPT defines the services included in the CPT surgical package. It also provides rules on bundling and unbundling that must be followed.

CPT Surgical Package

All CPT surgery codes include the **surgical package**, also known as the *global surgical concept*. The surgical package includes specific services, in addition to the operation, which

Integumentary System	10021–19499
Musculoskeletal System	20000–29999
Respiratory System	30000–32999
Cardiovascular System	33010–39599
Digestive System	40490–49999
Urinary System	50010–53899
Male Genital System	54000–55980
Female Genital System	56405–58999
Maternity Care and Delivery	59000–59899
Endocrine System	60000–60699
Nervous System	61000–64999
Eye and Ocular Adnexa	65091–68899
Auditory System	69000–69979
Operating Microscope	69990

Figure 19-7 ■ Subsections within the Surgery section.

cannot be billed separately. These services, outlined in the CPT Surgery Section guidelines include the following:

- One related E&M encounter on the date immediately prior to or on the date of procedure, subsequent to (following) the decision for surgery
- Preparing the patient for surgery including local infiltration, topical anesthesia
- Performing the operation, including normal additional procedures, such as debridement
- Evaluating the patient in the postanesthesia recovery area
- Immediate postoperative care, including dictating operative notes, talking with the family and other physicians
- Writing orders
- Typical postoperative followup visits for normal uncomplicated care

The **global period** refers to the number of days surrounding a surgical procedure during which all services relating to that procedure—preoperative, during the surgery, and postoperative—are considered part of the surgical package. Medicare defines postoperative followup periods of 0, 10, or 90 days, based on the type of procedure.

Third-party payers have varying definitions of what constitutes a surgical package and varying policies about what is in the surgical package, including the number of followup days. Therefore, it is important to ask about the surgical package criteria when certifying for surgery with third-party payers. By doing so, the office knows in advance which services may or may not be billed separately in addition to the surgical procedure.

The surgical package does not include certain services. Code these services separately for reimbursement in addition to the surgical package fee:

- Complications, exacerbations, recurrence, requiring additional services

- Ongoing care (other than the surgical procedure) for the condition for which a procedure was performed
- Care for coexisting conditions or injuries
- Supplies beyond the usual

Bundled Codes

In addition to the surgical package, CPT codes may include multiple procedures that are commonly performed together. Many surgical code descriptions include phrases, such as *with* or *only*, to identify incidental services included or excluded from a particular code. For example, code *31535 Laryngoscopy, direct, operative, <u>with</u> foreign body removal.*

When a description includes the phrase *with or without*, it means that the same code should be reported regardless of whether the identified incidental service was provided or not. For example, code *58150 Total abdominal hysterectomy (corpus and cervix), <u>with or without</u> removal of tube(s), <u>with or without</u> removal of ovary(s).*

The CPT subsection notes and guidelines may indicate that a particular code includes certain related or supporting procedures. **Unbundling** occurs when separate procedures are reported that should have been included under a bundled code. This practice is illegal and results in denial of a claim and, possibly, fines.

Example: CPT Surgical Package

Dr. O'Neil performed the surgery for a cholecystectomy. He monitored the patient in the recovery room and provided postoperative care instructions to the patient and family. He later saw the patient for postoperative followup one week and four weeks after the procedure. All services are included in the CPT surgical package, so Dr. O'Neil bills one code.

47600 Cholecystectomy.

Coding for Radiology (70010–79999)

The codes in the Radiology section report radiological services performed by or supervised by a physician. The process of performing a radiology examination includes several steps:

- **Order the examination**—A physician or other qualified health professional writes an order for the test, often as part of an E&M encounter. There is no code for ordering a radiological examination because it is included in the other services provided by the ordering physician. When the physician orders a radiology service that will be performed at another facility, do not assign a code from the 70000 series for the service.
- **Perform the actual imaging**—The radiological examination itself is reported by the provider or facility that actually provides the service using the 70000 series of codes. Creating the image, including personnel and equipment, is the **technical component** of a radiology code. When

PROCEDURE 19-1 Code for a Procedure

Theory and Rationale

Proper procedure coding in the medical office facilitates timely payment of providers' claims. Therefore, medical assistants must be familiar with the steps involved in locating and assigning proper procedure codes.

Materials

- CPT coding manual
- Superbill/encounter form
- Patient's chart

Competency

1. On the superbill, locate the procedure code the physician has circled.
2. Identify the primary and secondary services or procedures performed, as stated in the medical record.

3. Locate the Main Term in the Index.
4. Review any modifying terms or instructional notes associated with the Main Term.
5. Identify the preliminary code(s) associated with the most appropriate modifying term(s).
6. Locate the preliminary code(s) in the Tabular List.
7. Interpret the conventions used in the Tabular List.
8. Select the code with the highest level of specificity.
9. Review the code for appropriate bundling, add-on codes, and quantity.
10. Determine if modifiers are required.
11. Verify the final code against the documentation.
12. Assign the code.

only the technical component is provided, the facility appends the modifier -TC.

- **Analyze and report on the examination results**—A qualified physician reviews the image results and writes a report that details the findings. This is the **professional component** of a radiology code and is bundled into the same 70000 series code used to report performing the test. When a physician provides only the professional component, the medical assistant appends the modifier −26.

When a physician provides both the technical and professional components of a radiology service, the medical assistant bills the full code from the 70000 series with no modifiers.

Example: Professional and Technical Components

The physician takes a chest X-ray (single view) in the office to assess whether a patient has pneumonia. The physician provides the equipment and the technician, and interprets the results. The medical assistant assigns CPT code 71010 *Radiologic examination, chest; single view, frontal* with no modifiers, because the physician provided both the technical and professional components.

The Radiology section is divided by modality, or imaging method (Table 19-6). Each modality subsection is further divided by anatomic site.

Some radiological procedures, such as X-rays, are coded based on the number of views taken of the anatomic site. Each view is an image made from a different direction or angle, such as anterior and posterior (A/P). When reviewing the codes for a particular procedure, be sure that the number of views identified in the code description matches the number of views documented in the chart or report.

To locate codes for radiology procedures, look up the modality or imaging method as the Main Term and the anatomic site as the modifying term.

TABLE 19-6 Radiological Modalities (Methods)	
Method	**Description**
Computerized tomography (CT)	A 3-dimensional image created using X-rays to make a series of cross-sectional images in an area of the body.
Fluoroscopy	A real-time, moving X-ray image, usually viewed on a monitor.
Magnetic resonance imaging (MRI)	An image created using powerful magnets and radio waves.
Mammography	An image of the breasts, or mammary glands, created using low-dose X-rays.
Positron emission tomography (PET)	An image created using a radioactive substance called a tracer to show how organs and tissues are functioning.
Radiation oncology	A form of cancer treatment that uses high-energy ionizing radiation to shrink or kill tumors. Also called radiation therapy.
Ultrasound (US)	An image created using sound waves, useful to view soft structures within the body.
X-ray	A picture created using radiation particles, used primarily for solid structures within the body.

Example: Coding for Radiology

A patient is seen for an X-ray consisting of two views of one knee. In the Index, look up *X-ray*, then locate the modifying term *Knee 73560–73564, 73580*. Refer to the Tabular List to review codes 73560 through 73564 and code 73580. Select the code for the correct number of views: *73560 Radiologic examination, knee; 1 or 2 views*.

Coding for Pathology and Laboratory (80047–89398)

The codes in the Pathology/Laboratory section (80000 series of codes) cover services provided by physicians or by technicians under the supervision of a physician. The process of performing a laboratory test includes several steps:

- **Order the test**—A physician or other qualified health professional writes an order for the test, often as part of an E&M encounter. Do not code for writing orders.

- **Obtain and handle the sample**—The collection method used to obtain the sample, such as a biopsy, venipuncture, capillary stick, or arterial puncture, is coded separately. Codes in the 36400–36425 series are used to report obtaining of blood samples.

- **Perform the actual test**—The test itself is reported using the 80000 series of codes. Performing the test, including personnel and equipment, is the technical component of a laboratory code.

- **Analyze and report on the test results**—A qualified physician reviews the test results and writes a report that details the findings. This is the professional component of a laboratory code and is bundled into the same 80000-series code used to report performing the test.

The Pathology and Laboratory section is divided by type of test (Table 19-7), the type of specimen, and the substance being tested for. To locate a CPT for a laboratory or pathology procedure, look up the name of the test, the substance tested for, or the type of specimen in the Index. Procedures and services are listed in the Index under the following types of Main Terms:

- Name of the test, such as urinalysis, drug test
- Procedure, such as hormone assay or fine needle aspiration
- Abbreviations, such as CBC, RBC, TLC
- Panel of tests, under Blood Tests
- Type of specimen, such as blood or urine

The Pathology and Laboratory section provides codes for organ or disease-oriented panels 80047–80076 series. A **panel** is a group of tests ordered together to detect particular diseases or malfunctioning organs. When a panel is reported, all of the listed tests must have been performed with no substitution. If all the tests listed in the panel code are not performed, then the individual CPT codes for each test should be listed, not the code for the panel. Panels were developed for coding purposes and should not be interpreted as clinical standards for testing.

TABLE 19-7 Types of Laboratory Tests

Type of Test	Description
Chemistry	Quantitative tests for the amount of a substance contained in a specimen
Microbiology	Tests that identify the presence and type of microorganisms in a specimen
Hematology	Blood tests to determine cell counts of various types of blood cells
Immunology	Tests on antigens, allergens, or antibodies
Cytopathology	The microscopic examination of cells from anywhere in the body to detect conditions and determine if neoplasms are benign or malignant
Pathology	The visual examination of body structures or tissue, with or without a microscope

Example: Disease-oriented Panels

The physician marks the encounter form for 80051 *Electrolyte Panel*. The medical assistant checks the documentation to confirm that the each of the following tests were performed:

82374	Carbon dioxide
82435	Chloride
84132	Potassium
84295	Sodium

The medical assistant enters CPT code 80051 in Item 24D on the CMS-1500 form.

Some medical practices have laboratory equipment and perform their own testing. In-office labs must be certified by the Clinical Laboratory Improvement Amendment (CLIA) of 1988, which awards three levels of certification. The lowest level allows in-office certified labs to perform dipstick urinalysis and urine pregnancy. If the medical practice does not have a lab but obtains the specimen for the lab, the venipuncture code 36415 may be billed for obtaining the blood sample. As in every medical setting, the Occupational and Safety and Health Administration (OSHA) regulates safety.

Although Medicare does not allow physicians to bill for lab work they did not perform, other third-party payers do. When a medical practice has a contract with a lab and pays the lab for the work, the medical practice may bill for the tests reported. The modifier –90 is attached to the code for the lab test. On the CMS-1500, Item 20 must be checked "Yes" and the fee that the medical practice pays the lab must be entered under "Charges" in Item 24F. Finally, Item 32 must report the name, address, and NPI of the laboratory.

When the medical office collects a specimen to be sent to an outside lab for processing, code only the specimen collection and handling.

Example: Specimen Collection and Handling

The office draws blood for a metabolic panel and sends it to an outside lab for processing.

> 36415 Collection of venous blood by venipuncture
>
> 99000 Handling and/or conveyance of specimen for transfer from the office to a laboratory

When the medical office collects a specimen and processes it in the office, code the specimen collection and the test itself.

Example: In-office Lab Tests

The office draws blood for a CBC with differential, and processes it in the in-house lab.

> 36415 Collection of venous blood by venipuncture
>
> 85025 Blood count; complete (CBC), automated (Hgb, Hct, RBC, WBC and platelet count) and automated differential WBC count

Coding for Medicine (90281–99199; 99500–99602)

The Medicine section of the CPT manual contains codes for reporting diagnostic testing, non-invasive or minimally invasive procedures (procedures that do not require a surgical incision), and treatments for all areas of medical practice, as well as some nonphysician providers. Examples include vaccines, psychiatry, ophthalmology, cardiology, allergy, neurology, infusion therapy, audiology, and physical and occupational therapy.

Codes in this section are, in general, divided by medical specialty. To locate a code in the Index, look up the name of the procedure, such as electrocardiogram, or the condition for which it is provided.

Immunizations and Vaccinations

Immunizations and vaccinations are a service commonly provided in medical offices. Immunizations require two codes, one for administering the immunization and the other for the particular vaccine or toxoid that is given (**Figure 19-8** ■). The codes for administering the vaccines are divided based on the age of the patient and whether or not counseling was provided to parents of children. Add-on codes are provided when more than one immunization is administered at the same encounter.

To locate codes for administration of the vaccine, look for the MainTerm *Immunization Administration* in the Index. To locate codes for the product administered, look in the Index for the name of the product, such as *DTaP* or *Typhoid*. You may also look up the Main Term *Vaccines*, then select the appropriate modifying term for the specific product.

Assigning CPT Codes

Instructions: Underline the Main Term. Use the CPT manual to look up each condition in the Index, then verify it in the Tabular List. Write the code on the line provided.

Example: *29086* <u>Finger</u> cast

1. _____ Excision of pilonidal cyst, extensive

2. _____ Excision of a 1.5 cm tumor of the subcutaneous tissue on the face

3. _____ Routine 12-lead EKG with interpretation and report

4. _____ Transvaginal ultrasound on a pregnant female with real time image documentation

5. _____ Urinalysis, by dip stick, non-automated, without microscopy

6. _____ Biopsy of the vestibule of the mouth

7. _____, _____ Suture of two digital nerves in the foot (2 codes)

8. _____ Intracapsular cataract extraction with insertion of intraocular lens prosthesis (1-stage procedure)

9. _____ Incision and drainage of an abscess on the eyelid

10. _____ Quantity _____ Wheelchair management, assessment, and training, 30 minutes

The Healthcare Common Procedure Coding System (HCPCS)

The **Healthcare Common Procedure Coding System (HCPCS)**, pronounced "Hick Picks," is a set of codes developed and maintained by CMS for the reporting of professional services, nonphysician services, supplies, durable medical equipment (**DME**), and injectable drugs. HCPCS codes are divided into two levels.

CPT codes are HCPCS **Level I codes** for professional services.

Level II codes are alphanumeric codes that begin with a letter, followed by four numbers, for example, A4356. Typically,

> 90471 Immunization administration
> 90710 Measles, mumps, rubella, and varicella vaccine (MMRV), live, for subcutaneous use

Figure 19-8 ■ Coding for immunizations.

when professionals refer to "HCPCS codes," they are referring to Level II codes. Level II codes cover supplies, DME, drugs, nonphysician providers, and certain physician services for Medicare and Medicaid. When CPT and HCPCS codes exist for the same service, with the same description, use the CPT code. When procedure descriptions differ, use HCPCS Level II codes, because these codes are required by Medicare and Medicaid. They have been mandated as a HIPAA uniform code set for all insurance carriers, but implementation is in progress. Be sure to check with private carriers to verify if they accept HCPCS Level II codes. Reimbursement for supplies and equipment is usually faster when HCPCS codes are used, because these codes are more specific than the generic CPT code for supplies, which is 99070. A list of the categories in Level II appears in Table 19-8. Level II codes are updated on a quarterly basis; the manual is published annually in October. Quarterly updates are available on the CMS Web site at www.cms.gov.

The HCPCS Level II coding manual contains an Index and a Tabular Listing. As with the other coding manuals, use the Index first to locate the item or service, then refer to the Tabular List to verify. Many DME manufacturers print a suggested HCPCS code on the item packaging. This is a useful aid, but always verify the HCPCS code in the manual. Many entries in the manual also contain cross-reference information to Medicare reimbursement rules for the specific item or service.

HCPCS Level II also contains alphanumeric modifiers that can be used with either Level I CPT codes or Level II codes. The most commonly used modifiers are those that designate specific anatomical sites of procedures and nonphysician provider types (Table 19-9). Many additional modifiers exist for specific Medicare and Medicaid reimbursement situations. One of the most important of these is the modifier -GA,

TABLE 19-8 Level II HCPCS Codes

Service	Code Range
Transportation services	A0021–A0999
Medical and surgical supplies	A4206–A7509
Miscellaneous and experimental	A9000–A9999
Enteral and parenteral therapy	B4000–B9999
Temporary hospital outpatient PPS	C1300–C9899
Dental procedures	D0000–D9999
Durable medical equipment (DME)	E0100–E9999
Procedures and services, temporary	G0008–G9156
Alcoholic and drug abuse treatment services	H0001–H0237
Drugs administered other than oral method	J0120–J8499
Chemotherapy drugs	J8501–J9999
Temporary codes for DMERCS	K0000–K9999
Orthotic procedures	L0000–L4999
Prosthetic procedures	L5000–L9999
Medical services	M0000–M0301
Pathology and laboratory	P0000–P9999
Temporary codes	Q0035–Q9968
Diagnostic radiology services	R0000–R5999
Private payer codes	S0000–S9999
State Medicaid agency codes	T1000–T9999
Vision	V0000–V2999
Hearing services	V5000–V5999

TABLE 19-9 HCPCS Modifiers Used for Medical Office Services

Modifier	Description
AH	Clinical psychologist
AJ	Clinical social worker
E1	Upper left eyelid
E2	Lower left eyelid
E3	Upper right eyelid
E4	Lower right eyelid
F1	Left hand, second digit
F2	Left hand, third digit
F3	Left hand, fourth digit
F4	Left hand, fifth digit
F5	Right hand, thumb
F6	Right hand, second digit
F7	Right hand, third digit
F8	Right hand, fourth digit
F9	Right hand, fifth digit
FA	Left hand, thumb
GA	Signed advance beneficiary notice (ABN) form on file (for Medicare patients)
LT	Left side
PC	Professional courtesy
RT	Right side
SA	Nurse practitioner with physician
TC	Technical component

Source: www.cms.gov

which indicates that a Medicare Advanced Beneficiary Notice (ABN) form was signed by the patient when a covered service is expected to be denied. Through experience, medical assistants become familiar with the specific requirements for their medical office.

Exercise 19-7
HCPCS Coding

Instructions: Underline the Main Term. Use the HCPCS manual to look up each condition in the Index, then verify it in the Tabular List. Write the code on the line provided.

Example: *L0120* Contour cervical collar

1. _____Spenco removable foot insert, molded to patient model

2. _____Lightweight wheelchair with detachable arms and swing-away detachable, elevating leg rest

3. _____Eye patch

4. _____Infusion set for external insulin pump, needle type

5. _____Anterior chamber intraocular lens

Ensuring Proper Reimbursement

To receive proper payment for medical services, physician offices must keep adequate, accurate, and complete patient medical and billing records. The adage, "If it isn't charted, it wasn't done," applies. Medical offices must keep accurate and thorough documentation of all patient encounters for legal purposes and in order to perform accurate and complete procedure coding.

Proper coding begins with the right tools: a current year CPT coding manual, a HCPCS manual, and a medical dictionary. Outdated coding tools can provide outdated codes, and outdated codes risk claim delay or denial. With the right tools on hand, every service or procedure must be documented in electronic or paper form before any claims are sent to insurance companies. When medical assistants are asked to code charts with incomplete service or procedure documentation, they should route the charts back to the health care providers who performed the services with a query. While rerouting may delay insurance claim submission, in the long run it is faster and more effective than submitting inaccurate or incomplete claims.

Medical assistants may work in offices that use certified coders to assign and audit procedure codes. Because this chapter provides an introduction to procedure coding, medical assistants should be aware of coding situations that require the attention of a certified coder. Examples of such situations include those requiring multiple CPT codes, complex operative procedures, and those with many choices in the CPT Tabular List.

Reporting incorrect procedure codes on an insurance claim can create problems such as improper reimbursement, fraud, and inaccurate patient medical history. Whenever medical assistants are unsure of how to select a code, they should reach out to their supervisor or a certified coder. Awareness of special coding situations enables medical assistants to show their professionalism by recognizing when additional expertise is required.

Critical Thinking Question 19-2

Refer back to the case study at the beginning of the chapter. Assuming Lydia complied with Dr. Anderson's request to bill Medicare for higher codes, what might Medicare do, and why?

Critical Thinking Question 19-3

Referring to the case study at the beginning of the chapter, how could Lydia describe upcoding to Dr. Anderson?

In Practice

During the five years Audrey has worked for Dr. Suarez, the physician has often asked her to bill for services he did not perform. Audrey has never objected, in part because she feels patients are unharmed by the practice. She also believes she is blameless, because she receives no additional money from the process.

One day Audrey arrives at work to find that Dr. Suarez has been arrested. Later, the physician is convicted and sentenced to two years in jail. The office closes, and Audrey loses her job. Audrey begins a job search but finds that her association with Dr. Suarez is affecting her negatively. In fact, several potential employers have turned her away as a result. One of those employers said, "I'm sorry, but we just can't trust someone who worked for a doctor involved in insurance fraud." How could Audrey have avoided this situation?

REVIEW

Chapter Summary

- The CPT coding manual is designed to standardize the coding process by requiring health care providers to choose a procedure code based on the explicit description.
- CPT is a listing of five-character alphanumeric codes and descriptions used to report outpatient medical services and procedures.
- With the passage of Medicare and Medicaid in 1965, industry recognized the need to standardize the description of health care services.
- Today, the CPT manual lists over 8,800 codes which are updated annually to clarify code descriptions and incorporate new technologies and equipment.
- The challenge in procedural coding is to find the most appropriate and accurate code for each patient encounter.
- Medical assistants need to become familiar with the organization of the CPT manual so that they can find needed information quickly.
- A list of commonly used symbols, modifiers, and place-of-service codes appears inside the front cover of the CPT manual.
- The Tabular List is a numerical listing of all CPT codes, divided into Category I, Category II, and Category III.
- The CPT manual has several appendices, which provide additional reference information.
- The Index lists procedures and services in the CPT manual alphabetically by Main Term and modifying terms that aid in locating the most appropriate code or range of codes.
- Accurate procedure coding consists of three basic steps: 1) abstract procedures from the patient's medical record; 2) look up the procedure(s) in the Index; and 3) select and verify the code in the Tabular List.

- Medical assistants abstract clinical information from the medical record in order to code for services and the reasons they were provided.
- Using the Index involves determining the Main Term, modifying terms, and codes or code ranges.
- All codes must be verified in the Tabular List to ensure that the description accurately describes the service provided.
- Coding for surgery requires adhering to the CPT surgical package and following rules on bundling and unbundling.
- Modifiers are two-digit suffixes used with CPT codes to report a service or procedure that has been modified by some specific circumstance without altering or modifying the basic definition or CPT code.
- Evaluation and Management (E&M) codes describe patient encounters with a physician for the evaluation and management of a health problem.
- Coding for E&M services requires five steps: 1) identify the type of service; 2) determine the key components and contributing factors; 3) compare the final code with the documentation; 4) identify bundled and separately billable services; and 5) append modifiers, if needed.
- The Healthcare Common Procedure Coding System (HCPCS) provides codes for reporting nonphysician services, supplies, or durable medical equipment (DME), and certain physician services for Medicare and Medicaid.
- To receive proper payment for medical services, physician offices must keep adequate, accurate, and complete patient medical and billing records.
- Reporting incorrect procedure codes on an insurance claim can create problems such as improper reimbursement, fraud, and inaccurate patient medical history.

Chapter Review

Multiple Choice

1. Procedure codes are always _____ digits long.
   a. three
   b. four
   c. five
   d. six
   e. seven

2. Which section of the CPT manual should be consulted first, when assigning a code?
   a. Index
   b. Tabular list
   c. Table of contents
   d. Appendix A
   e. Appendix B

3. "Standardized" procedural coding means that every health care provider:
   a. uses the same code to describe the same service
   b. references the same manual to look up codes
   c. employs only registered or certified medical assistants as coders
   d. charges the same price for the same service
   e. all of the above

4. The "CPT" acronym stands for:
   a. Correct Procedural Terminology
   b. Current Procedural Terminology
   c. Correct Payment Terminology
   d. Current Physician Terminology
   e. Current Professional Terminology

5. The portion of a test or procedure in which a qualified physician interprets the results and writes a report is called:
   a. technical component
   b. professional component
   c. global package
   d. bundling
   e. results reporting

True/False

T F **1.** E&M codes are rarely used in health care.

T F **2.** When the CPT Index lists only one code after the Main Term, the code must be verified in the Tabular List.

T F **3.** The time a physician spends with a patient is the most important factor in code selection.

T F **4.** An indented code must be billed together with the parent code.

T F **5.** All payers follow the same definition of the surgical package.

Short Answer

1. When do new CPT codes take effect each year?
2. What are the four levels of history and physical examination for E&M codes?
3. What are the four levels of decision making for E&M codes?

4. What is the general purpose of modifiers?
5. What does it mean to "unbundle" codes?
6. Explain the use of the semicolon in the CPT Tabular List.
7. When multiple procedures are performed on the same day, how should they appear on the CMS-1500 billing form?
8. What is the CPT surgical package and how does it affect billing?
9. Explain what is meant by "upcoding."
10. Describe the relationship between accurate documentation and proper reimbursement.

Coding Exercises

Underline the Main Term. Use the CPT manual to look up each condition in the Index, then verify it in the Tabular List. Write the code on the line provided.

1. _____Extracapsular cataract removal with insertion of intraocular lens prosthesis (1-stage procedure), using the phacoemulsification technique
2. _____Tonsillectomy and adenoidectomy for a 13-year-old patient
3. _____Laparoscopic control of an upper GI hemorrhage
4. _____CT scan, bone density study
5. _____Office visit for a 45-year-old male, last seen 5 years ago, who came in due to visible hematuria. The physician provided a detailed history, a detailed examination, and medical decision making of low complexity.

Research

1. Interview a person who works in the billing office of a local medical office. How does that office handle the process of procedural coding? Do the physicians assign the codes? Do the medical assistants assign the codes?
2. Go to your state's Department of Health Web site. What resources are available for providers who have questions about proper coding?
3. Look at your state's Medicaid Web site. What are some of the rules Medicaid applies regarding the use of procedure codes?

Practicum Application Experience

Willie Harrison, a Medicare-covered patient, arrives at Dr. Annissette's office, and the physician removes two skin tags from Willie's neck. After the procedure, the physician circles one procedure code on the superbill and writes "× 2" next to it to indicate the medical assistant should charge for two procedures. What is the proper way for the medical assistant to code for this service, including the quantity?

Resource Guide

AAPC (formerly known as the American Academy of Professional Coders)
2480 South 3850 West, Suite B
Salt Lake City, UT 84120
Phone: (800) 626-2633
http://www.aapc.org

American Health Information Management Association (AHIMA)
233 N. Michigan Avenue, 21st Floor
Chicago, IL 60601-5809
Phone: (800) 335-5535
http://www.ahima.org

American Medical Association (AMA)
515 N. State Street
Chicago, IL 60610
Phone: (800) 621-8335
http://www.ama-assn.org

Center for Medicare and Medicaid Services (CMS)
7500 Security Boulevard
Baltimore, MD 21244
Phone: (877) 267-2323
http://www.cms.gov

20

Billing, Collections, and Credit

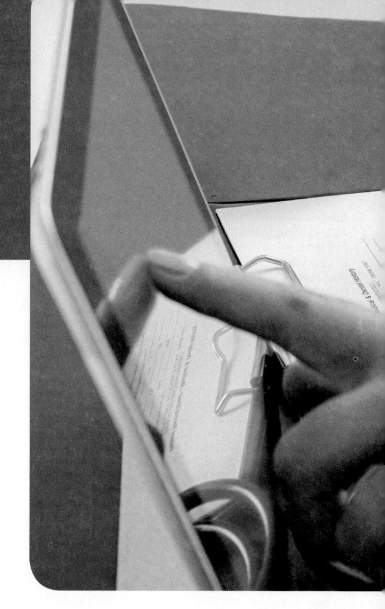

Case Study

Read the following case study and answer the critical thinking questions presented throughout the chapter.

Millie Alonso owes $550 for services her young son received, but she has made no payments for 2 months. As a result, her account now appears as past due. The certified medical assistant must call Millie to determine when she will send payment, either in full or by installment. The assistant knows that the office maximum allowed balance owing is $500 and that the minimum monthly payment is $50.

Objectives

After completing this chapter, you should be able to:

20.1 Define and spell the key terminology in this chapter.

20.2 Identify the three types of payment typically made in the medical office.

20.3 Discuss how a computerized medical billing system is used in the medical office, and list desired features.

20.4 Outline how professional fees are determined, and create a fee schedule.

20.5 Understand how physicians contract to become participating providers, and how that benefits patients in that insurance plan.

20.6 Discuss how to communicate medical office credit and collection policies to patients.

20.7 List information required on patient registration forms, and verify patient identification.

20.8 Manage accounts receivables.

20.9 Describe the various types of collection issues in managed care.

20.10 List and describe collection and credit laws that pertain to the medical practice.

20.11 Research collection agencies, and describe their pros and cons.

20.12 Describe the medical assistant's role when account overpayments are made.

20.13 Describe how small claims court works for the medical office, and discuss the pros and cons of using this method to collect past-due accounts.

Key Terminology

accounts receivables (AR)—money owed the medical practice

aging report—documentation of the money owed the medical office and how long accounts have been outstanding

certified letter—postal service letter that the recipient must sign for upon receipt

collection agency—company that pursues overdue accounts for a fee

community property laws—legislation that deems one spouse financially responsible for the other spouse's debts

dual fee schedule—facility or health care provider with two fees for the same service

Fair Debt Collection Practices Act (FDCPA)—law that dictates how debts may be collected

fee schedule—list of services and their fees

geographical practice cost index (GPCI)—Medicare system of adjusting fees based on the area in which the health care provider practices

hardship agreement—agreement a patient signs to indicate an inability to pay full health care costs due to financial hardship

insurance fraud—illegal act by a health care provider involving an insurance company

national conversion factor—number released by Medicare each year that determines fee schedules for all health care services

national standard—point of reference for developing charges for health care services used throughout the United States

Omnibus Budget Reconciliation Act (OBRA)—legislation passed by Congress in 1989 to calculate health care service fees by formula

patient billing statements—monthly statements sent to patients who have an outstanding balance

post—to add charges or payments to a patient's account

professional courtesy—to give a patient a discount, or free service, due to the fact that the patient is a health care professional

Red Flags Rule—rule passed in January 2008 by the Federal Trade Commission, along with other governmental agencies, to help prevent identity theft

relative value unit (RVU)—numeric value assigned by Medicare to formulate fee schedules for health care providers

tickler file—tool for tracking future events, such as patient appointments

uncollectible—account believed never to be paid

write off—to remove a balance from a patient account

Abbreviations

AR—accounts receivable

CMS—Centers for Medicare and Medicaid Services

CPT—Current Procedural Terminology

FDCPA—Fair Debt Collection Practices Act

GPCI—geographic price cost index

HIPAA—Health Insurance Portability and Accountability Act

NSF—nonsufficient funds

OBRA—Omnibus Budget Reconciliation Act

RBRVS—resource-based relative value scale

RVU—relative value unit

Certification Exam Coverage

AAMA (CMA) Exam Coverage:
- Accounts receivable
  - Billing procedures
    - Itemization
    - Billing cycles
  - Aging/collection procedures
    - Collection agencies
    - Consumer protection acts

AMT (CMAS) Exam Coverage:
- Fundamental financial management
  - Manage accounts receivable
  - Understand professional fee structures
  - Understand credit arrangements

- Patient accounts
  - Manage patient accounts/ledgers
  - Manage collections in compliance with state and federal regulations

AMT (RMA) Exam Coverage:
- Coding
  - Process insurance payments and contractual write-off amounts
  - Track unpaid claims
  - Generate aging reports
- Financial bookkeeping
  - Understand terminology associated with medical financial bookkeeping

AAMA (CMA) certification exam topics are reprinted with permission of the American Association of Medical Assistants.

AMT (CMAS) certification exam topics are reprinted with permission of American Medical Technologists.

AMT (RMA) certification exam topics are reprinted with permission of American Medical Technologists.

Certification Exam Coverage (continued)

- Patient billing
  - Maintain and explain physician's fee schedules
  - Collect and post payments
  - Manage patient ledgers and accounts
  - Understand and prepare *Truth in Lending* statements
  - Prepare and mail itemized statements
  - Understand and employ available billing methods
  - Understand and employ billing cycles
- Collection
  - Prepare aging reports and identify delinquent accounts
  - Perform skip tracing
  - Understand application of the Fair Debt Collections Practices Act
  - Identify and understand bankruptcy and small claims procedures
  - Understand and perform collections procedures
- Fundamental medical office accounting procedures
  - Employ appropriate accounting procedures
    - Computerized
  - Perform daily balancing procedures

- Prepare monthly trial balance
- Apply accounts receivable and payable principles
- Banking procedures
  - Prepare and make bank deposits
  - Maintain checking accounts
  - Reconcile bank statements
  - Understand check processing procedures and requirements
    - Nonsufficient funds (NSF)
- Financial mathematics
  - Understand and perform appropriate calculations related to patient and practice accounts

NCCT (NCMA) Exam Coverage:
- General office procedures
  - Patient instruction
- Bookkeeping
  - Record keeping
  - Preparing and collecting patient accounts

Competency Skills Performance

1. Prepare an accounts receivable trial balance.
2. Explain professional fees to a patient.
3. Call a patient regarding an overdue account.
4. Send a patient a billing statement.
5. Post a nonsufficient funds check.
6. Post an adjustment to a patient account.
7. Post a collection agency payment.
8. Process a patient refund.
9. Process an insurance company overpayment.

Introduction

To stay in business, the medical office must be financially sound. Service fees, a vital facet of an office's success, must be in line with federal and local laws, as well as consistent from patient to patient. In health care, billing, collections, and credit are best undertaken equitably and communicated about openly.

Identifying Payment Basics

Patients typically make three types of payment in the medical office: 1) cash, 2) check, or 3) debit or credit card. Some medical offices use prepaid cards or health care finance cards that patients apply for just for payment of their medical bills. With cash payments, medical assistants should write receipts both for patients and the office. Keeping a copy of the receipt in the medical office helps discourage stealing by the office staff. With a paper trail, medical assistants or office managers can easily track all office cash. In the event the patient has a dispute about the amount of cash payment made, both the office and the patient will have a copy of the receipt for reference.

When patients offer personal checks as payment, the medical assistant must verify that the amount written out in words on the check matches the amount written in numerals. Assistants must also ensure that checks are dated and signed. When an assistant takes a check from a party other than the patient, the assistant should request the check writer's photo identification to verify the writer's identity. Many medical offices do not accept third-party checks. A third-party check is written on an account owned by someone other than the patient. When checks are for large amounts, the assistant should call the issuing bank to ensure funds are available. When a check is marked

"Payment in Full," the assistant must verify that the check is for the full amount owed by the patient. When it is not, patients might later have a legal argument that no additional payment is required.

Depending on the number and dollar amount of credit card charges, the medical office pays bank fees in the amount of 1 to 3 percent of charges for debit or credit card payments when they accept credit card payments from patients. Some offices use check-verification systems that, while costly, guarantee checks. Some of these systems simply check to see if patients have written bad checks. Others are more sophisticated, holding the patient's bank funds until the check clears. As these systems become more sophisticated, however, their cost increases.

Computerized Billing Systems

While computerized medical billing systems vary, most allow staff to:

- **Post** charges and payments to patient accounts
- Print insurance billing forms and patient billing forms
- Create **aging reports** that document the money owed to the medical office by patients and how long the account has been outstanding

Billing systems with basic features, such as reports, are affordable for most medical offices. Higher-level features increase the price of billing systems. Some billing systems, for example, offer integrated electronic appointment books. Others send insurance claims electronically and receive insurance payments electronically. Some billing systems even allow remote access, which means health care teams can access their billing systems when out of the office. To ensure that the office receives the software package it needs, the medical assistant or office manager should research a number of options.

Most medical billing programs offer a wide variety of reports that provide information such as all patients with birthdays in any given month, or all female patients over age 40 who have not had a mammogram in the past year. These features are useful in marketing services for the medical office.

Fee Schedules

In 1989, the U.S. Congress passed the **Omnibus Budget Reconciliation Act** (**OBRA**), in part to require that physician reimbursement for Medicare services be based on a **fee schedule** (**Figure 20-1** ■). Fee schedules set maximum amounts for services using the resource-based relative value scale (**RBRVS**), which is designed to reduce Medicare costs and establish a **national standard** for payments to physicians. This national standard is itself organized with a separate fee for each Current Procedural Coding (**CPT**) code used for patient visits.

Medicare service fees are calculated based on the five following factors:

- Service intensity

AUDIOLOGY SERVICES		
Screening audio air only	92551	$38.00
Pure tone air	92552	$37.00
Pure tone air and bone	92553	$50.00
Comprehensive audio	92557	$101.00
Loudness balance test	92562	$38.00
Tone decay	92563	$41.00
Tympanography	92567	$40.00
Acoustic reflex	92568	$42.00
Reflex decay	92569	$43.00
Visual reinforced audio	92579	$78.00
Brain stem audiogram	92585	$327.00

Figure 20-1 ■ Sample fee schedule.

- Time needed for the service
- Skills needed to perform the service
- Practice's overhead
- Practice's malpractice premiums

Physicians' fees are adjusted according to a **geographical practice cost index** (**GPCI**), which factors in the differing health care costs across the United States. Together these factors determine a health care provider's **relative value unit** (**RVU**). The RVU was devised by the Centers for Medicare and Medicaid Services (**CMS**) as a way for physicians to create a fee schedule for the services they render. RVUs take into account three factors: how much work by the physician is involved in performing the service, what sort of expertise the physician needs to have in order to perform the service, and the cost of the physician's malpractice insurance policy.

Each year, Medicare assigns a **national conversion factor** that is multiplied by the RVU. The national conversion factor is a number released by Medicare each year that determines fee schedules for all health care services. The national conversion factor is multiplied by the physician's RVU for any given service or procedure to determine the allowed fee for that service. For example, imagine CPT code 99205 has an RVU of 4.78 for a health care provider practicing in the Los Angeles area, and the national conversion factor is 37.5623. This would make the Medicare allowed charge for this service $179.55 (4.78 × 37.5623 = $179.55). Because most health insurance plans base their fee schedules on the Medicare fee schedule, the Medicare allowed charge is typically considered the maximum charge any insurance plan will allow for any given service or procedure. **Dual fee schedules**, which impose different fees on different patients, are fraudulent. Exceptions to this would be fee schedules that are contracted between providers and managed care insurance companies.

In Practice

Dr. Bowman wants to raise his prices for certain services. He tells his medical assistant he fails to understand why insurance companies do not pay him more simply because he has begun charging more. What can the medical assistant say about fee schedule determination?

Participating Provider Agreements

Most patients with private health insurance are covered by managed care plans. As a condition of participation, managed care plans credential health care providers and require those providers to apply. When providers agree to participate in managed care plans, they agree to accept predetermined fee schedules. Some managed care plans also dictate the type of medications that are covered on the plans and the types of specialist referrals providers are allowed to make.

Participating provider agreements range from several pages long to small-book size. Though it might be time consuming, physicians should read their agreements in full. Once providers have signed with plans, they are obligated to see patients with that coverage for the agreed-upon fees, which might be lower than providers are willing to accept.

The best way to review participating provider agreements is with a highlighter. Medical assistants should highlight all areas of interest or concern, especially any details about fee schedules or provider care restrictions, and then review the highlighted areas with the physicians. Objections to any item may be grounds for declining plan participation.

Credit and Collections

The best way to ensure that patients pay their bills properly is to discuss the medical office's credit and collection policies before services are rendered. Medical assistants should discuss all fees and outline all payment policies. When patients will make regular payments on their balances, for example, medical assistants should provide written contracts that stipulate the payment amounts and due dates (**Figure 20-2 ■**). Such contracts avoid confusion and reduce or eliminate patient questions.

To further ensure that payment terms are clear, many medical offices include important financial information in their office brochures and send these brochures, along with registration paperwork and fee and credit policies, before patients arrive for their first visit. Well-informed patients help

May 21, 20xx

I, [patient's name], agree to pay Monroe Family Practice $100 every 2 weeks until my $800 balance is paid in full. I understand that finance charges will not accrue while I am making these payments and that if I stop making payments before my balance is paid in full finance charges will begin to accrue on the remaining balance.

Patient Signature   Date

_____

Witness Signature   Date

_____

Figure 20-2 ■ Sample payment contract.

avoid collection problems. Copayments, for example, should be paid at visit check-in.

The following payment policies should be included in an introductory brochure:

- Requirement for payment at the time of service, if any
- Allowable time frame for payment (e.g., within 30 days)
- Guidelines for insurance claim submission on patient's behalf
- Time the medical office will carry an outstanding balance
- Credit limit extended to patients
- Percentage of finance charges that will accrue on a balance and when they will start to accrue (e.g., after 30 days, after 60 days)
- Point at which accounts are turned over to collection agencies
- Process for assigning benefits to the provider

Each state has a statute of limitations that sets the maximum time in which health care providers can collect patient

TABLE 20-1	Statutes of Limitations on Health Care Debts		
State	**Number of Years**	**State**	**Number of Years**
AL	6	MT	8
AK	3	NE	5
AZ	6	NV	6
AR	5	NH	3
CA	4	NJ	6
CO	6	NM	6
CT	6	NY	6
DE	3	NC	3
D.C.	3	ND	6
FL	5	OH	15
GA	6	OK	5
HI	6	OR	6
ID	5	PA	4
IL	10	RI	10
IN	10	SC	3
IA	10	SD	6
KS	5	TN	6
KY	15	TX	4
LA	10	UT	6
ME	6	VA	5
MD	3	VT	6
MA	6	WA	6
MI	6	WI	6
MN	6	WV	5
MS	3	WY	10
MO	10		

debts. Because Medicare and many managed care insurance companies prohibit providers from billing patients until insurance companies have issued explanations of benefits outlining the amounts patients owe, it is crucial to bill insurance providers soon after the service is provided so that the patient portion can be billed in a timely manner. Table 20-1 outlines the number of years from the patient's last date of service or last billing statement that a health care provider may send a bill to a patient.

Critical Thinking Question 20-1

Referring back to the case study at the beginning of the chapter, would Millie be more or less likely to have a balance due if someone in the medical office had discussed a payment plan when services were rendered? Why?

Medical offices should predetermine the amount of credit they are willing to extend to patients, document the amount in policies, and apply the policies equitably. The health care provider may not pick and choose the patients who will receive an extension of credit. The credit extension policy must apply to every patient in the facility.

Verifying Patient Identification

When a new patient visits the medical office, the medical assistant must copy some sort of photo identification, like the patient's driver's license, and the patient's insurance cards, front and back (**Figure 20-3** ■). This documentation confirms the patient's identity and can help the assistant track the patient for collection purposes.

As part of the drive to combat identity theft, the federal government instituted the **Red Flags Rule** in 2003. Portions of this law have been implemented in the years since then, with mandates for many organizations and industries, including health care, to verify patient identity. In order to comply with this rule, health care facilities are now asking patients to present photo identification upon arrival for services. In the event the patient is unable to produce such identification, the medical facility may refuse to see the patient, unless there is a life-threatening condition present.

Medical offices should request certain pieces of information on their patient registration forms to make tracking patients, and therefore debt collection, easier. For example, offices should request the name and telephone number of the patient's employer, as well as the names and numbers of emergency contacts who do not live with the patient. When contacting a patient at her place of employment, the medical office staff will want to be careful to protect patient privacy. The reason for the call should not be divulged to anyone other than the patient. If a message must be left, the name of the caller, the name of the physician or clinic, and telephone number are all that can be given. Emergency contact information provides another option for contacting the patient when her account becomes past due and she cannot be reached at home. The patient's bill must not be discussed with the emergency contact person, however, in order to

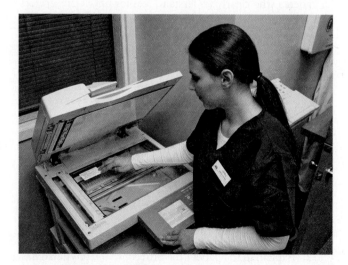

Figure 20-3 ■ The medical assistant should make a copy of both sides of the patient's insurance card.

Source: *Dylan Malone.*

maintain patient privacy. Discussing the patient's bill with anyone other than the patient or the patient's spouse (in a community property state) would be a violation of HIPAA protection. Even in a community property state, the spouse may not be told the type of services rendered or the diagnosis for which the patient was seen—only the amount of the bill can be discussed along with a way to set up payment arrangements.

Managing Accounts Receivable

Any successful medical office must manage its **accounts receivable (AR)**, which is the money owed the office from all sources, including patients, insurance companies, worker's compensation, Medicare, and Medicaid. Accounts receivable management, which entails documenting how

PROCEDURE 20-1 Prepare an Accounts Receivable Trial Balance

Theory and Rationale

By preparing an accounts receivable trial balance, the medical assistant is able to determine if there is any discrepancy between the daily journal and the ledger or the patient accounts.

Materials

- Patient accounts in computerized format
- Computer
- Fee slips for services rendered to the patients for the day
- Calculator
- Pen

Competency

1. Calculate the total of the charges on the fee slips for the day.
2. Using the computer, calculate the total of the charges posted to patient accounts for the day.
3. Compare the total of the charges from the fee slips to the total of the charges in the computer.
4. If the balances do not match, calculate the totals a second time to verify you added them correctly.
5. If the balances continue to differ, go through the fee slips to see where the error in entry has occurred.
6. Correct the entry error and calculate the totals again.
7. If the balances continue to differ, go through the above steps until they match.

PROCEDURE 20-2 Explain Professional Fees to a Patient

Theory and Rationale

Patients who clearly understand fees for physician services are better equipped to make health care choices and to understand their bills. When a patient does not understand the fees he incurs in the medical facility, this confusion can lead to nonpayment of the bill.

Materials

- Patient medical record
- Copy of office fee schedule
- Blue or black pen
- Payment contract

Competency

1. Find a private location to sit with the patient.
2. Explain to the patient the procedure the physician has prescribed.

3. Explain to the patient the fee for the procedure.
4. Explain to the patient any insurance coverage for the fee.
5. Explain to the patient the payment amount and deadline.
6. Secure an agreement from the patient about the payment date.
7. Enter the payment agreement and arrangements on the payment contract.
8. On the payment contract, obtain the patient's signature and sign as the witness.
9. Answer any questions the patient might have about the fee or the procedure.
10. Place the payment agreement in the patient's financial record.

much money is owed the office, by whom, and for how long, is a weighty task and so must be done regularly and thoroughly.

As mentioned earlier, medical billing computer programs can run reports, some on accounts receivable accounts. *Aging reports* are important to accounts receivable management for a number of reasons. The accounts receivable aging report will list the names of patients who have outstanding accounts and the age of the accounts. When physicians wish to take business loans, for example, banks will request documentation on accounts receivable accounts. Physicians with high or old accounts receivable balances are considered a greater risk to insure, as the older the account balance, the less likely it will be paid. Medical assistants will commonly consult the accounts receivable report to determine the patient accounts that are past due and that require further collection activity.

The most effective way to collect money on past due accounts is to speak with the patient while he is in the office. When face-to-face communication is not possible, the next most effective method is to call the patient, but from a private office location to safeguard patient confidentiality. Medical assistants making such calls must pay strict attention to the law regarding collections and must document all calls and conversations, as well as any patient messages, in the patient's financial records. Table 20-2 outlines procedures for telephone collection calls.

When a patient has a past due account and moves out of the area or changes her phone number, the medical assistant may use the Internet to search for the patient's new location. This is a process known as *skip tracing*.

Collection in Managed Care

Some medical offices collect entire first-day visit fees from patients, but that practice is not recommended if the patient is covered by managed care. Some managed care plans strictly govern how much money, if any, providers may collect from

patients. When offices participate with Medicare, for example, providers are disallowed from charging patients for covered services at the time of service. Instead, those providers must bill Medicare and then bill the patients for the portions Medicare determines those patients owe. For patients who have no insurance coverage for their health care needs, medical offices may request a full or partial payment at the time of service. Many offices offer cash discounts for patients who pay in full up front rather than carry a balance and make monthly payments.

When speaking with patients about fees or payments, it is important to remember that people tend to associate payment with value. When medical assistants act embarrassed about fees, or fail to ask for payment, they give the impression that the physician's services lack value.

Forgiving Deductibles or Copayments

Because it is a violation of a federal law entitled the Hill-Burton Act, it is illegal, and in fact considered **insurance fraud**, for a health care provider to forgive a patient's deductible or copayment. When a patient cannot pay his bill and the physician agrees to treat him for lesser or no fees, the patient must sign and date a **hardship agreement** letter for his file (**Figure 20-4** ■). The hardship letter becomes part of the patient's permanent medical record. Hardship agreements are typically based on the patient's income level. In many medical facilities, patients in need of discounts due to inability to pay will be required to provide proof of income. Physicians may use hardship information to determine the amount of discount the patient is to receive.

In many medical facilities, the billing staff stays up-to-date on current local and national programs that may assist patients who are unable to pay their medical bills for services, as well as for medications. In these cases, the patient is typically referred to the staff member who handles these patient

TABLE 20-2 Dos and Don'ts for Collection Telephone Calls	
Do	**Don't**
• Call the patient from a private location in the medical office. • Call the patient between 8:00 A.M. and 9:00 P.M. • Verify the patient's identity. Be respectful, polite, and professional. • Tell the patient the reason for the call. • Keep the conversation short and to the point. • Document any promises the patient makes. • Follow up on any of the patient's promises.	• Call the patient from a location where other patients can overhear. • Call the patient if the patient requests not to be called. • Speak with anyone except the patient or the patient's parent or guardian about the patient's bill. • Call repeatedly if the patient fails to answer or return messages. • Become angry if emotions rise. • Make promises that cannot be kept, such as reducing the bill. • Converse about topics other than the subject of the call. • Neglect to document all parts of the conversation with the patient.

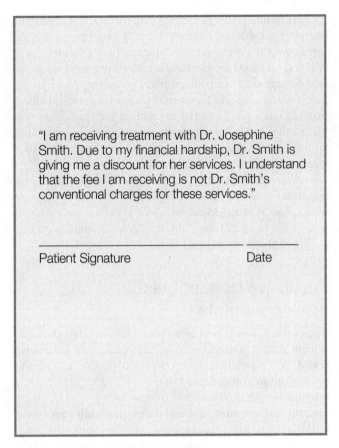

"I am receiving treatment with Dr. Josephine Smith. Due to my financial hardship, Dr. Smith is giving me a discount for her services. I understand that the fee I am receiving is not Dr. Smith's conventional charges for these services."

_____   _____
Patient Signature   Date

Figure 20-4 ■ Sample hardship agreement.

assistance programs; the patient will often need to fill out paperwork to apply for the program.

Patients Who File for Bankruptcy

Patients who are unable to pay their medical bill may file for bankruptcy. A Harvard study performed in 2011 found that inability to pay medical bills is the leading cause of bankruptcy filings, affecting nearly 2 million Americans each year. Depending upon the type of bankruptcy the patient files, the medical office might or might not be repaid any of the amount outstanding on the patient's account. Since bankruptcy is designed to protect debtors from further collection activity, the medical office may no longer contact the patient for payment of their account once the patient has filed a bankruptcy claim.

Professional Courtesy

Physicians who treat other physicians or other health care providers for free or at greatly reduced fees extend what is called **professional courtesy**. Such courtesy is often extended to family or friends of the physician or health

care provider, to the family of other physicians or healthcare provider, even to such professional associates as the physician's attorney or accountant. When a professional courtesy is given to a patient, that amount may not be charged and collected from the patient's insurance carrier. In other words, only the actual amount that has been charged to the patient may be billed to the insurance carrier.

In cases of professional courtesy, accurate patient charts are vital to avoid the appearance of fraud or impropriety. Medical assistants should have any patients in these situations sign professional courtesy agreements, such as, "I understand Dr. Jones is giving me a professional courtesy discount for services rendered." Waiving copayments, coinsurance, and deductibles is frowned upon by managed care and insurance companies. The existence of copayments, coinsurance, and deductibles is designed to create a system where the patient shares in the cost of his or her medical care. When the medical facility chooses to waive those fees, it may be seen as fraudulent by the insurance carriers. Without proper documentation from the patient indicating that the waiver is due to a financial hardship or professional courtesy, physicians risk losing their preferred provider status with insurance carriers, if caught waiving those amounts due.

Patient Billing Statements

Medical offices should set aside a day each month to send **patient billing statements** to patients with balances due (**Figure 20-5** ■), preferably after the first of the month when rent and mortgages are typically due. Patient billing statements that arrive mid- to late-month are more likely to be paid in a timely fashion.

While patient billing statements are one means of securing payment, collecting patient copays at the time of office visit is far more cost-effective. Monthly billing statements have been shown to cost about $8 per month per bill. To provide incentive, health care providers can offer discounts, called "cash discounts," to patients who pay their bills in full. The amount of the discount should be based on how much it costs the provider to collect an unpaid bill, or to bill the patient's insurance. Any cash discount policies must be clearly documented and applied and offered fairly to all patients. Any cash discounts must be accurately noted in the patients' financial files.

Many medical offices outsource their patient billing to outside companies. In these cases, the charges and diagnoses are sent to the outside agency and the patient's insurance is billed. Once payment is received from the insurance carrier, any balance due is then billed by the outside agency to the patient. Patients who call to discuss their balances may be directed to the outside billing agency.

Heritage Park Women's Clinic
14 Heritage Way
Heritage Park, IN   12345

Lillian Vidali
2715-16th Drive SW
Heritage Park, IN   12345

STATEMENT

CLOSING DATE	PREVIOUS BALANCE	BALANCE DUE
10/2/xx	0	20.00

NOTE: ALL PAYMENTS AND CHARGES POSTED AFTER THE ABOVE CLOSING DATE WILL APPEAR ON THE NEXT STATEMENT.

AMOUNT PAID $ _____

BANKCARD PAYMENT AUTHORIZATION	☐ VISA	☐ M/C

VISA M/C ACCOUNT NUMBER

CARDHOLDER SIGNATURE   EXP. DATE

PLEASE DETACH AND **RETURN** THIS STUB WITH YOUR PAYMENT TO INSURE PROPER CREDIT

RETAIN THIS PORTION FOR YOUR RECORDS.

DATE OF SERVICE	DOCTOR / CPT CODE	DESCRIPTION	CHARGES	CREDITS
9/7/xx	Wilson/99211	Office Visit	62.00	
9/20/xx	Wilson	Insurance payment 9/7/xx		42.00

PAST DUE				CURRENT	BALANCE DUE
0	0	0	0	20.00	20.00
OVER 120 DAYS	OVER 90 DAYS	OVER 60 DAYS	OVER 30 DAYS	0 - 30 DAYS	

COMMENTS: Payment due by 11/10/xx

Figure 20-5 ■ Sample patient billing statement.

Critical Thinking Question 20-2

Refer back to the case study at the beginning of the chapter. Should medical offices have policies to offer discounts to patients like Millie when those patients agree to pay their full bills via credit card during collection calls? Why?

Collecting from patients who are in the office is the most effective way to collect payment. When patients with past due accounts are due in for appointments, medical assistants should ask the receptionist to route those patients to the billing department before those patients receive treatment. In private areas out of the hearing of other patients the assistants can remind the patients of their balances. When patients cannot provide payment in full, the assistants should make payment arrangements with the patient.

Dismissing Patients Due to Nonpayment

When patients are chronically late with payments or refuse to pay at all, providers can dismiss those patients from care with a **certified letter. Figure 20-6** ■ provides an example of a dismissal letter to a patient. Providers must give patients at least 30 days to receive care, but after that period, providers are no longer bound to provide treatment. Physicians who do not honor this commitment may be sued for patient abandonment. Patients should be dismissed only after physicians have given their consent and a signed receipt verifying that the patient received the certified letter has been filed in the patient's permanent medical records.

Charging Interest on Medical Accounts

Medical providers who wish to charge interest on past-due balances must be sure to check the laws in their state. Any change in financial policy, including the decision to charge interest on overdue accounts, requires providers to prominently post written notices in the office at least 30 days before the changes occur.

▶▶▶ Pulse Points

Billing for the Physician's Friends and Family

Medicare prohibits physicians from billing for the treatment they provide their immediate relatives or household members. Immediate relatives include the physician's spouse, parents, children, siblings, grandparents, grandchildren, stepparents, stepsisters, stepbrothers, and stepchildren. Household members include anyone living in the same home as the physician, like a nanny, maid, butler, chauffer, medical caregiver, or assistant. Boarders—people who rent rooms from physicians—are not considered household members.

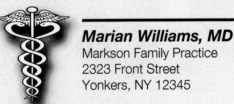

Marian Williams, MD
Markson Family Practice
2323 Front Street
Yonkers, NY 12345

Joseph Paterniti
41 Bronxville Ave
Yonkers, NY 12345

January 31, 20xx

Dear Mr. Paterniti:

Our office has tried several times to contact you regarding your outstanding balance with us. Because we have failed to reach you, I must dismiss you as a patient. Please find a new physician and notify this office within 30 days if you would like your medical records transferred. If you need care within the next 30 days, you may still patronize this office. After 30 days, you will be disallowed from making another appointment with us.

Sincerely,

Marian Williams, MD

Figure 20-6 ■ Sample dismissal letter.

PROCEDURE 20-3 Call a Patient Regarding
an Overdue Account

Theory and Rationale

Even with the most efficient administrative staff, every medical office has patients who are slow to pay and long overdue accounts. These accounts require medical assistants to act, such as by calling the patients. These telephone calls must be made professionally and documented appropriately.

Materials

- Telephone
- Electronic patient ledger
- Blue or black pen

Competency

1. Dial the patient's home telephone number.
2. If you reach the patient:
   a. Identify yourself and the name of your clinic, and state the reason for the call.
   b. Ask the patient when payment on the outstanding bill will be made.
   c. If the patient agrees to pay via credit card, take the credit card information over the telephone, verify the amount to be charged, charge the credit card, and mail the patient a receipt.
   d. If the patient agrees to mail payment to the office, secure a date by which the payment is to be received and note the date in the patient's electronic billing ledger.
   e. If the patient expresses an inability to make a payment at this time, secure a date by which the patient expects to be able to make a payment, and note the date in the patient's electronic billing ledger.
3. If unable to reach the patient, leave a message that discloses no personal information about the patient's care in the office.
4. Note the message in the patient's electronic billing ledger.

Addressing Checks That Fail to Clear

When patients provide "bounced" or nonsufficient funds (**NSF**) checks, which are checks drawn on insufficient funds, most banks charge the medical office a fee. As a result, offices can legally charge patients a fee in turn. Most banks will redeposit NSF checks only once, so when a check cannot be redeposited, the medical assistant must contact the patient to inform him of the returned check and communicate the fee charged by the office. In such a conversation, the assistants should determine the date by which the patient will send a replacement payment. At the end of the interaction, the assistant should make any relevant notations in the patient's billing ledger.

In order to reduce the number of NSF checks received, medical offices may choose to pay for a check verification system that electronically verifies that funds are available in the patient's account at the time the check is received.

Contacting Nonpaying Patients

When a patient fails to pay her monthly bill by the date due, the medical assistant should try to contact the patient regarding payment. Unless the patient has instructed otherwise, it is legal to contact her at her place of employment. Once the assistant reaches the patient, the MA should communicate the outstanding balance and ask when payment may be expected. When a patient agrees to a date and

amount, the assistant should make notations in a **tickler file**. Serving as a reminder, a tickler file facilitates followup should payment fail to arrive when expected. Tickler files can be manual, such as index cards in a small box, or electronic. Many medical software programs have such reminder mechanisms.

In addition to making notes in a tickler file, the assistant should follow up in writing with the patient. Letters should outline conversation details, including the amount owed on the account, the agreed-upon payment amount and due date, and any followup actions in the event of nonpayment. Many medical offices send a return envelope with these letters to give the patient an easy way to mail the payment to the office.

HIPAA Compliance

HIPAA regulations prevent members of the health care team from leaving messages with live parties or on voicemail when those messages might violate patient confidentiality. It is inappropriate, for example, to mention that a message is about a past due balance. An appropriate message is, "This is Ceila from Dr. Stewart's office. I need to leave a message for John Cooper to call me at (425) 555-9899." Document all phone calls in the patient's financial ledger.

Critical Thinking Question 20-3

Refer to the case study at the beginning of the chapter. Imagine that Millie agrees to pay $100 on her credit card now and $100 per month for the next 4 months. What is the best means the medical assistant has for tracking this agreement?

Sending Patients Collection Letters

When a patient continues to be delinquent in his account, the medical assistant can send the patient a letter stating the amount owed and the requested payment terms. **Figure 20-7** ∎ gives an example. Some offices have their office managers,

clinic directors, or health care providers try to contact the patients. Whatever procedure an office follows, the medical assistant must be sure to consistently and carefully apply the same guidelines to all patients.

When a patient ignores the medical office's efforts to collect on the account, the office may send the patient's account to a collection agency, write off the balance, or take the patient to small claims court. All these options require the physician's consent, however.

When an office chooses a **collection agency** to collect past due accounts, the collection agency must be reputable. Other medical offices are a good source for agency references. Collection companies should actively pursue accounts, not harass or offend patients. Such agencies must also abide by federal guidelines for debt collection. The **Fair Debt Collection Practices Act (FDCPA)** was enacted to eliminate abusive, deceptive, and unfair collection practices. This law

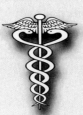

Russ Bowman, RMA (AMT)
Markson Family Practice
2323 Front Street
Yonkers, NY 12345

Joseph Paterniti
41 Bronxville Ave
Yonkers, NY 12345

January 31, 20xx

Dear Mr. Paterniti:

It has come to my attention that your account is now past due. We received the last payment on your account on [date of last payment]. To render your account current, we must receive your payment by [date 10 days from the letter's date].

If you cannot meet this deadline, please contact this office immediately to make other arrangements. If we do not receive your payment or fail to hear from you by the date listed previously, we will refer your account to a third-party collection agency.

Sincerely,

Russ Bowman, RMA (AMT)

Figure 20-7 ∎ Sample collection letter to a patient.

PROCEDURE 20-4 Send a Patient Billing Statement

Theory and Rationale

Nearly every medical office sends monthly billing statements to patients with outstanding balances. These billing statements must comply with the Health Insurance Portability and Accountability Act (**HIPAA**) and be sent on or near the same day each month. In order to be HIPAA compliant, the statement must be sent in a security envelope (one that does not allow for the contents to be viewed without opening the envelope).

Materials

- Computer with medical billing software
- Printer

Competency

Computerized billing: in the billing software, follow the appropriate steps to print a patient billing statement.

1. Once printed, verify that the information on the bill is correct.
2. Place the copy of the bill into an envelope.
3. Stamp the envelope and place it in the mail.

PROCEDURE 20-5 Post a Nonsufficient Funds Check

Theory and Rationale

When medical offices receive nonsufficient (NSF) checks from patients, those checks must be handled according to office policy and with respect for the patients. As with any patient conversations about finances, discussions about NSF checks must be clearly noted in a patient's financial records.

Materials

- Check returned due to NSF
- Computer with medical billing software

Competency

1. Verify that you have located the correct patient in the medical billing system.
2. Enter the NSF check and any fees into the patient's account.
3. Notify the patient via phone that the check was returned. Indicate any corresponding fees.
4. Secure a date by which a replacement payment will be received.
5. In the patient's ledger, note the outcome of the conversation.

---

applies to all consumer debt for personal, family, or household purposes. The following are highlights of the federal Fair Debt Collection guidelines:

Medical offices must:

- Threaten to take only action that is legal or intended to come to fruition. For example, offices that threaten to sue patients for nonpayment must be willing and able to file lawsuits or face harassment accusations.
- Accurately represent themselves and the amounts patients owe.
- Make collection phone calls after 8:00 a.m. and before 9:00 p.m. unless directed otherwise by patients.
- Stop calling about accounts upon request by the patient. Continued calling would be considered harassment.

Other federal laws govern how collections may proceed against the patient who owes for medical care. The Equal Credit Opportunity Act prohibits credit discrimination on the basis of race, color, religion, national origin, sex, marital status, age, or because the patient is on public assistance (Medicaid). This law provides the consumer with protection from unlawful credit practices.

The Federal Truth in Lending Act provides protection for consumers by requiring that they be told the exact finance charge being imposed, the amount financed, and the total number of payments the consumer is expected to make to pay off the debt.

Once an account goes to collection, offices typically write off the balance owed. Collection agencies typically charge percentage fees for their services. The standard rate is 33 percent of the amount owed. Therefore, if a patient owes $99 when the office sends the account to collections, the provider is paid $66.00 when the collection agency collects the account in full ($99.00 − $33.00). Some collection agencies charge a flat dollar amount to collect accounts,

PROCEDURE 20-6 Post an Adjustment to a Patient Account

Theory and Rationale

Once medical offices have sent an account to a collection agency, the balance of the account is typically written off. To effect this change, medical assistants must post adjustments to those accounts.

Materials

- Medical billing software

Competency

1. Locate the correct patient ledger in the computer.
2. Enter the adjustment as a debit or a credit.
3. In the patient's financial record, note the reason for the adjustment.

PROCEDURE 20-7 Post a Collection Agency Payment

Theory and Rationale

When a collection agency sends the medical office a payment on an account, the medical assistant must properly post the payment and make appropriate debit adjustments.

Materials

- Calculator
- Computer
- Collection agency payment

Competency

1. Find the patient's account in the computer.
2. Verify that the patient account is correct.
3. Post the payment, choosing "collection payment" as the payment source.
4. If applicable, enter any adjustment due to the collection agency's fee.
5. Verify the payment amount and adjustment.
6. Save all changes.

---

which is most cost-effective for large accounts. To maximize their collections efforts, medical offices can use multiple collection agencies.

Uncollectible Accounts

Some offices choose to **write off** accounts deemed **uncollectible** to maintain patient relations. Patients may have legitimate reasons for nonpayment, such as the death of a spouse or the loss of a job. Writing off the account balance is legal and should only be done with the physician's approval. When the medical office chooses to write off the balance a patient owes, the medical assistant must send the patient a letter to that effect (**Figure 20-8** ■). A copy of the letter should reside in the patient's file.

Collecting from Estates

Patients sometimes die with a balance owed to the medical office. Providers may choose to forgive the balance if the

deceased was unmarried, for example, or lacked assets. When the provider chooses to pursue the amount owed, however, the medical assistant should send statements to the estate of the deceased in the following format:

Estate of [patient's name]
c/o [name of patient's spouse or next of kin]
Patient's last known address

In return, the person handling the estate of the deceased should contact the medical office to arrange for payment. If the office receives no response, the medical assistant can contact the County Recorder's Office in the Probate Department of the Superior Court in the county where the deceased resided. This office should provide the name of the estate's executor. If the office receives no response from the estate's executor, the assistant should gather the proper forms from the county clerk's office to file a claim against the estate for the amount owing. In general, medical offices have from 2 to 36 months to act, depending upon state law. While a claim remains outstanding, the assistant should continue sending the estate's executor monthly billing statements.

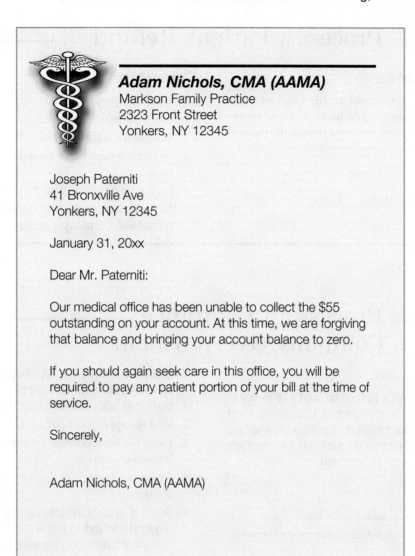

Adam Nichols, CMA (AAMA)
Markson Family Practice
2323 Front Street
Yonkers, NY 12345

Joseph Paterniti
41 Bronxville Ave
Yonkers, NY 12345

January 31, 20xx

Dear Mr. Paterniti:

Our medical office has been unable to collect the $55 outstanding on your account. At this time, we are forgiving that balance and bringing your account balance to zero.

If you should again seek care in this office, you will be required to pay any patient portion of your bill at the time of service.

Sincerely,

Adam Nichols, CMA (AAMA)

Figure 20-8 ■ Sample letter forgiving a patient balance.

Overpaying on Accounts

Account overpayments can occur for a number of reasons, including when patients overpay on their accounts or when insurance policies pay unexpectedly high amounts or when patients have multiple policies that together pay more than owed. When overpayments occur, careful review is needed to identify the party to receive the refund.

One common reason for an overpayment of a patient account is the presence of dual insurance coverage. As an example, a patient with dual coverage might believe she has to pay her insurance copayment when she comes to the medical office for care. Once the primary insurance is billed, the balance is sent to the secondary insurance company. In many cases, the secondary company pays the copayment amount, and if the patient has already paid this as well, a credit will now exist on the account.

Collections Through Small Claims Court

Small claims court is yet another option for collecting on past due accounts. To pursue a small claims suit, the balance owed by the patient must fit the "small claim" criteria, which is typically the dollar amount of the claim, in the state where the provider's office is located. The most common amount for small claims court is claims under $5,000. If the claim is for more than that amount, the provider would need to bring suit against the patient in regular court.

Depending on the laws in the state where the medical assistant works, the assistant may be able to file claims online or through the mail. Some states require claims to be filed in person at the local county courthouse. All methods incur a cost at the time of filing. Though the notice may be

PROCEDURE 20-8 Process a Patient Refund

Theory and Rationale

When a patient balance is overpaid, a credit balance results. Research is needed to return credit balances to the appropriate parties. When a patient is owed a refund, the medical assistant must know how to post the refund.

Materials

- Computer with medical billing software

Competency

1. Locate the proper patient ledger in the billing software.
2. Enter the refund amount.
3. Choose the adjustment code for "Refund to Patient."
4. Obtain a refund check from the physician or office manager.
5. Send the refund check to the patient.
6. In the patient ledger, note the party receiving the refund and the number of the refund check.

PROCEDURE 20-9 Process an Insurance Company Overpayment

Theory and Rationale

When a credit appears on a patient account due to insurance company overpayment, the medical assistant must process the refund to the company. The medical assistant must carefully review the file to determine the appropriate insurance company to receive the refund.

Materials

- Computer with medical billing software
- Copies of insurance companies' explanation of benefits

1. Using the insurance companies' explanation of benefits, determine which company is the patient's primary insurance carrier and which is secondary.
2. Find the appropriate patient ledger in the computer.
3. Using the appropriate code, enter the refund to the insurance company.
4. Obtain a refund check from the physician or office manager.
5. Send a note to the insurance company explaining the reason for the refund, as well as copies of the primary and secondary insurance companies' explanations of benefits.

sent to the patient via certified mail, some offices choose to have the patient served with the notice in person. Notice of the suit must be served on the patient by someone who does not work in the medical office. Often, offices hire companies specializing in this task.

When small claims cases enter court, staff from the medical office must appear to testify. The office representative will need a copy of the patient's account ledger and any documentation proving the health care provider treated the patient. Any signed documentation indicating the patient agreed to pay an outstanding bill is also important to bring. Typically, in small claims court, the health care provider's office need only prove that the patient was treated and that the patient knew of the charges for the service. Providers

often win judgment in these cases, and patients are ordered to pay their bills.

When a patient fails to pay the amount ordered, the physician may opt to garnish the patient's wages. To do this, the physician will need to obtain a court order, which is then presented to the patient's employer. The Consumer Credit Protection Act protects consumers from being fired due to their wages being garnished. This federal wage requirement also limits the amount of an employee's earnings that may be garnished in any one week. In states with **community property laws**, a patient's spouse is also responsible for the bills. As a result, a spouse's wages can also be garnished. To act appropriately, medical assistants must check the laws in their state.

REVIEW

Chapter Summary

- The best computerized medical billing systems provide basic functionality, like payment posting and reporting, as well as any advanced features that support the office's business objectives.
- Professional fees are determined by a set of defined criteria so medical offices can operate within a fair and consistent fee schedule.
- A medical office's accounts receivable department is vital to securing payment for services rendered.
- Because fees are a crucial facet of an office's business success, collection policies are important.
- Collection agencies should be fair and equitable while being effective.

- Out of professional courtesy, physicians may sometimes treat patients they know personally without charging the patient for the service, or for a reduced fee.
- Hardship discounts are reserved for those who most need them. They are typically given to patients who need the care but are unable to afford the cost. These cases are typically granted on a case-by-case basis.
- When otherwise able patients fail to honor their financial obligations, small claims courts can help medical offices collect their past-due accounts.

Chapter Review

Multiple Choice

1. A physician might decide to give a professional courtesy discount to:
   a. Another physician
   b. A patient who claims a hardship
   c. A patient who is friends with the receptionist
   d. A patient who demands a professional courtesy
   e. None of the above

2. Each month, each patient statement costs about $_____ to send.
   a. 5
   b. 6
   c. 7
   d. 8
   e. 9

3. Health care providers can discount their services _____ percent for patients who pay in full at the time of service.
   a. 5
   b. 10
   c. 15
   d. 20
   e. 25

4. The most effective way to collect money from patients who owe is:
   a. Over the telephone
   b. In person in the office
   c. Through the mail
   d. By hiring a collection agency
   e. Going to the patient's home

5. Which of the following is illegal under the Fair Debt Collection Act?
   a. Refusing to self-identify to patients
   b. Calling patients at their homes
   c. Threatening to send patients to collections and then doing so
   d. Refusing to let patients know what their charges are for
   e. All of the above

True/False

T F 1. Medical billing software is often capable of providing lists of patients by demographics, such as all women over the age of 40.

T F 2. Most health insurance plans base their fee schedules on the Medicare fee schedule.

T F 3. A medical office can choose which patients will receive credit.

T F 4. Legally, health care providers can forgive patients' copays or deductibles.

T F 5. Dismissing patients from care due to nonpayment is legal.

T F 6. The interest rate on medical accounts is the same in all states.

T F 7. All collection agencies charge a 33 percent fee to collect accounts.

T F 8. Small claims court is an option for collecting on past-due accounts.

Short Answer

1. What is an accounts aging report?
2. Why is it important to analyze participating provider agreements before deciding to become a participating provider?
3. What are *accounts receivable* in the medical office?
4. What is a hardship agreement, and how is it used in the medical office?
5. What is a professional courtesy?
6. What is a tickler file, and why would it be useful in a medical office?
7. What is the purpose of sending an office brochure to new patients before those patients first visit the office?

8. How should a medical office handle a situation in which a patient dies while owing an outstanding balance to the office?

Research

1. Interview a person who works in the billing department of a local medical office. What kind of training has the person had before taking the job?
2. Research the various collection agencies in your area that handle medical accounts. How do they compare to one another?
3. Research the laws in your state regarding collecting medical debts.

Practicum Application Experience

Martina Sylvan, a patient in Dr. DaSilva's office, owes $652 on her account. The medical assistant must contact Martina regarding her outstanding balance and set up a payment plan. When the assistant reaches Martina via telephone, Martina says she has no extra money to pay her bill at this time. How should the medical assistant handle this situation?

Resource Guide

Federal Deposit Insurance Corporation
http://www.fdic.gov/

Federal Trade Commission
600 Pennsylvania Avenue, N.W.
Washington, D.C. 20580
Phone: (202) 326-2222
www.ftc.gov

Managed Outsource Solutions (provides both domestic and offshore outsourcing services)
Phone: (918) 451-8175
http://www.managedoutsource.com

21

Payroll, Accounts Payable, and Banking Procedures

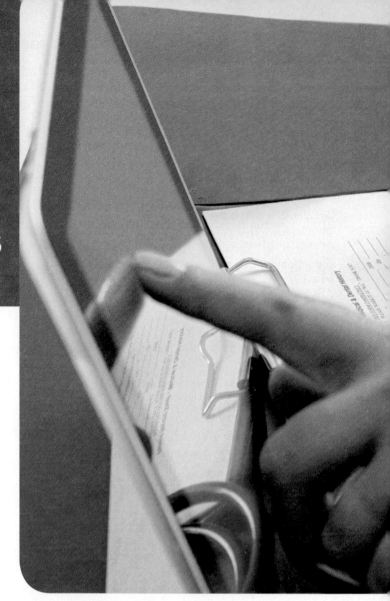

Case Study

Read the following case study and answer the critical thinking questions presented throughout the chapter.

Francie, who works as the medical office's receptionist, recently married a man with three children. Francie asks the medical assistant, who is in charge of payroll, to help her change her tax deductions so that fewer taxes are taken from her paycheck. Prior to her marriage, Francie did not have any children. Because she was single with no dependents, Francie did not claim any exemptions for her federal tax withholding from wages earned.

Objectives

After completing this chapter, you should be able to:

21.1 Define and spell the key terminology in this chapter.

21.2 Discuss the history of payroll in the United States and present day employment issues.

21.3 Discuss the payroll processing function in the medical office.

21.4 Describe the components of, and how to create, a new employee record.

21.5 Update employee records.

21.6 Describe the purpose of the W4 form.

21.7 Record employees' work hours.

21.8 Calculate payroll.

21.9 List the types of deductions.

21.10 Describe the use of software to calculate payroll.

21.11 Discuss the process to follow when employees' wages are garnished.

21.12 Describe the function of accounts payable in the medical office.

21.13 Prepare a deposit slip.

21.14 Access bank accounts via the Internet.

21.15 Describe how to manage the petty cash fund.

21.16 Describe how to reconcile a monthly bank statement.

Competency Skills Performance

1. Create a new employee record.
2. Calculate an employee's payroll.
3. Pay an office supply invoice.
4. Write checks to pay bills.
5. Complete a deposit slip.
6. Account for petty cash.
7. Reconcile a bank statement.

Key Terminology

auditors—those who review personal or corporate bank or tax records on behalf of an agency such as the Internal Revenue Service (IRS)

charitable contributions—cash or other donations given to charitable organizations

Circular E—yearly booklet published by the IRS that outlines the federal tax deductions to be taken from individuals' wages depending on marital status and number of exemptions

deductions—number of allowances to be withheld from wages

endorsement stamp—rubber tool that imprints a receiving agency's banking information

Fair Labor Standards Act (FLSA)—law passed by U.S. Congress in 1938 to address employment issues like federal minimum wage

Federal Insurance Contributions Act (FICA)—law that addresses Social Security withholding taxes

Federal Unemployment Tax Act (FUTA)—law that addresses federal unemployment tax withholdings

garnish—to withhold wages from an employee's paycheck due to a court order

gross pay—amount earned before taxes or deductions are subtracted

net pay—amount remaining after deductions and taxes are subtracted

outsource—to send to another business for completion

overtime—wages paid beyond 40 hours in a work week, at a rate 1.5 times the normal rate for that employee

payroll—process of calculating the amounts employees receive for their work

payroll taxes—monies withheld from wages for federal income tax, Social Security, and Medicare obligations

personnel file—set of employment-related documents for an employee, including an original application, federal withholding requests, and dates and copies of evaluations

quarterly payroll reports—documents that specify the taxes withheld from wages quarterly

security envelope—nontransparent envelope

Social Security Act—law passed by the U.S. Congress in 1935 to provide workers and their families financial security post-retirement

time clock—piece of equipment that records employees' arrival and departure times for payroll purposes

unemployment insurance—program that pays employees who have lost their jobs

W-2 form—U.S. federal form that annually documents the wages employees drew the previous year

W-4 form—U.S. federal form that indicates employees' marital status and federal tax exemptions

wages—monies paid for work performed

withholding allowances—number of exemptions on federal tax forms

Abbreviations

FICA—Federal Insurance Contributions Act

FLSA—Fair Labor Standards Act

FUTA—Federal Unemployment Tax

HIPAA—Health Insurance Portability and Accountability Act

IRS—Internal Revenue Service

Certification Exam Coverage

AAMA (CMA) Exam Coverage:

- Bookkeeping principles
  - Daily reports, charge slips, receipts, ledgers, etc.
    - Charges, payments, and adjustments
    - Identifying and correcting errors
- Accounting and banking procedures
  - Accounts payable
    - Ordering goods and services
    - Monitoring invoices
    - Tracking merchandise
  - Banking procedures
    - Processing accounts receivable
    - Preparing bank deposits

- Employee payroll
  - Calculating wages
  - Payroll forms
- Bookkeeping principles
  - Daily reports, charge slips, receipts, ledgers, etc.
    - Charges, payments, and adjustments
    - Identifying and correcting errors
- Petty cash

AMT (CMAS) Exam Coverage:

- Fundamental financial management
  - Understand basic principles of accounting
  - Perform bookkeeping procedures including balancing accounts

AAMA (CMA) certification exam topics are reprinted with permission of the American Association of Medical Assistants.

AMT (CMAS) certification exam topics are reprinted with permission of American Medical Technologists.

- Perform financial computations
- Manage accounts payable
- Prepare monthly trial balance (reports)
- Understand basic audit controls
- Banking
  - Understand banking services and procedures (accounts, lines of credit, checking endorsements, deposits, reconciliation, and statements)
  - Manage petty cash
- Payroll
  - Prepare employee payroll and reports
  - Maintain payroll tax deduction procedures and records
- Human Resources*
  - Manage staff payroll and scheduling

AMT (RMA) Exam Coverage:
- Financial bookkeeping
  - Endorsements
    - Process payables and practice obligations
    - Understand and maintain disbursement accounts

- Employee payroll
  - Understand hourly and salary payroll procedures
  - Understand and apply payroll withholding and deductions
  - Prepare and maintain payroll tax deduction/withholding records
  - Prepare employee tax forms
  - Prepare quarterly tax forms and deposits
- Understand terminology pertaining to payroll and payroll tax

NCCT (NCMA) Exam Coverage:
- Bookkeeping
  - Basic banking
  - Basic accounting
  - Record keeping

Introduction

In health care, payroll, accounts payable, and banking procedures are vital to office functioning. The payroll function involves keeping accurate records on employees. Accounts payable involves paying the office bills for rent, utilities, and supplies. Banking procedures involve balancing the office checking account and filing the appropriate quarterly and yearly statements with state and federal agencies.

Many large medical offices hire outside firms to help them complete their financial procedures; smaller offices tend to rely on their physicians or office managers for these tasks. Whether accounting, banking, and payroll procedures are outsourced or completed in house, medical assistants should understand how those procedures work.

Processing Payroll

Given its role in the financial stability of its employees, payroll in the medical office is vital. As computer technology has advanced, payroll's function has been transformed.

The History of Payroll

When the 16th Amendment to the Constitution passed in 1913, Congress gained the ability to impose a federal income tax on individuals and corporations. Each year when they filed their income tax returns, employees paid the federal government directly. By 1918, the government was collecting just over $1 billion each year as a result. By 1920, that figure had risen to $5.4 billion. When World War II began and employment increased, taxes climbed to $7.3 billion annually.

In 1935, Congress passed the **Social Security Act** to provide workers and their families financial security. Congress followed that legislation with the **Fair Labor Standards Act (FLSA)** in 1938. This act addressed several worker-related issues, including a federal minimum wage that rises with the

---

* Note: Asterisked areas addressed by the Medical Office Management job function may or may not be performed by the Certified Medical Administrative Specialist at entry-level practice. Nevertheless, the competent specialist should have sound knowledge of these management functions at certification level.

AMT (RMA) certification exam topics are reprinted with permission of American Medical Technologists.

NCCT (NCMA) certification exam topics © 2013 National Center for Competency Testing. Reprinted with permission of NCCT.

inflation rate. As of 2013, the federal minimum wage was $7.25. Many states choose to enforce a minimum wage that is higher than the federal minimum wage. In addition to things like minimum wage, the FLSA requires employers to pay employees **overtime** earnings of 1.5 times normal hourly wages for any work completed beyond 40 hours in 1 week.

As the years passed, the government tried to remain vigilant to workers' needs, but many employees were finding it difficult to keep up with increasing taxes. Many individual taxpayers found it tough to pay their full tax bills at the end of each year. In 1943 withholding taxes on wages was introduced. Under this law, businesses were responsible for collecting employees' income taxes and sending those taxes to the government. Employers had to keep written records of all the taxes they withheld from employee pay, as well as records of those employees' addresses, employment dates, and wages. This legislation boosted the number of taxpayers yet further. By 1945, taxes collected had jumped to $43 billion.

Present-Day Employment Issues

Throughout the decades, the U.S. government has continued to use legislation to address employment issues. For example, the Social Security Act enacted in the mid-1930s has evolved over the years to a system that today has two main parts: 1) the elderly, survivors, and disability insurance, and 2) hospital insurance, known as Medicare. Two other laws address the payment of Social Security and Medicare taxes: 1) the **Federal Insurance Contributions Act (FICA)**, and 2) the **Federal Unemployment Tax Act (FUTA)**. FICA is the amount deducted from an individual's wages for Medicare and Social Security. Still other laws require **unemployment insurance**, a program for which employers make quarterly payments to their state and federal governments. Employees who lose their jobs may be eligible to collect from the unemployment insurance fund while they seek new employment. The Federal Unemployment Act provides for payments of unemployment compensation to workers who have lost their jobs. Many employers pay both a federal and a state unemployment tax for their employees. The employee, however, does not have unemployment taxes deducted.

When the FICA tax started, it was set at 1 percent. In 2007, given rising inflation, it rested at 7.65 percent. Of that 7.65 percent FICA tax, employees pay 6.2 percent of their gross income for Social Security and 1.45 percent for Medicare. All employers must match the 7.65 percent amount, creating a deposit for each employee of 15.3 percent of their gross payrolls. Not all income is subject to FICA tax, however. As of 2013, only the first $113,700 of an individual's wages is subject to FICA tax. The Medicare tax has no wage limit.

The federal agency responsible for enforcing income tax laws is the Internal Revenue Service (IRS). This agency has offices in every major city and employs over 15,000 **auditors**. Auditors are responsible not only for conducting tax audits but also for giving taxpayers federal tax advice. The federal income taxes an employer withholds from employees' pay

must be paid to the IRS each month. FICA taxes, like IRS income taxes, must be deposited monthly. Every business must file quarterly payroll reports to the IRS in which they account for all monies withheld as taxes and deposits made to the IRS of those taxes (**Figure 21-1 ■**). These forms are filled out quarterly and are filed with the appropriate amount due.

Many states have income taxes that are separate from and in addition to the federal income tax. State laws are similar to federal ones with regard to tax deductions and deposits. To comply with state tax laws, employers must withhold specified amounts and file reports quarterly.

In addition to income taxes, most states have laws that require employers to provide employees with coverage should those employees become injured on the job. This coverage, known as workers' compensation, is used for medical care, lost wages, or death benefits. In many states, the employee pays a portion of the workers' compensation premium, but the employer generally funds the larger share. Employers in high-injury-risk industries like construction or mining pay higher premiums than those in low-risk businesses like insurance processing or data entry. However, even employers in low-risk industries will pay higher premiums if many of their employees are injured on the job.

Payroll Processing

Today, **payroll** processing involves far more than paycheck issuance. Various laws and regulations govern just about every phase of payroll, from calculating employees' deductions and the taxes to be withheld from employees' **gross pay** to maintaining and reporting payroll records. The local and national laws impacting payroll practices can continue to change, so it is crucial for the staff member responsible for the medical office's payroll function to track those changes.

Many large offices now use computer software for their payroll functions, but some still calculate payroll manually. Still other offices **outsource** their payroll function to parties like accountants. In large and small medical offices alike, the member of the health care team who processes payroll is assigned a wide range of duties, including:

- Staying current with state and federal laws for **payroll taxes**
- Keeping written records of employees' hours and wages
- Computing the taxes and other **deductions** to be taken from employees' paychecks
- Documenting the **wages**, deductions, and **net pay** for each employee
- Preparing and distributing paychecks to employees
- Calculating payroll taxes and depositing the funds
- Preparing **quarterly payroll reports**

Creating New Employee Records

For each new employee, the medical office should create a **personnel file** with all of the employee's employment-related documentation, such as the job application, résumé,

Form **941 for 2014:** **Employer's QUARTERLY Federal Tax Return**   950114
(Rev. January 2014)   Department of the Treasury — Internal Revenue Service

OMB No. 1545-0029

Employer identification number (EIN) ☐☐ – ☐☐☐☐☐☐☐

Name *(not your trade name)*

Trade name *(if any)*

Address
Number   Street   Suite or room number

City   State   ZIP code

Foreign country name   Foreign province/county   Foreign postal code

Report for this Quarter of 2014
(Check one.)

☐ **1:** January, February, March

☐ **2:** April, May, June

☐ **3:** July, August, September

☐ **4:** October, November, December

Instructions and prior year forms are available at *www.irs.gov/form941*.

Read the separate instructions before you complete Form 941. Type or print within the boxes.

Part 1: **Answer these questions for this quarter.**

1 **Number of employees who received wages, tips, or other compensation for the pay period including:** *Mar. 12* (Quarter 1), *June 12* (Quarter 2), *Sept. 12* (Quarter 3), or *Dec. 12* (Quarter 4)   **1**

2 **Wages, tips, and other compensation** **2**

3 **Federal income tax withheld from wages, tips, and other compensation** **3**

4 **If no wages, tips, and other compensation are subject to social security or Medicare tax**   ☐ Check and go to line 6.

	Column 1		Column 2
5a Taxable social security wages . .		× .124 =	
5b Taxable social security tips . . .		× .124 =	
5c Taxable Medicare wages & tips. .		× .029 =	
5d Taxable wages & tips subject to Additional Medicare Tax withholding		× .009 =	

5e **Add Column 2 from lines 5a, 5b, 5c, and 5d** **5e**

5f **Section 3121(q) Notice and Demand—Tax due on unreported tips** (see instructions) . .   **5f**

6 **Total taxes before adjustments.** Add lines 3, 5e, and 5f **6**

7 **Current quarter's adjustment for fractions of cents** **7**

8 **Current quarter's adjustment for sick pay** **8**

9 **Current quarter's adjustments for tips and group-term life insurance** **9**

10 **Total taxes after adjustments.** Combine lines 6 through 9 . . . .   **10**

11 **Total deposits for this quarter, including overpayment applied from a prior quarter and overpayments applied from Form 941-X, 941-X (PR), 944-X, 944-X (PR), or 944-X (SP) filed in the current quarter** **11**

12 **Balance due.** If line 10 is more than line 11, enter the difference and see instructions . . .   **12**

13 **Overpayment.** If line 11 is more than line 10, enter the difference ☐ Check one: ☐ Apply to next return. ☐ Send a refund.

▶ **You MUST complete both pages of Form 941 and SIGN it.**   Next ▶

For Privacy Act and Paperwork Reduction Act Notice, see the back of the Payment Voucher.   Cat. No. 17001Z   Form **941** (Rev. 1-2014)

Figure 21-1 ■ A 941 Employer's Quarterly Federal Tax Return.

Source: www.irs.gov.

950214

Name *(not your trade name)*	Employer identification number (EIN)

Part 2: **Tell us about your deposit schedule and tax liability for this quarter.**

If you are unsure about whether you are a monthly schedule depositor or a semiweekly schedule depositor, see Pub. 15 (Circular E), section 11.

14   Check one: ☐ **Line 10 on this return is less than $2,500 or line 10 on the return for the prior quarter was less than $2,500, and you did not incur a $100,000 next-day deposit obligation during the current quarter.** If line 10 for the prior quarter was less than $2,500 but line 10 on this return is $100,000 or more, you must provide a record of your federal tax liability. If you are a monthly schedule depositor, complete the deposit schedule below; if you are a semiweekly schedule depositor, attach Schedule B (Form 941). Go to Part 3.

☐ **You were a monthly schedule depositor for the entire quarter.** Enter your tax liability for each month and total liability for the quarter, then go to Part 3.

Tax liability: Month 1   [.   ]

Month 2   [.   ]

Month 3   [.   ]

Total liability for quarter   [.   ]   **Total must equal line 10.**

☐ **You were a semiweekly schedule depositor for any part of this quarter.** Complete Schedule B (Form 941), Report of Tax Liability for Semiweekly Schedule Depositors, and attach it to Form 941.

Part 3: **Tell us about your business. If a question does NOT apply to your business, leave it blank.**

15   If your business has closed or you stopped paying wages . . . .   ☐ Check here, and

enter the final date you paid wages   [/   /   ] .

16   If you are a seasonal employer and you do not have to file a return for every quarter of the year   . .   ☐ Check here.

Part 4: **May we speak with your third-party designee?**

Do you want to allow an employee, a paid tax preparer, or another person to discuss this return with the IRS? See the instructions for details.

☐ Yes.   Designee's name and phone number   [   ]   [   ]

Select a 5-digit Personal Identification Number (PIN) to use when talking to the IRS.   [ ] [ ] [ ] [ ] [ ]

☐ No.

Part 5: **Sign here. You MUST complete both pages of Form 941 and SIGN it.**

Under penalties of perjury, I declare that I have examined this return, including accompanying schedules and statements, and to the best of my knowledge and belief, it is true, correct, and complete. Declaration of preparer (other than taxpayer) is based on all information of which preparer has any knowledge.

✗   **Sign your name here**   [   ]

Print your name here   [   ]

Print your title here   [   ]

Date   [/   /   ]

Best daytime phone   [   ]

Paid Preparer Use Only   Check if you are self-employed   . . .   ☐

Preparer's name	[ ]	PTIN	[ ]
Preparer's signature	[ ]	Date	[/ /]
Firm's name (or yours if self-employed)	[ ]	EIN	[ ]
Address	[ ]	Phone	[ ]
City	[ ]	State [ ]	ZIP code	[ ]

Figure 21-1 ■ (continued)

PROCEDURE 21-1   Create a New Employee Record

Theory and Rationale

As each new staff member is added to the medical facility, a new employee record must be created. Much of what is contained in the record is mandated by local and federal law. The medical assistant must be aware of the paperwork needed and must comply with all laws regarding the maintenance of these records.

Materials

- Pen
- Paper
- Employee file
- Copy machine

Competency

1. Ask the new employee to bring the following items with them on their first day of employment:
   a. Picture identification or other proof of ability to work in the United States.
   b. Social Security card.
   c. Copies of any certifications or professional licenses.
2. Photocopy any documents the employee has brought for the employee record.
3. Give the employee a W-4 IRS form to complete to indicate the number of exemptions to be claimed.
4. Place the employee's résumé and application into the employee record.
5. Give the employee an I-9 form to complete to verify citizenship.

---

credentials, licensing and insurance information, I-9, and references. To prove their identities at hire, all new employees must provide a copy of their driver's license or other photo identification, as well as copies of their Social Security card. In lieu of a Social Security card, employees may provide a copy of their valid passport as a means of identification.

The Social Security card contains a unique number for every individual. This nine-digit number follows the individual throughout his or her life and cannot be used by another person. Many states provide forms for parents to apply for a Social Security number for their newborns, while still in the hospital post-birth. Parents will be unable to claim their child(ren) on their annual tax returns without a valid Social Security number for each child. In many states, employers are required to submit information on new hires to the state. This is done in order to determine if there are any outstanding orders for payment due from the employee. Most commonly, those outstanding orders are for back child support. In the event an employee is found to have such an outstanding order for payment, the medical office will be directed on how to deduct amounts owed from the employee's wages.

Updating Employee Records

Personnel records should reflect all changes to employment status, such as pay raises, evaluations, disciplinary actions, marital status changes, tax exemptions, and continuing education credits, as those changes occur. Employee records should also include copies of such items as employees' cardiopulmonary resuscitation (CPR) certifications and malpractice insurance documents. In short, personnel records should be accurate, up-to-date pictures of employees.

All personal employee information in the medical office, including payroll information, must be kept confidential and in a place where only authorized personnel can access it.

Under no circumstances should unauthorized parties be allowed access to personal employee information. Employees, however, must be allowed to view their personnel files and to request corrections as needed.

Critical Thinking Question 21-1

Referring back to the case study presented at the beginning of this chapter, what should the medical assistant do with Francie's employee file now that she has provided new information?

The W-4 Form

Every new employee must complete an **IRS W-4 form**, or Employee's Withholding Allowance Certificate, which shows the employer the number of **withholding allowances** the employee is claiming (**Figure 21-2 ■**). This number determines the amount, if any, to be withheld from the employee's earnings each payroll period. Exemptions are claimed for the number of dependents an employee supports, such as children, or a spouse who does not work outside the home. As a general rule, the more exemptions claimed on the W-4 form, the lower the amount of federal taxes that will be withheld. In some cases, employees may choose to claim no exemptions, which will cause the maximum amount of federal taxes to be withheld. In other cases, an employee may claim to be exempt from federal tax withholding. This might be done if the employee does not expect to have any federal tax liability in that year. No matter how many exemptions an employee claims, or how much federal tax is withheld from his wages, he will need to file a federal tax return, after which he might end up receiving a refund for overpayment or be required to pay tax in the event of an underpayment.

Form W-4 (2014)

Purpose. Complete Form W-4 so that your employer can withhold the correct federal income tax from your pay. Consider completing a new Form W-4 each year and when your personal or financial situation changes.

Exemption from withholding. If you are exempt, complete **only** lines 1, 2, 3, 4, and 7 and sign the form to validate it. Your exemption for 2014 expires February 17, 2015. See Pub. 505, Tax Withholding and Estimated Tax.

Note. If another person can claim you as a dependent on his or her tax return, you cannot claim exemption from withholding if your income exceeds $1,000 and includes more than $350 of unearned income (for example, interest and dividends).

Exceptions. An employee may be able to claim exemption from withholding even if the employee is a dependent, if the employee:

• Is age 65 or older,

• Is blind, or

• Will claim adjustments to income; tax credits; or itemized deductions, on his or her tax return.

The exceptions do not apply to supplemental wages greater than $1,000,000.

Basic instructions. If you are not exempt, complete the **Personal Allowances Worksheet** below. The worksheets on page 2 further adjust your withholding allowances based on itemized deductions, certain credits, adjustments to income, or two-earners/multiple jobs situations.

Complete all worksheets that apply. However, you may claim fewer (or zero) allowances. For regular wages, withholding must be based on allowances you claimed and may not be a flat amount or percentage of wages.

Head of household. Generally, you can claim head of household filing status on your tax return only if you are unmarried and pay more than 50% of the costs of keeping up a home for yourself and your dependent(s) or other qualifying individuals. See Pub. 501, Exemptions, Standard Deduction, and Filing Information, for information.

Tax credits. You can take projected tax credits into account in figuring your allowable number of withholding allowances. Credits for child or dependent care expenses and the child tax credit may be claimed using the **Personal Allowances Worksheet** below. See Pub. 505 for information on converting your other credits into withholding allowances.

Nonwage income. If you have a large amount of nonwage income, such as interest or dividends, consider making estimated tax payments using Form 1040-ES, Estimated Tax for Individuals. Otherwise, you may owe additional tax. If you have pension or annuity iincome, see Pub. 505 to find out if you should adjust your withholding on Form W-4 or W-4P.

Two earners or multiple jobs. If you have a working spouse or more than one job, figure the total number of allowances you are entitled to claim on all jobs using worksheets from only one Form W-4. Your withholding usually will be most accurate when all allowances are claimed on the Form W-4 for the highest paying job and zero allowances are claimed on the others. See Pub. 505 for details.

Nonresident alien. If you are a nonresident alien, see Notice 1392, Supplemental Form W-4 Instructions for Nonresident Aliens, before completing this form.

Check your withholding. After your Form W-4 takes effect, use Pub. 505 to see how the amount you are having withheld compares to your projected total tax for 2014. See Pub. 505, especially if your earnings exceed $130,000 (Single) or $180,000 (Married).

Future developments. Information about any future developments affecting Form W-4 (such as legislation enacted after we release it) will be posted at www.irs.gov/w4.

Personal Allowances Worksheet (Keep for your records.)

A   Enter "1" for **yourself** if no one else can claim you as a dependent . . . . **A** _____

B   Enter "1" if: { • You are single and have only one job; or
• You are married, have only one job, and your spouse does not work; or
• Your wages from a second job or your spouse's wages (or the total of both) are $1,500 or less. } . . **B** _____

C   Enter "1" for your **spouse.** But, you may choose to enter "-0-" if you are married and have either a working spouse or more than one job. (Entering "-0-" may help you avoid having too little tax withheld.) . . . . **C** _____

D   Enter number of **dependents** (other than your spouse or yourself) you will claim on your tax return . . . . **D** _____

E   Enter "1" if you will file as **head of household** on your tax return (see conditions under **Head of household** above) . . **E** _____

F   Enter "1" if you have at least $2,000 of **child or dependent care expenses** for which you plan to claim a credit . . . **F** _____
    (**Note.** Do **not** include child support payments. See Pub. 503, Child and Dependent Care Expenses, for details.)

G   **Child Tax Credit** (including additional child tax credit). See Pub. 972, Child Tax Credit, for more information.
    • If your total income will be less than $65,000 ($95,000 if married), enter "2" for each eligible child; then **less** "1" if you have three to six eligible children or **less** "2" if you have seven or more eligible children.
    • If your total income will be between $65,000 and $84,000 ($95,000 and $119,000 if married), enter "1" for each eligible child . . . **G** _____

H   Add lines A through G and enter total here. (**Note.** This may be different from the number of exemptions you claim on your tax return.) ▶ **H** _____

For accuracy, complete all worksheets that apply.
- If you plan to **itemize** or **claim adjustments to income** and want to reduce your withholding, see the **Deductions and Adjustments Worksheet** on page 2.
- If you are **single and have more than one job** or are **married and you and your spouse both work** and the combined earnings from all jobs exceed $50,000 ($20,000 if married), see the **Two-Earners/Multiple Jobs Worksheet** on page 2 to avoid having too little tax withheld.
- If **neither** of the above situations applies, **stop here** and enter the number from line H on line 5 of Form W-4 below.

------ **Separate here and give Form W-4 to your employer. Keep the top part for your records.** ------

Form W-4
Department of the Treasury
Internal Revenue Service

Employee's Withholding Allowance Certificate

▶ Whether you are entitled to claim a certain number of allowances or exemption from withholding is subject to review by the IRS. Your employer may be required to send a copy of this form to the IRS.

OMB No. 1545-0074

2014

1 Your first name and middle initial   Last name   **2** Your social security number

Home address (number and street or rural route)

3 ☐ Single ☐ Married ☐ Married, but withhold at higher Single rate.
Note. If married, but legally separated, or spouse is a nonresident alien, check the "Single" box.

City or town, state, and ZIP code

4 If your last name differs from that shown on your social security card, check here. You must call 1-800-772-1213 for a replacement card. ▶ ☐

5 Total number of allowances you are claiming (from line **H** above **or** from the applicable worksheet on page 2)   **5**

6 Additional amount, if any, you want withheld from each paycheck . . . . **6** $

7 I claim exemption from withholding for 2014, and I certify that I meet **both** of the following conditions for exemption.
    • Last year I had a right to a refund of **all** federal income tax withheld because I had **no** tax liability, **and**
    • This year I expect a refund of **all** federal income tax withheld because I expect to have **no** tax liability.
If you meet both conditions, write "Exempt" here . . . . ▶ **7**

Under penalties of perjury, I declare that I have examined this certificate and, to the best of my knowledge and belief, it is true, correct, and complete.

Employee's signature
(This form is not valid unless you sign it.) ▶   Date ▶

8 Employer's name and address (Employer: Complete lines 8 and 10 only if sending to the IRS.)   **9** Office code (optional)   **10** Employer identification number (EIN)

For Privacy Act and Paperwork Reduction Act Notice, see page 2.   Cat. No. 10220Q   Form **W-4** (2014)

Figure 21-2 ■ W-4 form.

Source: www.irs.gov.

Form W-4 (2014)

Deductions and Adjustments Worksheet

Note. Use this worksheet *only* if you plan to itemize deductions or claim certain credits or adjustments to income.

1	Enter an estimate of your 2014 itemized deductions. These include qualifying home mortgage interest, charitable contributions, state and local taxes, medical expenses in excess of 10% (7.5% if either you or your spouse was born before January 2, 1950) of your income, and miscellaneous deductions. For 2014, you may have to reduce your itemized deductions if your income is over $305,050 and you are married filing jointly or are a qualifying widow(er); $279,650 if you are head of household; $254,200 if you are single and not head of household or a qualifying widow(er); or $152,525 if you are married filing separately. See Pub. 505 for details	**1**	$ _____

2   Enter: { $12,400 if married filing jointly or qualifying widow(er) / $9,100 if head of household / $6,200 if single or married filing separately } . . . . . . **2** $ _____

3   **Subtract** line 2 from line 1. If zero or less, enter "-0-" . . . . **3** $ _____

4   Enter an estimate of your 2014 adjustments to income and any additional standard deduction (see Pub. 505)   **4** $ _____

5   **Add** lines 3 and 4 and enter the total. (Include any amount for credits from the *Converting Credits to Withholding Allowances for 2014 Form W-4* worksheet in Pub. 505.) . . . . **5** $ _____

6   Enter an estimate of your 2014 nonwage income (such as dividends or interest) . . . . . **6** $ _____

7   **Subtract** line 6 from line 5. If zero or less, enter "-0-" . . . . **7** $ _____

8   **Divide** the amount on line 7 by $3,950 and enter the result here. Drop any fraction . . . . **8** _____

9   Enter the number from the **Personal Allowances Worksheet, line H**, page 1 . . . . . . **9** _____

10   **Add** lines 8 and 9 and enter the total here. If you plan to use the **Two-Earners/Multiple Jobs Worksheet**, also enter this total on line 1 below. Otherwise, **stop here** and enter this total on Form W-4, line 5, page 1 **10** _____

Two-Earners/Multiple Jobs Worksheet (See *Two earners or multiple jobs* on page 1.)

Note. Use this worksheet *only* if the instructions under line H on page 1 direct you here.

1   Enter the number from line H, page 1 (or from line 10 above if you used the **Deductions and Adjustments Worksheet**)   **1** _____

2   Find the number in **Table 1** below that applies to the **LOWEST** paying job and enter it here. **However,** if you are married filing jointly and wages from the highest paying job are $65,000 or less, do not enter more than "3" . . . . **2** _____

3   If line 1 is **more than or equal to** line 2, subtract line 2 from line 1. Enter the result here (if zero, enter "-0-") and on Form W-4, line 5, page 1. **Do not** use the rest of this worksheet . . . . **3** _____

Note. If line 1 is **less than** line 2, enter "-0-" on Form W-4, line 5, page 1. Complete lines 4 through 9 below to figure the additional withholding amount necessary to avoid a year-end tax bill.

4   Enter the number from line 2 of this worksheet . . . . **4** _____

5   Enter the number from line 1 of this worksheet . . . . **5** _____

6   **Subtract** line 5 from line 4 . . . . **6** _____

7   Find the amount in **Table 2** below that applies to the **HIGHEST** paying job and enter it here . . . . **7** $ _____

8   **Multiply** line 7 by line 6 and enter the result here. This is the additional annual withholding needed . . **8** $ _____

9   Divide line 8 by the number of pay periods remaining in 2014. For example, divide by 25 if you are paid every two weeks and you complete this form on a date in January when there are 25 pay periods remaining in 2014. Enter the result here and on Form W-4, line 6, page 1. This is the additional amount to be withheld from each paycheck **9** $ _____

Table 1

Married Filing Jointly		All Others	
If wages from **LOWEST** paying job are—	Enter on line 2 above	If wages from **LOWEST** paying job are—	Enter on line 2 above
$0 - $6,000	0	$0 - $6,000	0
6,001 - 13,000	1	6,001 - 16,000	1
13,001 - 24,000	2	16,001 - 25,000	2
24,001 - 26,000	3	25,001 - 34,000	3
26,001 - 33,000	4	34,001 - 43,000	4
33,001 - 43,000	5	43,001 - 70,000	5
43,001 - 49,000	6	70,001 - 85,000	6
49,001 - 60,000	7	85,001 - 110,000	7
60,001 - 75,000	8	110,001 - 125,000	8
75,001 - 80,000	9	125,001 - 140,000	9
80,001 - 100,000	10	140,001 and over	10
100,001 - 115,000	11		
115,001 - 130,000	12		
130,001 - 140,000	13		
140,001 - 150,000	14		
150,001 and over	15		

Table 2

Married Filing Jointly		All Others	
If wages from **HIGHEST** paying job are—	Enter on line 7 above	If wages from **HIGHEST** paying job are—	Enter on line 7 above
$0 - $74,000	$590	$0 - $37,000	$590
74,001 - 130,000	990	37,001 - 80,000	990
130,001 - 200,000	1,110	80,001 - 175,000	1,110
200,001 - 355,000	1,300	175,001 - 385,000	1,300
355,001 - 400,000	1,380	385,001 and over	1,560
400,001 and over	1,560		

Privacy Act and Paperwork Reduction Act Notice. We ask for the information on this form to carry out the Internal Revenue laws of the United States. Internal Revenue Code sections 3402(f)(2) and 6109 and their regulations require you to provide this information; your employer uses it to determine your federal income tax withholding. Failure to provide a properly completed form will result in your being treated as a single person who claims no withholding allowances; providing fraudulent information may subject you to penalties. Routine uses of this information include giving it to the Department of Justice for civil and criminal litigation; to cities, states, the District of Columbia, and U.S. commonwealths and possessions for use in administering their tax laws; and to the Department of Health and Human Services for use in the National Directory of New Hires. We may also disclose this information to other countries under a tax treaty, to federal and state agencies to enforce federal nontax criminal laws, or to federal law enforcement and intelligence agencies to combat terrorism.

You are not required to provide the information requested on a form that is subject to the Paperwork Reduction Act unless the form displays a valid OMB control number. Books or records relating to a form or its instructions must be retained as long as their contents may become material in the administration of any Internal Revenue law. Generally, tax returns and return information are confidential, as required by Code section 6103.

The average time and expenses required to complete and file this form will vary depending on individual circumstances. For estimated averages, see the instructions for your income tax return.

If you have suggestions for making this form simpler, we would be happy to hear from you. See the instructions for your income tax return.

Figure 21-2 ■ (continued)

To ensure timely payroll processing, employees must complete and sign their W-4 forms before their first payroll period. As employees experience life changes, such as marriage or children, their withholding allowances will change. To keep their payroll up to date, the medical office should require employees to notify their personnel department or payroll staff of any such changes.

When an employee wishes to change her withholding allowance, she must complete and sign a new W-4 form. W-4 changes should take effect in the next payroll period. When the medical office outsources its payroll function, W-4 changes might be delayed. In this case, the office should notify the affected employee.

Critical Thinking Question 21-2

Referring to the case study at the beginning of the chapter, what does the office manager need to do to help Francie ensure that withholding allowances are processed properly?

Critical Thinking Question 21-3

Refer to the case study at the beginning of this chapter. Because the medical assistant, and not an outside agency, handles the medical office's payroll, what can the assistant tell Francie about the time it will take to change her payroll deductions?

Recording Employees' Work Hours

To meet FLSA requirements for overtime pay, employers must accurately record the hours their employees work. For all employees, salaried and hourly, employers must also send their state premiums to cover worker's compensation insurance. These premiums are based on the number of hours all covered employees worked in each quarter.

Calculating Payroll

Employers have varied ways to track employees' work hours. Some employers use **time clocks** that stamp employees' cards at the beginning and end of shifts (**Figure 21-3** ■). Other employers direct employees to track their hours on timesheets they submit when each pay period ends.

Employees Paid on an Hourly Basis

The gross earnings of an employee paid hourly are calculated by multiplying the number of regular hours worked by the employee's hourly rate. Any overtime hours are calculated by multiplying the overtime hours worked by 1.5 times the employee's hourly rate. When an employee works partial hours, some employers round those hours to the nearest half hour; others round to the nearest quarter hour. **Figure 21-4** ■ shows how hourly payroll is calculated.

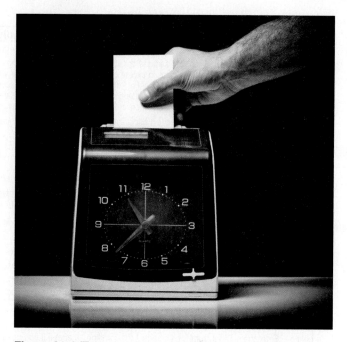

Figure 21-3 ■ An employee uses a time clock to document the time he arrives at work.
Source: Fotolia © tiero.

Salaried Employees

The gross earnings of a salaried employee remain the same each pay period, no matter how many hours are worked, up to 40 hours in 1 week. In general, when salaried employees work more than 40 hours in a week, they must be paid overtime for each hour over 40, unless that employee is considered an exempt salaried employee. Overtime pay is calculated based on an hourly rate, which is calculated by dividing the employee's salaried amount by the number of hours in the pay period. **Figure 21-5** ■ provides an example of how salaried payroll is calculated.

Ortiz's regular hourly rate is $15.00, and his regular hours per week are 40. In the past 2-week payroll period, Ortiz worked 84 hours. To calculate Ortiz's gross earnings, multiply his regular hours by his hourly wage (80 × $15.00 = $1,200.00). Next, calculate his overtime earnings by calculating his overtime hourly rate (1.5 × $15.00 = $22.50) and then multiply his overtime rate by his overtime hours ($22.50 × 4 = $90.00). Finally, add the amount Ortiz earned in regular hours with the amount he earned in overtime hours to determine his gross earnings for the payroll period ($1,200.00 + $90.00 = $1,290.00).

Figure 21-4 ■ Employee scenario: How hourly payroll is calculated.

Molly is a salaried employee paid $1,000.00 for each 2-week payroll period. In this pay period, Molly worked 85 hours. Calculating Molly's overtime pay entails first determining her normal hourly wage by dividing her $1,000.00 salary by the 80 hours in the 2-week pay period ($1,000.00/80 hours = $12.50 per hour). Next, determine Molly's overtime rate by multiplying 1.5 by her normal hourly rate (1.5 × $12.50 = $18.75) and then multiplying that figure by the 5 extra hours she worked during the pay period ($18.75 × 5 hours = $93.75). Finally, add Molly's base salary to her overtime hours to determine her gross earnings total for the pay period ($1,000.00 + $93.75 = $1093.75).

Figure 21-5 ■ Employee scenario: How salaried payroll is calculated.

Payroll Deductions

Some payroll deductions, like the federal withholding and FICA taxes discussed earlier, are mandated by law. Other deductions, like those for health and life insurance or disability policies, are voluntary. Medical offices should give new employees lists of voluntary deductions so those employees can choose to participate if desired.

Employees may elect to have some payroll deductions taken from their wages prior to being taxed on those wages. These deductions are covered under federal law, and typically apply to out of pocket health care and daycare expenses. By having these deductions subtracted from the pre-tax wages, the employee is not taxed on the amounts deducted.

The Circular E

When employers calculate payroll manually, medical assistants need an IRS publication called the **Circular E** (**Figure 21-6** ■). This publication, revised annually, tells employers how much federal tax to withhold for each employee. Married and single employees appear in separate tables, as do weekly, biweekly, semimonthly, and monthly pay periods. To use the Circular E form properly, medical assistants need employees' completed W-4 forms. The following scenario highlights the use of the Circular E:

Danesha is married and claims four withholding allowances from her payroll. Her gross earnings this biweekly payroll period are $855.00. To determine the federal tax to withhold from Danesha's earnings, consult the married persons, biweekly payroll period chart (**Figure 21-7** ■). Move down the left column to Danesha's wages, and then move across the row to the number for people claiming four exemptions. This amount is the federal tax to withhold from Danesha's earnings.

To determine an employee's FICA withholding amount, the medical assistant must first multiply the employee's gross

earnings from regular and overtime pay by 6.2 percent for Social Security. Next, the assistant must multiply the employee's gross earnings by 1.45 percent for Medicare withholding. When the assistant works in a state with state and local income taxes, she will consult state and local reference tables to determine state and local taxes. Tax payments from the medical office may be made online, through the mail, or in person at the medical office provider's bank.

Other Deductions

To determine total deductions from employees' payrolls, amounts for items like worker's compensation insurance, health insurance, retirement plans, and **charitable contributions** must be calculated and added to federal and state or local taxes. Many employers offer services to employees, such as gym membership at a discount or medical insurance benefits for the employee's spouse and/or children. Some employers may offer a charitable contribution match to employees who choose to donate part of their wage to a charity. Once all deductions are subtracted, the balance, called the net payroll or *take-home pay*, is the amount the employee will receive in a check.

Using Software to Calculate Payroll

For employers who calculate payroll using computer software, payroll is far simpler than for those who choose the manual option. Although payroll software requires employers to set up each new employee, it streamlines the process of entering an employee's hours and calculating the employee's withholdings. Many such software packages also print payroll checks, quarterly payroll tax reports, and W-2 forms.

W-2 forms (**Figure 21-8** ■) outline employees' wages and the federal taxes withheld for the previous year. Because employees need these forms to file their personal taxes, federal law requires employers to send these forms to employees postmarked no later than January 31.

Garnishing Wages

Employees' wages may be **garnished**, or taken, for many reasons. Wages may be garnished to repay loans, fulfill child or spousal support, or pay monetary judgments against employees. Medical assistants who handle payroll must keep accurate records of all garnishment requests that arise from court orders. These court orders specify the amount to be taken from an employee's gross wages, as well as the party who is to receive that amount. Occasionally, a percentage of an employee's gross wages, rather than a set dollar amount, is garnished. Separate checks for garnished amounts must be sent to the agency on the court order. Whenever a medical assistant mails a check to an agency, an insurance carrier, or a patient, she should use a **security envelope** to mask the contents. When wages are garnished, corresponding deductions appear on the employee's payroll sheet. The employee receives the balances of her wages, which are less other deductions and taxes.

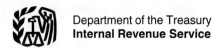

Department of the Treasury
Internal Revenue Service

Publication 15
Cat. No. 10000W

(Circular E), Employer's Tax Guide

For use in **2014**

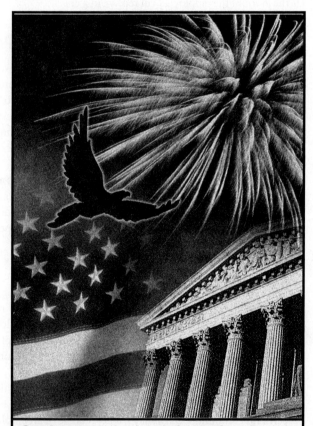

Get forms and other Information faster and easier by

Internet at IRS.gov

Dec 18, 2013

Contents

Future Developments

For the latest information about developments related to Publication 15 (Circular E), such as legislation enacted after it was published, go to *www.irs.gov/pub15*.

What's New

Social security and Medicare tax for 2014. The social security tax rate is 6.2% each for the employee and employer, unchanged from 2013. The social security wage base limit is $117,000.

The Medicare tax rate is 1.45% each for the employee and employer, unchanged from 2013. There is no wage base limit for Medicare tax.

Figure 21-6 ■ The Circular E IRS table is used to find the correct amount of federal withholding tax for an employee.

Source: www.irs.gov.

MARRIED Persons—WEEKLY Payroll Period

(For Wages Paid through December 2014)

And the wages are–		And the number of withholding allowances claimed is—										
At least	But less than	0	1	2	3	4	5	6	7	8	9	10
		The amount of income tax to be withheld is—										
$800	$810	$79	$68	$56	$45	$34	$26	$19	$11	$3	$0	$0
810	820	80	69	58	46	35	27	20	12	4	0	0
820	830	82	71	59	48	36	28	21	13	5	0	0
830	840	83	72	61	49	38	29	22	14	6	0	0
840	850	85	74	62	51	39	30	23	15	7	0	0
850	860	86	75	64	52	41	31	24	16	8	1	0
860	870	88	77	65	54	42	32	25	17	9	2	0
870	880	89	78	67	55	44	33	26	18	10	3	0
880	890	91	80	68	57	45	34	27	19	11	4	0
890	900	92	81	70	58	47	35	28	20	12	5	0
900	910	94	83	71	60	48	37	29	21	13	6	0
910	920	95	84	73	61	50	38	30	22	14	7	0
920	930	97	86	74	63	51	40	31	23	15	8	0
930	940	98	87	76	64	53	41	32	24	16	9	1
940	950	100	89	77	66	54	43	33	25	17	10	2
950	960	101	90	79	67	56	44	34	26	18	11	3
960	970	103	92	80	69	57	46	35	27	19	12	4
970	980	104	93	82	70	59	47	36	28	20	13	5
980	990	106	95	83	72	60	49	38	29	21	14	6
990	1,000	107	96	85	73	62	50	39	30	22	15	7
1,000	1,010	109	98	86	75	63	52	41	31	23	16	8
1,010	1,020	110	99	88	76	65	53	42	32	24	17	9
1,020	1,030	112	101	89	78	66	55	44	33	25	18	10
1,030	1,040	113	102	91	79	68	56	45	34	26	19	11
1,040	1,050	115	104	92	81	69	58	47	35	27	20	12
1,050	1,060	116	105	94	82	71	59	48	37	28	21	13
1,060	1,070	118	107	95	84	72	61	50	38	29	22	14
1,070	1,080	119	108	97	85	74	62	51	40	30	23	15
1,080	1,090	121	110	98	87	75	64	53	41	31	24	16
1,090	1,100	122	111	100	88	77	65	54	43	32	25	17
1,100	1,110	124	113	101	90	78	67	56	44	33	26	18
1,110	1,120	125	114	103	91	80	68	57	46	34	27	19
1,120	1,130	127	116	104	93	81	70	59	47	36	28	20
1,130	1,140	128	117	106	94	83	71	60	49	37	29	21
1,140	1,150	130	119	107	96	84	73	62	50	39	30	22
1,150	1,160	131	120	109	97	86	74	63	52	40	31	23
1,160	1,170	133	122	110	99	87	76	65	53	42	32	24
1,170	1,180	134	123	112	100	89	77	66	55	43	33	25
1,180	1,190	136	125	113	102	90	79	68	56	45	34	26
1,190	1,200	137	126	115	103	92	80	69	58	46	35	27
1,200	1,210	139	128	116	105	93	82	71	59	48	36	28
1,210	1,220	140	129	118	106	95	83	72	61	49	38	29
1,220	1,230	142	131	119	108	96	85	74	62	51	39	30
1,230	1,240	143	132	121	109	98	86	75	64	52	41	31
1,240	1,250	145	134	122	111	99	88	77	65	54	42	32
1,250	1,260	146	135	124	112	101	89	78	67	55	44	33
1,260	1,270	148	137	125	114	102	91	80	68	57	45	34
1,270	1,280	149	138	127	115	104	92	81	70	58	47	35
1,280	1,290	151	140	128	117	105	94	83	71	60	48	37
1,290	1,300	152	141	130	118	107	95	84	73	61	50	38
1,300	1,310	154	143	131	120	108	97	86	74	63	51	40
1,310	1,320	155	144	133	121	110	98	87	76	64	53	41
1,320	1,330	157	146	134	123	111	100	89	77	66	54	43
1,330	1,340	158	147	136	124	113	101	90	79	67	56	44
1,340	1,350	160	149	137	126	114	103	92	80	69	57	46
1,350	1,360	161	150	139	127	116	104	93	82	70	59	47
1,360	1,370	163	152	140	129	117	106	95	83	72	60	49
1,370	1,380	164	153	142	130	119	107	96	85	73	62	50
1,380	1,390	166	155	143	132	120	109	98	86	75	63	52
1,390	1,400	167	156	145	133	122	110	99	88	76	65	53
1,400	1,410	169	158	146	135	123	112	101	89	78	66	55
1,410	1,420	170	159	148	136	125	113	102	91	79	68	56
1,420	1,430	172	161	149	138	126	115	104	92	81	69	58
1,430	1,440	173	162	151	139	128	116	105	94	82	71	59
1,440	1,450	175	164	152	141	129	118	107	95	84	72	61
1,450	1,460	176	165	154	142	131	119	108	97	85	74	62
1,460	1,470	178	167	155	144	132	121	110	98	87	75	64
1,470	1,480	179	168	157	145	134	122	111	100	88	77	65

$1,480 and over	Use Table 1(b) for a **MARRIED person** on page 43. Also see the instructions on page 41.

Publication 15 (2014)

Figure 21-7 ■ This chart from the Circular E shows the correct amount of withholding tax for this employee.

Source: www.irs.gov.

22222	Void ☐	a Employee's social security number	For Official Use Only ▶ OMB No. 1545-0008		

b Employer identification number (EIN)		1 Wages, tips, other compensation	2 Federal income tax withheld
c Employer's name, address, and ZIP code		3 Social security wages	4 Social security tax withheld
		5 Medicare wages and tips	6 Medicare tax withheld
		7 Social security tips	8 Allocated tips
d Control number		9	10 Dependent care benefits
e Employee's first name and initial Last name Suff.		11 Nonqualified plans	12a See instructions for box 12 C o d e
		13 Statutory employee ☐ Retirement plan ☐ Third-party sick pay ☐	12b C o d e
		14 Other	12c C o d e
			12d C o d e
f Employee's address and ZIP code			

15 State Employer's state ID number	16 State wages, tips, etc.	17 State income tax	18 Local wages, tips, etc.	19 Local income tax	20 Locality name

Form **W-2** Wage and Tax Statement   **2014**   Department of the Treasury—Internal Revenue Service
Copy A For Social Security Administration — Send this entire page with   **For Privacy Act and Paperwork Reduction**
Form W-3 to the Social Security Administration; photocopies are **not** acceptable.   **Act Notice, see the separate instructions.**
Cat. No. 10134D
Do Not Cut, Fold, or Staple Forms on This Page

Figure 21-8 ■ W-2 Form.
Source: www.irs.gov.

PROCEDURE 21-2 Calculate an Employee's Payroll

Theory and Rationale

Depending on the size of the medical office, the medical assistant may perform the employee payroll function. This function must be performed while paying strict attention to the state and national laws governing payroll.

Materials

- Calculator
- Employee's W-4 form
- IRS Circular E list of federal tax deduction amounts
- Record of number of hours the employee worked
- Employee's payroll record

Competency

1. Calculate the number of hours the employee worked during the payroll period.
2. For an hourly employee, calculate the employee's gross wage by multiplying the number of hours worked in the payroll period by the employee's hourly wage.
3. If the employee worked any overtime hours, first multiply the employee's hourly wage by 1.5 and then multiply that amount by the employee's overtime hours.
4. Consult the employee's W-4 form to determine filing status (i.e., married or single) and the number of deductions.
5. Consult the IRS Circular E form to determine the amount to be withheld from the employee's gross wages.
6. Deduct the federal withholding tax from the Circular E form from the employee's gross payroll.
7. Multiply the employee's gross payroll amount by 6.2 percent to determine the FICA (Social Security) to withhold from the employee's payroll.
8. Multiply the employee's gross payroll amount by 1.45 percent to determine the Medicare tax to withhold from the employee's payroll.
9. Consult the employee's file to determine any other deductions (e.g., health insurance or retirement contributions) to withhold from the employee's payroll.
10. Determine the net payroll by subtracting all deductions from the gross payroll.

Accounts Payable

The accounts payable function in the medical office is similar to the way people handle their finances in their homes: bills come in and must be paid. In the medical office, bills might include rent, utilities, insurance, and supplies. Some accounts are paid in single installments, whereas others are paid monthly or on other, similarly regular schedules. The medical assistant in charge of the accounts payable function must determine the accuracy of bills before making payment, and must keep accurate records of all checks going out.

Several suppliers offer discounts for bills paid by a set date, typically 10, 15, or 30 days after supplies ship. Other suppliers offer discounts when supplies are paid by credit card rather than invoiced. To take advantage of such discounts, medical assistants should research the policies of suppliers and vendors.

The Checkbook Register

Whether medical offices keep their checkbook registers electronically or manually, those registers must be accurate and clear as to payment purpose and receiver. Clarity, like the availability of the information, is especially important when the IRS conducts an audit. To ensure clarity, checkbook registers should have columns with labels such as "Utilities," "Payroll," and "Clinical Supplies." Categorized expenditures help offices track their payments. The following is a list of some common expenditure categories:

- **Rent**—fee for office space
- **Utilities**—cost of electric, telephone, Internet, and gas services

- **Payroll**—wages paid to employees
- **Taxes**—monies paid to city, state, or federal agencies
- **Office supplies**—costs of items like pens, paper, and envelopes
- **Clinical supplies**—cost of items for clinical activities (e.g., gowns, syringes, and lab supplies)
- **Maintenance**—expenditures for repairs or cleaning staff and equipment maintenance and upkeep
- **Continuing education**—tuition for professional classes for physicians and staff
- **Insurance**—cost of office's liability insurance
- **Travel**—expenses for office-related travel (e.g., travel to seminars)
- **Marketing**—price of office advertising

Ordering and Receiving Supplies

Before ordering medical office supplies, the health care team should thoroughly investigate the suppliers and their policies. For example, staff should try to uncover any hidden costs, determine shipping costs, explore the possibility of bulk-rate discounts, and examine companies' return policies. For large purchases, the office might want to ask suppliers for references as an added investigative step.

When supplies arrive in the office, staff should check the packing slip to verify the order. Any invoices should be routed to the accounts payable office.

 PROCEDURE 21-3 Write Checks to Pay Bills ———————————

Theory and Rationale

In the medical office, bills (accounts payable) must be paid in a timely manner. The medical assistant who performs this function must understand how to use the checkbook register to pay the bills, as well as the importance of accuracy in this function.

Materials

- Office checkbook register
- Bills to be paid
- Blue or black pen
- Calculator

Competency

1. Verify the bill is accurate and that the supplies or services were received.
2. Determine if the company offers a discount if the bill is paid by a certain date. If so, pay the bill by the discount due date to obtain the discount.
3. Complete the check, providing the date, name of the vendor or supplier, and check amount.
4. On the invoice, write the date, check number, and payment amount.
5. File the invoice.
6. Give the check to the physician or office manager for signature.
7. In the checkbook register, note the payment category, date, and amount of the check.

PROCEDURE 21-4 Pay an Office Supply Invoice

Theory and Rationale

Many suppliers ask for payment upon receipt and mark their invoices accordingly. The medical assistant must know how to pay these invoices in a timely manner.

Materials

- Office supply invoice
- Office checkbook and checkbook register
- Blue or black pen
- Calculator

Competency

1. Verify that the supplies on the invoice were received, that inventory was taken of the supplies, and that the supplies were distributed in the office appropriately.

2. Determine whether the supplier offers a discount if the bill is paid by a certain date. If so, pay the bill by the discount due to obtain the discount.

3. Write a check for the supplies, providing the date, supplier name, and check amount.

4. Give the check to the physician or office manager for signature.

5. In the office checkbook register, note the payment, including the supply category, the date, and the amount of the check

6. Mail the payment to the supplier.

Preparing a Deposit Slip

At the end of each business day, medical offices should deposit their daily receipts (**Figure 21-9** ■). Such deposits include cash and personal checks collected from patients, usually for copays, and insurance and patient payments received in the mail. Patients might sometimes fund their services through traveler's checks, which are purchased while traveling as a safe alternative to cash. Other checks that may be presented for payment in the medical office are cashier's checks, certified checks, counter checks, or money orders. These forms of payment are typically purchased by the patient from their local bank or another financial institution. All forms of payment are deposited with the daily receipts. Computerized offices can

 PROCEDURE 21-5 Complete a Deposit Slip

Theory and Rationale

In the medical office, part of keeping accurate records is completing the deposit slip correctly and accurately. This function is typically handled at the end of the business day so that the deposit can be taken to the bank after the office has closed.

Materials

- Calculator
- Deposit slip
- Printout from the electronic or manual billing system showing amount received for the day
- Pen
- Endorsement stamp

Competency

1. Check to see that all checks have been properly endorsed.

2. Total all cash receipts.

3. On the line marked "cash" on the deposit slip, list the cash receipt total.

4. On the deposit slip, list each check individually by bank routing number or name of the patient or insurance company.

5. Total the checks.

6. On the appropriate line of the deposit slip, list the check total.

7. Total the checks and cash.

8. On the appropriate line of the deposit slip, list the checks and cash total.

9. Attach the deposit slip, cash, and checks with a paperclip.

10. Place the paper clipped deposit in an envelope.

11. Take the deposit to the bank.

12. Obtain a receipt.

13. Return to the office.

14. Using the receipt, record the deposit amount in the clinic checkbook register.

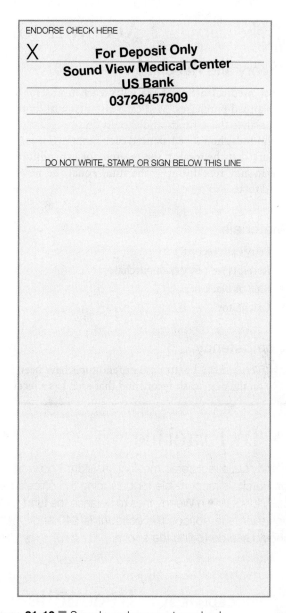

Figure 21-9 ■ Sample deposit slip.

print the days' collection using the medical office software. Such reports, which detail the day's receipts, should cross-check against the money to be deposited.

The medical assistant who is responsible for preparing deposits must ensure that the amounts the computer indicates as the daily collection matches the deposit amount. When these figures fail to match, the assistant must search for and rectify the error. Only when figures match may deposit slips be prepared.

Endorsement Stamps

Medical offices use **endorsement stamps** to endorse the back of all checks they receive (**Figure 21-10** ■). This stamp list the office's name, the bank's name, and the office's account number at the bank. The phrase "For Deposit Only" should also appear on the stamp. Checks stamped in this manner are difficult for unauthorized parties to cash. The "deposit only" stamp is known as restrictive endorsement.

HIPAA Compliance

Any document containing patient information, including a personal check, is considered confidential. As a result, documents like these must be kept out of the view of other patients or staff who lack the authority to access confidential patient information.

Accessing Bank Accounts via the Internet

Most banks now allow users to access their bank accounts and complete banking functions, like paying bills, via the Internet. This benefits both the patient and the medical office. In order to access these features, the medical office or patient must have a computer with access to the Internet. This service is convenient, because it is available 24 hours a day, 7 days a week, and medical offices may receive payments from patients by mail. The medical assistant should post these payments, identified with patient account or identification number, as they would post conventional hard-copy checks. Many medical offices

Figure 21-10 ■ Sample endorsement on check.

today provide patients with the opportunity to pay outstanding accounts over the office's Web site, via a secure portal.

Petty Cash

Most medical offices keep petty cash funds, small amounts of money to fund spur-of-the-moment costs like out-of-stock office supplies or postage. A petty cash fund is typically set up with a base amount of money. When money is taken from petty cash, receipts or vouchers in the amounts paid, and the reason for the expenditure, should replace the money in the fund. Each month, petty cash funds should be balanced, which entails ensuring that the total of the receipts for expenditures and the money remaining in the fund equals the assumed total of the petty cash fund. Petty cash funds are typically started with a certain amount of money and payments from the fund are recorded in a ledger.

PROCEDURE 21-6 Account for Petty Cash

Theory and Rationale

Most medical offices have petty cash funds for small, unplanned purchases. Medical assistants must know how to balance these funds and should do so regularly. Petty cash funds should be balanced each month. The MA must ensure that the total of the receipts for expenditures and the money remaining in the fund equal the petty cash fund total.

Materials

- Petty cash record
- Receipts for petty cash purchases
- Blue or black pen
- Calculator

Competency

1. Verify that all petty cash expenditures have been listed on the petty cash record and that each has a receipt.

2. Subtract all expenditures from the petty cash balance.
3. Enter the new balance on the petty cash record.
4. Count the money in petty cash.
5. Verify that the petty cash amount matches the resulting amount in step 2.
6. If the amounts do not match, verify that all subtraction was done accurately and that all receipts were entered in the petty cash record.
7. Once the account balances, obtain a check for the total expenditures from the physician or office manager.
8. Cash the check at the bank.
9. Enter the money in the petty cash record.

 ## In Practice

Wendy Lu, a registered medical assistant who works for Dr. Patch, is responsible for balancing the office's petty cash fund. When Wendy tries to balance the fund today, however, she notices the account is $40 short. What should she do to find the error?

Reconciling Bank Statements

Medical assistants, physicians, office managers, or outside companies may be responsible for reconciling the medical office's bank statements. The bank statement is a document that outlines the deposits made and monies withdrawn from the bank account over the past month. Online banking is also

 PROCEDURE 21-7 Reconcile a Bank Statement

Theory and Rationale

The medical office's bank statement must be balanced monthly to ensure the account balance is accurate and error free.

Materials

- Bank statement
- Checkbook register
- Calculator
- Blue or black pen

Competency

1. Comparing the bank statement to the checkbook register, make a check mark next to each check processed by the bank.

2. Write the ending balance on the bank statement.
3. Add any deposits made since the bank statement was printed.
4. Subtract any checks not yet processed when the bank statement was printed.
5. Add any interest awarded by the bank.
6. Subtract any bank service fees taken by the bank.
7. If the resulting balance fails to match the balance in the checkbook register, verify that steps 1 through 6 were performed correctly.
8. If the balances still do not match, check for addition or subtraction errors in the checkbook register.

a convenient option because it allows whomever is reconciling the bank statement to view the office's banking activities in real time. Offices need not wait for statements to arrive or call banks with payment or deposit questions when using online banking.

The reconciliation of medical office bank statements resembles the reconciliation of personal bank statements. Once the office's bank statement arrives from the bank, the staff member in charge of reconciliation must check off on the office's book register the checks and deposits listed as processed on the statement. Next, staff should add the end-of-month balance on the statement to any outstanding deposits in the office's checkbook register. From that number, any outstanding checks must be deducted. The resulting number should match the amount in the office's checkbook register. If the numbers do not match, the medical assistant will need to verify the deposits and payments that were made in order to identify the discrepancy.

REVIEW

Chapter Summary

- Payroll is a critical function in the medical office. The payroll function involves keeping accurate records on all employees.
- Manual and computerized payroll systems are both employed in health care, though the latter tend to offer greater ease and convenience.
- In the medical office, accounts payable serves to secure the monies that keep the business functioning.
- When it comes time to deposit any payments received, checks must be endorsed properly following a documented procedure.

- Medical office payments are deposited according to a set procedure.
- Petty cash is a valuable tool the medical office can use for unexpected, though minor, purchases.
- The individual charged with reconciling the office's monthly bank statement should do so in a way that ensures an accurate result. The medical office's bank statement should be balanced monthly to ensure that the account balance is accurate and free of errors.

Chapter Review

Multiple Choice

1. In what year did Congress pass legislation requiring that federal income taxes be paid?
   a. 1893
   b. 1903
   c. 1913
   d. 1923
   e. 1933

2. As of 2009, the federal minimum wage was:
   a. $5.25
   b. $6.25
   c. $7.25
   d. $8.25
   e. $9.25

3. Worker's compensation covers:
   a. Work time lost due to injury
   b. Medical expenses incurred due to illness not injury related
   c. Medical insurance premiums
   d. Copays for medical visits
   e. All of the above

4. Overtime is paid at _____ times the hourly rate.
   a. 1.25
   b. 1.5
   c. 1.75
   d. 2
   e. 2.5

True/False

T F 1. Employers use the IRS Circular E form to determine the federal withholding taxes to be withheld from employees' wages.

T F 2. Employers must track the hours their employees work, whether those employees are salaried or hourly.

T F 3. Another term for *gross pay* is *net pay*.

T F 4. All employers must match the Social Security and Medicare taxes withheld from employees' payrolls.

T F **5.** Medical office collections should be deposited daily.

T F **6.** All states in the United States have state income taxes.

Short Answer

1. Name three items that should be in every employee's personnel file.
2. When choosing new suppliers for the medical office, what kinds of questions should be asked?
3. What does it mean to endorse a check?
4. Why is it important to endorse checks soon after they arrive in the medical office?
5. Name a common purchase made with petty cash.
6. Describe some desirable characteristics in medical assistants who handle office payroll or accounts payable functions.
7. Why would patients pay for their visit to the physician with traveler's checks?
8. Define the term *accounts payable*.
9. Explain what it means to garnish an employee's wages.
10. Explain how a time clock is used.

Research

1. Interview the office manager of a local medical office. Ask the manager if the function of payroll is handled within the medical office or if it is handled by an outside firm.
2. Look at the IRS Web site. What information is contained there that might be helpful to the medical office with regard to processing payroll?
3. Research the laws regarding the garnishment of wages in your state.

Practicum Application Experience

A recently hired medical assistant has been asked to visit the manager's office on his first day so that the manager can set up an employee file. What type of information should the assistant bring to expedite this task?

Resource Guide

Payroll-Taxes.com
14350 North 87th Street, Suite 170
Scottsdale, AZ 85260
Phone: (480) 596-1500
Fax: (480) 991-0572
http://www.payroll-taxes.com

Quickbooks Payroll
Phone: (888) 729-1996
http://www.quickbooks.com

22

Managing the Medical Office

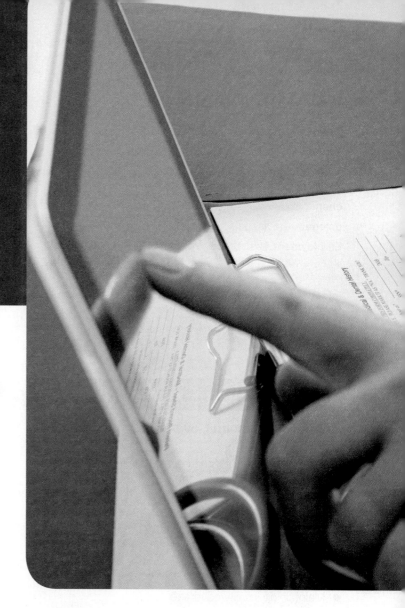

Case Study

Read the following case study and answer the critical thinking questions presented throughout the chapter.

Juanita Ryan is the office manager at Valley View Medical Clinic, which has three physicians, one of whom arrives late every morning and returns late after lunch. Juanita has spoken with the physician, Dr. Whittier, several times. Patients are angry and frustrated by their long waits.

Objectives

After completing this chapter, you should be able to:

22.1 Define and spell the key terminology in this chapter.

22.2 Describe the characteristics and responsibilities of an effective office manager.

22.3 Define different management leadership styles.

22.4 Explain how to conduct an effective staff meeting, how to write a staff meeting agenda, and discuss items that should be included.

22.5 Explain the medical office manager's role in hiring, training, and supervising staff in the medical office.

22.6 Discuss how to overcome scheduling issues.

22.7 Explain how to conduct employee evaluations.

22.8 Discuss the steps to effectively discipline and terminate staff.

22.9 Define sexual harassment and discuss the medical office manager's role with regard to sexual harassment policy in the medical office.

22.10 List employment resources available to employees.

22.11 Describe the process involved in providing employee references.

22.12 Describe the team effort involved in improving quality and managing risk in the medical office.

22.13 Describe incident reporting in the medical office, including staff training on these procedures.

22.14 Discuss the use of personal protective equipment in the medical office.

22.15 Describe the appropriate disposal of hazardous waste.

22.16 Develop employee safety protocol for the medical office.

Key Terminology

adverse outcome—unfavorable treatment result

agenda—list of items to be addressed during a meeting

body language—set of nonverbal actions that communicate what a person is thinking or feeling

chemical waste—wasted drugs, cleaning solutions, germicides

delegate—to assign a task to another individual

Employment Assistance Programs (EAPs)—resources, such as counseling and drug or alcohol rehabilitation, for those in personal crises

infectious waste—any item exposed to bodily fluids or any laboratory cultures or blood products

radioactive waste—any waste contaminated with radioactive material

sentinel event—an occurrence involving death or serious physical or psychological injury, or the risk thereof

sexual harassment—unwanted sexual attention or comments in the workplace

solid waste—paper, cans, cups and other garbage from nonclinical areas

Abbreviations

ADA—Americans with Disabilities Act

ADEA—Age Discrimination in Employment Act

EAP—Employee Assistant Program

EEOC—Equal Employment Opportunity Commission

MSDS—Material Safety Data Sheet

Certification Exam Coverage

AAMA (CMA) Exam Coverage:

- Physical environment
  - Arrangement of furniture, equipment and supplies
  - Facilities and equipment
    1) Maintenance and repair
    2) Safety regulations
       a) Occupational Safety and Health act (OSHA)
       b) Centers for Disease Control and Prevention (CDC) guidelines
       c) Americans with Disabilities Act (ADA)

- Maintaining liability coverage
  - Types of coverage
  - Record keeping

- Time management
  - Establishing priorities
  - Managing routine duties

AMT (CMAS) Exam Coverage:

- Fundamental financial management
  - Understand physician/practice/owner compensation provisions
  - Manage other financial aspects of office management

- Office communications
  - Facilitate staff meetings and in-service, and ensure communication of essential information to staff

- Business organization management
  - Manage medical office business functions
  - Manage office mailing and shipping services

- Manage outside vendors and supplies
- Manage contracts and relationships with associated health care providers
- Comply with licensure and accreditation requirements

- Human Resources*
  - Manage/supervise medical office staff
  - Conduct performance reviews and disciplinary action
  - Manage staff recruiting in compliance with state and federal laws
  - Orient and train new staff
  - Manage employee benefits

- Safety
  - Maintain office safety, maintain office safety manual, and post emergency instructions
  - Observe emergency safety requirements
  - Maintain records of biohazardous waste, hazardous chemicals (Material Safety Data Sheets), and safety conditions
  - Comply with Occupational Safety and Health Act (OSHA) guidelines and regulations

- Physical office plant
  - Maintain office facilities and environment

- Risk management and quality assurance
  - Understand and employ risk management and quality assurance concepts

AAMA (CMA) certification exam topics are reprinted with permission of the American Association of Medical Assistants.

AMT (CMAS) certification exam topics are reprinted with permission of American Medical Technologists.

Note: Asterisked areas addressed by the Medical Office Management job function may or may not be performed by the Certified Medical Administrative Specialist at entry-level practice. Nevertheless, the competent specialist should have sound knowledge of these management functions at certification level.

AMT (RMA) Exam Coverage:
- Interpersonal relations
  - Employer/administration
  - Co-workers
  - Vendors
  - Business associates
  - Observe and respect cultural diversity in the workplace

NCCT (NCMA) Exam Coverage:
- General office procedures
  - Patient instruction
  - Organizational skills

Competency Skills Performance

1. Direct a staff meeting.
2. Write a job description.
3. Conduct an interview.
4. Call employee references.
5. Perform an employee evaluation.
6. Discipline an employee.
7. Terminate an employee.
8. File a medical incident report.
9. Use personal protective equipment.
10. Develop an exposure control plan.
11. Use proper lifting techniques.

Introduction

A skilled office manager is vital to the success of the ambulatory health care office. Often, office managers are medical assistants who prefer to complete administrative tasks, but it is also common to find office managers who lack clinical training. Sometimes, physicians act as their own office managers, but such arrangements fail to use physicians' time most efficiently. In some offices, clinical office managers direct the clinical portions while administrative office managers oversee administrative duties. Whatever the arrangement, as office leader, the office manager oversees and facilitates all office activities.

Characteristics of the Medical Office Manager

Successful office managers know that being a leader involves more than simply telling others what to do. Good leaders lead by example and encourage those they manage to do the best jobs they can do.

As office lead, the medical office manager must be able to multitask, which means being able to manage several people as well as several projects at the same time. Office managers must have excellent communication skills and the ability to project confidence. The following is a list of the traits office managers must possess:

- Excellent organizational skills
- Flexibility
- Patience
- Honesty
- Excellent communication skills
- Good listening skills
- Ability to resolve conflict
- Support for all office personnel

Responsibilities of the Office Manager

The office manager may be called on to handle any number of situations in the medical office. Unresolvable disputes between staff are just one example. When such a dispute arises, the office manager must remain objective and fair and listen to both parties in an attempt to reach a mutual and fair solution. Office managers may also be called upon to address patient complaints. To address complaints in a fair and timely fashion, the office manager needs top-notch communication skills.

In general, the medical office manager must be able to **delegate** as well as oversee tasks. One person alone cannot complete all tasks in a busy medical practice, so knowing how and to whom to hand off tasks is a sign of true efficiency. The following is a list of some of the many responsibilities that are typically given to the medical office manager and that are discussed in this chapter. These duties will vary depending upon the type and size of practice.

- Conducting effective staff meetings
- Staffing the medical office
- Scheduling staff
- Conducting performance evaluations
- Disciplining and terminating staff
- Addressing sexual harassment in the medical office

AMT (RMA) certification exam topics are reprinted with permission of American Medical Technologists.

NCCT (NCMA) certification exam topics © 2013 National Center for Competency Testing. Reprinted with permission of NCCT.

- Providing employees with employment resources
- Providing employee references
- Improving quality and managing risks in the medical office
- Ensuring the proper use of protective equipment and the proper disposal of hazardous waste in the medical office
- Ensuring employee safety

In Practice

Carrie is an administrative medical assistant working the medical office's reception desk. Mrs. Carnes enters the office and begins to loudly complain about a bill she has received. She demands that Carrie explain why the bill is so high. During the exchange, several other patients in the reception room watch Carrie for her reaction. What should Carrie do to defuse this scene?

Leadership Styles

Leadership takes one of six basic styles. Managers generally tailor their leadership style to the situation at hand.

- **Autocratic style**—The leader makes all decisions without seeking input. This style works best in emergencies, when orders must be given quickly and followed exactly.
- **Democratic style**—The leader tends to ask for opinions and/or advice before making decisions and may seek consensus or retain sole decision-making authority.
- **Laissez-faire style**—The leader tends to allow others to make their own decisions, becoming involved only when absolutely needed.
- **Pacesetting style**—The leader expects and models excellent work ethics and self-direction. The leader sets the pace of the work, by demonstrating the pace desired.
- **Coaching style**—The leader takes the time to allow employees to think up solutions on their own, then guides them in learning the best processes. This style is used when the manager wishes to build up the skill set of an employee, perhaps with the idea that the employee will one day be a leader himself.
- **Coercive style**—The leader encourages employees by manipulating them into doing what the leader wants done. This style works best with employees who do not speak up for themselves and prefer to go along with the direction of the leader.

It is important for medical office managers to adopt different leadership styles in response to varying situations.

Constant use of the autocratic leading style, for example, may inspire staff to resign or resist making decisions on their own. The laissez-faire style, in contrast, may disorganize the office when used all the time. The ability to balance all these styles is critical to addressing issues on a case-by-case basis.

Critical Thinking Question 22-1

Refer back to the case study presented at the beginning of this chapter. As the office manager, how should Juanita address Dr. Whittier's tardiness?

Conducting Effective Staff Meetings

Staff meetings should be scheduled regularly in the medical office (**Figure 22-1** ■). During the business day, staff are often too busy to communicate with each other effectively, and miscommunication and errors can result. Regular staff meetings with all staff present can help keep the lines of communication open between coworkers. When staff meetings are scheduled outside normal office hours or during lunch times, all in attendance must be compensated. This communicates to staff that the meetings, and their time, are both valuable to the office—and paying staff for the time spent working is mandated by law.

Typically, office managers or physicians lead staff meetings. Some offices find that alternating the staff meeting leader encourages full staff participation, confirms that all staff are members of the health care team, and underscores that each staff member's participation is valuable.

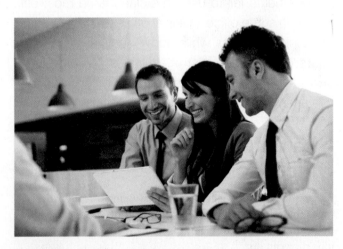

Figure 22-1 ■ Staff meetings should be scheduled regularly in the medical office.
Source: Fotolia © Bartłomiej Szewczyk.

Referring to the case study at the beginning of the chapter, how could Juanita use a staff meeting to address the issue of Dr. Whittier's tardiness?

Robert's Rules of Order

Robert's Rules of Order is a book intended for groups wishing to follow parliamentary procedure for meetings. Originally published in 1876, this book is now in its 11th edition. The purpose of *Robert's Rules of Order* is to maintain control of the meeting and to allow for debate, with each person speaking the same language in terms of how the meeting is run. The use of this process allows for a constructive meeting, with each member encouraged to participate.

Creating Staff Meeting Agendas

To be maximally effective, a staff meeting should have a clear start and end time and follow a well-organized **agenda** that staff receives before the meetings commences. The following are examples of items that might appear on a staff meeting agenda:

- Report on activities or projects since the last staff meeting
- Report on upcoming activities or projects
- Review of schedules for the upcoming week/month
- Review of any concerns from staff

Staff-meeting agendas notify attendees of discussion topics so those attendees can come prepared to participate. For each item on the agenda, a designated amount of time should be determined (**Figure 22-2 ■**). Following the scheduled agenda is easier to do when the amount of time allocated to each item is listed ahead of time. Generally, meeting leaders prepare agendas, which should be followed as strictly as possible to honor time and other commitments.

Part of many staff meetings is the ability for each staff member to bring up issues or announcements that they feel the group would be interested in knowing about or addressing.

Occasionally, attendees raise topics not on the agenda. When this occurs, the staff-meeting leader should determine whether there is time to discuss the topic. If not, the topic should be deferred to the next staff meeting and listed on the next agenda. One method of working through issues as a group is to use a process called *brainstorming*. This is a process where each member of the team should feel comfortable commenting on the issue at hand. For example, if the issue of how to best market a new provider to the clinic were raised, members of the team might each mention their ideas, without worrying that the idea hasn't been thoroughly thought through beforehand. Ideas that are found to have good potential may be discussed further, or added to another meeting agenda.

Staff Meeting Minutes

Staff-meeting minutes serve as a written account of meeting discussions. Such accounts are important for several reasons. First, staff members who cannot attend can review them and catch up on missed material. Second, minutes are written accounts that cannot easily be misinterpreted or forgotten. Finally, staff can use meeting minutes as a reference when composing the agenda for subsequent meetings. The following items should appear in staff-meeting minutes:

- List of all staff members at the meeting
- List of all staff members absent from the meeting
- Date and times the meeting began and ended
- Brief description of each discussed item
- Brief description of any action taken at the meeting, including any staff member assignments
- List of any items to be deferred to the next staff meeting
- Signature of the person taking the minutes

A person other than the staff-meeting leader should record the meeting's minutes. Staff should take turns assuming recording duties to encourage full team participation, just as they take turns leading the staff meeting. Whoever records a meeting's minutes should type and distribute those minutes to all staff, including those not in attendance. A copy should also appear in the office notebook as documentation of the meeting's events.

March 16, 20xx
10:00 a.m.

- Report on activities or projects since the last staff meeting – 10 minutes
- Report on upcoming activities or projects – 15 minutes
- Review schedules for the upcoming months – 10 minutes
- Review any concerns from staff – 25 minutes

Figure 22-2 ■ Sample staff meeting agenda.

Refer to the case study at the beginning of the chapter. Imagine that the chronically late physician, Dr. Whittier, fails to attend the staff meeting at which the issue is addressed. How should Juanita inform him of the staff meeting's discussion?

PROCEDURE 22-1 Direct a Staff Meeting

Theory and Rationale

The office manager is often responsible for directing the medical office staff meeting. The office manager should project authority while including all staff.

Materials

- Blue or black pen
- Paper
- Clock or watch to keep time
- Staff meeting agenda

Competency

1. Before the staff meeting, create an agenda of the meeting's discussion topics.

2. Start the meeting on time.
3. Note which staff are in attendance and which are absent.
4. Discuss the agenda items one at a time, being mindful of the time.
5. When non-agenda items arise, determine if they should be included in this meeting or moved to the next.
6. Address any issues or concerns that arise.
7. End the meeting at the prearranged time.

Staffing the Medical Office

One of the most important parts of the office manager's job is staffing the medical office. Staffing involves discussing staffing needs with physicians, writing job descriptions and the employee handbook, recruiting and interviewing candidates, evaluating employees' performances, scheduling staff shifts, and handling any disciplinary or termination actions.

Writing Job Descriptions

Every position in the medical office must have a clear and concise description. A job description outlines the duties and expectations of a position and helps the office manager both interview potential employees and evaluate existing ones. Every job description should include the following items:

- Title of the job
- Name of the supervisor for this position
- Summary of the positions duties
- Required hours for the position
- Position's location, when the business has multiple locations
- Any employment requirements (e.g., cardiopulmonary [CPR] certification or malpractice insurance)
- Any physical requirements (e.g., lifting, standing, sitting, or walking)
- Summary of the office's evaluation process

The job-description format may vary from office to office, but within an office, that format should be consistent. **Figure 22-3** ■ shows a sample job description.

Creating Job Advertisements

Attracting and hiring the best employees starts with placing an effective advertisement for the job. To be effective, a job ad need not include in-depth information about the position. Instead, it should list a handful of the duties required, as well as any certification or experience stipulations. While many employers add terms like "friendly," "team player," and "professional" to their ads, these are characteristics to be uncovered in interviews, not necessarily items that should appear in the job ad. **Figure 22-4** ■ is an example of an effective job placement ad.

Recruiting and Interviewing Candidates

Medical offices can recruit new employees in various ways, but the most common is through local employment offices, private job-listing agencies, and local newspapers. Many medical offices post openings with local colleges, especially those with accredited medical assisting programs. Today, most medical offices have a Web site, and it is the most common avenue employers take to find new employees, as job placement ads may be posted at no additional cost to the employer. Potential employees in the area who desire to work for a particular medical office may look to the office's Web site for employment opportunities. When an office posts a job placement advertisement on its own Web site, candidates can often apply online, through the Web site interface.

To collect applications from candidates, offices might ask applicants to mail or fax their résumé or submit their application online. Once offices receive applications and resumes, office managers can review them for suitability. Typically, managers will discard any applicants who fail to meet the qualifications. Because résumés and applications reflect the candidates who submit them, office managers also often discard any applications with poor grammar or typographical errors.

Once the office manager has identified a pool of potential candidates, she will schedule those applicants for in-person

Administrative Medical Assistant Job Description

Administrative Duties

❑ Answers telephone calls and assesses urgency of call.
  • Provides assistance or directs caller to appropriate person, contacting physician/nurse directly for urgent needs.
  • Provides assistance to other receptionists in screening patient calls.
❑ Provides specialized information related to section, policies, procedures, insurance and services.
  • Assists patients with the completion of forms.
  • Builds monthly provider master schedules and clinic calendars from established sources and verifies provider sessions worked. Modifies master schedules to accommodate time off, extra patients, hospital emergencies, etc.
  • Creates patient bump lists as necessary due to last-minute provider callouts.
  • Schedules patient appointments and resolves scheduling conflicts.
  • Notifies patients of changes/cancellations and prioritizes urgency of appointments for rescheduling.
  • Receives patients and visitors. Secures names and needs and directs accordingly.
  • Updates patient information and verifies insurance information, level of services, and tracks referrals when necessary.
  • Initiates billing process by completing patient encounter forms and accepts and processes fee-for-service payments.
  • Books diagnostic tests and specialized appointments for patients at hospitals and other medical facilities and ensures that patients are provided with necessary paperwork and specialized instructions for procedures.
  • Schedules surgical procedures for patients. Coordinates available dates for surgery and scheduling of pre- and post-operative exams and lab work.
  • Obtains and distributes necessary paperwork and maintains system to track completion.
  • Coordinates surgery schedule changes as necessary.
  • Schedules and coordinates departmental meetings, classes, clinics, conferences, etc.
  • Utilizes computer input and retrieves data. Merges and manipulates data to generate complex reports. Compiles and maintains clinical and patient statistical data and produces summaries and reports.
  • Keyboards correspondence, clinical information, reports, publicity material, educational handouts, etc. Composes general written material.
  • Obtains patient charts, medical records, and lab reports, and verifies for completeness.
  • Sorts, screens, and distributes incoming mail. Prioritizes and ensures completion of medical forms by clinical staff.
  • Establishes and maintains filing systems.
  • Maintains inventory of administrative office supplies and educational material
  • Ensures adequate coverage of reception desk.

Figure 22-3 ■ Sample job description.

Certified or registered medical assistant wanted full time in busy pediatrics office. Two-plus years experience working with children and current CMA (AAMA) or RMA (AMT) certification required. Position includes clinical and administrative duties, as well as laboratory skills. Please e-mail resume to srangel@monroefp.com.

Figure 22-4 ■ Sample job placement ad.

interviews. Because first impressions are important, the office manager uses the interview to assess an applicant's appearance and confidence as well as his professional qualifications. To remain consistent from candidate to candidate, the manager should use a preprinted list of questions and tailor any other questions as needed. The following are some common questions to ask a job candidate:

● Why do you want to work in this office?
● Do you have the skills needed to perform this job?
● Why did you leave your last position?
● How do you respond to pressure?
● What is your desired salary?

PROCEDURE 22-2 Write a Job Description

Theory and Rationale

The medical office manager must compose a job description for every position in the medical office. To avoid confusion between employer and employee, these descriptions must be accurate and thorough.

Materials

- Computer with word-processing software
- List of skills needed for the position
- List of duties required for the position

Competency

1. Create a title for the job position.
2. List the name of the supervisor for the position.

3. Create a summary description of the position's duties.
4. List the hours required of the position.
5. List the location of the position, when it varies.
6. List any employment requirements (e.g., certification, malpractice insurance).
7. List any physical requirements for the position (e.g., lifting, excessive sitting or standing).
8. Describe the evaluation process for the position.
9. Review the job description for accuracy, as well as with the physician if needed.

Because office managers often interview multiple applicants for a position, they should take notes during each interview. In addition to observing the applicant's clothing and appearance, the manager should capture the applicant's responses and his positive or negative behaviors.

Avoiding Illegal Interview Questions

As the party in charge of employment practices, the office manager must know state and federal laws regulating employees, among them Title VII of the Civil Rights Act, the Americans with Disabilities Act (**ADA**), and the Age Discrimination in Employment Act (**ADEA**). According to agencies like the U.S. Equal Employment Opportunity Commission (**EEOC**), which enforces many similar laws, employers may not discriminate in their hiring, promotion, pay, benefits, retirement plan, discipline, or firing practices. Questions that address employee safety or suitability, however, are appropriate in interviews. For example, when a position will expose a candidate to medications that are hazardous to an unborn fetus, the employer may ask a female candidate about pregnancy. The following are questions to avoid in interviews:

- What is your race or ethnic background?
- What country are you from?
- What is/are your religion/religious beliefs?
- What is your gender?
- How old are you?
- Do you have any disabilities (*Note:* Disabilities prohibiting job performance are legally addressed.)
- What is your marital status?
- What political party do you belong to, or What are your political beliefs?

- What is your sexual orientation?
- Are you pregnant or thinking of becoming pregnant? (*Note:* This question may be asked if the employee will be exposed to chemicals hazardous to an unborn child.)

Calling for Employment References

Employee references, like employee credentials, are critical tools in the staffing process. During the interview, the office manager should ask whether she may call the applicant's previous employers for references. Reference information usually appears on an applicant's résumé or application, but when it does not, the manager should ask the applicant to supply the information. An applicant who resists such a request might be hiding negative information about previous employment.

▸▸ Pulse Points

Checking Credentials

Before an applicant is offered a position in the medical office, the office manager must check the applicant's credentials by calling state licensing agencies or certification registries. For example, certified medical assistant (CMA) (AAMA) certification status can be verified by calling (800) ACT-AAMA. Simply asking a prospective employee to provide certification information fails to suffice, because some applicants might be dishonest.

Open-ended questions, not those answered with just "yes" or "no," are appropriate when calling for employment references, because they tend to provide more useful information.

PROCEDURE 22-3 Conduct an Interview

Theory and Rationale

Medical office managers are typically responsible for interviewing prospective employees. Those managers must do so legally and with the aim of finding the best candidates.

Materials

- Pen
- Applicant's resume

Competency

1. Before meeting the applicant, read the résumé.
2. Highlight any areas of concern or interest on the résumé.
3. Highlight résumé items such as experience that apply to the position being filled.
4. Greet the applicant while making direct eye contact.

5. Use a firm handshake with the applicant.
6. Lead the applicant to a private room.
7. Show the applicant where to sit for the interview.
8. Ask the applicant about the potential to perform the job.
9. Review any areas of concern highlighted on the résumé.
10. Review the job description
11. Verify the applicant's ability to perform the required tasks.
12. Ask the applicant if he or she has any questions about the office or physicians.
13. Take note of any pertinent information.
14. Provide a decision date for the position.
15. Thank the applicant, and escort the applicant out of the office.

For example, an office manager might ask the former employer to describe the applicant's work habits rather than simply asking whether the applicant worked for the organization. Behavioral-based questioning is often used in interviewing potential staff today. These questions ask the candidate to describe a situation or event when a particular trait or skill was needed. An example of a behavioral-based question would be, "Tell me about a time when you were involved with a team to work on a project." The idea behind behavioral-based interviewing is that the employer will learn how the candidate reacted in a particular situation or environment, which may give insight into how that candidate would perform in the office setting, if hired.

 ## Pulse Points

Calling the Employee's Current Employer

Some applicants are employed when they interview for a new position and do not notify their current employer of their plan to work elsewhere. As a result, office managers should not call an applicant's current employer unless the applicant states that doing so is acceptable. A candidate should offer to have the current employer called for a reference, in the event that candidate becomes a final candidate for the position.

PROCEDURE 22-4 Call Employee References

Theory and Rationale

The medical office manager may uncover useful information from an applicant's former employer. The key is to ask the correct questions about the employee's history with his or her previous employer.

Materials

- Telephone
- Employee résumé
- Pen

Competency

1. Call the applicant's previous employer.
2. Ask to speak with the office manager or supervisor.

3. Identify yourself and give the reason for your call.
4. Ask the previous employer open-ended questions about the employee.
5. Ask the previous employer if the employee would be eligible for rehire.
6. Ask specifics as to the employee's job duties and job performance.
7. Ask the previous employer for any other relevant information.
8. Note all of the previous employer's statements.
9. Thank the previous employer.

TABLE OF CONTENTS

Figure 22-5 ■ Sample employee handbook Table of Contents.

Hiring New Staff

Once new staff has been hired, the office manager should create an employee file for the new hire. This file, which must be kept strictly confidential, will house the employee's evaluations and other work-related documentation. When a new staff member arrives for work, she should be given a copy of the office's employee handbook or policy manual. This book should outline all office policies, including those for benefits, dress code, and disciplinary action. The contents of the employee handbook should list the topics contained within (**Figure 22-5** ■).

Many offices require new employees to sign a form stating they have received a copy of their office's policies and that they agree to abide by those policies. Medical offices also often run criminal background checks on new staff and require those staff to undergo drug testing. For drug testing to occur, an applicant must sign a consent form (**Figure 22-6** ■).

Training New Staff

As a lead employee in the medical office, the office manager may be charged with overseeing new staff training. While another staff member typically completes the training, the office manager must ensure that the training has been completed and that the new staff member is clear about employment expectations. A detailed, up-to-date office policy manual facilitates such training.

Supervising Staff

Well-trained employees who clearly understand expectations ease the office manager's task of office supervision. Depending

I, a current employee of The Marysville Clinic ("the Company"), understand that the use of drugs, alcohol, and other controlled substances by employees creates a dangerous work environment. In consideration for my desire for a safe work environment, I give my consent for the Company to conduct the drug tests it considers necessary as outlined in its Drug Test policy. I hereby allow the Company to take the necessary specimens from me to test for any controlled substance, and I authorize the laboratory or medical personnel retained by the Company for these tests to release the results to the Company for whatever use the Company deems appropriate. Further, I release the laboratory or medical personnel conducting the drug test, the Company, and the Company's employees, directors, officers, and successors from any liabilities, claims, and causes of action, known or unknown, contingent or fixed, that may result from this drug test. I agree not to file any lawsuit or other action to assert a claim.

I have read and understood this agreement, and I sign this without any coercion or duress by any individual or institution.

Print Name	Signature	Date

Figure 22-6 ■ Sample consent form for drug testing.

on their work styles and personalities, staff require varying amounts of the manager's time in this arena. Some employees work well with little supervision; others require more oversight. The office manager must determine the best supervision method for each office employee.

Overcoming Scheduling Issues

The office manager must create and adhere to a fair policy to ensure that staff are scheduled properly and patient and physician needs are met. When an employee approaches the office manager with a request for a schedule change, the manager must balance the needs of all employees when honoring such a request. To avoid miscommunication, employees should submit their time-off requests in writing within a certain time frame, such as at least two weeks prior to the time requested off. **Figure 22-7** ■ is a sample form for this task.

Performance Evaluations

To monitor an employee's job performance and help the employee improve as needed, the office manager should evaluate the employee yearly. Yearly evaluations help keep employees apprised of job expectations, and help to build and maintain confidence and morale; the employee's salary should also be reviewed.

New employees should be evaluated frequently in their first year, perhaps at 30, 60, and 90 days, and then again on their one-year anniversary. Evaluations should be a positive experience for the employee, not simply a forum for raising

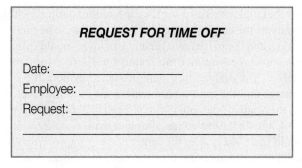

REQUEST FOR TIME OFF

Date: _____

Employee: _____

Request: _____

_____

Figure 22-7 ■ Time off request.

new problems or issues. Well-managed offices bring an issue to the employee's attention as soon as possible after the issue arises. The evaluation is not the place for an employee to hear about a new issue—whether good or bad. The evaluation is a time to review the employee's performance over a period of time.

To lay the groundwork for an evaluation, the office should give employees self-evaluation forms to complete before their evaluations occur. Correspondingly, office managers should prepare written evaluations and distribute copies to employees. Originals should reside in employees' files. Once evaluation meetings take place, office managers and employees should review the evaluations and discuss any areas of concern.

Typically, an employee evaluation includes an assessment of the employee's performance in his position in the office, including any attendance or tardiness issues that might have arisen since the last evaluation. The evaluation should include going over the employee's job description and an analysis of

 PROCEDURE 22-5 Perform an Employee Evaluation

Theory and Rationale

The medical office manager must evaluate all office employees at least once per year. Typically, evaluations fall on or near the anniversary of the employee's date of hire.

Materials

- Employee evaluation form
- Pen

Competency

1. Before the evaluation meeting, ask the employee to complete a self-evaluation form on job performance. Be sure to include job performance goals for the next year.
2. Meet with the employee at a prearranged time and in a private room.

3. Compare the employee's self-evaluation form with your evaluation.
4. Address any discrepancies between the two evaluations.
5. Address any areas of concern in performance or behavior.
6. Review the goals of the last evaluation and discuss progress toward those goals.
7. Review the goals set for the next evaluation, and set timelines as needed.
8. Discuss any pay raise associated with the employee's performance.
9. Have the employee sign the employee evaluation.
10. Place the evaluation in the employee's personnel file.
11. Raise any concerns about the performance evaluation with the physician.

how the employee is meeting the expectations outlined within. Any items the employee needs to work on should be noted in writing, and the office manager and employee should come up with an agreed-upon time frame for those issues to be resolved. The evaluation should be signed by both the office manager and the employee; a copy is given to the employee and the original goes into the employee's file. If any issues were brought up in the evaluation, the office manager and employee should meet again after the target date for improvement has passed in order to review the progress that has been made.

Disciplining and Terminating Staff

Employee handbooks should clearly identify situations mandating employee discipline. For example, patient or coworker abuse, or use of an illegal substance may be cause for immediate termination. Excessive tardiness or poor job performance, in contrast, may be cause for discipline or termination.

When staff must be disciplined, the office manager should act as soon as possible. Delays may be viewed as endorsements of unacceptable behavior, not only by the employee committing the infraction, but by the rest of the staff. Employee morale could plummet as a result. Before disciplining an employee, the office manager should gather all facts relevant to the case. When an employee has been excessively tardy, for example, the office manager should list all the dates the employee has been late, in addition to documentation of any other conversations the manager has had with the employee about tardiness.

Meetings on disciplinary issues should occur in private, and the office manager should remain professional and calm. A first offense may comprise a verbal warning that should be noted in the employee file. Serious infractions, like breaching patient confidentiality, require a written warning that outlines the offense and the action the offending employee must take (**Figure 22-8** ■). Employees should sign any written warning and receive a copy. Originals should reside in the employee file.

To prepare for the often difficult task of terminating an employee, an office manager should keep a clear timeline in the employee's file of warnings that were given and disciplinary actions that were taken. These types of documents, like clear office policies, both ease the difficult event and help safeguard the office from a wrongful termination lawsuit.

When an employee is terminated, her or she should be taken to a private location and advised of the reasons. The manager should regain all keys and other items owned by the office, and should escort the employee while he or she obtains any personal items in the office. When all property has been properly returned, the manager should escort the employee from the building. To ensure the privacy of the employee, the manager should not discuss the termination with other members of the staff.

Sexual Harassment in the Medical Office

Title VII of the Civil Rights Act protects employees against sexual harassment. **Sexual harassment** is legally defined as unwanted sexual advances, requests for sexual favors, and other verbal or physical conduct of a sexual nature, whether intentional or unintentional where:

- An individual's employment hinges upon participating in the sexual activity
- The conduct of an individual causes a hostile, humiliating, or offensive work environment for another individual

Sexual harassment is illegal in all workplaces and the medical office is no exception. In order for the conduct to be considered sexual harassment, it must be unwelcome. While there are many examples of conduct that could be construed as sexual harassment, examples include:

- Unwelcome sexual advances, including gestures, whistling, or comments
- Sexual jokes, either written or spoken
- Gossip regarding an individual's sex life
- Comments about an individual's body
- Displaying sexually explicit photographs, objects, or cartoons
- Questions about an individual's sexual experiences or activities

If an employee feels he or she has been sexually harassed, he or she must bring the problem to the attention of the office manager or supervisor. The office manager or supervisor must then take immediate action to investigate the claim and take proper action by educating, disciplining, or even terminating the offender. If, after receiving a complaint and verifying the validity of the complaint, the office manager or supervisor does not take action, the complaining employee may then file a lawsuit against the employer for allowing a hostile work environment to continue.

Employment Resources

Employment Assistance Programs (**EAPs**) are resources for people in personal crisis, such as counseling and drug or alcohol rehabilitation; EAPs are common in large medical offices and hospitals. Available resources should be outlined in office policies, and office managers should keep a list of resources as added reference. While any referral should appear in an employee's personnel file, all such information must be kept confidential.

Employee assistance programs often include resources for the following:

- Domestic violence
- Divorce/separation

Date: June 21, 20xx

Employee: Sara Brown

Infraction: On the following dates, the employee was more than 10 minutes late for her shift:

    5/21/20xx

    5/25/20xx

    6/10/20xx

    6/19/20xx

According to office policy regarding tardiness, any employee who is late four or more times in a month will incur disciplinary action in the form of a written warning. If, after this initial warning, the employee is more than 10 minutes late for a shift in the next 2 weeks, the employee will experience a second disciplinary action of a 1-week, nonpaid employment suspension.

Signature of Employee _____ Date_____

Signature of Office Manager_____ Date_____

Figure 22-8 ◾ Sample warning of disciplinary action.

- Substance abuse
- Workplace violence
- Handling traumatic events
- Sexual assault or violence
- Emotional distress
- Financial concerns
- Concerns about raising children or caring for aging parents

Providing Employee References

When a staff member leaves the office's employ, the office manager might receive a request for a reference from a potential new employer. For legal reasons, the office must follow strict, consistent policies in this arena. For example, an office manager must give a reference for all employees, not just a

PROCEDURE 22-6 Discipline an Employee

Theory and Rationale

The medical office manager must adhere to office policies for staff discipline. Staff discipline must be done in a private location, and copies of all documents must be signed by the employee and the office manager and placed in the employee's permanent file.

Materials

- Pen
- Paper

Competency

1. Verify all facts before meeting with the employee.
2. Write a disciplinary notice that contains the reason for the discipline and the action to be taken by the office and/or by the employee as a result.
3. Request a meeting with the employee.

4. Hold the meeting in a private room.
5. Let the employee know the reason for the meeting.
6. Discuss the disciplinary action being levied on the employee.
7. Discuss your expectations of the employee.
8. Discuss the outcome if the employee's behavior does not change.
9. Ask the employee to sign the disciplinary statement.
10. If the employee refuses to sign the statement, make a note on the statement of "Contents reviewed with employee. Employee refused to sign." Affix your signature and date the document.
11. Place the statement in the employee's personnel record.
12. Agree to a future date on which you will meet with the employee to discuss progress.
13. Inform the physician of the meeting's outcome.

PROCEDURE 22-7 Terminate an Employee

Theory and Rationale

While employee termination is generally difficult, the office manager is obligated to undertake the task professionally, respectfully, and legally.

Materials

- Pen
- Paper

Competency

1. Take the employee to a private room.
2. Discuss the reason for termination.

3. Ask the employee to return any office items, such as keys or identification badges.
4. Escort the employee to the workstation to collect personal belongings.
5. Escort the employee from the building.
6. If the employee is loud or abusive, ask the employee to leave immediately and inform the employee that personal belongings will be sent.
7. Note the meeting's outcome in the employee's personnel file.
8. Notify the physician of the meeting's outcome.

select few, and must share facts only, not speculation or opinions. Office policy should dictate what information is to be given to potential employers.

References might include only the dates employees worked in the office, the employee's job title, and any provable information in the employee's file. Managers can share when former employees have stolen, for example, but only when such events have been proven. Inaccurate information can damage a former employee and subject the office to a lawsuit. Similarly, a positive reference for an undeserving employee is grounds for legal action if a potential employer hires an employee with a proven record of stealing from the office and the office manager did not disclose that information when called for a reference.

Improving Quality and Managing Risk in the Medical Office

As health care consumers, patients face a wide array of choices. As in all other businesses, quality customer service is crucial to the success of a medical office. Patients who are treated respectfully and equitably communicate positive information about the office and will likely stay with those offices long term. Research has shown that patients rate their health care higher simply because they felt staff cared about them and took the time to listen to their concerns. Improving quality in the medical office includes looking for ways to improve the patient's experience in the medical office. This includes making sure patients do not wait for long periods for their appointment, explaining charges to patients before a service is performed, and maintaining patient confidentiality in all aspects of patient care.

Critical Thinking Question 22-4

Referring back to the case study at the beginning of the chapter, how could Juanita communicate to the chronically tardy physician the potential impact of his actions on patient care?

Creating a Quality Improvement Program

Quality improvement programs that focus on patients' emotional and physical health are vital to the success of any health care practice. Such programs should be implemented whenever health care employees notice areas or situations that, when improved, would raise patient satisfaction or safety. When staff members notice broken chairs or hallway carpet that has begun to unravel, they should raise the possible safety hazard with the appropriate parties. The following is a list of other issues for quality improvement review:

- Patient wait times
- Insurance company rejections of certain services or procedures
- Equipment needs
- Health Insurance Portability and Accountability Act (HIPAA) violations
- Collection practices
- Office remodeling
- Patient flow in the office
- Office waste
- Staffing
- Personal use of office telephones or computers

Health care staff should work as a team to solve problems immediately through quality improvement programs, which can be very simple. One common office problem is patient wait time. When offices receive complaints about patient wait times, those offices should mobilize teams quickly to solve the problem by studying appointment times or discussing outcomes with physicians. When long patient wait times are allowed to continue, patients may seek care elsewhere.

Working to Ensure Patient Safety

Medical errors are the fourth leading cause of death in the United States with four times as many errors happening in the ambulatory care setting than in the hospital setting, adjusting for the volume of patients seen. Every member of the health care team is responsible for patient safety, which means medical assistants should speak up when they see potential risk factors. For example, when a physician orders medications that the medical assistant believes to be incorrect, the assistant is responsible for clarifying the medication order before the medication is administered. This should be done only outside of the patient's hearing range.

Patient trust is a vital stepping-stone to patient safety. Patients who trust their health care providers become partners in their own safety. To participate in the patient partnership, medical assistants should listen to patients' questions and learn to recognize the **body language** that alerts them to a patient's unspoken messages. To make this task easier, the assistant should sit next to the patient or his family, whenever appropriate (**Figure 22-9** ■), and try to anticipate the patient's questions. As much as possible, assistants should provide the

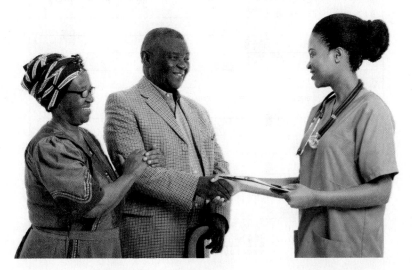

Figure 22-9 ■ The medical assistant should be ready to speak to the patient's family, if necessary.
Source: Fotolia © Michael Jung.

answers to commonly asked questions. It is also helpful for assistants to use touch appropriately to show concern and to speak in a patient's native language when possible, or to arrange for an interpreter if needed. To ensure communication is understood, the medical assistant should ask the patient and his family to repeat the discussion in his own words. Respecting the patient's decision and maintaining the patient's confidence is part of advocating for patients in health care.

Reporting Office Incidents

Occasionally, **adverse outcomes**, which are events that were unexpected or that are the result of an error on the part of one or more persons on the health care team, occur in the medical office. Occurrences involving death or serious physical or psychological injury, or risk thereof, are called **sentinel events**. The Joint Commission (TJC) describes sentinel events as ones in which injuries occurred, or could have occurred, in a medical setting. The following are possible sentinel events that might be encountered in ambulatory care:

- Incorrect medication administration
- A patient fall in the office
- Missing prescription pads or medications
- Incorrect or absent patient instructions following procedures
- Needle stick injuries to staff
- Inappropriate handling of patient laboratory supplies

When sentinel events occur, the medical office must document and report those events properly, not to blame or punish employees but to aid in prevention. Offices that strive to use errors as learning experiences rather than punishment tools promote a culture in which employees feel safe enough to self-report errors.

To report sentinel events, every office should fully complete sentinel reporting forms or incident report forms, using word processing software or blue or black ink (**Figure 22-10** ■). No areas should remain blank. When an area on the form does not apply, the medical assistant should enter "Not Applicable" or "NA." While sentinel reports should reside in a master

INCIDENT REPORT

Name of injured party _____ Date _____

Address _____ Telephone _____

_____

The injured party was: ☐ Employee   ☐ Patient   ☐ Other _____

Date of accident/incident _____   Time of incident _____

Where did incident occur? _____

Names of witnesses (include titles):

_____   _____

_____   _____

What first aid/treatment was given at the time of the incident?

_____

_____

Who administered first aid? _____

Briefly describe the incident. _____

_____

_____

_____

_____

Names of employees present at time of incident/injury:

_____

_____

Follow-up: What steps have been taken to prevent a similar accident? _____

_____

_____

_____

Date _____   Employee's signature _____

Date _____   Supervisor's signature _____

Figure 22-10 ■ Sample incident report.

PROCEDURE 22-8 File a Medical Incident Report

Theory and Rationale

In the medical office, staff members must file reports for incidents in which patients or employees are injured or could have been injured. Medical facilities that are TJC-certified are required to file incident reports. Medical clinics that are not TJC-certified may be required to do so by the department of health in the state where the practice is located.

Materials

- Incident report form
- Black or blue ink pen
- Patient's chart

Competency

1. Complete all areas of the incident report form using only facts, not opinions or judgments. For inapplicable areas, enter "NA" or "Not applicable."
2. Sign and date the form.
3. Give the form to the office manager or office director.
4. Participate in any educational meetings to determine how similar events could be avoided.

---

incidents report file, copies should not appear in an employee's file or in a patient's medical record, nor should copies leave the medical office.

In Practice

Martika is a medical assistant in a busy office. On her second day on the job, she slips in some liquid spilled on the floor on her way to the lab. She lands on her back and needs a few moments to catch her breath before rising. Another medical assistant enters the lab just as Martika is getting to her feet. After Martika recounts the events, the medical assistant tells her she must complete an incident report. Martika responds that she believes doing so will jeopardize her new job. What should the second medical assistant do?

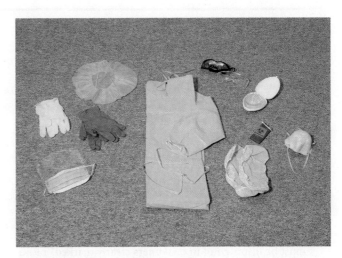

Figure 22-11 ■ Sample protective equipment found in the medical office.

Using Protective Equipment

Most medical offices perform procedures that require staff to use or wear personal protective equipment (**Figure 22-11** ■). For example, whenever health care employees may be exposed to a patient's bodily fluids, those employees must don gloves and possibly eye shields. Employees who X-ray patients must wear radiation badges to assess their possible X-ray exposure (**Figure 22-12** ■). Employers must supply any needed protective equipment, and clean and dispose of it per OSHA regulations.

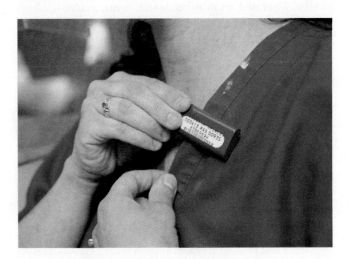

Figure 22-12 ■ Radiation exposure badge.

PROCEDURE 22-9 Use Personal Protective Equipment

Theory and Rationale

Any employee asked to perform a task that might involve contact with a dangerous material must be given the proper personal protective equipment, as well as instructions on the equipment's proper use.

Materials

- Latex or non-latex gloves

Competency

1. Wash hands.
2. Holding the rim of the left glove with the right hand, pull on the left glove.
3. Holding the rim of the right glove with the left hand, pull on the right glove.

4. Smooth both gloves onto the hands.
5. If, after application, the glove rips or is found to be defective, discard the glove and don a new pair. Gloves begin to deteriorate after 15 minutes.
6. To remove the gloves, with the right hand pinch the center of the left glove and pull off the left glove.
7. Hold the left glove in the right hand.
8. With the exposed left hand, cautiously place the first two fingers of the left hand under the rim of the right glove.
9. Push the right glove off over the left glove, turning the right glove inside out.
10. Place the removed gloves in the proper disposal container.
11. Wash hands.

Disposing of Hazardous Waste

Each year, health care facilities create 3.2 million tons of hazardous waste in the four following categories:

- **Solid**—paper, cans, cups, and other garbage from non-clinical office areas.
- **Chemical**—wasted drugs, cleaning solutions, and germicides. These items must be disposed of according to Occupational Safety and Health Association (OSHA) guidelines.
- **Radioactive**—any waste contaminated with radioactive material. Most common in oncology practices, this waste must be disposed of in containers clearly marked "radioactive" and removed only by licensed facilities.
- **Infectious**—any garbage exposed to bodily fluids or any laboratory cultures or blood products. These items must be separated from other waste items, placed in bags clearly labeled as biohazardous waste, and removed by a licensed medical waste removal company.

Though some hazardous waste may be disposed of through local garbage services, all must be disposed of according to federal and local law. On a federal level, medical offices must abide by OSHA guidelines in disposing of hazardous medical waste. These rules are in addition to any state or local laws the medical office must follow. OSHA requires medical offices to dispose of hazardous medical waste in the following manner:

- The waste must be placed into a container that is closable.
- The container must be designed to contain all of the contents and prevent leakage of fluids during handling, storage, transport, or shipping.

- The container must be labeled or color-coded, noting the contents are hazardous.
- The container must be closed prior to removal to prevent spillage of contents during handling, storage, transport, or shipping.
- If outside contamination occurs, the first container must be placed within a second container that meets all of the listed standards.

▸▸▸ Pulse Points

Material Safety Data Sheet (MSDS)

A Material Data Safety Sheet (**MSDS**) is required for any material(s) kept in the medical office that can cause harm to a person. Materials that can burn or cause respiratory issues, for example, require an MSDS. These sheets must be kept in the office and employees must be informed and trained on the use of these potentially dangerous products.

Ensuring Employee Safety

Just as patient safety demands constant attention in the medical office, so does employee safety. As a preventive step, all staff must remain vigilant to situations that can lead to employee injury. For example, staff should keep current on the maintenance and repair of office equipment and ensure that all employees are properly trained in the equipment's use. Attention to proper lifting techniques and office ergonomics also helps avoid injuries and lost time in the workplace.

PROCEDURE 22-10 Develop an Exposure Control Plan

Theory and Rationale

OSHA requires all medical offices to have exposure control plans that list all personal protective equipment in the office and information regarding its use, as well as information on what the employee is to do in the event of exposure.

Materials

- List of personal protective equipment in the office
- Training manual

Competency

1. List each piece of personal protective equipment in the office.

2. List the situations when each piece of equipment should/must be used.

3. Hold an in-office training session to review each item and to discuss its use.

4. Demonstrate each item's use.

5. Discuss how the office can reduce or eliminate exposure in the office.

6. Discuss the steps the employees should take in the event of exposure.

7. Document everything discussed at the meeting, and distribute copies to all staff.

 PROCEDURE 22-11 Use Proper Lifting Techniques

Theory and Rationale

Proper lifting techniques help prevent injuries in the medical office. Any employee who must lift supplies or patients must be properly trained to avoid injury.

Materials

- Item to lift

Competency

1. Examine the item to be lifted.

2. While bending at the knees, not the waist, with feet shoulder-width apart, grasp the item with both hands (**Figure 22-13a** ■).

3. Stand with the item held close to the body (**Figure 22-13b** ■).

4. Place the item down, bending at the knees, not at the waist, and keeping the back straight.

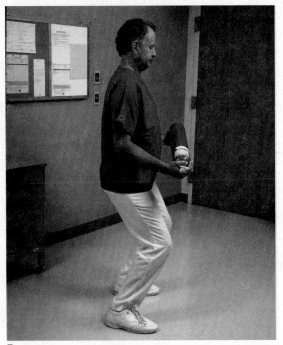

A   B

Figure 22-13 ■ (a) When picking up a heavy item, the back should remain straight while the knees are bent; (b) keeping the back straight, use the leg muscles to return to a standing position.

REVIEW

Chapter Summary

- An effective medical office manager demonstrates a range of high-level skills, including communication and organizational skills, and possibly clinical aptitude.
- Because health care situations dictate the appropriate management style, office managers must be able to assess situations and adapt accordingly.
- Effective staff meetings, often led by office managers, usually result from planning that includes detailed, accurate agendas.
- Job descriptions are important when medical offices are recruiting staff. Job descriptions include a list of the required duties the employee is expected to perform in addition to the hours and days the employee is expected to work.
- Offices can advertise for staff in a number of places, from conventional newspapers and Web sites to agencies and colleges.
- Effective job placement ads give an overview of job responsibilities.
- Effective interviews uncover the issues and characteristics untouched by résumés. These characteristics might include noticing that an applicant is nervous or overly talkative or is perhaps wearing unprofessional attire to the interview.
- When interviewing job candidates, employers must be careful to remain within ethical and legal boundaries.
- It is wise for hiring offices to check an applicant's professional credentials, as well as references.

- Once they are hired, medical office staff are effectively managed with organization, equity, and open communication.
- Employment policies that outline issues such as the terms for employee discipline or termination are valuable tools for offices.
- Employee evaluations are critical ways to ensure that employees remain fulfilled and productive as they progress.
- When a medical office must provide an employee reference, it should again remain within legal boundaries to remain professional and appropriate.
- Quality improvement programs are designed to keep the medical office a high-functioning, safe entity. Quality improvement programs include looking for ways to improve patient satisfaction in the medical office.
- All members of the health care team are accountable for quality improvement and patient safety outcomes.
- To help keep patients and health care staff safe, offices should report injury incidents properly.
- Medical office protective equipment is designed to safeguard those providing patient care.
- The proper disposal of hazardous waste is just one way to help ensure medical employee safety. This disposal is regulated by OSHA on the federal level and by state and local laws.

Chapter Review

Multiple Choice

1. Each year, the United States creates _____ tons of hazardous waste.
   a. 3,200
   b. 300
   c. 320
   d. 3.2 million
   e. 3.2 billion

2. The _____ leader is laid back and becomes involved only when needed.
   a. Autocratic
   b. Democratic

   c. Laissez-faire
   d. Pacesetting
   e. None of the above

3. What is the main purpose of reporting sentinel events in the medical office?
   a. To fire employees who were involved in the event
   b. To provide an experience from which the office can learn how to prevent a similar event in the future
   c. To protect the office in the event a patient files a lawsuit

d. To communicate to patients the event that took place in the medical office
e. None of the above

4. Why are employee evaluations necessary?
   a. To monitor an employee's performance
   b. To communicate with the employee any areas that need to be addressed
   c. To document any agreements made with the employee regarding job performance
   d. To give the employee a written document outlining her perceived performance within the medical office
   e. All of the above

5. Before conducting drug testing on employees, employers must do which one of the following?
   a. Get the employee's written permission
   b. Not charge the employee for the testing
   c. Give the employee the result of the testing
   d. All of the above
   e. None of the above

True/False

T F **1.** Quality improvement programs are used to improve an office's targeted areas.

T F **2.** The medical assistant is not responsible for alerting the office to a piece of broken equipment.

T F **3.** When giving a reference for a former employee, who was fired, the office manager should tell the potential employer why the employee was fired even when lacking proof.

T F **4.** To be the most effective, an office manager should learn to tailor her leadership style to the situation.

T F **5.** Only top-level management should attend staff meetings.

T F **6.** In small medical offices, it is appropriate for the physician-employer to require employees to supply their own protective equipment, such as examination gloves.

T F **7.** Each job description should outline the duties and physical requirements of the position.

T F **8.** Because a résumé and an application reflect on an applicant, office managers often discard applications with poor grammar or typographical errors.

T F **9.** When giving a reference for a former employee, it is important to have a set policy and to follow it closely.

Short Answer

1. Explain why a medical office manager must have outstanding communication skills.
2. What does it mean to delegate tasks?
3. What is the purpose of a staff meeting agenda?
4. What method might an office manager use to fill a vacant position in the medical office?
5. How can an office check a medical assistant's credentials?
6. Define the term "adverse outcome."

Research

1. What classes might you take at your local community college in order to obtain the skills needed to seek employment as a medical office manager?
2. Refer to page 453 and answer each of the questions as if you were interviewing for a position. How might you improve your answers?
3. Research online for information on how employees in the health care setting might work to ensure patient safety.

Practicum Application Experience

While patient Monica Schneider is in Dr. Garcia's examination room, she trips over an exposed carpet seam and falls. Afterward, she complains that her knee hurts where it hit the floor. What should the medical assistant do? What suggestions could the assistant make to prevent similar occurrences?

Resource Guide

Americans with Disabilities Act
Phone: (800) 514-0301
www.ada.gov

Centers for Medicare and Medicaid Services
7500 Security Boulevard
Baltimore, MD 21244
http://www.cms.hhs.gov/HIPAAGenInfo/

Employee Assistance Programs Online (an agency that provides links to employee assistance programs online)
http://www.eap-sap.com/

The Joint Commission
One Renaissance Blvd.
Oakbrook Terrace, IL 60181
Phone: (630) 792-5000
http://www.jointcommission.org/sentinel_event.aspx/

U.S. Department of Justice
950 Pennsylvania Avenue, NW
Washington, DC 20530-0001
Phone: (202) 514-2000
http://www.usdoj.gov/

U.S. Department of Labor
Frances Perkins Building,
200 Constitution Avenue, NW
Washington, DC 20210
Phone: (866) 4-USA-DOL
www.dol.gov

OSHA
http://www.osha.gov/SLTC/healthcarefacilities/index.html

23

Marketing the Medical Office

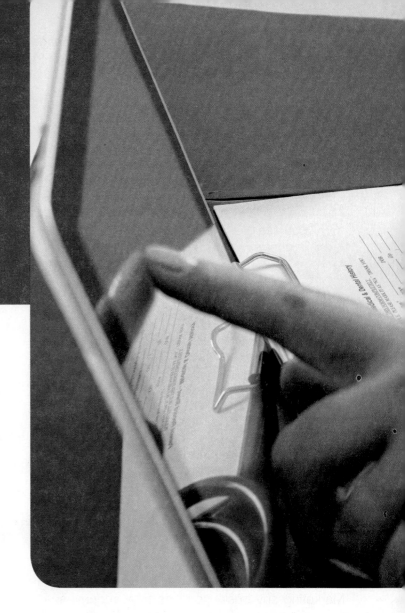

Case Study

Read the following case study and answer the critical thinking questions presented throughout the chapter.

Harold Price is the medical office manager for a large cardiology practice. The physicians in his clinic have asked Harold to put together a marketing plan and to present his ideas to them at the next department meeting. Harold is not sure what type of marketing would be best for this office, and he isn't sure what patients in the local area would want.

Objectives

After completing this chapter, you should be able to:

23.1 Define and spell the key terms in this chapter.

23.2 Describe the task of funding a marketing initiative.

23.3 Understand how to market to a practice's demographic.

23.4 Discuss the importance of researching the strengths, weaknesses, and opportunities of a medical practice.

23.5 Determine what to look for when researching the competition.

23.6 Describe how the Internet can be used for marketing purposes.

23.7 List the items available on a robust clinic Web site.

23.8 Describe how direct mail advertising works.

23.9 Describe the purchase of mailing lists as an advertising option for the medical office.

23.10 Understand how the Welcome to the Neighborhood program works within communities.

23.11 Describe the role of the medical office manager in setting up free or low-cost screenings.

23.12 List the steps involved at screening events.

23.13 Explain how social media sites can be used in advertising.

23.14 Define focus groups, and describe their use.

23.15 Understand how local businesses might be targeted for marketing purposes.

23.16 Describe possible venues for educational speaking engagements, and discuss the role of the medical office manager in planning for these events.

23.17 Describe how to use telephone books as advertising sources.

23.18 Describe on-hold messaging and explain how it is used.

23.19 Discuss the use of surveys in determining patients' satisfaction with their health care.

23.20 Explain how patients might be used as sources of advertising.

23.21 Describe how writing articles for local newspapers or periodicals is a form of marketing, and list members of the medical team who could be involved in this advertising.

23.22 Explain how to target local media for advertising.

23.23 Describe the benefits of hiring a marketing consultant.

Key Terminology

demographic—statistical data of a population, such as age, gender, education, income, and ethnicity

direct mail advertising—a form of advertising that is mailed directly to homes

focus group—a representative group of individuals brought together and questioned about their ideas on new products or services

marketing budget—the amount of money allocated by a company to promote its products or services

marketing firm—an organization hired to design a marketing plan

marketing plan—a comprehensive plan that outlines a business's overall marketing objectives in a given period

return on investment—the amount of profit an investment returns after implementation

screenings—events held to offer free services to individuals, such as blood pressure testing

search engine optimization—the process of affecting the visibility of a Web site or a Web page in a search engine's search

social media site—Web site where people can share information, interact, and communicate with each other

Introduction

Marketing any business takes time, money, and a good deal of preparation. Health care is no exception. Though any member of the medical office team can be involved with marketing initiatives in the medical office, in offices where there is a designated medical office manager, that person is typically the one leading the marketing efforts. The best preparation for beginning any marketing initiative is a properly prepared **marketing plan**, which is a comprehensive plan that outlines a business's overall marketing objectives in a given period. A strong marketing plan helps the medical office manager stay on schedule and spend allocated funds appropriately. Any marketing initiative, whether designed to start a new practice or bring new business into an existing practice, should be undertaken only after investigation of a number of factors. The medical office manager should work in concert with the physicians or with the owners of the business, if not the physicians.

Funding a Marketing Initiative

The clinic's **marketing budget**—the amount of money allocated by a company to promote its products or services—outlines the costs of the marketing initiatives that are planned. These funds may be allocated to hiring a **marketing firm**—a company that can compose and carry out a marketing plan—or they may be budgeted toward other endeavors developed in-house. Although the marketing budget should be determined before setting out to market the practice, no business should set this number in stone. The amount budgeted might need to be flexible as needs or opportunities arise.

▸▸▸ Pulse Points

Marketing Initiatives

Marketing initiatives can be very expensive, depending upon the type and amount of advertising desired. Television commercials, for example, are very costly to produce. Part of designing a marketing plan should include information on costs, in order to determine where the budget is best spent to reach the desired group of potential patients for the health care facility.

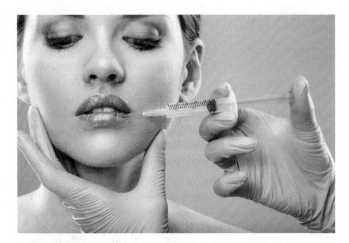

Figure 23-1 ■ A plastic surgeon may choose to market facial cosmetic surgery in a community where this service may be popular.
Source: Fotolia © Yriy Shevtsov.

To determine the **return on investment,** which is the amount of money brought in after a marketing initiative, the medical office manager should perform a prospective view for the marketing plan. This should include the number of patients expected to be reached by the plan and the dollars those patients will bring in once they come in for care. This number will vary according to the type of practice and care offered. For example, a plastic surgeon might choose to market a particular product or service, such as hair replacement, laser surgery, or botox injections (**Figure 23-1** ■).

Knowing the amount of money the service brings in, the medical office manager will be able to determine how much money the marketing plan should return for the dollars invested. In some cases, the amount of money brought into the practice will vary depending on patient needs. If, for example, a family practice physician is marketing for new patients, the amount of money each patient brings in will vary according to the type of care required by each individual.

Critical Thinking Question 23-1

Refer back to the case study at the beginning of the chapter. What do you think are the pros and cons of hiring a marketing firm to prepare a clinic's marketing plans?

Understanding the Demographic

Before undertaking any marketing plan, the medical office manager should determine the target audience. Determining the **demographic,** or makeup, of the population that the office marketing plan is intended to target is the process of looking at specifics such as age and number of children a person in a particular area would likely have. If the clinic is located in an area where the main demographic is blue collar workers, the manager might think about marketing services that are of interest to working families, such as sports physicals, or

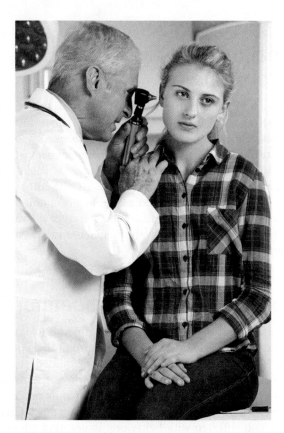

Figure 23-2 ■ The marketing plan might include marketing sports or back-to-school physicals in an area that is populated with families.
Source: Fotolia © Monkey Business.

back-to-school physicals (**Figure 23-2** ■). In an area that is populated with a large number of patients over the age of 60, the medical office manager might wish to market services such as osteoporosis or prostate screenings.

The type and method of advertising should be considered along with the demographic of patients being targeted. For example, many young families are on the go and might be best reached by advertisements on the side of buses or printed in school brochures. Elderly patients might be best reached with mailers sent directly to the home or via flyers placed in the local pharmacy or in local senior centers.

▶▶▶ Pulse Points

Targeting Specific Demographics

Marketing plans may be devised to target certain demographics at different times of the year. Flu shots, for example, may be marketed in the fall and winter, whereas back-to-school physical exams may be marketed in the summer months. October is breast cancer awareness month, making September and October prime months for a marketing plan to bring in patients for routine mammograms.

Researching Strengths, Weaknesses, and Opportunities

The medical office manager will want to market those areas where the practice is doing well and is able to handle increased business. For example, if a family practice has recently lost one of its two pediatricians, and getting an appointment with the remaining pediatrician presents a challenge, this would not be the time to market care related to children. On the other hand, if the practice has just received a large shipment of influenza vaccine and has the staff available to administer the vaccine, this is the perfect time to advertise influenza vaccines to the community (**Figure 23-3** ■).

Researching the Competition

Part of researching the practice's strengths and weaknesses should include a broader look at the surrounding community. The medical practice manager should determine where the competition is strong and where their weaknesses lie. For example, if the only other family practice in town has a physician who is well known for his ability to work with children with behavioral issues, this might not be an area in which competing practices would want to market. Spending dollars on marketing in an area where the competition has a strong foothold is not typically a wise decision.

Researching the competition includes activities such as noticing the advertising other organizations do, and the types of demographics they target. Research should include looking through local newspapers for advertisements, as well as encouraging staff members to bring in any direct-mail advertising they are receiving in their homes.

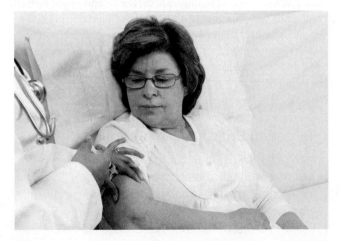

Figure 23-3 ■ The manager should market those areas where the practice is able to handle increased business, for example, administering influenza vaccines.
Source: Fotolia © Fernando Madeira.

Using the Internet for Marketing

The Internet can be a strong tool for medical office advertising. Many practices manage their own Web sites and others purchase space on a community site. There are many places to purchase advertising on the Internet. The medical office manager should research the options and do a cost comparison to determine which one, if any, is appropriate for the practice and the marketing plan intended.

Search engine optimization (SEO) is the process of making changes to a company's Web site content so that the site will come up at the top of a results list during an Internet search; SEO is an option many businesses choose to pursue. Businesses, including health care facilities, can also buy advertisements directly from Internet search engines. These advertisements appear on the main page of the search engine once certain terms are entered for a search. For example, if a potential patient is searching for a pediatrician in Portland, Oregon, she might go to an Internet search engine and type in "pediatrician in Portland, Oregon." An advertisement paid for by a pediatrics practice in Portland, Oregon, will appear on the right side of the screen, bringing in potential new patients to the practice (**Figure 23-4** ■).

A Robust Web Site

Most businesses today have their own Internet Web site. A site might be developed entirely by someone in the practice, such as the medical office manager or one of the physicians, or a company might be hired to design and manage the site. Many practices today have very robust Web sites on which patients are able to request or even schedule appointments, pay bills, and find answers to medical questions. Other items commonly found on a medical clinic's Web site include:

● Biographies of the individual physicians. This sometimes includes video segments of physicians discussing their care philosophies.

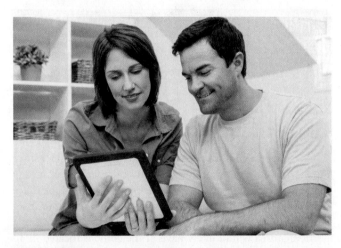

Figure 23-4 ■ Many patients today use the Internet to locate a new provider.
Source: Fotolia © Darren Baker.

- Insurance information, including the types of insurance plans accepted.
- Locations and hours sites are open for care. This typically includes driving directions and parking information.
- A list of job opportunities available at the medical facility.

Keeping the office's Internet Web site up to date and accurate is a very important key to the site being used successfully. As information about the practice, its providers, additional locations, and so on, changes, the Web site should be updated as well. Just like any other business, the medical office should work to keep its Web site fresh and attractive.

Critical Thinking Question 23-2

Refer to the case study at the beginning of the chapter. What other elements do you think a clinic's robust Web site should contain?

Direct Mail Advertising

Direct mail advertising is any form of print advertising that is sent via the mail directly to individuals' homes. Marketing companies exist that provide direct mail services. These companies have a database of information specific to the target market (e.g., potential customer names, phone numbers, e-mail addresses, traits) and are able to address marketing messages directly to the targeted audience. Medical office managers may choose to contract with one of these companies to prepare a direct-mail advertisement. Often, these advertisements are sent in an envelope along with the ads of other companies. They are mailed to households in a desired zip code area, typically one that is within a certain driving distance to the business.

Other direct marketing initiatives include e-mail, interactive customer websites, promotional letters, and cell phone texting (**Figure 23-5 ■**).

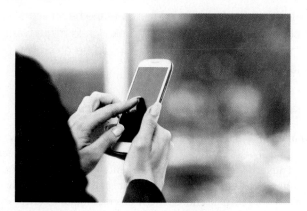

Figure 23-5 ■ Medical offices are able to extend their marketing initiatives to potential new patients via text messaging.

Purchasing Mailing Lists

Some health care facilities may choose to send direct mail advertisements themselves directly to households, rather than through a direct-mail marketing firm. Mailing lists can be purchased from marketing firms. With this marketing option, the medical office manager should work with the physicians to determine the type of advertisement desired and the demographic to be targeted. A budget should be created for the artwork and printing of the piece to be mailed. Postage must be taken into consideration as well.

Welcome to the Neighborhood

Most communities have a city- or county-funded committee whose function it is to provide information to new members of the community. Often, this function lies with the Chamber of Commerce or another similar department within the community government. These committees typically provide materials to people who are buying a home in the area or even to those who are newly renting their home. The materials usually include information on the location of libraries and other public facilities. Inside these "Welcome to the Neighborhood" packets, advertisement space is often sold to businesses in the community. Knowing that new residents will need to begin care with a physician or dentist, this can be an excellent opportunity to spend advertising dollars in an area that has a good return on the investment.

Offering Screenings

Many health care providers offer free **screenings** in their community as a way to bring in new patients. These screenings range from tests for scoliosis (abnormal curvature of the spine) to vision, to blood pressure checks, and more. When setting up free or even low-cost screenings, the medical office manager should determine the proper venue for the screening event. The event may take place in the clinic, but this might not be the best option for bringing in walk-up traffic. Often, screenings are planned in local malls, at fairs, or at other community events. The medical office manager should arrange to rent the space and to have appropriate supplies available for use at the screenings.

Some form of patient history form is filled out by the patient at a screening event. The purpose of the history form is not only to collect basic information about the patient but also to gather contact information from the patient for future marketing endeavors. After the screening is done, the physician or other medical staff can offer additional services to the patient, if needed. The patient's mailing address can be added to a list of patients who will receive flyers or brochures in the future.

In order for screenings to be most successful, part of the marketing plan should include advertising the upcoming screening. Placing flyers in the area where the screening will be held is a fairly inexpensive way to advertise the event. In some cases, other types of advertising, such as radio, newspaper, or Internet advertising, may bring in more people to the screening event.

Critical Thinking Question 23-3

Referring to the case study at the beginning of the chapter, what other ideas do you have for Harold with regard to screenings? What demographic should he target for those screenings? How would Harold figure out what demographic to target?

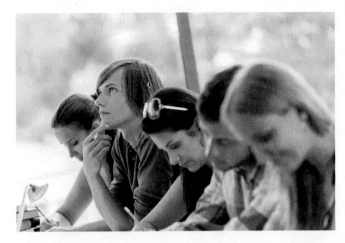

Figure 23-6 ■ Focus groups are commonly used to test new marketing ideas in a community.
Source: Fotolia © CandyBox Images.

Social Media Sites

Social media sites are Internet Web sites, such as Facebook, where individuals interact on a social level; these sites are becoming a popular method for medical offices to market their services, offering the ability to set up a page at no cost, where marketing information about the business can be published. Articles written by providers or staff and news items about the clinic can be shared in this public format. These sites also offer paid advertising spots on the social media site's home page. When a user types in a certain word or phrase, the social media site's search engine will automatically bring up advertisements that appear to fit with the search item. For example, if a user types in the words "low back pain," a paid advertisement for a local chiropractor might appear on the user's screen.

Critical Thinking Question 23-4

Refer to the case study at the beginning of the chapter. In what ways could Harold use social media sites for advertising? What kind of advertising have you seen on these sites?

Using Focus Groups

A **focus group** is a representative group of individuals brought together and questioned about their ideas on new products or services (**Figure 23-6** ■). In health care, these groups are typically one of two kinds. The first is a focus group of existing patients in the facility. These groups are asked to provide their opinions on types of care or to share their feelings about how physicians should interact with their patients. The second type of focus group consists of individuals who are not currently patients in the clinic. With this group, the goal is to survey the members to determine what kinds of services would be valuable to the group and what it would take to lure the members away from their current health care provider.

Using focus groups is common in marketing other businesses, and the feedback gained is typically very valuable. Although this is not an expensive form of marketing, it does take time to set up the groups. Space for the meetings must be arranged, and the members are often given a thank-you gift for their attendance. Focus groups should consist of a variety of people from the same demographic of people who live in the clinic's community. For example, if the clinic is located in a community that houses mostly elderly patients, a high percentage of the focus group members should be elderly patients. Having a focus group of young parents of young children would not provide the medical office with appropriate information about desired services in the community.

Critical Thinking Question 23-5

Referring back to the case study at the beginning of the chapter, what topics do you think Harold might want a focus group to discuss? How would he determine the topics?

Targeting Local Businesses

Many health care providers reach out to market directly to local businesses in their community. This is a form of direct-mail advertising in that advertisements may be sent to local businesses as an attempt to bring in new patients. Medical office managers may choose to use this method to contact local businesses about setting up private health screening events, or to make an offer to have one of the physicians give a presentation on workplace ergonomics. This type of advertising is very inexpensive in that the costs involved are confined to materials and postage and to the time required to follow up on offers to perform screenings or give educational presentations.

Offering Educational Speaking Engagements

Many physicians offer to give educational speaking engagements in their communities. These engagements may be targeted to local businesses, as mentioned above, or they may be targeted toward local community groups. As an example, a physician might give an educational talk about exercising to elderly patients at a local senior center or one about proper nutrition at a local diet center.

Physicians have also offered their services at local colleges, especially in vocational programs such as nursing or medical assisting. In these settings, physicians may speak about their particular profession or on a particular subject matter, such as how to deal with noncompliant patients.

Educational talks might also be offered to other medical practices in the community. This is most commonly done in specialty practices where the physicians wish to bring in referrals from primary care providers in the community. The medical office manager working with a specialty practice can set up this kind of talk by putting together a letter from the physicians in the practice with an offer to come and speak on an educational topic. Following up on the letters with a personal telephone call, either from the manager or one of the physicians, is one way to increase the likelihood of the offer being accepted.

Critical Thinking Question 23-6

Refer to the case study at the beginning of the chapter. What educational topics can you think of that a physician might want to discuss at a public speaking engagement? How would Harold come up with those topics? What might he consider about the targeted demographic?

Telephone Books as Advertising Sources

With the popularity and ease of use of the Internet, many people today forego owning or using telephone books or directories. This form of advertisement was one of the sole ways of reaching potential new patients for the medical practice prior to the advent of the Internet. Advertising in the telephone directory is still done by medical practices, though it is not recommended as a primary source of advertising. Just as with all forms of print advertising, the price is determined by the size of the advertisement and its placement.

On-Hold Messaging

Medical clinics today frequently include advertising messages in their telephone systems. These messages are heard by callers who are placed on hold. On-hold messaging can be purchased from a vendor, or clinics can design and record their own. Because the caller is a captive audience during the hold time, this is a perfect opportunity to market items that might be of interest to the caller. New services in the clinic, the availability of a new provider, or expanded office hours are all examples of advertising information that can be included in the on-hold message. Recordings for callers on hold should be professionally recorded. Callers listening to static, or a poorly recorded message might not stay on the line to listen to the message.

Offering Exceptional Customer Service to Keep Patients Satisfied

Patient satisfaction is looked at closely by most providers and clinics today. Patients are health care consumers and if they are not satisfied with all aspects of their care, they may choose to seek care elsewhere. Companies such as Press Ganey exist to provide services related to surveying patients on their satisfaction with care. These surveys are then compared to national averages to provide medical clinics with information on how well they are doing at providing satisfying care to their patients.

Because satisfied patients not only stay with their facility but also refer new patients to it, this area deserves focus and attention, regardless of the size of the clinic. Patient satisfaction concerns both the patient's clinical experience as well as how the patient was made to feel while she was in the office. The following are examples of survey questions asked of patients regarding their satisfaction with a particular medical visit. Patients are typically asked to rate areas such as these on a scale of 1 to 5, with 1 being very unhappy and 5 being extremely satisfied.

- How do you feel about the amount of time you were on hold before your call was answered?
- Do you feel you were greeted in a friendly manner by the receptionist?
- How do you feel about the amount of time you waited to be taken back to the exam room after checking in?
- Do you feel the medical assistant or nurse showed genuine concern for you?
- How do you feel about the amount of time the physician spent in the exam room with you?

Many medical clinics use their own form of survey to collect information about patient satisfaction. These may take the form of postcards or other forms given to patients with a request they be filled out and returned to the clinic in a postage-paid envelope.

After gathering information about patient satisfaction, medical office managers should share the information with staff and providers. By sharing the information in a department meeting, a discussion can be started on how to work on areas that need improvement.

Critical Thinking Question 23-7

Refer to the case study at the beginning of the chapter. What techniques do you think the medical office manager might talk to his staff about for raising patient satisfaction? How might a focus group help in determining the areas the office staff might want to focus on for raising patient satisfaction?

Patients as Advertising Tools

Patients who are very satisfied with their care will often refer their family and friends for care in the same facility. On the other hand, patients who are unhappy with their care will also discuss that fact with their family and friends, creating a negative effect on earning new business. Because patients are a form of advertisement—both good and bad—medical office managers should address patient concerns and complaints in a timely manner.

Many medical offices offer free screenings or discounts on services or visits for those patients referred in by a current patient. Those patients making the referral may also receive a complimentary or discounted service. The patients currently being seen in the medical office are often the best source of advertisement for the practice.

Writing Articles for Local Newspapers or Periodicals

Most communities have a local newspaper in which the news of the day is published. Often, these periodicals are open to publishing articles written by physicians. This is a form of free advertisement in that it costs the office nothing to pursue this option; the only costs incurred are those of the physician's time in writing the article. These articles can be written on particular topics, or they can be written in a question-and-answer format. For the latter, the questions could be those the physician has answered in her own practice, or they could be questions submitted to the periodical for answers.

Other members of the medical team may be involved in this form of advertising, with nurses or medical assistants writing articles about caring for patients with particular illnesses, or the medical office manager writing an article about how patients may be more involved in their care.

A blog is another idea for writing articles. A blog is a Web page on which an individual records opinions, links to other sites, and more on a regular basis. Just as when the physician or one of the medical team members writes a print article, a blog located on the clinic's Web site is a great informational tool that can act as an advertisement for new patients. Blogs can be written to discuss current trends in health care, treatments, or even opinions on health care policy.

Targeting the Local Media

Whenever a new development occurs in the medical practice, it provides a great opportunity to seek free advertisement with the local media. Examples include the addition of a new physician in the practice, a staff member who recently earned a new degree or certification, or the purchase of a new piece of equipment. These events may be submitted in the form of a press release to local newspapers or to the media as suggestions for news stories.

Hiring a Marketing Consultant

For clinics with larger budgets for advertising, a marketing consultant or marketing firm may be hired. These companies offer all of the services listed in this chapter, taking the work of researching products and competition, for example, off the shoulders of the medical office manager or physicians. If this method of setting up a marketing program is chosen, time should be spent first in researching the best firm. A company that has a good history of working with health care facilities, and one that freely provides contact information for some of its clients, is a good place to start.

REVIEW

Chapter Summary

- Before beginning any marketing initiative, it is important to acknowledge the funds that will be allocated for this purpose. The amount may be fluid, but should not be surpassed without good reason.

- By understanding the demographic in the clinic's area, the medical office manager is better able to target the most effective advertising to the target audience.

- Spending time researching a practice's strengths, weaknesses, and opportunities in the community will save the practice money by targeting advertising dollars appropriately.
- By researching the competition in the local area, the medical practice is able to highlight areas where advancements may be made.
- Many practices today use the Internet as a marketing tool. This is done in a variety of ways, some of which are more expensive than others.
- Many practices today have a very robust Web site for marketing their practice. These Web sites offer the ability to make appointments and pay bills online.
- Direct-mail advertising is the function of sending advertising pieces directly to the homes of the targeted audience.
- By purchasing mailing lists, medical practices are able to send their own direct mail pieces.
- Many medical offices use direct mail to target advertising to newcomers to the community.
- By offering screenings, medical practices are able to solicit new business from targeted audiences.
- Social media sites such as Facebook offer new marketing opportunities to medical practices.
- Focus groups may be used to understand how best to market products to a particular demographic in the practice's area.
- By targeting local businesses, medical practices may be able to garner new business.

- Offering educational speaking events to businesses or community centers is one way for the medical practice to attract new patients.
- Telephone books were once one of the only ways to advertise to consumers. Today, this form of advertisement is not the only way to reach the public in the community.
- On-hold messaging can be used to advertise to patients as they hold the line when calling the medical office.
- By giving patients excellent customer service, medical offices are able to retain loyal patients, as well as build their practice base.
- Patients who have received excellent customer service are a good source of advertising. These patients will tell their family and friends about their care, bringing in new business to the medical office.
- Many physicians or other office staff write articles for local periodicals. This service to the community is often a good source of new business for the clinic.
- When new events occur in the medical practice, it is a good idea to notify the local media. Stories that run in the media about positive events are good advertising for the clinic.
- Some clinics choose to hire marketing consultants to assist with their marketing needs.

Chapter Review

Multiple Choice

1. Which of the following best defines a *demographic*?
   a. The statistical data of a population, such as age, gender, and education
   b. The number of physicians who work in an office
   c. The amount of time allotted for a particular health care service
   d. The medications prescribed for a certain condition
   e. The location of the medical practice

2. Welcome to the Neighborhood packets are typically sent to which of the following?
   a. Established residents who live close to the medical clinic
   b. Employees of the medical clinic
   c. Patients taking a certain medication
   d. Residents who have recently moved into the community
   e. Residents who have recently left the community

3. Which of the following would be appropriate for an educational speaking engagement?
   a. A senior's group
   b. The medical office staff
   c. Family of the physicians
   d. Former patients
   e. Visitors from out of town

4. Which of the following is the more expensive form of advertising?
   a. Speaking engagements
   b. Writing an article in the local newspaper
   c. Patients speaking to their friends
   d. Internet advertisements
   e. Word of mouth

5. Which of the following would be appropriate for free screenings?
   a. Blood pressure
   b. Physical exams
   c. Liver function testing
   d. Treadmill stress tests
   e. X-ray testing

6. Which of the following is appropriate for a focus group?
   a. Deciding on the name for a new clinic
   b. Determining a fee schedule for a new practice
   c. Choosing a candidate for a reception position
   d. Recruiting for a new physician
   e. Determining topics for a newsletter

7. Which of the following stories might the local news media be interested in?
   a. New state-of-the-art equipment that no other medical practice in town has
   b. Newly hired receptionist
   c. Recently redone fee list
   d. New furniture in the medical practice
   e. A recent remodel of the medical office

8. Which of the following is considered a social media site?
   a. Local newspaper
   b. Online message board for parents of small children
   c. Facebook
   d. Community bulletin board
   e. E-mail

9. Which of the following best describes the concept of *return on investment*?
   a. The amount of money spent on advertising
   b. The amount of money paid by patients for a particular service
   c. The amount of money paid to staff to work at a screening event
   d. The amount of money earned compared to the amount of money spent on a marketing initiative
   e. The amount of money left over after an advertising campaign

10. What is the best reason for researching the competition before embarking on a marketing initiative?
    a. To make sure you are targeting an area where they are weak
    b. To give them competition in an area where they are strong
    c. To get an idea on how much money the competition is spending on marketing
    d. To understand how the competition's marketing plan is working for them
    e. To underscore the competition

True/False

Determine if each of the following statements is true or false.

T F 1. Once set, the marketing budget should never be adjusted.

T F 2. The Internet can be a strong tool for medical office advertising.

T F 3. The most lucrative form of advertising today is the telephone book advertisement.

T F 4. Whenever a new development occurs in the medical practice, it is a great opportunity to seek free advertisement with the local media.

T F 5. A strong marketing plan helps the medical office manager stay on schedule and spend allocated funds appropriately.

T F 6. Patient satisfaction is looked at closely by most providers and clinics today.

T F 7. Focus groups should be made up only of patients who are currently being treated in the clinic.

T F 8. For clinics with large budgets for advertising, a marketing consultant or marketing firm may be hired.

T F 9. The medical office manager will want to market those areas where the practice is doing well and is able to handle increased business.

T F 10. Articles in the local newspaper do not have to be written by the physician; they may be written by other members of the office staff.

Short Answer

1. Explain the advantages to performing an analysis of the demographic prior to making decisions about a marketing initiative.
2. Why might a medical office choose to purchase a mailing list for a marketing campaign?
3. How does paying attention to patient satisfaction play into the role of marketing in the medical office?
4. Explain how a focus group might be used to determine the best marketing campaign for a medical office.
5. How does the use of social media fit into marketing in the medical office?

Research

1. Review marketing materials from a local medical office in your area. What is it about the materials that strikes you? What demographic of patients do you think the material is targeting?
2. Using the Internet, look up the Web sites of three or four medical offices in your local area. How are they using their Web sites to market their services?
3. Thinking about the type of medical services you personally need or search for, what type of marketing materials do you believe would work best for a medical office that wishes to target individuals like you in their marketing campaign?

Practicum Application Experience

Jason Smith is the medical office manager in an orthopedics office. The physicians in his office specialize in treating sports injuries. What kind of marketing materials might Jason suggest to the physicians? What demographic would he want to focus upon? What type of marketing (direct mail, social media, etc.) would likely be most effective in targeting patients who have experienced a sports injury?

Resource Guide

Marketing strategies for medical offices
www.physiciannews.com

Physician News Digest
http://www.physiciansnews.com/category/business-law/

MedNet Technologies
www.mednet-tech.com

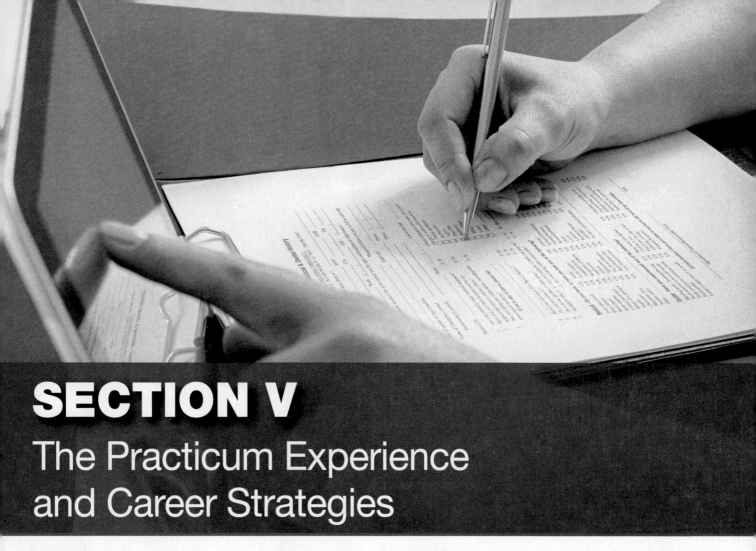

SECTION V
The Practicum Experience and Career Strategies

My name is Francis Wilkes, and I am a recent graduate of an administrative medical assisting program. After completing my practicum experience, I got right to work conducting my job search. I began by preparing a strong résumé and cover letter, and I searched newspapers and worked with my medical assisting program to see if any job listings were posted.

While conducting my search, I learned that many health care organizations list current job openings on their Web site. I found that an administrative medical assistant position was open at a local medical office, just twenty minutes from my home. I completed the online application for the position, uploaded a copy of my résumé and cover letter, and was granted an interview!

I found that preparing and dressing appropriately were very important to the job interview. I also wanted to ensure that I presented the right image to my prospective employer by maintaining eye contact, speaking to her directly, and conveying confidence. I took notes throughout the interview, and was able to ask questions. After the interview, I immediately followed-up with a hand-written thank-you note. Three days later, I was offered the position.

There are many opportunities available for medical assistants today, both in traditional medical offices and in nontraditional settings such as insurance companies. My advice to those searching for their first job, or to those switching jobs, is to make a great first impression on potential employers by writing cover letters and résumés that really stand out.

24 The Practicum Experience and Competing in the Job Market

24

The Practicum Experience and Competing in the Job Market

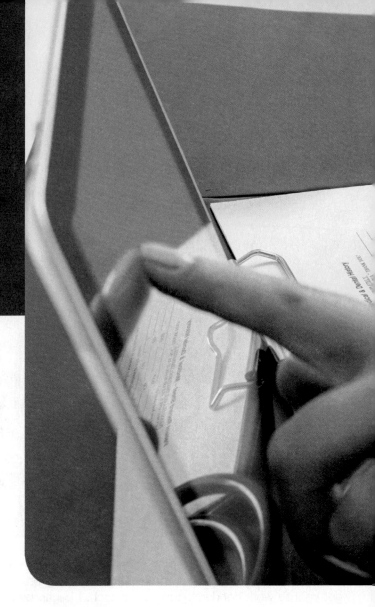

Case Study

Read the following case study and answer the critical thinking questions presented throughout the chapter.

Karim Yousef, a certified medical assisting graduate seeking employment in health care, lacks personal transportation. Because Karim must rely on public transportation, he has arrived late to a few interviews. As he prepares his cover letter and résumé in response to administrative medical assisting job postings, he is trying to determine the most pertinent information to include in these important documents. Karim knows he should include information about his training and experience in the workforce, but he is unsure if he should include information about his short-term employment periods, or that his employment was terminated due to tardiness with his last two employers.

Objectives

After completing this chapter, you should be able to:

24.1 Define and spell the key terminology in this chapter.

24.2 Discuss the practicum experience, including its benefits for the medical assistant, practicum site, and medical assisting program.

24.3 Prepare an attractive and effective résumé.

24.4 Write an effective cover letter, and discuss the importance of using cover letters.

24.5 Discuss varied places to look for employment as a medical assistant.

24.6 Complete an employment application.

24.7 List the Dos and Don'ts of an effective interview.

24.8 Discuss the importance of body language and proper dress while interviewing.

24.9 Explain how to follow up with a medical office after an interview.

24.10 Develop a plan of action for changing jobs.

Competency Skills Performance

1. Write a résumé.
2. Compose a cover letter.
3. Follow up with an employer after an interview.

Key Terminology

advocate—to defend the rights of others; one who defends or acts on behalf of another

cover letter—document that accompanies a résumé to a prospective employer

interview—meeting, usually face to face, between an employer and an applicant

mentor—person who supervises an practicum in a health care facility; also called a preceptor

practicum—final phase of the medical assisting education in an accredited program; consists of hands-on work in a medical office for a specified number of hours

preceptor—person who supervises an practicum in a health care facility; also called a mentor

résumé—document outlining a job applicant's education and job experience

Certification Exam Coverage

AAMA (CMA) Exam Coverage:
- Job readiness and seeking employment
  - Résumé and cover letter development
  - Methods of job searching
- Personnel records
- Performance evaluation
- Privacy

Introduction

The U.S. Department of Labor predicts that medical assisting will grow by 31 percent between 2010 and 2020, driven largely by the aging baby boomer generation. Because older patients tend to seek medical care more often than younger patients, medical offices will be expanding. Medical assisting positions, as a result, will be more and more plentiful and the scope of the position will expand. The scope of practice for any health care profession, including medical assisting, consists of the skills and competencies that the professional is licensed, certified, or trained to do. Typically, the scope of practice is defined by the Department of Health within each state. Already, medical assistants are employed in nontraditional organizations such as insurance companies and inpatient care facilities. The key to finding employment is to make a good impression on potential employers and write cover letters and résumés that stand out.

The Practicum Experience

Every accredited medical assisting program ends with a 60- to 240-hour **practicum program** that allows students to develop hands-on skills in medical offices. Practicum students are guests of the sponsoring medical offices. As such, students should behave as they would when hired: as professionals. In successful practicums, practicum sites, students, and medical assisting programs work together. Some medical assisting students find they are offered employment at their practicum site at the end of the practicum. The medical assisting student is not paid for the practicum work, but earns credit toward graduation from the medical assisting program.

Understanding the Practicum Site's Responsibilities

Practicum sites are responsible for giving medical assisting students forums in which to exercise their clinical and administrative skills. During practicums, medical assistants who work for the practicum sites, called **preceptors** or **mentors**, direct practicum students and serve as resources when questions or issues arise. Most practicum sites are well-versed in the responsibilities of practicums and take those responsibilities seriously.

AAMA (CMA) certification exam topics are reprinted with permission of the American Association of Medical Assistants.

HIPAA Compliance

Before launching practicums, medical offices should require students to sign a Health Insurance Portability and Accountability Act (HIPAA) agreement that states the students will share no personal patient information with anyone outside the offices.

Outlining the Student's Responsibilities

Practicum programs are an excellent place for students to showcase their skills to potential employers. To make their practicum experience as robust as possible, students should actively seek involvement in all their site's clinical and administrative procedures. While most offices allow practicum students to participate in all areas of patient care, patients must give their permission (**Figure 24-1 ■**).

Whatever duties they undertake, practicum students should remain professional, which means arriving on time, being prepared, and dressing in attire that meets the practicum site's requirements. Makeup and jewelry should be minimal, hair should be neat and away from the face, and clothing and shoes should be clean and in good repair.

Sometimes, when practicums are particularly successful, practicum sites offer students permanent positions upon program completion. When employment is not offered but the student is interested in working for his practicum site, the student should advise his preceptor of his desire and leave a copy of his résumé. Because the practicum site may be the first time the medical assisting student has worked in a health care setting, students should behave as if they are on a working

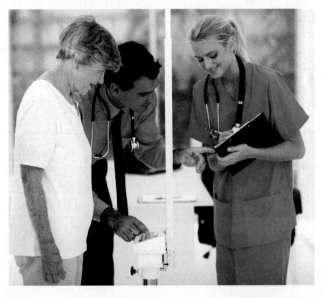

Figure 24-1 ■ During the practicum experience, the student medical assistant will both observe and participate in caring for patients.
Source: Fotolia © michaeljung.

interview for the entire experience. The manager of the practicum site could be a good professional reference for the student when seeking employment after the practicum experience is complete. Students should ask the manager of the practicum site for a letter of recommendation that can be included when applying for medical assisting positions after the practicum.

▸▶▶ Pulse Points

Asking Questions or Raising Concerns During the Practicum Experience

When a medical assisting student has a question or concern during the practicum and the mentor cannot address it, the student should raise the issue with the medical assisting practicum coordinator.

▸▶▶ Pulse Points

Asking Questions of the Physician in Front of the Patient

Medical assisting students should never question the decisions of a physician or other medical assistant in front of patients in the office. Instead, a student should pose questions outside patient's hearing to retain the respect health care professionals command.

The Responsibilities of the Medical Assisting Program

As **advocates** for practicum students, medical assisting practicum coordinators are primarily responsible for choosing appropriate practicum sites for students. In some medical assisting programs, the role of the practicum coordinator is held by a member of the faculty, or the program director. In other programs, the practicum coordinator is a separate position. With the help of the mentor, practicum coordinators should monitor the practicum process closely, making sure students succeed in this important last step in their education. To facilitate the monitoring process and observe students in the clinical environment, many practicum coordinators visit students on site. Many programs ask practicums to log their learning processes in weekly summaries or to meet periodically with the other practicum to share their experiences. Students should bring any concerns to the practicum coordinator's attention. In turn, coordinators should address student issues as soon as possible.

Writing an Effective Résumé

As a job applicant's first impression, the **résumé** is a critical tool in the job market (**Figure 24-2 ■**). Poorly written and prepared résumés suggest that their authors will similarly produce poor quality work in the medical office. As a result, many

RICHARD CORNELIUS, RMA (AMT)
1234, West Nile Street
Worcester, MA 12345
(808) 555-7890
richardc12345@sample.com

OBJECTIVE:
To obtain a challenging position in a medical setting that will allow me to gain experience working with a diverse and challenging population of patients.

EDUCATION:
Northridge Community College Medical Assisting Program, Northridge KY (September 1999–June 2001)

EXPERIENCE:
Williamsburg Women's Clinic, Northridge, KY (July 2001–January 2005): Clinical medical assistant

Martinville Pediatrics, Worcester, MA (March 2005–Present): Clinical medical assistant

ACTIVITIES:
Member of the PTA since 1997
Member of the AAMA

REFERENCES:
Excellent references are available upon request

Figure 24-2 ■ Sample résumé from a medical assistant.

employers discard résumés with poor grammar, typographical errors, or handwritten corrections. When medical assistants change phone numbers, for example, they should revise and reprint their résumés, not hand-mark changes. An applicant may be perfect for the job; however; a sub-par résumé will sacrifice employment opportunities.

Ideally, résumés are short, preferably one to two pages, and are impeccably written and presented. Instead of detailing all duties ever performed, résumés should summarize applicants' qualifications and experience and highlight experience most relevant to the open position. Résumés should include a telephone number that is attached to voicemail. Applicants need to be sure the message on the voicemail is one that is professional in nature. Having a small child record the message, or recording an outgoing message that contains unprofessional language might cause the potential employer to forego leaving a message, and discard the résumé. Résumés should also include a professional e-mail address. This e-mail account should be one the applicant checks on a regular basis. Using a pet name or other unprofessional wording in the email address can cause employers to believe the applicant is unprofessional. The following items should be included on the résumé:

- Name, address, telephone number, and e-mail address
- Educational background, in chronological order
- Licensures or certifications
- Work experience, including dates of employment and brief summaries of duties, in chronological order
- Reference information
- Any transferable skills or certifications

In addition to reviewing work history, the résumé should stress an applicant's skills and accomplishments. Duties performed in previous jobs should also be listed and briefly summarized in the résumé. Any perceived shortcomings, such as disabilities or missing skills, should only be raised in the interview. That way, the applicant can point out positive ways in which to address those issues. One of the most important pieces of information to include on the résumé is the objective statement. This statement should be short and to the point; a lengthy objective may be distracting on a résumé.

The objective should be personalized for the applicant as well as reflect on the position desired. For example, if the applicant is seeking employment with a pediatrics office, the objective might read, "To obtain a medical assisting position where my desire to work with children will be fulfilled."

Critical Thinking Question 24-1

Refer back to the case study presented at the beginning of the chapter. Should Karim note his lack of personal transportation on his résumé? Why or why not?

Accuracy is also crucial in résumé presentation. Applicants should never embellish résumé information. Falsifying applications or résumés is grounds for termination in most organizations. Instead of trying to capture an employer's attention with erroneous information, an applicant should focus on top-notch physical presentation to help get his résumé noticed. In general, however, applicants should defer to good taste and judgment. Résumés printed on lime green paper might get noticed, but résumés are traditionally an area where a more conservative approach is expected. Action words, in contrast, tend to capture the reader's attention in desired ways. While including references on the résumé is important, applicants will want to be sure that those references are aware of their inclusion on the résumé so that they are not surprised or caught off-guard when called by a potential employer. Appropriate references include former or current supervisors/managers and coworkers, former or current course instructors, as well as any professional reference that can speak to the applicant's

TABLE 24-1 Action Words

Achieved	Implemented
Attained	Monitored
Assisted	Organized
Awarded	Performed
Composed	Planned
Created	Prevented
Directed	Scheduled
Established	Screened
Handled	Witnessed

abilities in the workplace. Using family or friends as references should be done only if the applicant does not have any of the previously mentioned references available. Table 24-1 lists some action words applicants can use to reflect their skills and experiences properly on résumés.

Many companies offer professional résumé writing services. The fee charged by these companies is often worth the cost in that the résumé produced is one that is professionally done and more likely to stand out to the potential employer. Professional résumé-writing services will typically collect a copy of the individual's current résumé, as well as information regarding work history, hobbies, and volunteer work. **Figure 24-3** ■ contrasts a résumé composed by a recent

---

EMILY WHARTON, CMA (AAMA)
12345, Penny Lane
Grocer, WY 59098
(555) 567-9090
ewharton@email.com

OBJECTIVE:
To obtain a job as a medical assistant.

EDUCATION:
Smith Medical Assisting School–Grocer, WY

EXPERIENCE:
Burger Palace (February 2009–June 2009)

Bunches of Burgers (November 2009–March 2010)

Bushels of Tacos (August 2010–December 2010)

REFERENCES:
Mary Ann Debate (555) 453-9082
Joe Whittier (555) 210-9876

Figure 24-3a ■ Sample résumé created by the recent graduate.

EMILY WHARTON, CMA (AAMA)

12345, Penny Lane
Grocer, WY 59098
(555) 567-9090
ewharton@email.com

OBJECTIVE:

To use my customer service skills and medical assisting training in a position where I may provide outstanding service to the patients served.

EDUCATION:

Smith Medical Assisting School–Grocer, WY
Graduated with an Associates Degree in Technical Arts, Medical Assisting Certificate
Courses taken include: Medical Law and Ethics, Clinical and Laboratory Skills, Health Care Finances, and Communications
Skills obtained: All aspects of ambulatory care, as well as surgical assisting. Additional training received in taking radiographic images and creating casts for arms and legs.
Certified in AIDS prevention, Basic Life Support, and First Aid for the Health Care Professional

EXPERIENCE:

Food Service: (February 2009–December 2010)

Duties included: Cashiering, inventory, new employee training, customer service

Received Employee of the Month Award May 2009

PRACTICUM EXPERIENCE: Mount View Family Practice (2013)

Worked with patients ranging in age from birth to 90 years. Administered immunizations, assisted with minor surgeries, performed medical billing and coding, scheduled patient appointments for office as well as hospital procedures, performed inventory and stocking of supplies, performed EKGs, blood draws, and assisted with performing spirometry exams.

VOLUNTEER AND COMMUNITY SERVICE:

Midway Community for the Blind–lead field trips for blind children

Arlington Sands Community Center–lead crafting activities in this senior center

REFERENCES:

Mary Ann Debate (555) 453-9082
Joe Whittier (555) 210-9876

Figure 24-3b ■ Sample résumé created by a professional résumé writing service.

graduate (a), and the professional résumé composed by a résumé writing service (b).

There are many Web sites with useful information on composing a professional résumé. In addition, medical assistants may purchase books written to assist in writing a professional resume, designed to be noticed by the prospective employer.

Critical Thinking Question 24-2

Referring to the case study, Karim was fired from his last two jobs due to chronic tardiness. Should he mention those terminations in his résumé? Why or why not?

PROCEDURE 24-1 Write an Effective Résumé

Theory and Rationale

Every job search starts with a good résumé. Many employers see dozens of résumés for one open position in their organization. To secure an interview, the medical assistant need a professional résumé with the right information.

Materials

- Computer with word processing software

Competency

1. Choose a résumé template in the word-processing program.

2. Enter your name, address, telephone number, and e-mail address.

3. Enter an objective (e.g., "To obtain a position as a certified medical assistant in a medical practice where my skills can be used to their full potential").

4. Enter your educational background, including degrees, in chronological order.

5. Enter your employment history, including dates, in chronological order.

6. List references or a phrase like, "References available upon request."

7. Review the document for typographical errors.

8. Print the résumé on quality paper.

9. Review the résumé again for typographical errors.

Preparing a Cover Letter

Often, **cover letters** help job applicants secure opportunities to **interview**. Similar to résumés, cover letters are critical job-searching tools. Because cover letters can be critical to job searches, they should accompany all résumés, even those transmitted via e-mail. In addition, like résumés, they should be error-free and professionally presented.

Cover letters are the link between a résumé and an open job. As such, they should address open positions and explain why the applicant is the best candidate for the position. **Figure 24-4** ■ provides an example of a cover letter. Effective cover letters have headings with the applicant's full name, address, telephone number, fax number when appropriate, and e-mail address. As much as possible, the personal e-mail address should be professional. Potential employers are more likely to favor patricialocke12@sample.com over crazypatty@sample.com.

Joan Monson, CMA (AAMA)
2121 1st Avenue South
Seattle, WA 12345
Home Phone: (206) 555-9084
Mobile Phone: (206) 555-2434
e-Mail: joanmonson@direct.com

June 1, 20xx

Dear Ms. Nielsen:

I enclose my résumé in response to your ad for an administrative medical assistant skilled in pediatric medicine.

After working with children extensively for several years, I recently completed my associate degree and obtained a Certificate in Medical Assisting (CMA) distinction. I completed my practicum in a pediatric office, because I wish to continue applying my skills with children in the administrative environment.

As followup to this letter, I will call your office next week to determine if my qualifications meet your needs at this time, and to schedule an interview with you. Thank you for your time and consideration. I look forward to meeting you.

Sincerely,

Joan Monson, CMA (AAMA)

Figure 24-4 ■ Sample cover letter.

PROCEDURE 24-2 Compose a Cover Letter

Theory and Rationale

Every résumé should include a cover letter. As the personalized link between the résumé and the desired job, a cover letter allows the medical assistant to tell a potential employer why he or she should be chosen for an interview.

Materials

● Computer with word-processing software

Competency

1. Using the word-processing software, enter the date and name, company, and address of the letter's recipient.
2. Compose a letter that addresses the desired job qualifications and the reasons the employer should consider you for the position.
3. List any information that directly relates to your ability to perform the desired job.
4. Request an interview.
5. State that you will call the employer to follow up in a few days.

▶▶▶ Pulse Points

Fluency in Languages Other than English

Use the résumé to list fluency in languages other than English. Many medical offices, especially those in diverse neighborhoods, seek employees who are fluent in languages other than English.

Identifying Places to Look for Employment

Employment advertisements may appear in a number of venues, including newspapers and employment agencies. Medical assisting programs may also list job postings, and medical offices often advertise open positions on their Web sites. To cover all bases, medical assistants should send résumés and cover letters to offices that are not currently hiring. Those résumés may arrive just as open positions become available.

Most health care organizations list their current job openings on their Web site. A medical assistant seeking employment with that organization should visit the Web site of the organization and look up current listings. Typically, companies that list their job openings on their Web site include a link to apply for those jobs online. In this event, medical assistants can often fill out an application and upload a copy of their résumé and cover letter in application for the open position.

▶▶▶ Pulse Points

Use of Social Media Sites

Social media sites, such as Facebook, Twitter, and LinkedIn are useful tools in finding employment opportunities in medical facilities. Many employers place advertisements for open positions on their social media sites. Medical assistants should also place a notice of their desire to obtain a job on their own social media sites, as the notice may be seen by someone in the person's network who knows of an open position.

Critical Thinking Question 24-3

Refer to the case study at the beginning of the chapter. If Karim lacks personal transportation, how should he seek employment?

Completing Employment Applications

Employment applications are an effective way for employers to capture consistent information from all job applicants (**Figure 24-5** ■). As a result, many employers ask applicants to complete employment applications, even when those applicants have submitted a résumé.

Before providing any information on a job application, a candidate should carefully read all parts of the document, particularly the instructions. When it comes to entering information, all answers should be well thought out organized, and neatly written in black or blue ink. Every space should contain some type of information. When a section does not apply, applicants should enter "Not applicable" or "N/A." Errors should be neatly crossed through, not scribbled out. Even when applicants have already submitted a résumé, they should attach an additional copy to the application they turn in.

Many employers receive applications for employment only via their Web site. These employers will often allow for a résumé and cover letter to be uploaded electronically. Some employers will ask for a completed job application in addition to, or in place of, attaching a résumé. Applicants must be sure any information listed on applications is the same as listed on résumés. Discrepancies may be seen as the applicant's intent to mislead the potential employer.

The Successful Interview

When a résumé succeeds in capturing an employer's' attention, the applicant is generally called for an interview and asked for references. Potential employers may use the telephone or e-mail to contact the applicant. If necessary, applicants can use the cover letter to ask prospective employers not to contact their current places of employment.

APPLICATION FOR EMPLOYMENT

Mountain View Health Care Center is an equal opportunity employer and upholds the principles of equal opportunity employment. It is the policy of Mountain View Health Care Center to provide employment, compensation and other benefits related to employment based on qualifications and performance, without regard to race, color, religion, national origin, age, sex, veteran status or disability, or any other basis prohibited by federal or state law. As an equal opportunity employer, Mountain View Health Care Center intends to comply fully with all federal and state laws and the information requested on this application will not be used for any purpose prohibited by law. Disabled applicants may request any needed accommodation. This application is intended to allow you, the applicant, to provide Mountain View Health Care Center with the information and data so that your suitability and qualifications can be fairly determined for the position(s) for which you are applying. Please complete this application and answer all questions completely. Please print clearly in ink.

PLEASE PRINT CLEARLY—BE SURE TO SIGN THIS APPLICATION

Date

Name: Last   First   Middle

Social Security No.:   Home Phone:

Address:

         No.   -   Street

City   State   Zip

Have you been previously employed by Mountain View Health Care Center? ☐ Yes ☐ No
If "Yes", when?   In what capacity?

How did you learn of the position for which you are applying:
☐ Newspaper/Print Advertisement   ☐ Friend/Relative   ☐ Employment Agency   ☐ Job Service   ☐ Radio/TV Advertisement

EMPLOYMENT DESIRED

Position(s) applied for
Shift Preferences: ☐ First Shift – Days   ☐ Second Shift – Evenings   ☐ Third Shift – Nights
☐ Full-time   ☐ Part-time If "Part time", number of shifts/hours desired:
Date available to start   Salary requested

PERSONAL HISTORY

Are you a United States citizen or do you have an entry permit which allows you to lawfully work in the U.S.? ☐ Yes ☐ No
     If applicable, Visa Type: Immigration No.:
Are you at least 18 years old? ☐ Yes ☐ No

Are you able to perform all of the duties required by the position for which you are applying, without endangering yourself or compromising the safety, health, or welfare of the Patients or other Staff Persons? ☐ Yes ☐ No
     If "No," please explain:

EDUCATION

Name and Location Of School	Graduation Date	Course of Study/ Degree Issued
High School		
College		
Other		

LICENSURE/CERTIFICATION/REGISTRATION

Type of License/Certification	Registration Number

List any special skills or qualifications which you possess and feel are relevant to health care and the position for which you are applying.

Figure 24-5 ■ Sample employment application.

EMPLOYMENT HISTORY

Please give accurate and complete information. Start with present or most recent employer.

May we contact and communicate with your present employer? ☐ Yes   ☐ No

Employer	Telephone No.
Address	Employed from / to /
Name of Supervisor	Hourly Pay: Start Last
Position and Responsibilities	
Reason for Leaving	

- -

Employer	Telephone No.
Address	Employed from / to /
Name of Supervisor	Hourly Pay: Start Last
Position and Responsibilities	
Reason for Leaving	

- -

Employer	Telephone No.
Address	Employed from / to /
Name of Supervisor	Hourly Pay: Start Last
Position and Responsibilities	
Reason for Leaving	

- -

MILITARY SERVICE

Branch   From   To

What were your duties?

Did you receive any specialized training?   ☐ Yes   ☐ No
If "Yes", describe:

REFERENCES

Names of friends or relatives, if any, currently employed by Mountain View Health Care Center.

Name	Address	Phone
Name	Address	Phone

Names of co-workers (no relatives) you have worked with and whom we may contact for a reference.

Name	Address	Phone
Name	Address	Phone

Please read the following statements completely and carefully before you initial and sign your name.

The Applicant HEREBY CERTIFIES that the answers given on this Application For Employment, including any statements or answers provided by the Applicant during interview, are true and correct. The Applicant fully authorizes Mountain View Health Care Center to contact any references, past and present employers, persons, schools, law enforcement agencies and any other sources of information which may be relevant to the Applicant and this Application For Employment. It is understood and agreed that any misrepresentation, false statement, or omission by the Applicant will be sufficient reason for rejection of the Application For Employment or for dismissal from employment at any time, without recourse or liability to Mountain View Health Care Center.

I have read, understand and agree to the above statement.   (Please initial here). _____

SIGN HERE _____   DATE _____

Figure 24-5 ■ (continued)

When a potential employer calls to schedule an interview, the applicant is sometimes unavailable. Therefore, it is crucial for the applicants to record a professional outgoing voicemail message on the appropriate telephone. Mobile numbers are generally appropriate contact points for potential employers.

In Practice

Jerome is looking for employment as a medical assistant. He has submitted his résumé at several offices and has been waiting for telephone calls requesting interviews. When those calls come, the potential employers hear an unprofessional voicemail greeting left by Jerome and his roommate and decide to leave no message. What should Jerome do to increase his chances of gaining employment?

▶▶ Pulse Points

Using the Internet to Research a Candidate

Some employers today perform an online search for information about potential employees prior to hiring. Because information posted on the Internet is public, medical assistants should be careful that anything posted on Web sites, blogs, or social media sites is professional in nature.

Preparing for the Interview

The medical assistant will need to find out how long the commute to the interview will take. If there is time, making a trip prior to the interview is a good way for the medical assistant to gauge the amount of time needed to travel to the interview.

Before interviewing, the medical assistant should research the offices she will be visiting. Knowledge of the facility suggests interest in the practice and may win special attention from the employer. Assume, for example, an office is known for its success with a certain type of therapy. The applicant who asks about that therapy during the interview shows an interest and will likely stand out in the candidate pool. In addition to research, applicants should think of one or two appropriate questions to ask their prospective employer.

In general, questions about an office's history or industry trends are acceptable. Like doing research on the office beforehand, such questions demonstrate an applicant's interest and also prepare the applicant should the employer ask for questions when the interview closes. They also give an employer the chance to talk about their office.

The following are some things you should *not* do on the interview:

- Arrive with food or drink
- Cross the legs or arms
- Interrupt the employer while she is speaking
- Give one-word answers to questions
- Speak negatively of former employers
- Watch the clock

- Make jokes, especially off-color ones
- Arrive with a companion
- Request parking validation
- Ask about benefits, vacation pay, or time off
- Chew gum
- Answer cell phone or texts (your phone should be turned off during the interview)

Dressing for the Interview

When it comes time for the interview itself, several items are vital, including a working black or blue pen, a notepad, at least two copies of your résumé, and copies of reference letters, certifications, and awards. Appropriate dress is also a crucial part of the interview. Clothing should be clean and conservative as well as professional. Men should opt for a jacket and tie; women should wear clothing that fits properly and is cut modestly (**Figure 24-6 ■**). As a general rule, a professional image for an interview should be conservative in nature. Darker, nonpatterned colors are seen as more conservative, for example.

The applicant's personal hygiene, like her clothing, must be impeccable. Hands, nails, and teeth should be clean and groomed, and perfume and cologne should be nearly imperceptible. Smokers should try to erase all evidence of smoke on the clothing and the breath—all applicants should be pleasant and odor free. Men and women both should avoid large jewelry, although small earrings, necklaces, and wristwatches are appropriate when tasteful. Tattoos, whenever possible, should be covered; visible piercings, other than in the ears, are generally considered unprofessional

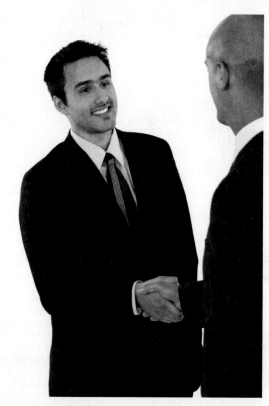

Figure 24-6 ■ Professional attire is appropriate for the medical office interview.
Source: Fotolia © auremar.

and should be removed prior to the interview. Women should take care that their blouse covers any cleavage and their skirts are of a conservative length. Shoes worn should also be conservative in nature, such as low heels or flat shoes.

Presenting the Right Image

At their initial meeting, the applicant should stand and shake the interviewer's hands. Eye contact should be direct when speaking; avoidance is viewed as deceptive. During the interview, applicants should strive to convey confidence. They should sit straight and speak in a calm, measured tone. Body language communicates a great deal to a prospective employer. Even when walking, applicants should maintain proper posture and avoid shuffling. When an applicant is prone to nerves, she can take notes to keep her hands busy (**Figure 24-7 ■**). At the end of the interview, the medical assistant should shake hands with the interviewer(s), thank them for their time and make a comment about looking forward to hearing from the interviewer(s) soon.

Common Interview Questions

While employers might ask specific questions about a candidates' experience and skills, there are some interview questions that are commonly asked. Medical assistants who have thought out how they might answer these common questions are better prepared for the interview. Some common questions include:

- Tell me why you want to work in health care.
- How would your coworkers (or supervisor) describe you?
- What would you say is your biggest weakness?
- Do you feel you work best alone, or in teams?
- What do you like to do in your free time?

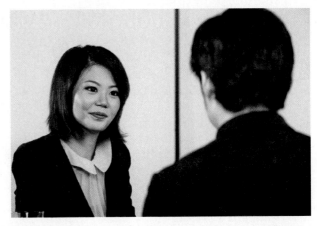

Figure 24-7 ■ The office manager interviews an applicant.
Source: Fotolia © Jenner.

Following Up After the Interview

Interview followup increases the likelihood of hiring. Followup both reminds the employer of the candidate and allows the candidate to ask questions, extend courtesies, and emphasize interest in employment. During the interview, the applicant should ask the interviewer for a date by which the decision for hiring will be made. The day after that date, the applicant should call the interviewer to whether a decision has been made and to inquire as to whether the interviewer has any additional questions of the applicant. The day after the interview is held, the candidate should send a handwritten thank-you note (**Figure 24-8 ■**).

Once a position has been offered to the medical assistant, a conversation regarding salary and benefits should ensue. At this point, the medical assistant might be able to negotiate terms of employment by asking for a higher salary, or additional vacation time, for example. These negotiations

---

September 4, 20xx

Dear Dr. Bryant:

Thank you for taking the time to interview with me on Monday. I enjoyed hearing about the advances you have made in the area of foot care for diabetic patients. As I stated during our meeting, I am very interested in working in the administrative area of your clinic and feel my qualifications are perfectly suited to what you are looking for in an administrative medical assistant.

If you would like to discuss the position further, I can be reached at (602) 555-0923. I welcome the opportunity to work with you in your clinic and hope that I will hear from you soon.

Sincerely,

Oksana Simonenko, CMA (AAMA)

Figure 24-8 ■ Sample interview thank you note.

PROCEDURE 24-3 Follow Up After an Interview

Theory and Rationale

Many medical offices interview several applicants for a single opening. To stand out in desired ways, medical assistants must find ways to make potential employers remember and want to hire them.

Materials

- Note card
- Blue or black pen

Competency

1. Handwrite or type a note to the interviewer.
2. Thank the person for the interview time.
3. List something about the position or office that inspires you to want to work there.
4. Express a desire to meet again.
5. Send the note immediately after the interview.

---

are typically done by medical assistants with more experience working in the medical field, or those who possess highly valued skills, such as fluency in multiple languages or training in a specialized area of health care.

Changing Jobs

Unlike 50 years ago, employees today tend to switch jobs every three to five years. As in all facets of medical assisting, it is impor-

tant to maintain professional protocol when leaving a job. To leave a position on good terms, the medical assistant should give the employer at least two weeks' notice in writing (four weeks if a supervisory position). During that period, it should be business as usual. Assistants should remain positive and continue performing their duties to the best of their abilities. They should clearly communicate the status of all projects, and they should also clean their workspace and return any office items. Finally, the assistant should ask the employer for a letter of recommendation (**Figure 24-9** ■).

November 11, 20xx

Re: Martin Hawkins, RMA (AMT)

To Whom It May Concern:

I have had the pleasure of working with Martin Hawkins from January 20xx to November 20xx when Martin and his family decided to relocate to Texas.

Martin has demonstrated a tremendous desire to learn, along with a drive to become the best he can be within his chosen profession within the health care field. His ability to work both alone and within groups is unsurpassed, and his attention to detail, especially in the area of patient confidentiality, will serve his future employer well.

I would highly recommend Martin Hawkins, RMA (AMT) for employment in a medical setting. He will make a valued asset to the medical office that recognizes his talents and abilities, and the patients he cares for will be fortunate to have him as their advocate.

Sincerely,

Sharon Tsete, MHA
Clinical Office Manager
Shoreline Family Medicine
(206) 555-9472

Figure 24-9 ■ Sample recommendation letter.

REVIEW

Chapter Summary

- An practicum program offers benefits for the medical assistant, the practicum site, and the medical assisting program.
- Attractive and effective résumés are critical tools for job seekers, whether those applicants are recently graduated students or established medical assistants.
- When résumés are clear, accurate, and written using action words, they can help medical assisting candidates secure jobs.
- Cover letters, like résumés, support job-searching initiatives by explaining to the potential employer the reasons why the applicant is right for the job.
- Medical assistants can search for job opportunities in varied places, such as newspapers, job fairs, local medical assisting programs, and on the Internet.

- Proper dress and body language are vital while interviewing.
- Interview followup can make the difference between a candidate securing the desired position or not. Followup techniques include sending a thank-you note to the potential employer and calling to see if the interviewer has any additional questions of the applicant.
- When a medical assistant decides to seek new employment, he should take all steps to leave his employer on good terms. Requesting a recommendation letter upon leaving the office may help secure a future position.

Chapter Review

Multiple Choice

1. During the practicum program, the student medical assistant should try to participate in areas devoted to:
   a. Administrative procedures
   b. Clinical procedures
   c. Administrative and clinical procedures
   d. Public relations
   e. None of the above

2. Which of the following is an "action" word?
   a. Monitored
   b. Willing
   c. Working
   d. Established
   e. All of the above

3. Which of the following is inappropriate for an interview?
   a. Three-inch pumps
   b. Necktie
   c. Suit jacket
   d. Modest attire
   e. All of the above

4. When job applicants change phone numbers, they should reflect the change on their résumés by:
   a. Crossing through the old number and handwriting the new one
   b. Whiting out the old number and handwriting the new one

   c. Placing a note over the old number about the change
   d. Retyping the number and reprinting the résumé
   e. None of the above

True/False

T F **1.** The U.S. Department of Labor predicts that medical assisting will grow by 31 percent between 2010 and 2020.

T F **2.** All practicum programs require 240 hours for accreditation.

T F **3.** Before witnessing patient procedures, the student medical assistant should ask for the patient's permission.

T F **4.** Before starting an practicum program, the student medical assistant should sign a HIPAA compliance form stating that she will disclose no patient information.

T F **5.** Sloppy and poorly written résumés suggest that work in the medical office will be similarly poor.

T F **6.** For medical assistants, scrubs are appropriate interview attire.

T F **7.** Résumés should reflect competencies such as fluency in sign language.

T F **8.** Attractive résumés gain attention through their appearance.

T F **9.** To gain attention, résumés should appear on bright paper, like bright pink or red.

T F **10.** It is acceptable to leave portions of employment applications blank.

T F **11.** Applicants who follow up with the employer after interviews are more likely to be hired.

Short Answer

1. Why is it important to get permission from professional references?
2. What is the purpose of the cover letter?
3. List several places the medical assistant may seek employment.

4. Why is it important to research offices before interviews?
5. Name several items that should not be taken to an interview.

Research

1. Looking at the jobs advertised for medical assistants in your area, what is the starting wage for a new medical assistant?
2. Search online for information on how to compose a professional résumé. What information did you find?
3. Ask one of your instructors to review your résumé and give you feedback on how you might improve it.

Practicum Application Experience

While the medical assisting student is completing an practicum in a family practice office, that assistant notices the physician appears to have made an error in a patient's medication. How should the assistant handle this situation?

Resource Guide

Absolutely Health Care (online community for posting résumés)
http://www.healthjobsusa.com/

Americans with Disabilities Act
http://www.ada.gov/workta.htm

Monster (Internet site for seeking employment)
www.monster.com

Indeed (Internet site for seeking employment)
www.indeed.com/

Appendix A

ICD-9-CM Diagnostic Coding

Introduction

ICD-9-CM provides the codes that identify all diagnoses physicians give patients. ICD-9-CM lists over 14,000 diagnostic codes in two volumes, plus a third volume that contains hospital inpatient procedure codes.

ICD-9-CM, implemented in 1979, was updated annually through October 1, 2013. At that time, updates ceased, in anticipation of ICD-10-CM being implemented on October 1, 2014. However, in April 2014, Congress delayed ICD-10-CM implementation until at least October 1, 2015. The exact implementation date had not been announced when this text went to press. ICD-9-CM will continue to be used as the HIPAA-mandated code set for diagnosis coding until ICD-10-CM is implemented. Medical assistants should use the edition of the ICD-9-CM that was in effect on the date of service.

Some payers that are not HIPAA-covered entities, such as worker's compensation and third-party liability carriers, will not be required to accept ICD-10-CM codes, so they may continue to use ICD-9-CM codes after ICD-10-CM implementation. It will be necessary to check with each individual carrier to learn which code set they will accept.

Organization of the ICD-9-CM Manual

Several companies publish the ICD-9-CM manual, so the exact order of information may vary, based on which publisher's book is used (Table A-1). A table of contents page near the front of the manual outlines the contents, organization, and page numbers of the ICD-9-CM.

The ICD-9-CM manual is separated into three volumes, as follows:

Volume I–Tabular List of Diseases

Volume II–Index to Diseases and Injuries

Volume III–Inpatient Procedures.

Each of the three ICD-9-CM volumes has a distinct purpose. Volume I is a Tabular List of diseases, Volume II is an alphabetic index of diseases, and Volume III is a Tabular List and alphabetic index of hospital procedures. Physicians use only Volumes I and II of ICD-9-CM. Hospitals use all three volumes.

In the physical organization of the manual, Volume II appears first, followed by Volume I, then Volume III. Many publishers print ICD-9-CM manuals for physician offices that contain only Volumes I and II, in order to save on cost. We first provide an overview of each volume in the order it appears in the book. Detailed coding instructions are presented later in this appendix. Each volume also uses a number of specialized rules, abbreviations, formatting, and symbols called conventions. These are described at the beginning of the manual. A key to selected symbols usually appears at the bottom of each page. The conventions and symbols are specific to each volume.

Introductory Material

The introductory material that appears at the beginning of the ICD-9-CM provides important information for medical assistants. Not only does it provide instructions on how to use ICD-9-CM, it also outlines the Official Guidelines for Coding and Reporting (OGCR), universal conventions, and publisher-specific conventions.

Official Guidelines for Coding and Reporting (OGCR)

The ICD-9-CM Official Guidelines for Coding and Reporting (OGCR) are rules that provide directions for how to code selected conditions and establish the rules for how to identify which diagnoses should be reported on a claim for any given patient. HIPAA requires that coders adhere to OGCR when assigning ICD-9-CM diagnosis codes. The OGCR also explain the conventions that are universal within the ICD-9-CM code set.

Conventions

Conventions are specialized rules, abbreviations, formatting, and symbols that alert users to important information. These are described at the beginning of the manual. A key to selected symbols usually appears at the bottom of each page. Official conventions are universal to all ICD-9-CM manuals while others are specific to each publisher.

Official ICD-9-CM Conventions Conventions that are an official part of the ICD-9-CM code set are explained in the OGCR and appear in Table A-2.

Publisher-Specific Conventions Publishers of the ICD-9-CM manual may use color-coding and special symbols to alert users to important information. Conventions that vary among publishers are publisher-specific conventions. Medical assistants can read the introductory material to learn about these conventions. A key that explains the conventions often appears at the bottom of the page in the Tabular List. Conventions are commonly used to indicate the following:

- New Code
- Revised Code
- Additional character(s) required
- Age-specific requirement
- Gender-specific requirement

TABLE A-1 Organization of the ICD-9-CM Manual

Type of Information	Name of Section	Purpose
Introductory Material	Preface Introduction How to Use the ICD-9-CM ICD-9-CM Official Conventions Additional Conventions ICD-9-CM Official Guidelines for Coding and Reporting	Information and rules on how to use the manual.
Volume II: Index	ICD-9-CM Index to Diseases (Index) ICD-9-CM Hypertension Table ICD-9-CM Table of Neoplasms ICD-9-CM Table of Drugs and Chemicals ICD-9-CM Index to External Causes	Alphabetical list of diseases and injuries, reasons for encounters, and external causes. Three tables provide quick look-ups for hypertension, neoplasms, and for drugs and chemicals causing injury. Coders must always reference one of these indices or tables when searching for a code.
Volume I: Tabular List	ICD-9-CM Tabular List of Diseases Supplementary Classification of External Causes of Injury and Poisoning (E000-E999) Appendix A: Morphology of Neoplasms Appendix B: Glossary of Mental Disorders (Deleted) Appendix C: Classification of Drugs by American Hospital Formulary Service Appendix D: Classification of Industrial Accidents According to Agency Appendix E: List of Three-digit Categories	Numerical list of diseases and injuries, reasons for encounters, and external causes. Provides additional instruction on how to use, assign, and sequence codes. Coders must always reference the Tabular List to verify a code, after consulting the Index, and before assigning the final code. The appendices provide reference information not needed by medical assistants on a daily basis.
Volume III:	Index to Hospital Inpatient Procedures Tabular List of Hospital Inpatient Procedures	Medical and surgical procedures reported by hospitals on inpatient claims.

TABLE A-2 ICD-9-CM Conventions

Convention	Meaning/Use
( ) Parentheses	**Tabular and Index:** Nonessential modifiers which describe the default variations of a term. These words are not required to appear in the documentation in order to use the code.
: Colon	**Tabular:** Appears after an incomplete term that requires one or more modifiers following the colon to be classified to that code or category.
[ ] Square brackets	**Tabular:** Synonyms, alternative wording, explanatory phrases. **Index:** Indicates sequencing on etiology/manifestation codes or other paired codes. The code in square brackets [ ] should be sequenced second.
And	**Tabular:** Means "and/or."
Boldface (Heavy type)	**Tabular:** Code titles. **Index:** Main Terms.
Code Also	**Tabular:** More than one code may be required to fully describe the condition.
Code First/Use Additional Code	**Tabular:** Provides sequencing instructions for conditions that have both an underlying etiology and multiple body system manifestations and certain other codes that have sequencing requirements.
Excludes	**Tabular:** Begins with the "Excludes" and identifies conditions that are not classified to the chapter, subchapter, category, subcategory, or specific subclassification code under which it is found.
Includes notes	**Tabular:** Begins with the word "Includes" and further defines, clarifies, or gives examples.
Italics (Slanted type)	**Tabular:** Exclusion notes, manifestation codes.
NEC	**Tabular and Index:** Not Elsewhere Classifiable. The medical record contains additional details about the condition, but there is not a more specific code available to use.
NOS	**Tabular:** Not Otherwise Specified. Information to assign a more specific code is not available in the medical record.
See	**Index:** It is necessary to reference another Main Term or condition to locate the correct code.
See Also	**Index:** Coder may refer to an alternative or additional Main Term if the desired entry is not found under the original Main Term.
With	**Tabular:** In a code title, means *both* or *together*

Volume II: *Index*

Volume II, which appears first in most ICD-9-CM coding manuals, contains three sections.

Section 1: Alphabetic Index to Diseases

Medical assistants use Section 1, the Alphabetical Index to Diseases (Index) as the first step in coding. Conditions, diseases, and reasons for seeking medical care are listed alphabetically by **Main Term** and **subterms** that aid in locating the most appropriate code. After identifying preliminary codes in the Index, they are verified in Volume I, the Tabular List. Final code selection should never be done based only on the Index. The Index contains two tables that have cross-tabbed index entries for hypertension and neoplasms. Detailed use of the Index and tables is described later.

Section 2: The Table of Drugs and Chemicals

Medical assistants use the Table of Drugs and Chemicals when a patient has been injured by a drug, chemical, biological, or other external agent. The table contains an alphabetical list of drugs and other chemical substances, cross-tabbed with a list of causes, to identify poisonings and external causes of drug-related adverse effects, such as drug-induced attempted suicide or an adverse reaction to penicillin. Detailed use of this table is discussed later.

Section 3: Alphabetic Index to External Causes of Injuries and Poisonings

When a condition is caused by an accident or other external event, supplemental codes describe the circumstances, such as a fall or motor vehicle accident. A separate index, referred to as the E-code index, provides an alphabetical list used to locate the external cause of an injury. Detailed use of the E-code index is described later.

Volume I: *Tabular List*

The Tabular List is divided into the main classification, supplementary classifications, and appendices.

Main Tabular List Classification (000-999)

The Tabular List is an alphanumerically sequenced list of all diagnosis codes, divided into 17 chapters based on cause, or etiology, and body system (Table A-3). After locating the diagnosis in the Index, medical assistants need to verify the code by referencing the Tabular List. Verifying a code means consulting the Tabular List to read detailed code descriptions, conventions, and instructional notes, and to assign additional specificity. Medical assistants need to know where to find the beginning of each chapter, because the beginning of the chapter provides global instructions that apply to all codes within the chapter. Each chapter begins with a heading

TABLE A-3 ICD-9-CM Tabular List

Chapter Number	Chapter Name	Code Range
1	Infectious and Parasitic Diseases	001–139
2	Neoplasms	140–239
3	Endocrine, Nutritional, and Metabolic Diseases and Immunity Disorders	240–279
4	Diseases of the Blood and Blood-Forming Organs	280–289
5	Mental, Behavioral, and Neurodevelopmental Disorders	290–319
6	Diseases of the Nervous System and Sense Organs	320–389
7	Diseases of the Circulatory System	390–459
8	Diseases of the Respiratory System	460–519
9	Diseases of the Digestive System	520–579
10	Diseases of the Genitourinary System	580–629
11	Complications of Pregnancy, Childbirth, and the Puerperium	630–679
12	Diseases of the Skin and Subcutaneous Tissue	680–709
13	Diseases of the Musculoskeletal System and Connective Tissue	710–739
14	Congenital Anomalies	740–759
15	Certain Conditions Originating in the Perinatal Period	760–779
16	Symptoms, Signs, and Ill-Defined Conditions	780–799
17	Injury and Poisoning	800–999
	Supplementary Classification of Factors Influencing Health Status and Contact with Health Services	V01–V91
	Supplementary Classification of External Causes of Injury and Poisoning	E800–E999
Appendix A	Morphology of Neoplasms	
Appendix B	Glossary of Mental Disorders	
Appendix C	Classification of Drugs by American Hospital Formulary Service	
Appendix D	Classification of Industrial Accidents	
Appendix E	List of Three-Digit Categories	

that states the chapter number and title. It can be helpful to place a self-adhesive tab on the first page of each chapter, to aid in locating it.

After locating the diagnosis in the appropriate index in Volume II, verify the code by referencing the Tabular List in Volume I. Volume I is a numerically-sequenced list of all diagnosis codes, divided into 17 chapters based on etiology of the disease or injury, as well as by location of the disease or injury on or in the body. Every chapter title describes the conditions within, followed by the range of three-digit codes within.

In addition to a title, each Volume I chapter has a subtitle in large print followed by a range of three-digit codes in that category. Each three-digit code describes a general disease; subsequent fourth and fifth digits add more specificity. Volume I identifies the number of digits needed for each code: three, four, or five.

Supplementary Classifications (E-codes and V-codes)

Following the 17 chapters listing codes 000-999, there are two sections with supplemental codes. The first of these, Supplementary Classification of Factors Influencing Health Status and Contact with Health Services, are commonly referred to as V-codes, because these codes begin with the letter "V" and range from V01 to V91. These codes classify the reason for care, other than an active illness. V-codes are located through the alphabetical index in Volume II, Section 1.

The second supplementary classification in Volume I is the Supplementary Classification of External Causes of Injury and Poisoning, commonly called E-codes, because these codes begin with the letter "E" and range from E800-E999. E-codes classify causes of injury and poisoning. E-codes are located through the index in Volume I, Section 2.

ICD-9-CM Appendices

Volume I of the ICD-9-CM book has five appendices. These appendices provide a clinical picture or further information about the patient's diagnosis. The appendices are used to further define the diagnosis, to classify new drugs, or to reference the type and cause of on-the-job injury the patient has sustained.

- **Appendix A: Morphology of Neoplasms**—This appendix provides "M" codes that indicate how neoplasms (tumors) have morphed to other body areas. M-codes are not used for billing; they are used only by tumor registries.
- **Appendix B: Glossary of Mental Disorders**—Appendix B was deleted from the ICD-9-CM coding manual on October 1, 2004, but a blank page still appears as a placeholder.
- **Appendix C: Classification of Drugs by American Hospital Formulary Service (AHFS)**—Each drug currently on the market appears here. This appendix is a cross-reference between the AHFS and the ICD-9-CM code for poisoning due to the drug.
- **Appendix D: Classification of Industrial Accidents**—This appendix lists reference information from the Statistics of

Employment used by labor statisticians in classifying on-the-job injuries. Injuries are classified by the type or place of accident. This information is not used in ICD-9-CM coding.
- **Appendix E: List of Three-Digit Categories**—All three-digit categories in the ICD-9-CM book appear here.

Volume III

Because Volume III of ICD-9-CM is used for inpatient procedure coding, medical assistants only use it if working in hospital settings. Though medical assistants may be hired by hospital-owned physician practices, the majority of hospitals hire professional certified coders to code inpatient charts.

Volume III contains an Index to Procedures, followed by the Tabular List of Procedures. Hospital procedure codes are three or four digits long, with a decimal point after the second digit, and range from 00.01 to 99.99. Physicians use the CPT® manual to code for procedures and services.

How to Assign ICD-9-CM Diagnosis Codes

Coding begins and ends with the patient's medical record. Medical assistants abstract information from the medical record in order to code for services and the reasons they were provided. Coding is to be performed to the highest level of certainty. All relevant information in the chart should be coded, but missing information should not be assumed or coded. Only conditions, diseases, and symptoms documented in the medical record can be coded and billed. If the medical record is incomplete or inaccurate, it should be corrected or amended, following proper procedures, before attempting to code.

Diagnosis coding involves three basic steps:

1. Identify the first-listed diagnosis.
2. Research the diagnosis in the Index.
3. Verify the code(s) in the Tabular List.

Several documents in the medical record contain information needed for coding. When coding for office-based or other outpatient services, medical assistants refer to the patient registration form, the encounter form, visit notes, lab and radiology reports, and to operative reports for outpatient procedures. When coding for services physicians provide to inpatients, medical assistants refer to the admitting history and physical (H&P), daily progress notes, operative reports, lab and radiology reports, and the discharge summary.

It is important to keep in mind that the diagnosis must describe 1) the reasons that the specific service was provided, and 2) related medical conditions that affect the specific service. Diagnosis codes should not repeat the patient's entire problem list. The problem list is a comprehensive list of all active conditions that often appears in the front of the medical record, but it does not document the reason(s) for a specific encounter.

Example: Code actively managed conditions

The physician sees a patient for a sinus infection who also has chronic gastric reflux. The physician prescribes an antibiotic for the sinus infection and inquires how the gastric reflux is doing, but does not further evaluate, treat, or manage it. The medical assistant should code only the sinus infection.

Example: Code all relevant medical conditions

A diabetic patient comes into the office for a burn on the hand. The physician treats the burn and indicates that the diabetes may slow the healing process and requires more frequent follow-up visits as a result. The medical assistant codes both the burn and the diabetes. The first listed diagnosis is the burn. The secondary diagnosis is diabetes.

The following coding steps provide the practical details medical assistants need to patiently and accurately execute the process. This discussion is oriented toward office-based coding.

Step 1. Identify the First-listed Diagnosis in the Medical Record

Medical assistants abstract information from the medical record in order to code for services and the reasons they were provided. Often the physician indicates a diagnosis code on the encounter form, but medical assistants may need to verify it against the medical record. Look for a definitive diagnostic statement by the physician regarding the reason for the visit (**Figure A-1** ■). The diagnosis may be indicated with the word *Impression* or, in SOAP notes, under *A (Assessment)*. This is the first-listed or primary diagnosis, the reason chiefly responsible for the services provided.

Uncertain or qualified diagnoses are those accompanied by terms such as *possible, probable, suspected, rule out (R/O),* or *working diagnosis*, indicating that the physician has not determined the root cause. For outpatient coding, do not use uncertain diagnoses. Instead, look for the patient's signs or symptoms that are part of the patient's chief complaint. The chief complaint is a statement in the patient's own words of the reason for the visit. Signs are indications of a condition that

---

the physician can observe or measure, such as a rash. Symptoms are indications reported by the patient that the physician cannot observe or measure, such as a headache.

Additional conditions or complaints become secondary diagnoses, which are coded in the same way as the primary, but listed after them on the CMS-1500 billing form. Signs and symptoms that are routinely associated with the first-listed diagnosis are not coded as secondary diagnoses.

Step 2. Research the Diagnosis in the Index

After determining the diagnosis in the patient's medical record, use the ICD-9-CM coding manual to assign the actual code number. The first step in using the coding manual is to identify the diagnosis in the Index. Using the Index involves three steps:

1. Locate the Main Term.
2. Read the subterms and modifiers.
3. Identify the preliminary code(s).

Locate the Main Term

Identify the word(s) from the first-listed diagnosis to be looked up as the Main Term in the Index (**Figure A-2** ■). The Main Term is always boldfaced with an initial capital letter. The Main Term may be any of the following:

- A condition, such as *Fracture*
- A disease, such as *Pneumonia*
- Reason for a visit, such as *Screening*
- Eponym (a disease or condition named after an individual), such as *Colles' fracture*
- Abbreviation or acronym, such as *AIDS*
- Nontechnical synonym (a word similar in meaning), such as *Broken* instead of fracture
- An adjective, such as *Twisted*

Some Main Terms are rather generic with pages of subterms, such as *Disease*, while others are quite specific with only a single code, such as *Duroziez's disease*.

Main Terms usually do not include anatomic sites. To locate a condition that affects a specific site, look up the condition itself as the Main Term. Then read the subterms to locate the anatomic site (**Figure A-3** ■).

Example: Anatomic sites

A medical assistant needs to code for an ankle sprain. She looks in the Index under *A* for the Main Term *Ankle*, and finds an entry with the cross reference *Ankle—see condition*. The condition is a sprain. She looks under *S* for the Main Term *Sprain* in the Index. Under *Sprain*, she locates the subterm, *ankle*. The subterm entry *ankle* provides additional subterms for the exact site and type of sprain.

---

fracture of left tibia
chest pain
sore throat
congestive heart failure
benign hypertension

Figure A-1 ■ Examples of diagnostic statements with Main Term underlined.

INDEX TO DISEASES AND INJURIES
A

AAT (alpha-1 antitrypsin) deficiency 273.4

AAV (disease) (illness) (infection) - see Human immunodeficiency virus (disease)
(illness) (infection)

Abactio - see Abortion, induced

Abactus venter - see Abortion, induced

Abarognosis 781.99

Abasia (-astasia) 307.9
  atactica 781.3
  choreic 781.3
  hysterical 300.11

Figure A-2 ■ Examples of Main Term entries in the Index to Diseases.

Leg - *see* condition

Stomach - *see* condition

Finger - *see* condition

Figure A-3 ■ Example of a cross reference for an anatomic site in the Index.

Read the Subterms and Modifiers

Modifiers and subterms provide additional information and variations on the condition described in the Main Term (**Figure A-4** ■).

Nonessential modifiers are words that appear in parentheses immediately after the Main Term. These words do not have to be present in the medical record in order to use the code, but if they are present, they confirm that the user has located the appropriate code. For example, the Main Term *Pneumonia* has many nonessential modifiers including *(acute)*, *(double)*, *(migratory)*, and others (**Figure A-5** ■).

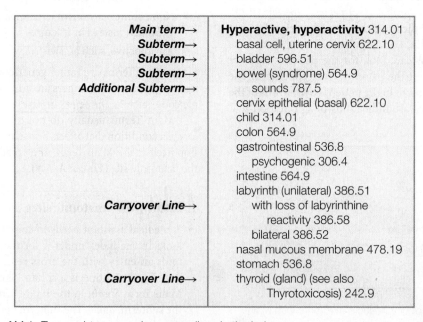

Main term→	**Hyperactive, hyperactivity** 314.01
Subterm→	basal cell, uterine cervix 622.10
Subterm→	bladder 596.51
Subterm→	bowel (syndrome) 564.9
Additional Subterm→	sounds 787.5
	cervix epithelial (basal) 622.10
	child 314.01
	colon 564.9
	gastrointestinal 536.8
	psychogenic 306.4
	intestine 564.9
	labyrinth (unilateral) 386.51
Carryover Line→	with loss of labyrinthine
	reactivity 386.58
	bilateral 386.52
	nasal mucous membrane 478.19
	stomach 536.8
Carryover Line→	thyroid (gland) (see also
	Thyrotoxicosis) 242.9

Figure A-4 ■ Example of Main Term, subterms, and carryover lines in the Index.

Pneumonia (acute) (double) (migratory) (purulent) (septic) (unresolved)

Figure A-5 ■ Example of Main Term with nonessential modifiers in the Index.

Pneumonia
anthrax 022.0 *[484.5]*

Figure A-6 ■ Example of the multiple coding convention in the Index.

Subterms are words indented two spaces under the bold-faced Main Term that further describe variations of the condition. Examples of types of subterms are:

- Etiology: Pneumonia, *allergic*
- Coexisting condition: Pneumonia, *with influenza*
- Anatomic site: Pneumonia, *interstitial*
- Episode: Pneumonia, *chronic*, or similar descriptors

Subterms often have additional levels of one or more of their own subterms, each of which are indented another two spaces.

Carryover lines are indented more than two spaces from the level of the preceding line. If the Main Term or subterm is too long to fit on one line, a carryover line is used. It is important to read carefully to distinguish between carry over lines and subterms.

Main terms or subterms may contain instructional notes, such as *see* or *see also*, which direct the user to other entries. For example, *Pneumonia, alveolar—see Pneumonia, other*. This instructs the user where to look for the code needed.

Entries under the Main Term may contain special formatting, such as slanted brackets, indicating that multiple coding may be required (**Figure A-6** ■). The second code in slanted brackets is required in addition to the first code to completely describe the condition. Multiple coding may also be indicated by instructional notes in the Tabular List to *Code first* a specific condition or to *Use additional code* to report an additional condition.

Identify the Preliminary Code(s)

When the appropriate subterms are located, the preliminary code(s) appears immediately to the right. It is helpful to jot down the appropriate codes before verifying in the Tabular List. Never use the Index to make the final code selection.

Step 3. Verify the Code in the Tabular List

The final step in coding is to verify the code in the Tabular List. To verify the code, read the detailed code description, interpret conventions and instructional notes, and assign the highest level of specificity. Verification requires five steps:

1. Locate the preliminary code(s) in the Tabular List.
2. Interpret the conventions and instructional notes.
3. Assign the highest level of specificity.
4. Compare the final code to the documentation.
5. Assign the code.

Locate the Preliminary Code(s) in the Tabular List

Look for the preliminary code number in the Tabular List which lists the code in alphanumeric order. The Tabular List contains 17 chapters based on etiology or the body system (Table A-3). Chapters are divided into sections with boldfaced or highlighted headings. Within the sections, the actual code numbers are tabulated in three levels: category (three-character entries), subcategory (four- and five-character entries), and codes (the most specific entry that requires no additional characters) (**Figure A-7** ■). It is helpful to learn the specific meanings of these designations, because the terms are used frequently in coding instructions.

Interpret the Conventions and Instructional Notes

Before verifying and finalizing the code, medical assistants must interpret the conventions presented with the code and its category. Tabular List conventions include punctuation, instructional notes, and symbols. Conventions may appear on the same line with the code, above it, below it, or at the beginning of a subcategory, category, section, or chapter. Look carefully for any information that may be relevant to the code selection. Additional information may direct you when to use a different code or an additional code, depending on your original diagnostic statement. In the Tabular List, the way in which punctuation is used has meaning (see Table A-2). Medical assistants should become familiar with these meanings.

Assign the Highest Level of Specificity

ICD-9-CM codes may be between 3 and 5 characters in length. There is no general rule regarding how many characters any given code will have. The number of characters is determined only after reading the instructional notes and conventions available in the category. Use the most specific code available in the Tabular List for the condition. Most coding manuals display a symbol or color-coding with entries that provide a more specific code (**Figure A-8** ■). Codes of the highest level of specificity may provide options for anatomic site, manifestations, and other details.

Compare the Final Code to the Documentation

As a final check, with coding manual instructions fresh in your mind, refer back to the original documentation and verify

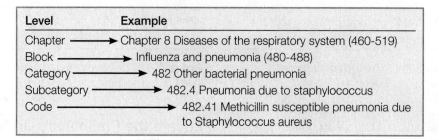

Level	Example
Chapter ⟶	Chapter 8 Diseases of the respiratory system (460-519)
Block ⟶	Influenza and pneumonia (480-488)
Category ⟶	482 Other bacterial pneumonia
Subcategory ⟶	482.4 Pneumonia due to staphylococcus
Code ⟶	482.41 Methicillin susceptible pneumonia due to Staphylococcus aureus

Figure A-7 ■ Organizational structure of ICD-9-CM chapters.

that all conditions of the code agree with the medical record. If a discrepancy arises, work through the process again from the beginning.

Assign the Code

Write down the final code where indicated on your worksheet or documentation. Be certain to proofread the number as you wrote or keyboarded it to avoid transcription errors that are easy to make.

Repeat this process for any additional codes required by the medical record.

Selecting a diagnosis code might seem like a long and tedious process at first. As medical assistants become familiar with the services and codes used by their medical office, coding becomes faster and easier, but accuracy and attention to detail is always paramount. Taking time and care to learn the fundamentals correctly helps create long-term success in the medical assistant's coding role.

Coding for Special Diagnostic Situations

As with any activity, there are always special situations that require additional information and knowledge. Diagnosis coding is the same. There are a number of conditions and

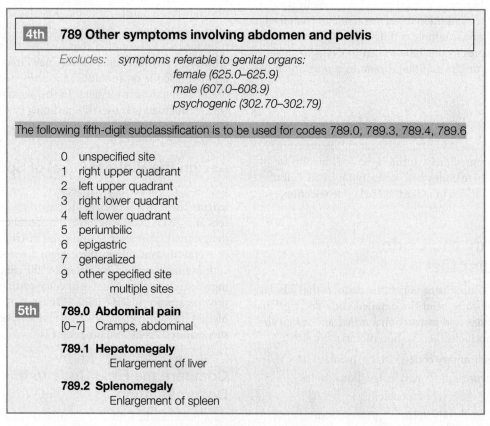

> **4th   789 Other symptoms involving abdomen and pelvis**
>
> Excludes: *symptoms referable to genital organs:*
> *female (625.0–625.9)*
> *male (607.0–608.9)*
> *psychogenic (302.70–302.79)*
>
> The following fifth-digit subclassification is to be used for codes 789.0, 789.3, 789.4, 789.6
>
> 0   unspecified site
> 1   right upper quadrant
> 2   left upper quadrant
> 3   right lower quadrant
> 4   left lower quadrant
> 5   periumbilic
> 6   epigastric
> 7   generalized
> 9   other specified site
>   multiple sites
>
> **5th   789.0 Abdominal pain**
> [0–7]   Cramps, abdominal
>
> **789.1 Hepatomegaly**
>   Enlargement of liver
>
> **789.2 Splenomegaly**
>   Enlargement of spleen

Figure A-8 ■ Examples of ICD-9-CM codes with varying number of characters.

circumstances that have unique tables, codes, and guidelines. An overview of these is provided in the remainder of the chapter.

Some conditions that frequently occur together may be described with a combination code. Careful reading of subterms in the Index and category *Includes* and *Excludes* notes in the Tabular List guide the medical assistant as to when a combination code is available. Combination code descriptions frequently contain specific words that indicate more than one condition is covered, such as *associated with, due to, secondary to, without, with, complicated by*, and *following*.

Medical assistants may work in offices that hire certified coders to assign and audit diagnosis codes. Whenever medical assistants are unsure of how to select a code, they should reach out to their supervisor or a certified coder. Reporting incorrect diagnosis codes on an insurance claim can create problems such as improper reimbursement, inaccurate patient medical history, and fraud. Awareness of special coding situations enables medical assistants to show their professionalism by recognizing when additional expertise is required.

Hypertension Table

Hypertension is a condition of elevated blood pressure over an extended period of time. It has been called *the silent killer* because it damages organs and causes numerous health issues without manifesting any symptoms until severe damage has occurred.

ICD-9-CM provides the Hypertension Table to aid in coding for hypertension. The Hypertension Table appears in the Index alphabetized under the letter H. **Figure A-9 ■** provides a complete listing of all conditions associated with hypertension. Four columns are shown:

- Hypertension/hypertensive condition
- Malignant
- Benign
- Unspecified

When there are no hypertensive conditions or manifestations, select a code from the first row, *Hypertension*. When a hypertensive condition or manifestation exists, locate the corresponding row in the first column. Then use the column *malignant, benign*, or *unspecified*, based on the documentation. Select the code where the row and column intersect. As with any other code, after the preliminary code has been identified in the Hypertension Table, verify the code in the Tabular List

Neoplasms

Neoplasm is the medical term for an abnormal growth of new tissue, often referred to as a tumor. Neoplasms can occur in any type of tissue anywhere in the body, and they can be either malignant or benign. Tumors that have cellular characteristics that cause them to invade adjacent healthy tissue or spread to distant sites are malignant, or life-threatening. The spreading of malignant neoplasm is called metastasis. Tumors that do not have these characteristics are benign. The Table of Neoplasms provides the index to the behaviors and anatomic sites of neoplasms (**Figure A-10 ■**).

The Table of Neoplasms lists the anatomical sites alphabetically. For each site, there are up to six possible codes, based on the type of neoplasm behavior.

Primary—Site of origin. Malignant neoplasms are coded as primary unless otherwise stated in the medical record.

Secondary—Site of metastasis, so stated in the medical record.

Ca in situ—Cells that have begun to change but have not yet invaded normal tissue, so stated in the medical record.

Benign—non-invasive.

Uncertain behavior—The pathologist clearly indicates that further study is needed before determining the benign or malignant behavior.

Unspecified—The medical record does not contain adequate description of the neoplasm, which may happen with a patient who has relocated and whose previous medical records are not yet available.

After determining the anatomic site and the type of behavior, select the code from the appropriate column, then verify it in the Tabular List.

Hypertension Table	Malignant	Benign	Unspecified
Hypertension, hypertensive (arterial) (arteriolar) (crisis) (degeneration) (disease) (essential) (fluctuating) (idiopathic) (intermittent) (labile) (low renin) (orthostatic) (paroxysmal) (primary) (systemic) (uncontrolled) (vascular)	401.0	401.1	401.9
with			
chronic kidney disease			
stage I through stage IV, or unspecified	403.00	403.10	403.90
stage V or end stage renal disease	403.01	403.11	403.91

Figure A-9 ■ Hypertension Table.

	Malignant					
	Primary	Secondary	Ca in situ	Benign	Uncertain Behavior	Unspecified
Neoplasm, neoplastic	199.1	199.1	234.9	229.9	238.9	239.9
abdomen, abdominal	195.2	198.89	234.8	229.8	238.8	239.8
cavity	195.2	198.89	234.8	229.8	238.8	239.8
organ	195.2	198.89	234.8	229.8	238.8	239.8
viscera	195.2	198.89	234.8	229.8	238.8	239.8
acoustic nerve	192.0	198.4	–	225.1	237.9	239.7
acromion (process)	170.4	198.5	–	213.4	238.0	239.2
adenoid (pharynx) (tissue)	147.1	198.89	230.0	210.7	235.1	239.0

Figure A-10 ■ Table of Neoplasms.

Example: Coding for neoplasms

Patient presents with primary carcinoma of the abdominal cavity. Carcinoma can be coded from the Table of Neoplasms. Locate the term *Abdomen*. Locate the column *Primary*. Select the code where the row and column intersect. Verify the code in the Tabular List.

> *ICD-9-CM Code:* 195.2 Malignant neoplasm of abdomen

V-Codes: Factors Influencing Health Status and Contact with Health Services

Not all patients who seek health care services have a specific disease or condition. They might receive services such as preventive care, therapy, followup, suture removal, or pregnancy supervision. They might have problems that require screening. They might carry certain risk factors or have a certain health status that affects treatment and require coding. All of these are examples of situations that require V-codes.

V-codes fall into one of three general categories: health status problems, encounter for certain services, or other health-related information relevant to the encounter. V-codes are indexed in the alphabetical index of Volume II. The V-code Tabular List appears in Volume I after category 999.

1. **Health Status Problems:** V-codes identify a problem that could affect a patient's overall health status but is not itself a current illness or injury. The V-code in this example is supplemental.

   Example: V-code for a health status problem
   A patient with strep throat needs an antibiotic, but is allergic to penicillin.
   > *ICD-9-CM Codes:* 034.0 Streptococcal sore throat
   > V14.0 Personal history of allergy to penicillin

2. **Services:** A V-code can be used to describe circumstances in addition to the illness or injury that prompted the patient's visit, such as encounters for antineoplastic therapy. The V-code is sequenced first because it is the main reason for the encounter. The disease is coded in addition to the V-code.

   Example: V-code to identify the reason for the encounter
   Patient is seen for chemotherapy to treat her colon cancer.
   > *ICD-9-CM Codes:* V58.11 Encounter for antineoplastic chemotherapy
   > 153.3 Malignant neoplasm of sigmoid colon

3. **Health-related information:** V-codes are used to describe certain facts that do not fall into the "problem" or "service" categories.

   Example: V-codes to identify health history
   A patient with a family history of colon cancer presents with rectal bleeding (569.3).
   > *ICD-9-CM Codes:* 569.3 Hemorrhage of rectum and anus
   > V16.0 Family history of malignant neoplasm of gastrointestinal tract

   Example: V-codes to identify exposure to a contagious disease
   A patient presents to a health care facility for care after having unprotected sex with a partner who has tested positive for human immunodeficiency virus (HIV).
   > *ICD-9-CM Code:* V01.79 Contact with or exposure to other viral diseases

Fractures

Fractures may be traumatic (due to injury) or pathological (due to disease). When coding fractures, the following information is required:

- Nature of fracture (traumatic or pathological)
- Anatomic site
- Type of fracture (transverse, spiral, comminuted, etc.)
- Open or closed

Search the Index for the Main Term *Fracture*. Locate subterms for the anatomic site and type of fracture. Verify the code in the Tabular List to confirm all details of the fracture and assign any additional digits required.

Example: Coding for fractures

A patient is treated for a fracture to the base of the skull. She has closed subdural hemorrhage and was unconscious for 2 hours.

> *ICD-9-CM Code:* 801.23 Fracture of base of the skull, closed with subarachnoid, subdural, and extradural hemorrhage, with moderate loss of consciousness.

E-Codes: External Cause of Illness or Injury

E-codes are a supplementary classification that describes the external cause of illness or injury. They are never the first-listed diagnosis and are never used alone. They must be preceded by a diagnostic code from 001 to 999.

Example: E-codes

A patient is being treated for a fractured ulna because he fell off a ladder.

> *ICD-9-CM Codes:* 813.22 Closed fracture of shaft of ulna (alone)
> E881.0 Accidental fall from ladder

Examples of when external cause codes are used include:

- A patient was involved in a motor vehicle accident.
- A patient was a pedestrian who was struck by a car while crossing the street.
- A patient fell off a ladder at home.
- A patient was injured as a result of a medical mistake, such as the physician operating on the wrong limb.
- A patient was bitten by a poisonous spider.
- A patient was knocked down at a sporting event.
- A patient was assaulted by another person.

E-codes have a separate index in Volume II, which begins after the alphabetic index and after the Table of Drugs and Chemicals. E-codes also have a separate Tabular List, which appears in Volume I after the V-codes.

Poisonings and Adverse Effects

When coding for drugs or chemicals that have caused poisonings or adverse reactions, the medical assistant needs to determine the type of drug or chemical involved, if the event was accidental or purposeful, and whether the substance was prescribed by a health care provider. Table A-4 outlines external causes, event descriptions, and ranges where codes can be found.

ICD-9-CM provides the Table of Drugs and Chemicals (**Figure A-11 ■**) to assist in coding these circumstances. It is a cross-tabulated index to the type of poisoning or adverse effect and the substance that caused them. Codes identify the substance used and the intent. Use this table as follows:

1. Locate the row in the Substance column that contains the name of the substance, listed alphabetically on the left side of the table.
2. For poisonings, select a code from the second column, Poisoning, *and* a second code that identifies the intent: accident, suicide attempt, assault, undetermined.
3. For reactions to drugs administered as prescribed, select a code from the column Therapeutic use.
4. Locate the preliminary code where the substance row and intent column intersect.
5. Verify the preliminary code in the Tabular List to identify the full code.
6. When more than one substance is involved, assign a separate code for each substance.
7. Assign additional codes to identify the condition that resulted from the use of the substance. When coding a poisoning, the poisoning code from the table is sequenced first, followed by the E-code for the substance, and finally the code(s) for the condition that resulted. When coding therapeutic use, sequence the condition (effect) code first, followed by the code from the table.

TABLE A-4 Poisonings and Adverse Effect Codes

External Cause	Code Description	Code Range
Poisoning	Assigned to a patient according to the classification of the drug or chemical in the poisoning.	960–989
Accidental	Used for accidental overdose, wrong substance given or taken, drug taken accidentally, or accidental use of a drug or chemical during a medical procedure.	E850–E869
Therapeutic use	Used for the external effect caused by a correct substance properly administered that caused an adverse or allergic reaction.	E930–E949
Suicide attempt	Used to report attempted suicide via drugs or chemicals.	E950–E959
Assault	Used to report a poisoning that was inflicted on another person with the intent to harm or kill.	E961–E962
Unknown	Used when the medical record is unclear whether the poisoning was intentional or accidental.	E980–E982

Substance	Poisoning	Accident	Therapeutic Use	Suicide Attempt	Assault	Undetermined
Antidepressants	969.00	E854.0	E939.0	E950.3	E962.0	E980.3
monoamine oxidase inhibitors (MAOI)	969.01	E854.0	E939.0	E950.3	E962.0	E980.3
specified type NEC	969.09	E854.0	E939.0	E950.3	E962.0	E980.3
SSNRI (selective serotonin and norepinephrine reuptake inhibitors)	969.02	E854.0	E939.0	E950.3	E962.0	E980.3
SSRI (selective serotonin reuptake inhibitors)	969.03	E854.0	E939.0	E950.3	E962.0	E980.3
tetracyclic	969.04	E854.0	E939.0	E950.3	E962.0	E980.3
tricyclic	969.05	E854.0	E939.0	E950.3	E962.0	E980.3
Antidiabetic agents	962.3	E858.0	E932.3	E950.4	E962.0	E980.4

Figure A-11 ■ Example of the Table of Drugs and Chemicals.

Burns

Burns may be caused by a source of heat or radiation or by a chemical. Both types are classified under the Main Term *Burn* in the Index. Codes for burns identify both the anatomic site and the degree (first, second, third).

Assign a code for the highest degree of burn at each site and an additional code for the extent of the total body surface area (TBSA) affected by third-degree burns. Codes for TBSA are based on the "rule of nines" in estimating the body surfaces involved, as illustrated in **Figure A-12** ■. Assign external cause codes where applicable.

Example: Coding for burns

A patient suffered third-degree burns to the back and the back of the left arm, and second-degree burns to the back of the left leg when she fell into a campfire.

> ***ICD-9-CM Codes:*** 942.34 Full-thickness skin loss [third degree, not otherwise specified] of back [any part]
> 943.39 Full-thickness skin loss [third degree, not otherwise specified] of multiple sites of upper limb, except wrist and hand
> 945.24 Blisters with epidermal loss due to burn (second degree) of lower leg

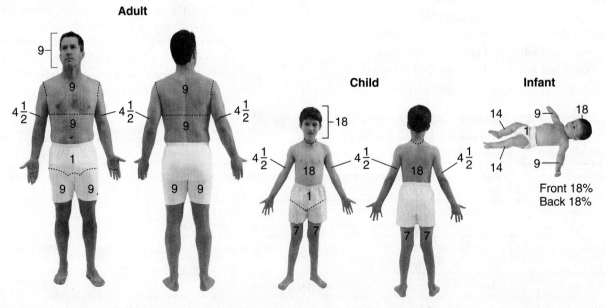

Note: Each arm totals 9% (front of arm $4\frac{1}{2}$ %, back of arm $4\frac{1}{2}$ %)

Figure A-12 ■ Rule of nines.

TABLE A-5 Coding for Stages of HIV/AIDS

Stage of Disease	ICD-9-CM Code
Exposure to HIV virus	V01.79 Contact with or exposure to other viral diseases
HIV testing	V73.89 Special screening examination for other specified viral diseases
Nonconclusive test results	795.71 Nonspecific serologic evidence of human immunodeficiency virus [HIV]
Confirmed HIV (seropositive)	V08 Asymptomatic human immunodeficiency virus [HIV] infection status
HIV counseling	V65.44 Human immunodeficiency virus (HIV) counseling
AIDS manifestations or illnesses	042 Human immunodeficiency virus [HIV] disease

948.32 Burn [any degree] involving 30–39 percent of body surface with third-degree burn, 20–29%

E897 Accident caused by controlled fire not in building or structure

E888.8 Other fall

HIV

Codes for HIV and AIDS differ based on the stage in the disease cycle, as summarized in Table A-5. In addition, assign codes for all AIDS-related illnesses.

Influenza

Influenza is a condition that medical assistants encounter frequently. Influenza is caused by one of several types of viruses, such as avian, novel A, H1N1, and swine, and may have manifestations that affect the respiratory system, digestive system, or heart. To code for influenza, locate the Main Term *Influenza*, then locate the subterm for the specific virus or *unidentified*, then locate the next level of subterm to identify the manifestations. Verify the code in the Tabular List.

Example: Coding for influenza

A patient presents with laryngitis that the physician diagnoses as an unidentified influenza virus.

ICD-9-CM Code: 487.1 Influenza with other respiratory manifestations

Obstetrics

Obstetric coding is one of the more complex areas of coding because multiple codes are required for anything other than a normal delivery of a single liveborn infant. All visits for supervision of a pregnancy require a V-code from the category V22 for a normal pregnancy or V23 for a high-risk pregnancy. These codes can be located in the Index under *Pregnancy, supervision.* Carefully review the subcategories to ensure correct code selection.

Complications of pregnancy are located in the Index under *Pregnancy, complicated by* or *Pregnancy, management affected by.* Chapter 11 of the Tabular List (630–679) contains the codes for complications of pregnancy, childbirth and the puerperium (six weeks after delivery). These codes are used only on the record of the mother. Most complications of pregnancy have a unique code from Chapter 11 that is to be used in place of, or in addition to, a code for the same condition in a nonpregnant person (Table A-6).

Example: Pregnancy-related condition

A pregnant woman, age 29, presents for a prenatal visit at 30 weeks of gestation. She has gestational diabetes (diabetes caused by pregnancy) that has been successfully controlled with diet. This is her first pregnancy.

ICD-9-CM Codes: V22.0 Supervision of normal first pregnancy

648.83 Abnormal glucose tolerance of mother, antepartum condition or complication

Example: Pre-existing condition affecting pregnancy

A pregnant woman, age 32, presents for monitoring of pre-existing Type I diabetes. This is her second pregnancy and she has completed 14 weeks of gestation.

TABLE A-6 Obstetrics Coding

Type of Encounter	Index Main Term and Subterms
Routine prenatal visit	**Index:** *Pregnancy, supervision*
Complications of pregnancy	**Index:** *Pregnancy, complicated by*
Normal delivery	**Tabular List:** 650 Normal delivery V27.0 Outcome of delivery, single liveborn
Delivery with complications	**Index:** *Delivery, complicated by* *Outcome of delivery* (Category V27)
Cesarean delivery	**Index:** *Delivery, cesarean* *Outcome of delivery* (Category V27)
Birth encounter for the newborn	Categories V30–V39 Liveborn infants according to place of birth and type of delivery **Index:** *Newborn, affected by*

ICD-9-CM Codes: 648.03 Antepartum diabetes mellitus 250.01 Diabetes mellitus without mention of complication, type I [juvenile type], not stated as uncontrolled

The birth episode requires codes for the delivery, any complications, and the outcome of delivery. A normal delivery is defined as a vaginal delivery needing minimal or no assistance, resulting in a single liveborn infant. Multiple births, cesarean sections, and complicated deliveries require multiple codes that describe all the circumstances. All delivery encounters require an additional code to identify the number of livebirths and stillbirths. These codes appear in category V27 and are indexed under the Main Term entry *Outcome of delivery.*

Example: Obstetrics coding

Delivery of twins by vaginal delivery with no antepartum or postpartum complication, both liveborn.

ICD-9-CM Codes: 651.01 Twin pregnancy, delivered, with or without mention of antepartum condition V27.2 Outcome of delivery, twins, both liveborn

A separate medical record is opened for all liveborn infants. The infant's record requires a code from the range V30–V39, which describes the location of birth and the existence of multiple liveborn or stillborn mates. For example, V31.00 Twin birth, mate liveborn, born in hospital, delivered without mention of cesarean section. Any other medical conditions of the infant are assigned additional codes to describe the problem.

Diabetes

Not only is diabetes mellitus (DM) a common condition, it causes and impacts many other conditions, so medical assistants frequently encounter the need to code for it. Medical assistants need to thoroughly review the medical record to abstract certain facts about patients' DM: whether it is type I, type II, or unspecified; whether it is stated as being uncontrolled; what complications exist.

To code for diabetes, locate the Main Term *Diabetes* in the Index. Select the appropriate subterm for the type of diabetes: *type I, type II,* or *secondary,* and a subterm for any manifestations. All diabetes codes must be verified in the Tabular List in order to assign the fifth digit and any additional codes for manifestations. Type I and type II usually lead to a code from category 250. Acute manifestations or complications are coded with subcategories 250.1 to 250.3. Chronic manifestations are coded with subcategories 250.4 through 250.9, based on body system affected. For all diabetes codes, the fifth digit identifies type of DM and whether or not it is uncontrolled. Secondary diabetes—diabetes caused by another condition—is coded from category 249.

If more than one body system is affected, use a code from each body system, and be certain the fifth digit is the same for all. For each body system with manifestation(s), an additional code is required to specify the nature of the manifestation. The most common manifestations are listed in the instructional notes within each subcategory. Verify the manifestation code where it originally appears within the Tabular List.

When a type II diabetic requires long-term insulin use, assign the additional code V58.67 to report this information.

Example: Diabetes coding

Type II DM, with long-term insulin use and associated glaucoma.

ICD-9-CM Codes: 250.50 Diabetes with ophthalmic manifestations, type II or unspecified type, not stated as uncontrolled
365.44 Glaucoma associated with systemic syndromes
V58.67 Long-term (current) use of insulin

Appendix B

Correlation of Text to Certification Exams, ABHES Competencies, and CAAHEP Standards

CMA (AAMA) Certification/Recertification Examination Content Outline

Competencies	Chapter Reference(s)
I. A-F General	
A. Medical Terminology	3, 7, Appendix C
1. Word building and definitions	3, 7, Appendix C
a. Basic structure	7, Appendix C
(1) Roots or stems	
(2) Prefixes	
(3) Suffixes	
(4) Abbreviations	
b. Surgical procedures	Appendix C
c. Diagnostic procedures	Appendix C
d. Medical specialties	3
2. Uses of terminology	Appendix C
a. Spelling	7, Appendix C
b. Selection and use (e.g., data entry, reports, records, documents, patient education, correspondence, medicolegal documentation, letters memos, messages, facsimiles)	7, Appendix C
c. Reference sources	7, Appendix C
D. Professionalism	3
1. Displaying professional attitude	3
a. Supporting professional organization	3
b. Accepting responsibility for own actions	3
2. Job readiness and seeking employment	24
a. Résumé and cover letter	24
b. Methods of job searching	24
c. Interviewing as a job candidate	24
3. Working as a team member to achieve goals	3, 5, 6
a. Member responsibility	3, 6
b. Promoting competent patient care	3, 5
c. Utilizing principles of group dynamics	6
E. Communication	6
1. Adapting communication according to an individual's needs	6
a. Blind	6
b. Deaf	6
c. Elderly	6
d. Children	6
e. Seriously ill	6
f. Mentally impaired	6

(continued)

Competencies	Chapter Reference(s)
g. Illiterate	6
h. Non-English speaking	6
i. Anxious	6
j. Angry/distraught	6
k. Culturally different	6
2. Recognizing and responding to verbal and nonverbal communication	6
a. Body language	6
b. Listening skills	6
c. Eye contact	6
d. Barriers to communication	6
e. Identifying needs of others	6
3. Professional communication and behavior	6
a. Professional situations	6
(1) Tact	
(2) Diplomacy	
(3) Courtesy	
(4) Responsibility/Integrity	
b. Therapeutic relationships	6
(1) Impartial behavior	
(2) Empathy/sympathy	
(3) Understanding emotional behavior	
4. Patient interviewing techniques	4, 6
a. Types of questions	6
(1) Exploratory	
(2) Open-ended	
(3) Direct	
b. Evaluating effectiveness	6
(1) Observation	
(2) Active listening	
(3) Feedback	
c. Legal restrictions	4, 6
5. Receiving, organizing, prioritizing, and transmitting information	9
a. Modalities for incoming and outgoing data (e.g., mail, fax, telephone, computer)	9
b. Prioritizing incoming and outgoing data (e.g., importance, urgency, recipient availability)	9
6. Telephone techniques	8
a. Incoming calls management criteria	8
(1) Screening	
(2) Maintaining confidentiality	
(3) Gathering data	
(4) Multiple-line competency	
(5) Transferring appropriate calls	
(6) Identifying caller, office, and self	
(7) Taking messages	
(8) Ending calls	

(continued)

Competencies	Chapter Reference(s)
b. Monitoring special calls	8
(1) Problem calls (e.g., unidentified caller, angry patient, family member)	
(2) Emergency calls	
7. Fundamental writing skills	7
a. Sentence structure	7
b. Grammar	7
c. Punctuation	7
F. Medicolegal guidelines and requirements	4
1. Licenses	4
a. Medical practice acts	4
b. Revocation/suspension of license	4
(1) Criminal/unprofessional conduct	
(2) Professional/personal incapacity	
2. Legislation	4, 5
a. Advance directives	4
b. Anatomical gifts	5
c. Reportable incidences	5
(1) Public health statutes (e.g., communicable diseases, vital statistics, substance abuse/chemical dependency, abuse against persons)	
(2) Wounds of violence	
d. Occupational Safety and Health Act (OSHA)	4
e. Food and Drug Administration (FDA)	4
f. Clinical Laboratory Improvement Act (CLIA '88)	4
g. Americans with Disabilities Act (ADA)	4
h. Health Insurance Portability and Accountability Act (HIPAA)	4
3. Documentation/reporting	4, 11, 17, 23
a. Sources of information	4
b. Drug Enforcement Administration (DEA)	4
c. Internal Revenue Service (e.g., personnel forms)	4
d. Employment laws	4
e. Personal injury occurrences	4
f. Workers' compensation	17
g. Medical records	11
(1) Patient activity	
(2) Patient care	
(3) Patient confidentiality	
(4) Ownership	
h. Personnel records	22
(1) Performance evaluation	
(2) Privacy	

(continued)

Competencies	Chapter Reference(s)
4. Releasing medical information	4, 11
a. Consent	4, 11
(1) Patient written authorization	
(2) Federal codes	
(a) Right to privacy	
(b) Drug and alcohol rehabilitation records	
(c) Public health and welfare disclosures	
(d) HIV-related issues	
(e) Subpoena duces tecum	
b. Rescinding authorization for release	11
5. Physician–patient relationship	4, 17
a. Contract	4
(1) Legal obligations	
(2) Consequences for noncompliance	
b. Responsibility and rights	4
(1) Patient	
(2) Physician	
(3) Medical assistant	
c. Guidelines for third-party agreements	17
d. Professional liability	4
(1) Current standard of care	
(2) Current legal standards	
(3) Informed consent	
e. Arbitration agreements	4
f. Affirmative defenses	4
(1) Statute of limitations	
(2) Comparative/contributory negligence	
(3) Assumption of risk	
g. Termination of medical care	4
(1) Establishing policy	
(2) Elements for withdrawal	
(3) Patient notification and documentation	
h. Medicolegal terms and doctrines	4
6. Maintaining confidentiality	4
a. Agent of physician	4
(1) Patient rights	
(2) Releasing patient information	
b. Intentional tort	4
(1) Invasion of privacy	
(2) Slander and libel	
7. Performing within ethical boundaries	5
a. Ethical standards	5
(1) AAMA Code of Ethics	
(2) AMA Code of Ethics	

(continued)

Competencies	Chapter Reference(s)
b. Patient rights	5
c. Current issues in medical bioethics	5
II. G-Q Administrative	4, 6, 8–16, 21, 22
G. Data Entry	
1. Keyboard fundamentals and functions	13
a. Alpha, numeric, and symbol keys	13
b. Tabulation	13
2. Formats	7
a. Letters	7
b. Memos	7
c. Reports	7
d. Envelopes	7
e. Chart notes	7
3. Proofreading	7
a. Proofreader's marks	7
b. Making corrections from rough draft	7
H. Equipment	8, 14
1. Equipment operation	8, 14
a. Calculator	14
b. Photocopier	14
c. Computer	14
d. Fax machine	14
e. Telephone services and features	8
f. Scanners	14
2. Maintenance and repairs	14
a. Contents of instruction manual	14
b. Routine maintenance	14
(1) Agreements	
(2) Warranty	
(3) Repair service	
3. Protection and safety	14
I. Computer Concepts	13
1. Computer components	13
a. Technology	13
b. Central processing unit (CPU)	13
c. Printer	13
d. Disk drive	13
e. Storage devices (e.g., hard drives, magnetic tapes, CD-ROMs, flash drives)	13
f. Operating systems	13
g. Basic commands	13
2. Computer applications	13
a. Word processing	13
b. Database (e.g., menu, fields, records, files)	13
c. Spreadsheets, graphics	13

(continued)

Competencies	Chapter Reference(s)
d. Electronic mail	13
e. Networks	13
f. Security/password	13
g. Medical management software	13
(1) Patient data	
(2) Report generation	
3. Internet services	13
J. Records management	11
1. Needs, purposes, and terminology of filing systems	11
a. Basic filing systems	11
(1) Alphabetic	
(2) Numeric/terminal digit	
(3) Subject	
b. Special filing systems	11
(1) Color-code	
(2) Tickler file	
(3) Electronic data processing files (EDP)	
(4) Cross-reference/master file	
2. Filing guidelines	11
a. Storing	11
b. Protecting/safekeeping	11
c. Transferring	11
3. Medical records (paper/electronic)	11, 12
a. Organization of patient's medical record	11,12
b. Types	11
(1) Problem-oriented	
(2) Source-oriented	
c. Collecting information	11, 12
d. Making corrections	11, 12
e. Retaining and purging	11
(1) Statute of limitations	
K. Screening and processing mail	7
1. U.S. Postal Service	7
a. Classifications	7
b. Types of mail services	7
2. Processing machine/meter	7
3. Processing incoming mail	7
4. Preparing outgoing mail	7
a. Labels	7
b. Optical character recognition (OCR) guidelines	7
L. Scheduling and monitoring appointments	10
1. Utilizing appointment schedules/types	10
a. Stream	10
b. Wave/modified wave	10

(continued)

Competencies	Chapter Reference(s)
c. Open booking	10
d. Categorization	10
2. Appointment guidelines	10
a. Appointment schedule matrix	10
b. Legal aspects	10
c. New/established patient	10
d. Patient needs/preference	10
e. Physician preference/habits	10
f. Facilities/equipment requirements	10
3. Appointment protocol	8, 9, 10
a. Follow-up visits	10
(1) Routine	
(2) Urgent	
b. Emergency/acutely ill	8, 10
c. Physician referrals	10
d. Cancellations/no-shows	9, 10
e. Physician delay/unavailability	9, 10
f. Outside services (e.g., lab, X-ray, surgery)	10
g. Reminders/recalls	10
(1) Appointment cards	
(2) Phone calls	
M. Resource information and community services	6, 15
1. Patient advocate	6, 15
a. Services available	6, 15
b. Appropriate referrals	6, 15
c. Follow-up	6, 15
N. *(Currently there are no items for this category)*	
O. Maintaining the office environment	4, 14, 16, 22
1. Physical environment	4, 14, 16, 22
a. Arrangement of furniture, equipment, and supplies	14, 22
b. Facilities and equipment	4, 14, 16, 22
(1) Maintenance and repair	
(2) Safety regulations	
(a) Occupational Safety and Health Act (OSHA)	
(b) Centers for Disease Control and Prevention (CDC) guidelines	
(c) Americans with Disabilities Act (ADA)	
(d) Fire regulations	
(e) Security systems	
2. Equipment and supply inventory	14
a. Inventory control	14
b. Purchasing	14
3. Maintaining liability coverage	22
a. Types of coverage	22
b. Recordkeeping	22

(continued)

Competencies	Chapter Reference(s)
4. Time management	3, 22
a. Establishing priorities	3, 22
b. Managing routine duties	3, 22
P. Office policies and procedures	15
1. Patient information booklet	15
2. Personnel manual	15
3. Policy and procedures manuals/protocols	15
Q. Practice Finances	21
1. Bookkeeping principles	21
a. Daily reports, charge slips, receipts, ledgers, etc.	21
(1) Charges, payments, and adjustments	
(2) Identifying and correcting errors	
b. Petty cash	21
2. Coding systems	18, 19, Appendix A
a. Types	18, 19, Appendix A
(1) Current Procedural Terminology (CPT)	
(2) International Classification of Diseases, Clinical Modifications (ICD-CM) (*current schedule*)	
(3) Healthcare Common Procedural Coding System (HCPCS Level II)	
b. Relationship between procedure and diagnosis codes	18, 19, Appendix A
3. Third-party billing	17
a. Types	17
(1) Capitated plans	
(2) Commercial carriers	
(3) Government plans	
(a) Medicare	
(b) Medicaid	
(c) Tricare	
(d) CHAMPVA	
(4) Prepaid HMO, PPO, POS	
(5) Workers' compensation	
b. Processing claims	17
(1) Manual and electronic preparation of claims	
(2) Tracing claims	
(3) Sequence of filing (e.g., primary vs. secondary)	
(4) Reconciling payments/rejections	
(5) Inquiry and appeal process	
c. Applying managed care policies and procedures	17
(1) Referrals	
(2) Precertification	

(continued)

Competencies	Chapter Reference(s)
d. Fee schedules	17
(1) Methods for establishing fees	
(a) Relative Value Studies	
(b) Resource-based Relative Value Scale (RBRVS)	
(c) Diagnosis Related Groups (DRGs)	
(2) Contracted fees	
4. Accounting and banking procedures	20, 21
a. Accounts receivable	20
(1) Billing procedures	
(a) Itemization	
(b) Billing cycles	
(2) Aging/collection procedures	
(a) Collection agencies	
(b) Consumer protection acts	
b. Accounts payable	21
(1) Ordering goods and services	
(2) Monitoring invoices	
(3) Tracking merchandise	
c. Banking procedures	21
(1) Processing accounts receivable	
(2) Preparing bank deposit	
5. Employee payroll	21
a. Calculating wages	21
b. Payroll forms	21
III. R-Z Clinical	14, 16
R. Principles of Infection control	16
1. Disposal of biohazardous material	16
2. Standard precautions	16
S. Treatment area	14
2. Restocking supplies	14
T. Patient preparation and assisting the physician	6
4. Patient education	6
a. Health maintenance and disease prevention	6
b. Use and care of patient equipment (e.g., wheelchair, crutches)	6
c. Instruction for procedure preparation	6
d. Patient administered medications	6
U. Patient history interview	11
1. Components of patient history	11
a. Personal data	11
b. Chief complaint	
c. Past, present, family, and social history	
d. Review of systems	
2. Documentation guidelines	3, 11

(continued)

Competencies	Chapter Reference(s)
X. Emergencies	16
1. Preplanned action	16
a. Policies and procedures	16
b. Legal implications and action documentation	
c. Equipment	
(1) Crash cart	
(2) Automated external defibrillator	
3. Emergency preparedness	16
Y. First aid	16
1. Identifying and responding to:	16
a. Bleeding/pressure points	16
b. Burns	16
c. Cardiac and respiratory arrest/CPR	16
d. Choking/Heimlich maneuver	16
e. Fractures	16
f. Poisoning	16
g. Seizures	16
h. Shock	16
i. Syncope	16
j. Wounds	16
Z. Nutrition	N/A
1. Basic principles	N/A
a. Dietary guidelines	N/A
b. Food nutrients (e.g., vitamins, minerals)	N/A
2. Special needs	N/A
a. Diets	N/A
b. Restrictions	N/A

Source: The CMA (AAMA) Certification/Recertification Examination Content Outline is reprinted with the permission of The American Association of Medical Assistants (AAMA).

American Medical Technologists Certified Medical Administrative Specialist (CMAS) Competencies and Examination Specifications

Competencies	Chapter Reference(s)
I. Medical Assisting Foundations (13% of exam)	Appendix C
A. Medical Terminology	Appendix C
1. Use and spell basic medical terms appropriately	Appendix C
2. Identify root words, prefixes, and suffixes	Appendix C
3. Define basic medical terms	Appendix C
C. Legal and Ethical Considerations	4, 5
1. Apply principles of medical law and ethics to the health care setting	4, 5
2. Recognize legal responsibilities of and know scope of practice for the medical administrative specialist	4
3. Know basic laws pertaining to medical practice	4
4. Know and observe basic disclosure laws (patient privacy, minors, confidentiality)	4
5. Know the principles of medical ethics established by the AMA	5
6. Recognize unethical practices and identify ethical responses for situations in the medical office.	5
D. Professionalism	3, 6
1. Employ human relations skills appropriate to the health care setting	3, 6
2. Display behaviors of a professional medical administrative specialist	3, 6
3. Participate in appropriate continuing education	3, 2
II. Basic Clinical Medical Office Assisting (8% of exam)	16
F. Medical Office Emergencies	16
1. Recognize and respond to medical emergencies	16
2. Employ first aid and CPR appropriately	16
3. Report emergencies as required by law	16
III. Medical Office Clerical Assisting (10% of examination)	9, 10
A. Appointment Management and Scheduling	9, 10
1. Schedule and monitor patient and visitor appointments	10
2. Address cancellations and missed appointments	9, 10
3. Prepare information for referrals and preauthorizations	9, 10
4. Arrange hospital admissions and surgery, and schedule patients for outpatient diagnostic tests	9, 10
5. Manage recall system and file	9
B. Reception	9
1. Receive and process patients and visitors	9
2. Screen visitors and vendors requesting to see physician	9
3. Coordinate patient flow into examining rooms	9
C. Communication	6, 7, 8, 9
1. Employ effective written and oral communication	6, 7
2. Address and process incoming telephone calls from outside providers, pharmacies, and vendors	8
3. Employ appropriate telephone etiquette when screening patient calls and addressing office business	8
4. Recognize and employ proper protocols for telephone emergencies	8
5. Format business documents and correspondence appropriately	7
6. Process incoming and outgoing mail	7, 9

(continued)

Competencies	Chapter Reference(s)
D. Patient Information and Community Resources	9, 10
1. Order and organize patient information materials	9
2. Maintain list of community referral resources	6
IV. Medical Records Management (14% of examination)	11, 12
A. Systems	11, 12
1. Demonstrate knowledge of, and manage patient medical records systems	11, 12
2. Manage documents and patient charts using paper methods	11
3. Manage documents and patient charts using computerized methods	12
B. Procedures	11, 12
1. File records alphabetically, numerically, by subject, and by color	11
2. Employ rules of indexing	11
3. Arrange contents of patients charts in appropriate order	11
4. Document and file laboratory results and patient communication in charts	11
5. Perform corrections and additions to records	11, 12
6. Store, protect, retain, and destroy records appropriately	11
7. Transfer files	11
8. Perform daily chart management	11
9. Prepare charts for external review and audits	11
C. Confidentiality	11, 12
1. Observe and maintain confidentiality of records, charts, and test results	11, 12
2. Observe special regulations regarding the confidentiality of protected information	11, 12
V. Health Care Insurance Processing, Coding, and Billing (17% of exam)	17, 18, 19, Appendix A
A. Insurance Processing	17
1. Understand private/commercial health insurance plans (PPO, HMO, traditional indemnity)	17
2. Understand government health care insurance plans (Medicare, Medicaid, Veteran's Administration, Tricare, use of Advance Beneficiary Notices)	17
3. Process patient claims using appropriate forms (including superbills) and time frames	17
4. Process Workers' Compensation/disability reports and forms	17
5. Submit claims for third-party reimbursements, including the use of electronic transmission methods	17
B. Coding	18, 19, Appendix A
1. Understand procedure and diagnosis coding	18, 19
2. Employ Current Procedural Terminology (CPT) and Evaluation and Management codes appropriately	19
3. Employ International Classification of Diseases 9 (ICD-9) codes appropriately	Appendix A
4. Employ Healthcare Financing Administration Common Procedure Coding System (HCPCS) codes appropriately	19
C. Insurance Billing and Finances	17
1. Understand health care insurance terminology (deductible, copayment, preauthorization, capitation, coinsurance)	17
2. Understand billing requirements for health care insurance plans	17
3. Process insurance payments	17
4. Track unpaid claims, and file and track appeals	17
5. Understand fraud and abuse regulations	17

(continued)

Competencies	Chapter Reference(s)
VI. Medical Office Financial Management (17% of exam)	20, 21, 22
A. Fundamental Financial Management	20, 21, 22
1. Understand basic principles of accounting	21
2. Perform bookkeeping procedures including balancing accounts	21
3. Perform financial computations	21
4. Manage accounts payable	21
5. Manage accounts receivable	20
6. Prepare monthly trial balance (reports)	21
7. Understand basic audit controls	21
8. Understand professional fee structures	20
9. Understand physician/practice owner compensation provisions	22
10. Understand credit arrangements	20
11. Manage other financial aspects of office management	22
B. Patient Accounts	20
1. Manage patient accounts/ledgers	20
2. Manage patient billing (methods, cycle billing procedures)	20
3. Manage collections in compliance with state and federal regulations	20
C. Banking	21
1. Understand banking services and procedures (accounts, lines of credit, checking endorsements, deposits, reconciliation, and statements)	21
2. Manage petty cash	21
D. Payroll	21
1. Prepare employee payroll and reports	21
2. Maintain payroll tax deduction procedures and records	21
VII. Medical Office Information Processing (7% of exam)	13
A. Fundamentals of Computing	13
1. Possess fundamental knowledge of computing in the medical office including keyboarding, data entry, and retrieval	13
2. Possess fundamental knowledge of PC-based environment	13
3. Possess fundamental knowledge of word processing, spreadsheet, database, and presentation graphics applications	13
4. Employ procedures for ensuring the integrity and confidentiality of computer-stored information	13
B. Medical Office Computer Applications	13
1. Employ medical office software applications	13
2. Use computer for billing and financial transactions	13
3. Employ e-mail applications	13, 20
VIII. Medical Office Management (14% of exam)	15, 21, 22
A. Office Communications*	22
1. Facilitate staff meetings and in-service, and ensure communication of essential information to staff	22
B. Business Organization Management*	22
1. Manage medical office business functions	22
2. Manage office mailing and shipping services	22
3. Manage outside vendors and supplies	22
4. Manage contracts and relationships with associated health care providers	22
5. Comply with licensure and accreditation requirements	22

(continued)

Competencies	Chapter Reference(s)
*C. Human Resources**	22
1. Manage/supervise medical office staff	22
2. Conduct performance reviews and disciplinary action	22
3. Maintain office policy manual	15
4. Manage staff payroll and scheduling	21
5. Manage staff recruiting in compliance with state and federal laws	22
6. Orient and train new staff	22
7. Manage employee benefits	22
D. Safety	16, 22
1. Maintain office safety, maintain office safety manual, and post emergency instructions	22
2. Observe emergency safety requirements	22
3. Maintain records of biohazardous waste, hazardous chemicals (Material Safety Data Sheets), and safety conditions	16, 22
4. Comply with Occupational Safety and Health Act (OSHA) guidelines and regulations	16, 22
E. Supplies and Equipment	14
1. Manage medical and office supply inventories and order supplies	14
2. Maintain office equipment and arrange for (and maintain records of) equipment maintenance and repair	14
F. Physical Office Plant	22
1. Maintain office facilities and environment	22
G. Risk Management and Quality Assurance	22
1. Understand and employ risk management and quality assurance concepts	22

Note: Asterisked areas addressed by the Medical Office Management job function may or may not be performed by the Certified Medical Administrative Specialist at entry-level practice. Nevertheless, the competent specialist should have sound knowledge of these management functions at certification level.

Source: The CMAS competencies and examination specifications are reprinted with the permission of the American Medical Technologists.

National Center for Competency Testing Medical Assistant Certification Exam Content Outline

Approximate % of Exam	Content Categories	Chapter References
10–12.5%	**Anatomy and Physiology**	N/A
	• Body systems and functions	N/A
	• Basic disease recognition	N/A
	• Bones	N/A
	• Body positioning for examination	N/A
	• Major muscles	N/A
18–20.5%	**Medical Office Management**	3, 4, 5, 6, 7, 8, 9, 10, 11, 12, 13, 14, 22
	• General Office Procedures (10–12.5%)	3, 4, 5, 6, 7, 8, 9, 10, 11, 12, 13, 14, 22
	1. Oral and written communication skills	6, 7, 8, 9
	2. Legal and professional concepts	3, 4
	3. Patient instruction	3, 4, 6, 7, 8, 9, 10, 20, 22
	4. Computers	12, 13
	5. Equipment operation and maintenance	14
	6. Organizational skills	3, 11, 22
	7. Cultural awareness	4, 5, 6, 9
	8. Medical record keeping	11, 12
	• Bookkeeping (4%)	20, 21
	1. Basic banking	21
	2. Basic accounting	21
	3. Record keeping	20, 21
	4. Preparing and collecting patient accounts	20
	• Insurance Processing (4%)	17, 18, 19
	1. Managed care models	17
	2. Insurance plans	17
	3. Referrals and precertification	17
	4. Filing claims	17
	5. Third party payers	17
	6. Basic procedural and diagnostic coding for reimbursement; DRGs	18, 19
12.5%	**Medical Procedures (including understanding Scope of Practice in all areas of medical procedures)**	16
	• Infection and Exposure Control	16
	1. Biohazardous waste disposal	16
	2. Exposure control	16
	3. Asepsis	16
	4. Personal protective equipment	16
	5. Universal precautions; blood and body fluids	16
	6. Sanitation, sterilization, and disinfection	16
	7. OSHA safety regulations	16

(continued)

Approximate % of Exam	Content Categories	Chapter References
10–12.5%	• **Patient Examination (Clinical Skills)**	N/A
	1. Patient history and screening; charting	N/A
	2. Basic patient examination skills; vitals, temperature; other measurements	N/A
	3. Assistance in minor surgical procedures	N/A
	4. Bandaging or dressing wounds; suture/staple removal	N/A
	5. Assistance with therapeutic modalities	N/A
	6. Vision testing (e.g., acuity; color blindness)	N/A
	7. Specialty testing (e.g., allergy)	N/A
	8. Recognition of normal and abnormal conditions; response (first aid, CPR)	N/A
	9. Patient instruction	N/A
	10. Comprehension of scope of practice (including state law)	N/A
10–12.5%	• **Phlebotomy**	N/A
	1. Venipuncture and capillary puncture	N/A
	2. Patient preparation and site selection/prep	N/A
	3. Safety and infection control, QC	N/A
	4. Equipment and tubes (types, uses, limitations, additives, collection amounts)	N/A
	5. Coagulation and anticoagulation	N/A
10–12.5%	• **Diagnostic Testing: ECG and other Lab Procedures**	N/A
	1. CLIA-waived lab testing, including QC and instrument maintenance	N/A
	2. Specimen collection (e.g., urine, throat, stool, wound, etc.)	N/A
	3. ECG (12-lead) testing, monitoring, troubleshooting	N/A
	4. Basic respiratory testing, treatment	N/A
10–12.5%	*Medical Terminology*	4, 5, 17, Appendix C
	1. Foundations of word structure (roots, prefixes, suffixes)	Appendix C
	2. Standard medical/pharmaceutical abbreviations and symbols	Appendix C
	3. Terms re: Insurance processing, anatomy and physiology, law, ethics	4, 5, 17, Appendix C
	4. Terms re: surgical procedures, common diseases, common pathology	Appendix C
10–12.5%	*Pharmacology*	N/A
	1. Use of Pharmaceutical Desk Reference (e.g., PDR and others)	N/A
	2. Basic drug calculations and metric conversions	N/A
	3. Pharmacology terms and abbreviations	N/A
	4. Legal prescription requirements for all drug schedules and classes	N/A
	5. Common drugs and their classifications/side effects/indications for use	N/A
	6. DEA regulations	N/A
	7. Safe preparation and administration of medications (e.g., oral, topical, subcutaneous, intramuscular) and other routes	N/A
100%	*Total*	

Source: The National Center for Competency Testing Medical Assistant Certification Exam Content Outline is reprinted with the permission of the National Center for Competency Testing.

Registered Medical Assistant Certification Examination Competencies and Construction Parameters

Registered Medical Assistant Competencies	Textbook Reference(s)
I. GENERAL MEDICAL ASSISTING KNOWLEDGE	N/A
A. Anatomy and Physiology	N/A
1. Body systems—identify the structure and function of the following systems:	N/A
a. Skeletal	N/A
b. Muscular	N/A
c. Endocrine	N/A
d. Urinary	N/A
e. Reproductive	N/A
f. Gastrointestinal	N/A
g. Nervous	N/A
h. Respiratory	N/A
i. Cardiovascular/circulatory	N/A
j. Integumentary	N/A
k. Special senses	N/A
2. Disorders and diseases—identify and define various:	N/A
a. Disease processes	N/A
b. Conditions or states of health	N/A
c. Health-related syndromes	N/A
3. Wellness	N/A
a. Identify nutritional factors that are required for or influence wellness	N/A
b. Identify factors associated with exercise that are required for or influence wellness	N/A
c. Identify factors associated with lifestyle choices that are required for or influence wellness	N/A
B. Medical Terminology	Appendix C
1. Word parts	Appendix C
a. Identify word parts: root, prefixes, and suffixes	Appendix C
2. Definitions	Appendix C
a. Define medical terms	Appendix C
3. Common abbreviations and symbols	Appendix C
a. Identify and understand utilization of medical abbreviations and symbols	Appendix C
4. Spelling	7, Appendix C
a. Spell medical terms accurately	Appendix C
C. Medical Law—identify and understand the application of:	4
1. Medical law	4
a. Types of consent used in medical practice	4
b. Disclosure laws and regulations (including HIPAA security and privacy acts, state and federal laws)	4
c. Laws, regulations, and acts pertaining to the practice of medicine	4
d. Scope of practice acts regarding medical assisting	4
e. Patient Bill of Rights legislation	4
2. Licensure, certification, and registration	4
a. Identify credentialing requirements of medical professionals	3, 4
b. Understand the application of the Clinical Laboratory Improvement Amendments of 1988 (CLIA '88)	4
3. Terminology	4
a. Define terminology associated with medical law	4

(continued)

Registered Medical Assistant Competencies	Textbook Reference(s)
D. Medical Ethics	3, 4, 5
1. Principles of medical ethics and ethical conduct:	3, 4, 5
a. Identify and employ proper ethics in practice as a medical assistant	5
b. Identify the principles of ethics established by the American Medical Association	5
c. Identify and understand the application of the AMA Patient Bill of Rights	4
d. Recognize unethical practices and identify the proper response	5
e. Recognize the importance of professional development through continuing education	3
E. Human Relations	3, 6
1. Patient relations	3, 6
a. Identify age-group specific responses and support	6
b. Identify and employ professional conduct in all aspects of patient care	3, 6
c. Understand and properly apply communication methods	6
d. Identify and respect cultural and ethnic differences	6
e. Respect and care for patients without regard for age, gender, sexual orientation, or socioeconomic level	6
2. Interpersonal relations	6, 22
a. Employ appropriate interpersonal skills with:	6, 22
1. Employer/administration	6, 22
2. Co-workers	6, 22
3. Vendors	6, 22
4. Business associates	6, 22
b. Observe and respect cultural diversity in the workplace	6, 22
F. Patient Education	6, 22
1. Patient instruction—identify and apply proper written and verbal communication to instruct patients in:	6, 22
a. Health and wellness	6
b. Nutrition	6
c. Hygiene	6
d. Treatment and medications	6
e. Pre- and postoperative care	6
f. Body mechanics	6
g. Personal and physical safety	6, 22
2. Patient resource materials	15
a. Develop, assemble, and maintain appropriate patient brochures and informational materials	15
3. Documentation	11, 12
a. Understand and utilize proper documentation of patient encounters and instruction	11, 12
II. ADMINISTRATIVE MEDICAL ASSISTING	4, 17, 18, 19
A. Insurance	17
1. Terminology	17
a. Identify and define terminology associated with various insurance types in the medical office	17
2. Plans	17
a. Identify and understand the application of government, medical, disability, and accident insurance plans	17

(continued)

Registered Medical Assistant Competencies	Textbook Reference(s)
b. Identify and appropriately apply plan policies and regulations for programs including:	4, 17
1. HMO, PPO, EPO, indemnity, open, etc.	17
2. Short-term and long-term disability	17
3. Family Medical Leave Act (FMLA)	4
4. Workers' Compensation	17
a. Complete first reports	17
b. Complete followup reports	17
5. Medicare (including Advance Beneficiary Notice [ABN])	17
6. Medicaid	17
7. CHAMPUS/Tricare and CHAMPVA	17
3. Claims	17
a. Complete and file insurance claims	17
1. File claims for paper and Electronic Data Interchange	17
2. Understand and adhere to HIPAA security and uniformity regulations	17
b. Evaluate claims responses	17
1. Understand and evaluate explanation of benefits	17
2. Evaluate claims rejection and utilize proper followup procedures	17
4. Coding	18, 19, Appendix A
a. Identify HIPAA-mandated coding systems and references	18, 19, Appendix A
b. Process insurance payments and contractual write-off amounts	17, 20
c. Track unpaid claims	17, 20
d. Generate aging reports	17, 20
B. Financial Bookkeeping	20
1. Terminology	20
a. Understand terminology associated with medical financial bookkeeping	20
2. Patient billing	20
a. Maintain and explain physician's fee schedules	20
b. Collect and post payments	20
c. Manage patient ledgers and accounts	20
d. Understand and prepare Truth in Lending Statements	20
e. Prepare and mail itemized statements	20
f. Understand and employ available billing methods	20
g. Understand and employ billing cycles	20
3. Collections	20
a. Prepare aging reports and identify delinquent accounts	20
b. Perform skip tracing	20
c. Understand application of the Fair Debt Collections Practices Act	20
d. Identify and understand bankruptcy and small claims procedures	20
e. Understand and perform collection procedures	20
4. Fundamental medical office accounting procedures	20
a. Employ appropriate accounting procedures	20
1. Pegboard/double entry	N/A
2. Computerized	20
b. Perform daily balancing procedures	20

(continued)

Registered Medical Assistant Competencies	Textbook Reference(s)
c. Prepare monthly trial balance	20
d. Apply accounts receivable and payable principles	20
5. Banking procedures	20, 21
a. Understand and manage petty cash account	21
b. Prepare and make bank deposits	20
c. Maintain checking accounts	20
d. Reconcile bank statements	20
e. Understand check processing procedures and requirements	20
1. Nonsufficient funds (NSF)	20
2. Endorsements	21
f. Process payables and practice obligations	21
g. Understand and maintain disbursement accounts	21
6. Employee payroll	21
a. Prepare employee payroll	21
1. Understand hourly and salary payroll procedures	21
2. Understand and apply payroll withholding and deductions	21
b. Understand and maintain payroll records	21
1. Prepare and maintain payroll tax deduction/withholding records	21
2. Prepare employee tax forms	21
3. Prepare quarterly tax forms and deposits	21
c. Understand terminology pertaining to payroll and payroll tax	21
7. Financial mathematics	20
a. Understand and perform appropriate calculations related to patient and practice accounts	20
C. Medical Receptionist/Secretarial/Clerical	9
1. Terminology	9
a. Understand and correctly apply terminology associated with medical receptionist and secretarial duties	9
2. Reception	9
a. Employ appropriate communication skills when receiving and greeting patients	9
b. Understand basic emergency triage in coordinating patient arrivals	9
c. Screen visitors and salespersons arriving at the office	9
d. Obtain patient demographics and information	9
e. Understand and maintain patient confidentiality during check-in procedures	9
f. Prepare patient record	9
g. Assist patients into examination rooms	9
3. Scheduling	10
a. Employ appointment scheduling system	10
1. Identify and employ various scheduling styles (wave, open, etc.)	10
b. Employ proper procedure for cancellations and missed appointments	10
c. Understand referral and authorization process	10
d. Understand and manage patient recall system	10
e. Schedule non-office appointments (hospital admissions, diagnostic tests, surgeries)	10

(continued)

Registered Medical Assistant Competencies	Textbook Reference(s)
4. Oral and written communication	6, 7, 8, 9
a. Employ appropriate telephone etiquette	8
b. Perform appropriate telephone	8
c. Instruct patients via telephone	8
d. Inform patients of test results per physician instruction	8
e. Receive, process, and document results received from outside provider	8
f. Compose correspondence employing acceptable business format	7
g. Employ effective written communication skills adhering to ethics and laws of confidentiality	7, 9
h. Employ active listening skills	6
5. Records and chart management	11, 12
a. Manage patient medical record system	11, 12
b. Record diagnostic test results in patient chart	11, 12
c. File patient and physician communication in chart	11, 12
d. File materials according to proper system	11
1. Chronological	11
2. Alphabetical	11
3. Problem-oriented medical records (POMR)	11
4. Subject	11
e. Protect, store, and retain medical records according to proper conventions and HIPAA privacy regulations	11, 12
f. Prepare and release private health information as required, adhering to state and federal guidelines	11, 12
g. Identify and employ proper documentation procedures adhering to standard charting guidelines	11, 12
6. Transcription and dictation	7
a. Transcribe notes from dictation system	7
b. Transcribe letter or notes from direct dictation	7
7. Supplies and equipment management	14
a. Maintain inventory of medical/office supplies and equipment	14
b. Coordinate maintenance and repair of office equipment	14
c. Maintain equipment maintenance logs according to OSHA regulations	14
8. Computer applications	13
a. Identify and understand hardware components	13
b. Identify and understand application of basic software and operating systems	13
c. Recognize software application for patient record maintenance, bookkeeping, and patient accounting system	13
d. Employ procedures for integrity of information and compliance with HIPAA security and privacy regulations	13
1. Encryption	13
2. Firewall software and hardware	13
3. Personnel passwords	13
4. Access restrictions	13
5. Activity logs	13
e. Maintain records of biohazardous waste and chemical disposal	13

(continued)

Registered Medical Assistant Competencies	Textbook Reference(s)
III. CLINICAL MEDICAL ASSISTING	4, 16
K. First Aid and Emergency Response	16
1. First aid procedures	16
a. Identify criteria for and steps in performing CPR and the Heimlich maneuver	16
b. Maintain emergency (crash) cart	16
c. Identify injuries, recognize emergencies, and provide appropriate response	16
2. Legal responsibilities	4, 16
a. Understand protection and limits of the Good Samaritan Act	4
b. Understand scope of practice when providing first aid	4, 16
c. Understand mandatory reporting guidelines and procedures	4

Note: The above table lists only those clinical competencies that apply to the administrative skills presented in this text.

Source: The Registered Medical Assistant Certification Examination Competencies and Construction Parameters are reprinted with the permission of American Medical Technologists (AMT).

ABHES Programmatic Education Standards for Medical Assisting

Competencies		Chapter Reference(s)
1. General Orientation	**Graduates will be able to:**	2, 3
a. Employment conditions	a. Describe the current employment outlook for the medical assistant	3
b. The allied health professions	b. Compare and contrast the allied health professions and understand their relation to medical assisting	3
c. Credentialing of the medical assistant	c. Describe medical assistant credentialing requirements and the process to obtain the credential. Comprehend the importance of credentialing	3
d. General responsibilities of the medical assistant	d. List the general responsibilities and skills of the medical assistant	2, 3
3. Medical Terminology	**Graduates will be able to:**	3, 7, Appendix C
a. Basic structure of medical words	a. Define and use entire basic structure of medical words and be able to accurately identify in the correct context (i.e., root, prefix, suffix, combinations, spelling, and definitions)	Appendix C
b. Word element combinations	b. Build and dissect medical terms from roots/suffixes to understand the word element combinations that create medical terminology	Appendix C
c. Medical terms for specialties	c. Apply various medical terms for each specialty	3, Appendix C
d. Acceptable medical abbreviations	d. Define and use acceptable medical abbreviations when appropriate and acceptable	7
4. Medical Law and Ethics	**Graduates will be able to:**	4, 5, 11, 12
a. Documentation	a. Follow documentation guidelines	11, 12
b. Federal and state guidelines	b. Institute federal and state guidelines when releasing medical records or information	4
c. Established policies	c. Follow established policies when initiating or terminating medical treatment	4
d. Liability coverage	d. Understand the importance of maintaining liability coverage once employed in the industry	4
e. Risk management	e. Perform risk management procedures	4

(continued)

Competencies		Chapter Reference(s)

f. Health laws and regulations
 	
    1. The scope of practice within the state of employment
    2. Delegation
	f. Comply with federal, state, and local health laws and regulations as they relate to health care settings
	    1. Define scope of practice for the medical assistant within the state that the medical assistant is employed.
	    2. Describe what procedures can and cannot be delegated to the medical assistant and by whom within various employment settings
		4

g. Ethics	g. Display compliance with Code of Ethics of the profession	5
5. Psychology of Human Relations	**Graduates will be able to:**	6
a. Abnormal behavior patterns	a. Respond appropriately to patients with abnormal behavior patterns	6

b. Terminally ill patients	b. Provide support for terminally ill patients
	    1. Use empathy when communicating with terminally ill patients
	    2. Identify common stages that terminally ill patients experience
	    3. List organizations/support groups that can assist patients and family members of patients experiencing terminal illnesses
		6

c. Patient advocacy	c. Intervene on behalf of the patient regarding issues/concerns that may arise (e.g., insurance policy information, medical bills, physician/provider orders)	6
d. Developmental stages of life	d. Discuss developmental stages of life	6
e. Working with diverse populations	e. Analyze the effect of hereditary, cultural, and environmental influences on behavior	6
7. Records Management	**Graduates will be able to:**	12, 13
a. Data entry skills	a. Perform basic keyboarding skills (i.e., Microsoft Word, etc.)	13
b. Office systems and software including electronic medical records	b. Utilize electronic medical records (EMR) and practice management systems	12, 13
c. Laws and regulations	c. Comply with federal, state, and local laws relating to exchange of information, and describe elements of meaningful use and reports generated	12
8. Administrative Procedures	**Graduates will be able to:**	6, 7, 10, 11, 12, 14, 17, 18, 19, 20, 21
a. Records management	a. Gather and process documents	11, 12

b. Financial practices	b. Perform billing and collection procedures
	    1. Accounts payable and accounts receivable
	    2. Post adjustments
	    3. Payment procedures (e.g., credit balance, non-sufficient funds, refunds)
		20, 21

c. Insurance and coding	c. Process insurance claims
	    1. Differentiate between procedures of private, federal, and state payers
	    2. Differentiate managed care (e.g., HMO, PPO, IPA including referrals and precertification)
	    3. Perform diagnostic and procedural coding
		17, 18, 19

d. Scheduling	d. Apply scheduling principles
	    1. Schedule in- and outpatient procedures
	    2. Admission or hospital procedures
		10

e. Office environment	e. Maintain inventory of equipment and supplies 1. Perform routine maintenance of administrative equipment	14
f. Communication	f. Display professionalism through written and verbal communications	6, 7

(continued)

Competencies		Chapter Reference(s)
10. Medical Office Laboratory Procedures	**Graduates will be able to:**	16
c. Biohazards	c. Dispose of biohazardous materials	16
11. Career Development	**Graduates will be able to:**	3, 23
a. Essentials for employment	a. Perform the essential requirements for employment such as résumé writing, effective interviewing, dressing professionally, time management, and following up appropriately	23
b. Professionalism	b. Demonstrate professional behavior	3, 23

Note: The above table lists only those clinical competencies that apply to the administrative skills presented in this text.

Source: The Accrediting Bureau of Health Education Schools (ABHES) Programmatic Evaluation Standards for Medical Assisting are reprinted by permission of ABHES.

CAAHEP Standards and Competencies Adopted by the 2009 Medical Assisting Education Review Board (MAERB)

Cognitive (Knowledge Base)	Chapter Reference(s)	Psychomotor (Skills)	Chapter Reference(s)	Affective (Behavior)	Chapter Reference(s)
I.C. Anatomy and Physiology	N/A	**I.P. Anatomy and Physiology**	N/A	**I.A. Anatomy and Physiology**	
				1. Apply critical thinking skills in performing patient assessment and care	6, 16
				2. Use language/verbal skills that enable patients' understanding	6
				3. Demonstrate respect for diversity in approaching patients and families	6
II.C. Applied Mathematics		**II.P. Applied Mathematics**	N/A	**II.A. Applied Mathematics**	N/A
1. Demonstrate knowledge of basic math computations	20, 21				
III.C. Applied Microbiology/Infection Control		**III.P. Applied Microbiology/Infection Control**		**III.A. Applied Microbiology/Infection Control**	
4. Identify personal safety precautions as established by the Occupational Safety and Health Administration (OSHA)	4, 16	1. Participate in training on Standard Precautions	16		
11. Describe Standard Precautions, including: a. Transmission based precautions b. Purpose c. Activities regulated	16	2. Practice Standard Precautions	16		

(continued)

Cognitive (Knowledge Base)	Chapter Reference(s)	Psychomotor (Skills)	Chapter Reference(s)	Affective (Behavior)	Chapter Reference(s)
13. Identify the role of the Centers for Disease Control and Prevention (CDC) and regulations in health care settings	5				
IV.C. Concepts of Effective Communication		**IV.P. Concepts of Effective Communication**		**IV.A. Concepts of Effective Communication**	
1. Identify styles and types of verbal communication	6	1. Use reflection, restatement and clarification techniques to obtain a patient history	6	1. Demonstrate empathy in communicating with patients, family and staff	6
2. Identify nonverbal communication	6	2. Report relevant information to others succinctly and accurately	6	2. Apply active listening skills	6
3. Recognize communication barriers	6	3. Use medical terminology, pronouncing medical terms correctly, to communicate information, patient history, data, and observations	6, Appendix C	3. Use appropriate body language and other nonverbal skills in communicating with patients, family, and staff	6
4. Identify techniques for overcoming communication barriers	6	4. Explain general office policies	15	4. Demonstrate awareness of the territorial boundaries of the person with whom communicating	6
5. Recognize the elements of oral communication using a sender–receiver process	6	5. Instruct patients according to their needs to promote health maintenance and disease prevention	6	5. Demonstrate sensitivity appropriate to the message being delivered	6
6. Differentiate between subjective and objective information	6	6. Prepare a patient for procedures and/or treatments	6	6. Demonstrate awareness of how an individual's personal appearance affects anticipated responses	6
7. Identify resources and adaptations that are required based on individual needs—i.e., culture and environment, developmental life stage, language, and physical threats to communication	6	7. Demonstrate telephone techniques	8	7. Demonstrate recognition of the patient's level of understanding in communications	6
8. Recognize elements of fundamental writing skills	7	8. Document patient care	7	8. Analyze communications in providing appropriate responses/feedback	6

(continued)

Cognitive (Knowledge Base)	Chapter Reference(s)	Psychomotor (Skills)	Chapter Reference(s)	Affective (Behavior)	Chapter Reference(s)
9. Discuss applications of electronic technology in effective communication	7	9. Document patient education	7	9. Recognize and protect personal boundaries in communicating with others	6
10. Diagram medical terms, labeling the word parts	Appendix C	10. Compose professional/business letters	7	10. Demonstrate respect for individual diversity, incorporating awareness of one's own biases in areas including gender, race, religion, age, and economic status	6
11. Define both medical terms and abbreviations related to all body systems	Appendix C	11. Respond to nonverbal communication	6		
12. Organize technical information and summaries	11, 12	12. Develop and maintain a current list of community resources related to patients' health care needs	15		
13. Identify the role of self-boundaries in the health care environment	3, 4	13. Advocate on behalf of patients	3, 6		
14. Recognize the role of patient advocacy in the practice of medical assisting	3, 6				
15. Discuss the role of assertiveness in effective professional communication	6				
16. Differentiate between adaptive and nonadaptive coping mechanisms	6				
V.C. Administrative Functions		**V.P. Administrative Functions**		**V.A. Administrative Functions**	
1. Discuss pros and cons of various types of appointment management systems	10	1. Manage appointment schedule, using established priorities	10	1. Consider staff needs and limitations in establishment of a filing system	11
2. Describe scheduling guidelines	10	2. Schedule patient admissions and/or procedures	10	2. Implement time management principles to maintain effective office function	9, 10
3. Recognize office policies and protocols for handling appointments	10	3. Organize a patient's medical record	11, 12		
4. Identify critical information required for scheduling patient admissions and/or procedures	10	4. File medical records	11		

Cognitive (Knowledge Base)	Chapter Reference(s)	Psychomotor (Skills)	Chapter Reference(s)	Affective (Behavior)	Chapter Reference(s)
5. Identify systems for organizing medical records	11, 12	5. Execute data management using electronic health care records such as the EMR	12		
6. Describe various types of content maintained in a patient's medical record	11, 12	6. Use office hardware and software to maintain office systems	13		
7. Discuss pros and cons of various filing methods	11	7. Use internet to access information related to the medical office	13		
8. Identify both equipment and supplies needed for filing medical records	11, 12, 14	8. Maintain organization by filing	11		
9. Describe indexing rules	11	9. Perform routine maintenance of office equipment with documentation	14		
10. Discuss filing procedures	11	10. Perform an office inventory	14		
11. Discuss principles of using electronic medical records (EMR)	12				
12. Identify types of records common to the health care setting	11				
13. Identify time management principles	3				
14. Discuss the importance of routine maintenance of office equipment	14				
VI.C. Basic Practice Finances		**VI.P. Basic Practice Finances**		**VI.A. Basic Practice Finances**	
1. Explain basic bookkeeping computations	21	1. Prepare a bank deposit	21	1. Demonstrate sensitivity and professionalism in handling accounts receivable activities with clients	20
2. Differentiate between bookkeeping and accounting	21	2. Perform accounts receivable procedures, including:	20		
3. Describe banking procedures	21	a. Post entries on a daysheet			
4. Discuss precautions for accepting checks	21	b. Perform billing procedures	20		
5. Compare types of endorsement	21	c. Perform collection procedures	20		

(continued)

Cognitive (Knowledge Base)	Chapter Reference(s)	Psychomotor (Skills)	Chapter Reference(s)	Affective (Behavior)	Chapter Reference(s)
6. Differentiate between accounts payable and accounts receivable	20, 21	d. Post adjustments	20		
7. Compare manual and computerized bookkeeping systems used in ambulatory health care	20	e. Process a credit balance	20		
8. Describe common periodic financial reports	21	f. Process refunds	21		
9. Explain both billing and payment options	20	g. Post nonsufficient fund (NSF) checks	20		
10. Identify procedure for preparing patient accounts	20	h. Post collection agency payments	20		
11. Discuss procedures for collecting outstanding accounts	20	3. Utilize computerized office billing systems	20		
12. Describe the impact of both the Fair Debt Collection Act and the Federal Truth in Lending Act of 1968 as they apply to collections	20				
13. Discuss types of adjustments that may be made to a patient's account	20				
VII.C. Managed Care/ Insurance		**VII.P. Managed Care/ Insurance**		**VII.A. Managed Care/ Insurance**	
1. Identify types of insurance plans	17	1. Apply both managed care policies and procedures	17	1. Demonstrate assertive communication with managed care and/or insurance providers	17
2. Identify models of managed care	17	2. Apply third-party guidelines	17	2. Demonstrate sensitivity in communicating with both providers and patients	17
3. Discuss workers' compensation as it applies to patients	17	3. Complete insurance claim forms	17	3. Communicate in language the patient can understand regarding managed care and insurance plans	17
4. Describe procedures for implementing both managed care and insurance plans	17	4. Obtain precertification, including documentation	17		
5. Discuss utilization review principles	17	5. Obtain preauthorization, including documentation	17		

(continued)

Cognitive (Knowledge Base)	Chapter Reference(s)	Psychomotor (Skills)	Chapter Reference(s)	Affective (Behavior)	Chapter Reference(s)
6. Discuss referral process for patients in a managed care program	17	6. Verify eligibility for managed care services	17		
7. Describe how guidelines are used in processing an insurance claim	17				
8. Compare processes for filing insurance claims both manually and electronically	17				
9. Describe guidelines for third-party claims	17				
10. Discuss types of physician fee schedules	17				
11. Describe the concept of RBRVS	17				
12. Define diagnosis-related groups (DRGs)	17				
VIII.C. Procedural and Diagnostic Coding		**VIII.P. Procedural and Diagnostic Coding**		**VIII.A. Procedural and Diagnostic Coding**	
1. Describe how to use the most current procedural coding system	19	1. Perform procedural coding	19	1. Work with physician to achieve the maximum reimbursement	19
2. Define upcoding and why it should be avoided	19	2. Perform diagnostic coding	18		
3. Describe how to use the most current diagnostic coding classification system	18				
4. Describe how to use the most current HCPCA coding	18				
IX.C. Legal Implications		**IX.P. Legal Implications**		**IX.A. Legal Implications**	
1. Discuss legal scope of practice for medical assistants	3, 4	1. Respond to issues of confidentiality	3, 4	1. Demonstrate sensitivity to patient rights	4
2. Explore issue of confidentiality as it applies to the medical assistant	4	2. Perform within scope of practice	4	2. Demonstrate awareness of the consequences of not working within the legal scope of practice	4
3. Describe the implications of HIPAA for the medical assistant in various medical settings	4	3. Apply HIPAA rules in regard to privacy/ release of information	4, 11	3. Recognize the importance of local, state, and federal legislation and regulations in the practice setting	4

(continued)

Cognitive (Knowledge Base)	Chapter Reference(s)	Psychomotor (Skills)	Chapter Reference(s)	Affective (Behavior)	Chapter Reference(s)
4. Summarize the Patient Bill of Rights	4	4. Practice within the standard of care for a medical assistant	4		
5. Discuss licensure and certification as it applies to health care providers	3, 4	5. Incorporate the Patient's Bill of Rights into personal practice and medical office policies and procedures	4		
6. Describe liability, professional, personal injury, and third-party insurance	4	6. Complete an incident report	4		
7. Compare and contrast physician and medical assistant roles in terms of standard of care	3	7. Document accurately in the patient record	11, 12		
8. Compare criminal and civil law as it applies to the practicing medical assistant	4	8. Apply local, state, and federal health care legislation and regulation appropriate to the medical assisting practice setting	4		
9. Provide an example of tort law as it would apply to a medical assistant	4				
10. Explain how the following impact the medical assistant's practice and give examples	4				
a. Negligence	4				
b. Malpractice	4				
c. Statute of limitations	4				
d. Good Samaritan Act(s)	4				
e. Uniform Anatomical Gift Act	4				
f. Living will/advanced directives	4				
g. Medical durable power of attorney	4				
11. Identify how the Americans with Disabilities Act (ADA) applies to the medical assisting profession	4				
12. List and discuss legal and illegal interview questions	4, 22				

(continued)

Cognitive (Knowledge Base)	Chapter Reference(s)	Psychomotor (Skills)	Chapter Reference(s)	Affective (Behavior)	Chapter Reference(s)
13. Discuss all levels of governmental legislation and regulation as they apply to medical assisting practice, including FDA and DEA regulations	5				
14. Describe the process to follow if an error is made in patient care	11, 12				
X.C. Ethical Considerations		**X.P. Ethical Considerations**		**X.A. Ethical Considerations**	
1. Differentiate between legal, ethical, and moral issues affecting health care	4, 5	1. Report illegal and/or unsafe activities and behaviors that affect health, safety, and welfare of others to proper authorities	4, 5	1. Apply ethical behaviors, including honesty/integrity in performance of medical-assisting practice	5
2. Compare personal, professional and organizational ethics	5	2. Develop a plan for separation of personal and professional ethics	5	2. Examine the impact personal ethics and morals may have on the individual's practice	4, 5
3. Discuss the role of cultural, social, and ethnic diversity in ethical performance of medical assisting practice	5			3. Demonstrate awareness of diversity in providing patient care	5
4. Identify where to report illegal and/or unsafe activities and behaviors that affect health, safety, and welfare of others	4				
5. Identify the effect personal ethics may have on professional performance	5				
XI.C. Protective Practices		**XI.P Protective Practices**		**XI.A. Protective Practices**	
1. Describe personal protective equipment	16	1. Comply with safety signs, symbols and labels	16	1. Recognize the effects of stress on all persons involved in emergency situations	16
2. Identify safety techniques that can be used to prevent accidents and maintain a safe work environment	16	2. Evaluate the work environment to identify safe vs. unsafe working conditions	16	2. Demonstrate self-awareness in responding to emergency situations	16

(continued)

Cognitive (Knowledge Base)	Chapter Reference(s)	Psychomotor (Skills)	Chapter Reference(s)	Affective (Behavior)	Chapter Reference(s)
3. Describe the importance of Material Safety Data Sheets (MSDS) in a health care setting	16	3. Develop a personal (patient and employee) safety plan	16		
4. Identify safety signs, symbols, and labels	16	4. Develop an environmental safety plan	16		
5. State principles and steps of professional/ provider CPR	16	5. Demonstrate proper use of the following equipment:	16		
6. Describe basic principles of first aid	16				
7. Describe fundamental principles for evaluation of a health care setting	16	b. Fire extinguishers	16		
8. Discuss fire safety issues in a health care environment	16	c. Sharps disposal containers	16		
9. Discuss requirements for responding to hazardous material disposal	16	6. Participate in a mock environmental exposure event with documentation of steps taken	16		
10. Identify principles of body mechanics and ergonomics	16	7. Explain an evacuation plan for a physician's office	16		
11. Discuss critical elements of an emergency plan for response to a natural disaster or other emergency	16	8. Demonstrate methods of fire prevention in the health care setting	16		
12. Identify emergency preparedness plans in your community	16	9. Maintain provider/ professional level CPR certification	16		
13. Discuss potential role(s) of the medical assistant in emergency preparedness	16	10. Perform first aid procedures	16		
		11. Use proper body mechanics	22		
		12. Maintain a current list of community resources for emergency preparedness	16		

Note: The above table lists only those clinical competencies that apply to the administrative skills presented in this text.

Source: The Core Curriculum for Medical Assistants Medical Assisting Education Review Board (MAERB) 2008 Curriculum Plan is reprinted with permission of MAERB.

Appendix C

Medical Terminology Word Parts

Medical terms are like individual jigsaw puzzles. Once you divide the terms into their component parts and learn the meaning of the individual parts, you can use that knowledge to understand many other new terms. Four basic component parts are used to create medical terms:

Root	The basic, or core, part that makes up the essential meaning of the term. The root usually, but not always, denotes a body part. Root words usually come from the Greek or Latin languages. For example, *bronch* is a root that means "the air passages in the lungs" or "bronchial tubes." *Cephal* means "head." An extensive list of root words is given on pp. 549–551.
Prefix	One or more letters placed before the root to change its meaning. Prefixes usually, but not always, indicate location, time, number, or status. For example, the prefix *bi-* means "two" or "twice." When *bi* is placed before the root *lateral* ("side"), to form *bilateral*, the meaning is "having two sides." An extensive list of prefixes is given on pp. 547–549.
Suffix	One or more letters placed after the root to change its meaning. Suffixes usually, but not always, indicate the procedure, condition, disorder, or disease. For example, the suffix *-itis* means "inflammation"—that is, damaged tissue that is red and painful. The medical term *bronchitis* means "inflammation of the bronchial tubes." Another example is the suffix *-ectomy*, which means "removal." Hence, *appendectomy* means "removal of the appendix." An extensive list of suffixes is given on pp. 551–552.
Combining vowel	A letter used to combine roots with other word parts. The vowel is usually an *o*, but sometimes it is an *a* or *i*. When a combining vowel is added to a root, the result is called a *combining form*. For example, in the word *encephalogram*, the root is *cephal* ("head"), the prefix is *en-* ("inside"), and the suffix is *-gram* ("something recorded"). These word parts are joined by the combining vowel *o* to make a word more easily pronounced. *Cephal/o* is the combining form. An *encephalogram* is an X-ray of the inside of the head.

Analyzing a Medical Term

You can often decipher the meaning of a medical term by breaking it down into its separate parts. Consider the following examples:

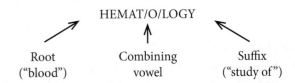

The term *hematology* is divided into three parts. When you analyze a medical term, begin at the end of the word. The ending is called the *suffix*. Almost all medical terms contain suffixes. The suffix in *hematology* is *-logy,* which means "study of." Now look at the beginning of the word. *Hemat* is the root word, which means "blood." The root word gives the essential meaning of the term.

The third part of this term, which is the letter *o,* has no meaning of its own, but is an important connector between the root (*hemat*) and the suffix (*logy*). It is the combining vowel. The letter *o* is the combining vowel usually found in medical terms.

Putting together the meanings of the suffix and the root, the term *hematology* means "the study of blood."

The combining vowel plus the root is called the combining form. A medical term can have more than one root word; therefore, there can be two combining forms. For example:

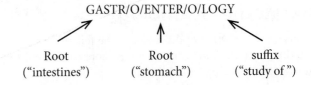

The two combining forms are *gastr/o* and *enter/o.* The entire term (reading from the suffix, back to the beginning of the term, and across) means "the study of the stomach and the intestines."

▶▶ Pulse Points

Prefix Guideline

A prefix does not require a combining vowel. Do not place a combining vowel between a prefix and a root word.

▸▸ Pulse Points

Word Part Guidelines

1. A single root word with a combining form cannot stand alone. A suffix must be added to complete the term.
2. The rules for the use of combining vowels apply when adding a suffix.
3. When a suffix begins with a consonant, a combining vowel such as *o*, is placed before the suffix.

Rules for Using Combining Vowels

1. A combining vowel is not used when the suffix begins with a vowel (*a-e-i-o-u*). For example, when *neur/o* (nerve) is joined with the suffix *-itis* (inflammation), the combining vowel is not used because *-itis* begins with a vowel. *Neuritis* (new-RYE-tis) is an inflammation of a nerve or nerves.
2. A combining vowel is used when the suffix begins with a consonant. For example, when *neur/o* (nerve) is joined with the suffix *-plasty* (surgical repair), the combining vowel *o* is used because *-plasty* begins with a consonant. *Neuroplasty* (NEW-roh-plas-tee) is the surgical repair of a nerve.
3. A combining vowel is always used when two or more root words are joined. As an example, when *gastr/o* (stomach) is joined with *enter/o* (small intestine), the combining vowel is used with *gastr/o*. *Gastroenteritis* (gas-troh-en-ter-EYE-tis) is an inflammation of the stomach and small intestine.

Suffixes and Medical Terms Related to Pathology

Pathology is the study of disease, and the following suffixes describe specific disease conditions. (A more complete list of suffixes appears on pp. 551–552.)

Suffix	Meaning
-algia	pain and suffering
-dynia	pain
-ectomy	surgical removal
-graphy	process of recording a picture or record
-gram	record or picture
-necr/osis	death (tissue death)
-scler/osis	abnormal hardening
-sten/osis	abnormal narrowing
-centesis	surgical puncture to remove fluid for diagnostic purposes or to remove excess fluid
-plasty	surgical repair
-scopy	visual examination with an instrument

The Double RRs Suffixes

The following suffixes are often referred to as the "double Rs."

-rrhage and -rrhagia	Bursting form; an abnormal excessive discharge or bleeding. *Note: -rrhage* and *-rrhagia* refer to the flow of blood.
-rrhaphy	To suture or stitch.
-rrhea	Abnormal flow or discharge; refers to the abnormal flow of most bodily fluids. *Note:* Although *-rrhea* and *-rrhage* both refer to abnormal flow, they are not used interchangeably.
-rrhexis	Rupture.

Contrasting and Confusing Prefixes

The following contrasting prefixes can be confusing. Study this list to make sure you know the differences between the contrasting terms. (A more complete list of prefixes appears on pp. 547–549.)

Ab- Means "away from." *Abnormal* means *not normal* or *away from normal.*

Ad- Means "toward" or "in the direction." *Addiction* means *drawn toward* or *a strong dependence on* a drug or substance.

Dys- Means "bad," "difficult," "painful." *Dysfunctional* means an organ or body that is not working properly.

Eu- Means "good," "normal," "well," or "easy." *Euthyroid* (you-THIGH-roid) means a normally functioning thyroid gland.

Hyper- Means "excessive" or "increased." *Hypertension* (high-per-TEN-shun) is higher than normal blood pressure.

Hypo- Means "deficient" or "decreased." *Hypotension* (high-poh-TEN-shun) is lower than normal blood pressure.

Inter- Means "between" or "among." *Interstitial* (in-ter-STISH-al) means between, but not within, the parts of a tissue.

Intra- Means "within" or "into." *Intramuscular* (in-trah-MUS-kyou-lar) means within the muscle.

Sub- Means "under," "less," or "below." *Subcostal* (sub-KOS-tal) means below a rib or ribs.

Supra- Means "above." *Supracostal* (sue-prah-KOS-tal) means above or outside the ribs.

Singular and Plural Endings

Many medical terms have Greek or Latin origins. As a result of these different origins, the rules for changing a singular word into a plural form are unusual. In addition, English endings have been adopted for some commonly used terms.

▶▶ Pulse Points

Using a Medical Dictionary

Learning to use a medical dictionary is an important part of mastering the correct use of medical terms. Some dictionaries use categories such as "Diseases and Syndromes" to group disorders with these terms in the titles. For example:

- Venereal disease would be found under "disease, venereal."
- Fetal alcohol syndrome would be found under "syndrome, fetal alcohol."

When you come across a term and cannot find it listed by the first word, the next step is to look under the appropriate category.

Guidelines to Unusual Plural Forms

Guideline	Singular	Plural
1. If the term ends in *a*, the plural is usually formed by adding an *e*.	bursa vertebra	bursae vertebrae
2. If the term ends in *ex* or *ix*, the plural is usually formed by changing the *ex* or *ix* to *ices*.	appendix index	appendices indices
3. If the term ends in *is*, the plural is usually formed by changing *is* to *es*.	diagnosis metastasis	diagnoses metastases
4. If the term ends in *itis*, the plural is usually formed by changing *is* to *ides*.	arthritis meningitis	arthritides meningitides
5. If the term ends in *nx*, the plural is usually formed by changes the *x* to *ges*.	phalanx meninx	phalanges meninges
6. If the term ends in *on*, the plural is usually formed by changing the *on* to *a*.	criterion ganglion	criteria ganglia
7. If the term ends in *um*, the plural is usually formed by changing the *um* to *a*.	diverticulum ovum	diverticula ova
8. If the term ends in *us*, the plural is usually formed by changing the *us* to *i*.	alveolus malleolus	alveoli malleoli

Basic Medical Terms

The following subsections discuss basic medical terms that are used to describe diseases and disease conditions, major body systems, and body direction.

▶▶ Pulse Points

Accuracy in Spelling

Accuracy in spelling medical terms is extremely important! Changing just one or two letters can completely change the meaning of the word—and this difference could literally be a matter of life or death for the patient.

Terms Used to Describe Diseases and Disease Conditions

The basic medical terms used to describe diseases and disease conditions are listed here.

- A *sign* is evidence of disease, such as fever, that can be observed by the patient and others. A sign is objective because it can be evaluated or measured by others.
- A *symptom,* such as pain or a headache, can only be experienced or defined by the patient. A symptom is subjective because it can be evaluated or measured only by the patient.
- A *syndrome* is a set of signs and symptoms that occur together as part of a specific disease process.
- *Diagnosis* is the identification of disease. To diagnose is the process of reaching a diagnosis.
- A *differential diagnosis* attempts to determine which of several diseases may be producing the symptoms.
- A *prognosis* is a forecast or prediction of the probable course and outcome of a disorder.
- An *acute* disease or symptom has a rapid onset, a severe course, and relatively short duration.
- A *chronic* symptom or disease has a long duration. Although chronic symptoms or diseases may be controlled, they are rarely cured.
- A *remission* is the partial or complete disappearance of the symptoms of a disease without having achieved a cure. A remission is usually temporary.
- Some diseases are named for the condition described. For example, *chronic fatigue syndrome* (CFS) is a persistent overwhelming fatigue that does not resolve with bed rest.
- An *eponym* is a disease, structure, operation, or procedure that is named for the person who discovered or described it first. For example, Alzheimer's disease is named for Alois Alzheimer, a German neurologist who lived from 1864 to 1915.
- An *acronym* is a word formed from the initial letter or letters of the major parts of a compound term. For example, the acronym AMA stands for American Medical Association.

Terms Used to Describe Major Body Systems

The following is a list of the major body systems and some common related combining forms used with each.

Major Structures and Body System	Related Roots with Combining Forms
Skeletal system	bones (oste/o) joints (arthr/o) cartilage (chondr/o)
Muscular system	muscles (my/o) ligaments (syndesm/o) tendons (ten/o, tend/o, tendin/o)
Cardiovascular system	heart (card/o, cardi/o) arteries (arteri/o) veins (phleb/o, ven/o) blood (hem/o, hemat/o)
Lymphatic and immune systems	lymph, lymph vessels, and lymph nodes (lymph/o), (lymphangi/o) tonsils (tonsill/o) spleen (splen/o) thymus (thym/o)
Respiratory system	nose (nas/o, rhin/o) pharynx (pharyng/o) trachea (trache/o) larynx (laryng/o) lungs (pneum/o, pneumon/o)
Digestive system	mouth (or/o) esophagus (esophag/o) stomach (gastr/o) small intestines (enter/o) large intestines (col/o) liver (hepat/o) pancreas (pancreat/o)
Urinary system	kidneys (nephr/o, ren/o) ureters (ureter/o) urinary bladder (cyst/o, visic/o) urethra (urethr/o)
Integumentary system	glands (aden/o) skin (cutane/o, dermat/o, derm/o) sebaceous glands (seb/o) sweat glands (hidraden/o)
Nervous system	nerves (neur/o) brain (encephal/o) spinal cord (myel/o) eyes (ocul/o, ophthalm/o) ears (acoust/o, ot/o)
Endocrine system	adrenals (adren/o) pancreas (pancreat/o) pituitary (pituit/o) thyroid (thyr/o, thyroid/o) parathyroids (parathyroid/o) thymus (thym/o)
Reproductive system	*Male:* testicles (orch/o, orchid/o) *Female:* ovaries (oophor/o, ovari/o) uterus (hyster/o, metr/o, metri/o, uter/o)

Terms Used to Describe Body Direction

Certain terms are used to describe the location of body parts relative to the trunk or other parts of the anatomy:

- *Ventral* (VEN-tral) refers to the front or belly side of the body or organ (*ventr* means "belly side" of the body and *al* means "pertaining to").
- *Dorsal* (DOR-sal) refers to the back of the body or organ (*dors* means "back of body" and *al* means "pertaining to").
- *Anterior* (an-TEER-ee-or) means situated in the front. It also means on the forward part of an organ (*anter* means "front" or "before" and *ior* means "pertaining to"). For example, the stomach is located anterior to (in front of) the pancreas. *Anterior* is also used in reference to the ventral surface of the body.
- *Posterior* (pos-TEER-ee-or) means situated in the back. It also means on the back portion of an organ (*poster* means "back" or "after" and *ior* means "pertaining to"). For example, the pancreas is located posterior to (behind) the stomach. *Posterior* is also used in reference to the dorsal surface of the body.
- *Superior* means uppermost, above, or toward the head. For example, the lungs are superior to (above) the diaphragm.
- *Inferior* means lowermost, below, or toward the feet. For example, the stomach is located inferior to (below) the diaphragm.
- *Cephalic* (seh-FAL-ick) means toward the head (*cephal* means "head" and *ic* means "pertaining to").
- *Caudal* (KAW-dal) means toward the lower part of the body (*caud* means "tail" or "lower part" of the body and *al* means "pertaining to").
- *Proximal* (PROCK-sih-mal) means situated nearest the midline or beginning of a body structure. For example, the *proximal* end of the humerus (the bone of the upper arm) forms part of the shoulder. Or, it may be easier for you to think of it as "closer to the origin of the body part or the point of attachment of a limb to the body trunk."
- *Distal* (DIS-tal) means situated farthest from the midline or beginning of a body structure. For example, the distal end of the humerus forms part of the elbow.
- *Medial* means the direction toward or nearer the midline. For example, the medial ligament of the knee is near the inner surface of the leg.

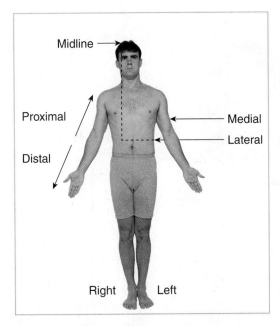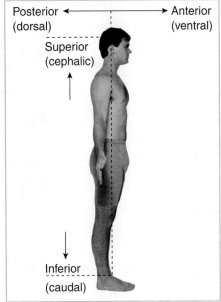

Figure C-1 ■ Directional anatomical terms.

- *Lateral* means the direction toward or nearer the side and away from the midline. For example, the lateral ligament of the knee is near the side of the leg.
- *Bilateral* means relating to, or having, two sides.

See **Figure C-1** ■.

Planes of the Body

Medical professionals often refer to sections of the body in terms of anatomical planes (flat surfaces). These planes are imaginary lines—vertical or horizontal—drawn through an upright body. The following terms are used to describe a specific body part (see **Figure C-2** ■):

- *Coronal plane (frontal plane)*: A vertical plane running from side to side; divides the body or any of its parts into anterior and posterior portions.
- *Sagittal plane (median plane)*: A vertical plane running from front to back; divides the body or any of its parts into right and left sides.
- *Axial plane (transverse plane)*: A horizontal plane; divides the body or any of its parts into upper and lower parts.

Prefixes, Root Words, and Suffixes

The most common medical prefixes, root words, and suffixes are listed here. Knowing these common prefixes, roots, and suffixes will help you decipher medical terms.

Prefixes

a	without or absence of
ab	from; away from
ad	to; toward
an	without or absence of
ante	before
anti	against
bi	two
bin	two
brady	slow
con	together
contra	against
de	from; down from; lack of
dia	through; complete; between; apart
dis	to undo; free from
dys	difficult; labored; painful; abnormal
ec	out
ecto	outside
endo	within
epi	on; upon; over
eso	inward
eu	normal; good
ex	outside; outward
exo	outside; outward
extra	outside of; beyond
hemi	half
hyper	above; excessive
hypo	below; incomplete; deficient
in	in; into; not
infra	under; below
inter	between
intra	within
mal	bad
meso	middle
meta	after; beyond; change
micro	small
multi	many

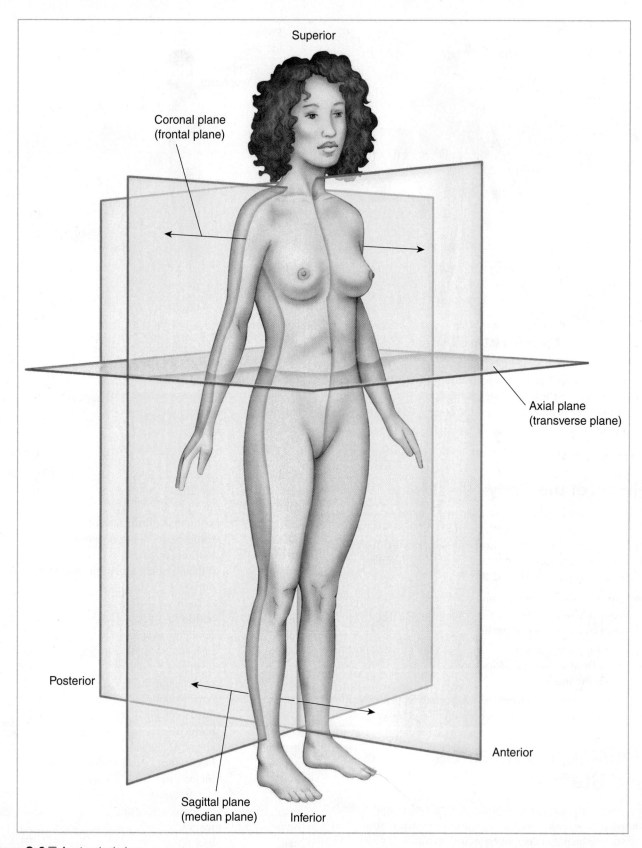

Figure C-2 ■ Anatomical planes.

neo	new
nulli	none
pan	all; total
para	outside; beyond; around
per	through
peri	surrounding (outer)
poly	many; much
post	after
pre	before; in front of
pro	before
quadri	four
re	back
retro	back; behind
semi	half
sub	under; below
super	over; above
supra	above; beyond; on top
sym	together; joined
syn	together; joined
tachy	fast; rapid
tetra	four
trans	through; across; beyond
tri	three
ultra	beyond; excess
uni	one

Root Words

abdomin	abdomen
aden	gland
adren	adrenal gland
adrenal	adrenal gland
aer	air; oxygen; gas
alveol	alveolus
angi	(blood) vessel; (lymph) vessel
ankyl	crooked; stiff; bent
appendic	appendix
arteri, arter	artery
arteriol	arteriole (small artery)
arthr	joint
ather	yellowish; fatty plaque
aur	ear
aut	self
bil	bile
bio	life
blephar	eyelid
bronch	airway; bronchus
bronchiol	bronchiole
burs	bursa
carcin	cancer
cardi	heart
caud	tail; toward lower part of the body
cephal	head
cerebell	cerebellum
cerebr	cerebrum; brain
cervic	neck; cervix

cheil	lip
chiro	hand
cholangi	bile duct
chole	gall; bile
chondr	cartilage
coccyg	coccyx; tailbone
col	colon; large intestine
conjunctiv	conjunctiva
corne	cornea
coron	heart; crown of the head
cost	rib
crani	cranium; skull
cutane	skin
cyan	blue
cyst	bladder; sac
cyt, cyte	cell
dacry	tears; tear duct
dactyl	fingers or toes
dent	tooth
derm	skin
dermat	skin
dipl	two; double
diverticul	diverticulum
dors	back (of the body)
duoden	duodenum
ectop	located away from usual place
edema	swelling
electr	electricity; electrical activity
encephal	brain
endocrin	endocrine
enter	intestines (usually small intestine)
epiglott	epiglottis
epitheli	epithelium
erythr	red
esophag	esophagus
esthesi	sensation; feeling; sensitivity
eti	cause (of disease)
exocrin	secrete out of
faci	face
fasci	fascia; fibrous band
fract	break; broken
galact	milk
gastr	stomach
ger	old age; aged
geront	old age; aged
gingiv	gums
glauc	gray
gloss	tongue
gluc	sweetness; sugar
glyc	sugar; glucose
glycos	sugar; glucose
gnos	knowledge; a knowing
gonad	gonad; sex glands
gyn	woman
gynec	woman
gyr	turning; folding

hem	blood	nyctal	night
hemat	blood	ocul	eye
hepat	liver	onc	tumor
hidr	sweat	onych	nail
hist	tissue	oophor	ovary
hom	same	ophthalm	eye
home	sameness; unchanging	or	mouth
hydr	water	orth	straight
hyster	uterus	oste	bone
ile	ileum	ot	ear
ili	ilium	ox	oxygen
immun	immune	palpat	touch; feel; stroke
irid	iris	pancreat	pancreas
kerat	horny tissue; hard	par, part	bear; give birth to; labor
kin	movement	parathyroid	parathyroid
kinesi	movement; motion	path	disease; suffering
labi	lips	pector	chest; muscle
lacrim	tear duct; tear	ped	child; foot
lact	milk	pelv	pelvis; pelvic bone
lapar	abdomen	pen	penis
laryng	larynx	perine	perineum
later	side	peritone	peritoneum
lei	smooth	petr	stone; portion of temporal bone
leuk	white	phac, phak	lens of the eye
lingu	tongue	phag	eat; swallow
lip	fat	phalang	finger or toe bone
lith	stone; calculus	pharyng	pharynx, throat
lob	lobe	phas	speech
lymph	lymph	phleb	vein
macr	abnormal largeness	phot	light
mamm	breast	phren	mind
mast	breast	physi	nature
meat	opening or passageway	pleur	pleura
melan	black	pneum	lung; air
men	menstruation	pneumat	lung; air
mening	meninges	pneumon	lung; air
ment	mind	pod	foot
mes, meso	middle	poli	gray matter
metr	uterus	polyp	polyp; small growth
mon	one	poster	back (of body)
morbid	disease; sickness	prim	first
muc	mucus	proct	rectum
my, myos	muscle	pseud	fake; false
myc	fungus	psych	mind
myel	bone marrow; spinal cord	pulmon	lung
myelon	bone marrow	py	pus
myring	eardrum	pyel	renal pelvis
narc	stupor; numbness	pylor	pylorus
nas	nose	pyr	fever; heat
nat	birth	quadr	four
necr	death (cells; body)	rect	rectum
nephr	kidney	ren	kidney
neur	nerve	retin	retina
noct	night	rhin	nose
nyct	night	sacr	sacrum fallopian (uterine)

salping	tube
sanit	soundness; health
sarc	flesh; connective tissue
scler	sclera; white of eye; hard
scoli	crooked; curved
seb	sebum; oil
seps	infection
sept	infection; partition; septum
sial	saliva
sinus	inus
somat	body
somn	sleep
son	sound
sopor	sleep
sperm	sperm, spermatazoa; seed
spermat	sperm, spermatazoa; seed
spher	round; sphere; ball
sphygm	pulse
spin	spine; backbone to
spir	breathe
splen	spleen
spondyl	vertebra; spinal or vertebral column
staphyl	grapelike clusters
stern	(breastbone)
steth	chest (muscles)
stoma	mouth; opening
stomat	mouth; opening
strab	squint; squint-eyed
synovi	synovia; synovial membrane
system	system
ten, tend	tendon
tendin	tendon
test	testis; testicle
therm	heat
thorac	thorax; chest
thromb	clot
thym	thymus gland; soul
thyr	thyroid gland
thyroid	thyroid gland
tom	cut; section
ton	tension; pressure
tone	to stretch
tonsill	tonsils
top	place; position; location
tox, toxic	poison; poisonous
trach, trache	trachea; windpipe
trachel	neck; neck-like
trich	hair
tubercul	little knot; swelling
tympan	eardrum; middle ear
ulcer	sore; ulcer
ungu	nail
ur	urine; urinary tract
ureter	ureter
urethr	urethra

uria	urination; urine
urin	urine or urinary organs
uter	uterus
uvul	uvula; little grape
vagin	vagina
valv	valve
valvul	valve
vas	vessel; duct
vascul	blood vessel; little vessel
ven	vein
versicul	seminal vesicles; blister
vertebr	vertebra; backbone
vesic	urinary bladder
vir	poison; virus
viril	masculine; manly
vis	seeing; sight
visc	sticky
viscer	viscera; internal organs sternum
viscos	sticky
vit	life
xanth	yellow
xen	strange; foreign
xer	dry
zygot	joined together

Additional Rootwords

caus	burning sensation; capable of burning
cusp	point; cusp
flexion	bending
genital	pertaining to birth
lumb	lumbar; loin region
mediastin	mediastinum
tens, tensi	pressure, force, stretching

Suffixes

Suffixes Meaning "Pertaining to"

ac
al, ine
ar, ior
ary, ory
eal, ous
ial
ic
ical, tic

Suffixes Meaning "Abnormal Conditions"

ago	abnormal condition, disease
esis	abnormal condition, disease
ia	abnormal condition, disease
iasis	abnormal condition, disease
ion	condition
ism	condition, state of abnormal condition
osis	disease

Common Suffixes Used in Medical Terminology

algia	pain, suffering
asthenia	weakness
cele	hernia, protrusion
centesis	surgical puncture to remove fluid
cidal	killing
clasia	break
clasis	break
clast	break
clysis	irrigating; washing
coccus	berry shaped (a form of bacterium)
crine	separate; secrete
crit	to separate
cyte	cell
desis	fusion; to bind; tie together
drome	run; running
ductor	to lead or pull
dynia	pain
ectasis	stretching out; dilation; expansion
ectomy	excision or surgical removal
ectopia	displacement
emesis	vomiting
emia	blood; blood condition
gen	producing, forming
genesis	producing; forming
genic	producing, forming
gnosis	a knowing
gram	record; X-ray
graph	instrument used to record
graphy	process of recording; X-ray filming
ictal	seizure; attack
ism	state of
itis	inflammation
lepsy	seizure
logist	specialist
logy	study of
lysis	destruction; reduce; separation
malacia	softening
mania	madness; insane desire
megaly	enlargement
meter	instrument used to measure
metry	measurement
morph	form; shape
oid, ode	resembling
oma	tumor; mass
opia	vision (condition)
opsy	to view
oxia	oxygen
paresis	slight paralysis
pathy	disease
penia	abnormal reduction in number; lack of

peps, pepsia	digestion
pexy	surgical fixation; suspension
phagia	eating; swallowing
philia	love
phily	love
phobia	abnormal fear of or aversion to specific objects or things
phonia	sound or voice
phoria	feeling
physis	growth
plasia	formation; development; a growth
plasm	growth; formation; substance
plasty	plastic or surgical repair
plegia	paralysis; stroke
pnea	breathing
porosis	lessening in density; porous condition
praxia	in front of; before
ptosis	drooping; sagging; prolapse
ptysis	spitting
rrhage	bursting forth, an abnormal excessive discharge or bleeding
rrhagia	bursting forth, an abnormal excessive discharge or bleeding
rrhaphy	to suture or stitch
rrhea	abnormal flow or discharge
rrhexis	rupture
schisis	split; fissure
sclerosis	hardening
scope	instrument used for visual exam
scopic	visual exam
scopy	visual exam with an instrument
sepsis	infection
sis	state of
spasm	sudden involuntary muscle contraction
stalsis	contraction; constriction
stasis	control; stop; standing still
stat	to stop
stenosis	narrowing; constriction
stomy	new artificial opening
therapy	treatment
tome	instrument used to cut
tomy	cutting into; surgical incision
tripsy	crushing
trophy	nourishment
ule	little
uria	urine; urination

Source: Adapted from Vines Allen, Deborah; Braceland, Ann; Rollins, Elizabeth; and Miller, Susan. Comprehensive Health Insurance: Billing, Coding, and Reimbursement, *2e. © 2013. Pearson Education. Upper Saddle River, NJ.*

Medical Assisting Task List

The various tasks that medical assistants perform include, but are not necessarily limited to, those on the following list.
The tasks presented in this inventory are considered by American Medical Technologists to be representative of the medical assisting job role. This document should be considered dynamic, to reflect the medical assistant's evolving role with respect to contemporary health care. Therefore, tasks may be added, removed, or modified on an on-going basis.

Medical Assistants that meet AMT's qualifications and pass a certification examination are **certified** as a Registered Medical Assistant (RMA).

I. GENERAL MEDICAL ASSISTING KNOWLEDGE

A. Anatomy and Physiology
1. Body systems
2. Disorders and diseases of the body

B. Medical Terminology
1. Word parts
2. Medical terms
3. Common abbreviations and symbols
4. Spelling

C. Medical Law
1. Medical law
2. Licensure, certification, and registration

D. Medical Ethics
1. Principles of medical ethics
2. Ethical conduct
3. Professional development

E. Human Relations
1. Patient relations
2. Interpersonal skills
3. Cultural diversity

F. Patient Education
1. Identify and apply proper communication methods in patient instruction
2. Develop, assemble, and maintain patient resource materials

II. ADMINISTRATIVE MEDICAL ASSISTING

A. Insurance
1. Medical insurance terminology
2. Various insurance plans
3. Claim forms
4. Electronic insurance claims
5. ICD-9/CPT Coding applications
6. HIPAA mandated coding systems
7. Financial applications of medical insurance

B. Financial Bookkeeping
1. Medical finance terminology
2. Patient billing procedures
3. Collection procedures
4. Fundamental medical office accounting procedures
5. Office banking procedures
6. Employee payroll
7. Financial calculations and accounting procedures

C. Medical Secretarial – Receptionist
1. Medical terminology associated with receptionist duties
2. General reception of patients and visitors
3. Appointment scheduling systems
4. Oral and written communications
5. Medical records management
6. Charting guidelines and regulations
7. Protect, store and retain medical records according to HIPAA regulations
8. Release of protected health information adhering to HIPAA regulations
9. Transcription of dictation
10. Supplies and equipment management
11. Medical office computer applications
12. Compliance with OSHA guidelines and regulations of office safety

III. CLINICAL MEDICAL ASSISTING

A. Asepsis
1. Medical terminology
2. State/Federal universal blood borne pathogen/body fluid precautions
3. Medical/Surgical asepsis procedure

B. Sterilization
1. Medical terminology associated with sterilization
2. Sanitization, disinfection, and sterilization procedures
3. Record keeping procedures

C. Instruments
1. Specialty instruments and parts
2. Usage of common instruments
3. Care and handling of disposable and re-usable instruments.

D. Vital Signs / Mensurations
1. Blood pressure, pulse, respiration measurements
2. Height, weight, circumference measurements
3. Various temperature measurements
4. Recognize normal and abnormal measurement results

E. Physical Examinations
1. Patient history information
2. Proper charting procedures
3. Patient positions for examinations
4. Methods of examinations
5. Specialty examinations
6. Visual acuity / Ishihara (color blindness) measurements
7. Allergy testing procedures
8. Normal / abnormal results

F. Clinical Pharmacology
1. Medical terminology associated with pharmacology
2. Commonly used drugs and their categories
3. Various routes of medication administration
4. Parenteral administration of medications (Subcutaneous, Intramuscular, Intradermal, Z-Tract)
5. Classes or drug schedules and legal prescriptions requirements for each
6. Drug Enforcement Agency regulations for ordering, dispensing, storage, and documentation of medication use
7. Drug Reference books (PDR, Pharmacopeia, Facts and Comparisons, Nurses Handbook)

G. Minor Surgery
1. Surgical supplies and instruments
2. Asepsis in surgical procedures
3. Surgical tray preparation and sterile field respect
4. Prevention of pathogen transmission
5. Patient surgical preparation procedures
6. Assisting physician with minor surgery including set-up
7. Dressing and bandaging techniques
8. Suture and staple removal
9. Biohazard waste disposal procedures
10. Instruct patient in pre- and post-surgical care

H. Therapeutic Modalities
1. Various standard therapeutic modalities
2. Alternative/complementary therapies
3. Instruct patient in assistive devices, body mechanics and home care

I. Laboratory Procedures
1. Medical laboratory terminology
2. OSHA safety guidelines
3. Quality control and assessment regulations
4. Operate and maintain laboratory equipment
5. CLIA waived laboratory testing procedures
6. Capillary, dermal and venipuncture procedures
7. Office specimen collection such as: Urine, throat, vaginal, wound cultures – stool, sputum, etc
8. Specimen handling and preparation
9. Laboratory recording according to state and federal guidelines
10. Adhere to the M A Scope of Practice in the laboratory

J. Electrocardiography
1. Standard, 12 Lead ECG Testing
2. Mounting techniques for permanent record
3. Rhythm strip ECG monitoring on Lead II

K. First Aid
1. Emergencies and first aid procedures
2. Emergency crash cart supplies
3. Legal responsibilities as a first responder

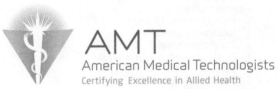

AMT
American Medical Technologists
Certifying Excellence in Allied Health

10700 W. Higgins Road Suite 150
Rosemont, Illinois 60018
Phone: (847) 823-5169
Fax: (847) 823-0458
www.amt1.com

How to Become a Successful Student

What Kind of Learner Are You?

In order to become a successful student, it is important to evaluate the type of learner you are. Following are the characteristics of the visual, auditory, and tactile learner.

The Visual Learner

- Tries to envision the word when spelling it out
- Dislikes listening for long periods of time
- Becomes distracted by movement when trying to concentrate
- May not remember names, but will typically remember faces
- Prefers face-to-face meetings
- Prefers to read or hear descriptions when learning new material
- Likes to look at pictures when learning new material

The Auditory Learner

- Tries to sound out the word when spelling it out
- Enjoys listening rather than talking
- Becomes distracted by sounds or noises when trying to concentrate
- Prefers the telephone to face-to-face meetings
- Prefers verbal instructions

The Tactile Learner

- Writes a word out when learning to spell it
- Uses gestures and expressive movements when talking
- Becomes distracted by activity when trying to concentrate
- Prefers to talk while participating in activities
- Is not necessarily a good reader—prefers stories that are action oriented
- Tends to figure things out as she goes along rather than reading directions

Skill Sets

Once you've realized the type of learner you are, take steps to use the skills you have in learning new material.

The Visual Learner Might Try:

- Looking at pictures or diagrams when learning new material
- Studying in a quiet room with no distractions
- Asking for descriptions or asking instructors to explain how a topic might apply in the real world. For example, "Would you demonstrate that skill to the class?"

The Auditory Learner Might Try:

- Reading aloud or taping his voice and playing it back to study new material
- Taping the instructor's lecture and replaying it later to study
- Studying in a quiet room with no distractions
- Working with study groups where students discuss the material they've learned

The Tactile Learner Might Try:

- Writing material down several times in order to memorize it
- Studying in a quiet area with no distractions
- Asking the instructor to give examples of how a topic is addressed. For example, "Would you allow the class to role-play that activity so we can see what it feels like?"
- Practicing activities or skills in order to commit them to memory

Time Management

One of the greatest difficulties for new students is time management and organization of priorities. For those students who have trouble in this area, the following steps might help:

- Set aside blocks of time for studying.
- Take periodic breaks when studying—get up and move around, get a drink, close your eyes for a few moments.
- Prioritize your assignments. Many students find it helpful to write down their assignments and place numbers next to each to indicate the order in which they need to be done.
- Study or read while doing other activities. Students can study or read while exercising, or at the gym.
- Review study material just prior to class on test day.
- Create to-do lists.
- Use a daily/weekly/monthly calendar. Write down dates of upcoming tests or project due dates, then backtrack to add in dates when certain stages of the project should be completed. For example, if a paper is due four weeks

from today, add a note to the calendar for one week from today that the outline should be completed, two weeks from today that the rough draft should be completed, and so on.

- Look for study partners for each class. Link up with study partners who are "good" students, not those who are not as dedicated as you are to learning the material. Spend time together each week going over the material from the class and studying or preparing for tests or projects.

Students should always be able to consult the course instructor for clarification of subject matter or for verification of course progress. Students must be aware of their progress in any given class and take an active part in assuring their own success.

Translation of English–Spanish Phrases

Would you prefer a morning or an afternoon appointment?
¿Preferiría una cita en la mañana o en la tarde?

Are you covered by medical insurance?
¿Tiene seguro médico?

Do you need directions to the office?
¿Necesita indicaciones para llegar a nuestra oficina?

Is your visit due to an accident?
¿Su visita está relacionada con algún accidente?

What is your home telephone number?
¿Cuál es el número de teléfono de su casa?

What is your work telephone number?
¿Cuál es el número de teléfono de su trabajo?

Your co-payment for today is $_____.
Su co-pago de hoy es $_____.

Please take a seat, the medical assistant will take you back in just a moment.
Por favor, tome asiento, el asistente médico lo atenderá en un momento.

Can you bring someone with you who speaks English?
¿Puede venir acompañado de alguien que hable inglés?

The doctor is running behind schedule, there will be a 20 minute wait.
El doctor está demorado, habrá una espera de veinte minutos.

Children may not be left unattended in the reception room.
No debe haber niños sin supervisión de un adulto en la sala de espera.

I need to take a photocopy of your driver's license.
Necesito fotocopiar su licencia de conducir.

Has someone referred you to our office?
¿Alguien le recomendó nuestra clínica?

Which doctor did you want to see?
¿Con qué doctor se quiere atender?

Is there a day of the week you would prefer for your appointment?
¿Prefiere algún día de la semana en particular para su cita?

Please bring your insurance information with you when you come in for your appointment.
Por favor traiga la información de su seguro médico cuando venga a su cita.

Please take this slip to the laboratory.
Por favor lleve esta hoja al laboratorio.

This form is our HIPAA privacy agreement.
Este es nuestro formulario de privacidad según la Ley de Portabilidad y Responsabilidad del Seguro de Salud (HIPAA)

I see that you are upset. Let me show you to a private room where we can talk.
Entiendo que esté molesto. Por favor, acompáñeme a una sala privada para que podamos dialogar.

This pamphlet contains written information about your condition.
Este panfleto contiene información escrita sobre su condición.

How long have you had problems with this?
¿Desde cuándo tiene este tipo de problema?

What is your name?
¿Cómo se llama?

Do you speak English?
¿Habla inglés?

Can you read English?
¿Puede leer en inglés?

Thank you
Gracias.

You are welcome.
De nada.

Please.
Por favor.

It is nice to meet you.
Encantado/a de conocerlo/a

abuse—with regard to billing practices, the improper behavior and billing practices that result in improper financial gain but are not fraudulent

abuse—the neglect, or physical, emotional, or financial misconduct of another

accept assignment—agreement by a physician to accept the amount approved by the insurance company as payment in full for a given service

accounts receivables (AR)—money owed the medical practice

accredited—endorsed by a reputable overseeing agency

Accrediting Bureau of Health Education Schools (ABHES)—agency that helps support the certification of medical assistants through program endorsement; accredits private and postsecondary institutions offering allied health education programs in medical assisting, medical laboratory technicians, and surgical technology programs

active listening—giving full attention during an exchange of information

active patient files—files for patients who have appointments or who have been in to see the physician recently

add-on code—a CPT code designated by the plus sign (+) that cannot be used alone; must be used with another CPT code

administrative—pertaining to office functions (e.g., computer operation, medical records management, coding, and billing)

administrative law—legislation passed by administrative governmental agencies

administrative skills—clerical-type responsibilities (e.g., typing, filing)

advance beneficiary notice—a form patients sign agreeing to pay for covered Medicare services that may be denied due to medical necessity or frequency

advance directives—documents that outline patients' wishes regarding health care should those patients be unable to speak for themselves

adverse outcome—unfavorable treatment result

advocate—to defend the rights of others; one who defends or acts on behalf of another

agenda—list of items to be addressed during a meeting

aging report—documentation of the money owed the medical office and how long accounts have been outstanding

allowed amount—the dollar amount for a service that an insurance company considers acceptable and uses to determine benefit payments

ambulatory care centers—health care clinics where patients are seen for short visits

American Association of Medical Assistants (AAMA)—national-level, professional association for medical assistants

American Medical Technologists (AMT)—national, professional association for medical technologists

American Red Cross—humanitarian organization that provides emergency assistance

Americans with Disabilities Act (ADA)—federal law that outlines appropriate treatment or accommodations for patients or employees with disabilities

anaphylaxis—severe, life-threatening allergic reaction

anatomy—study of the structure and organization of animals and plants

anesthesia—general or local loss of sensation induced by interventions or drugs to permit the performance of an otherwise painful procedure

annotation—process of reading a document and highlighting pertinent information

antisepsis—destruction of the microorganisms that produce sepsis or septic disease

appeal—request for review of a denied service or claim, in an attempt to see the insurance company's denial reversed or overturned

artificial insemination—fertilization of sperm and egg through a nonsexual process

assault—threat of causing physical harm to another without their consent

assess—to make a judgment about something

assignment of benefits—authorization by a patient for the insurance carrier to pay the health care professional directly rather than issuing monies to the patient

associate degree—degree awarded by community colleges after a roughly 2-year course of study

assumption of risk—defense to medical malpractice in which the provider must prove the patient was fully informed of a procedure's risks

astrology—study of how the planets and stars influence events and the lives and behaviors of individuals

attitude—state of mind; way of carrying one's self

audit—a review process that verifies that every detail of a CPT code is clearly documented in the medical record

auditors—those who review personal or corporate bank or tax records on behalf of an agency such as the Internal Revenue Service (IRS)

automatic dialer—telephone feature that dials numbers programmed into the system using codes

automatic routing unit—telephone equipment that allows callers to self-select their call destinations via an automated, electronic prompt system

autopsy—examination of a body after death to determine the cause of death

balance billing—billing a patient for the dollar difference between the provider's charge and the insurance approved amount; usually not permitted for participating providers

bar-code scanner—device that scans or views bar codes for transfer to attached computers

battery backup system—system that protects computers in the event of power surges or power outages

battery—act of harming another person without the person's consent

beneficiary—person who is eligible to receive benefits/services under an insurance policy

bilateral—on both sides of the body

bioethics—issues surrounding life-and-death situations in health care (e.g., cloning, artificial insemination, abortion)

birthday rule—a coordination of benefits rule which states that, when children are covered under the policies of both parents, the insurance policy of parent with the birthday earlier in the year is the primary insurance for the children; the insurance policy of the parent with the later birthday is the secondary insurance

body language—nonverbal means of communication (e.g., gestures, expressions)

body language—the process of communicating nonverbally through movements and gestures (e.g., facial expressions)

body—main portion of a business letter

brochure—document containing information about a topic

buffer time—an appointment scheduling method of leaving certain times of day open to accommodate situations such as patients who call for same-day appointments or physicians who need to catch up on charting

bundling—the act of combining multiple services under a single, all-inclusive CPT code and one charge

caduceus—emblem of the medical profession

call forwarding—telephone feature that forwards incoming calls to other numbers

capitation—a reimbursement method in which providers are paid set fees per month per member patients

category (CPT)—a division of a subheading within the CPT Tabular List

category (ICD-10-CM)—a three-digit code in ICD-10-CM Tabular List

Category I codes—CPT codes numbered 00100 to 99999 representing widely used services and procedures approved by the FDA

Category II codes—optional codes used to collect and track data for performance measurement; four numbers followed by the letter F, such as 1002F

Category III codes—temporary codes for data collection and tracking the use of emerging technology, services, and procedures; four numbers followed by the letter T, such as 0162T

certificate of coverage—a letter from the insurance company that provides proof of type and time frame of coverage when a patient terminates a health insurance policy

certified letter—postal service letter that the recipient must sign for upon receipt

certified medical assistant (CMA)—graduate of an accredited medical assisting program who has passed the certification examination of the American Association of Medical Assistants (AAMA)

CHAMPVA—a federal program that covers the health care expenses of the families of veterans with total, permanent, service-related, covered disabilities and the spouses and dependent children of veterans who died in the line of duty

chapter—one of 21 major sections of the ICD-10-CM Tabular List, organized by body system and etiology

charitable contributions—cash or other donations given to charitable organizations

checklist—list of activities or steps to take to perform a task

chemical waste—wasted drugs, cleaning solutions, germicides

chief complaint—statement in the patient's own words of the reason for seeking medical care

chiropractic—a system of complementary therapy that corrects misalignments of the joints, especially those of the spinal column

chloroform—early method of general anesthesia used to render a patient unconscious

Circular E—yearly booklet published by the IRS that outlines the federal tax deductions to be taken from individuals' wages depending on marital status and number of exemptions

civil law—legislation that governs actions between two or more citizens

clean claim—insurance claim with no data errors

clinical—pertaining to direct patient care (e.g., drawing blood samples, taking vital signs, assisting with surgery)

clinical skills—abilities gained through hands-on patient care

cloning—the process of producing an identical copy of something biological via DNA replication

closed patient files—files for patients who will not be returning to the clinic

closed-panel—an HMO in which physicians see only the patients of a specific HMO

close-ended question—question that can be answered with "yes" or "no"

closing—ending portion of a business letter

cluster scheduling—scheduling method that groups patients with similar appointments around the same time of day

code—the most specific entry that requires no additional characters

coinsurance—percentage of medical charges patients are responsible for according to their insurance plan contracts

collection agency—company that pursues overdue accounts for a fee

combination code—a single code that describes two or more conditions that frequently occur together

commercial law—legislation that governs business transactions

Commission on Accreditation of Allied Health Education Programs (CAAHEP)—agency supporting the process of medical assisting certification through program endorsement; accredits over 2,100 entry-level programs in 23 health science professions.

common descriptor—the portion of a standalone code before the semicolon that is shared with the indented codes that follow

common law—legislation derived from the Old English legal system that is based on precedence

community college—educational institution that provides 2-year undergraduate education

community property laws—legislation that deems one spouse financially responsible for the other spouse's debts

comparative negligence—defense to medical malpractice in which the physician proves the patient was partly responsible for the patient's injury

competency—skill in a defined area

computer peripherals—devices that connect to computers to add function or use

computer virus—program written to disrupt computer function

conference call—telephone feature that allows parties in different locations to participate in one call

confidentiality—state of privacy or secrecy

constitutional law—law outlined in the U.S. Constitution

contract law—legislation that relates agreements between two parties

contributing factors—three secondary criteria, in addition to the key components, that may influence the selection of an E&M code; include presenting problem, counseling/coordination of care, and physicians' face-to-face time with patients and families

contributory negligence—defense to medical malpractice in which the physician proves an injury would not have occurred if not for the patient's actions

conventions—coding rules, abbreviations, symbols, or formatting intended to ensure consistency in coding

conversion factor—a constant dollar value multiplied by the relative value unit to determine the price of individual services

coordination of benefits—the process of determining which insurance policy should be billed first, second, or third when a patient is covered by multiple policies

coordination of care—a contributory factor in E&M coding that describes physicians' work in arranging care with other providers

copayment—the established dollar amount per visit or service that patients are responsible for according to their insurance plan contracts

counseling—a contributory factor in E&M coding that describes physicians' discussions with patients and family members

courtesy—polite behavior

cover letter—document that accompanies a résumé to a prospective employer

covered—services potentially eligible for reimbursement

CPR mouth barrier—disposable barrier device used to prevent infection

crash cart—wheeled cart that contains emergency medical equipment

credibility— the quality of being worthy of trust; believable

criminal law—legislation that relates to crimes

cross-referencing—method of tracking and finding patient files for patients with multiple last names

Current Procedural Terminology—Level I of the HCPCS code set used to code procedures and services in outpatient health care settings

damages—money a patient is awarded for damages or injuries the patient sustained

deductible—monetary amount patients must pay to the provider for health care services before their health insurance benefits begin to pay

deductions—number of allowances to be withheld from wages

defamation of character—intentional false or negative statements about a person that causes damages

defibrillator—a device that delivers an electric shock to a patient

delegate—to assign a task to another individual

demographic—statistical data of a population, such as age, gender, education, income, and ethnicity

denied—a claim processed by an insurer and determined not eligible for payment

dependability—capable of being relied on

dependent—a family member or other individual who qualifies for coverage on the insured's policy

direct mail advertising—a form of advertising that is mailed directly to homes

direct telephone lines—telephone number that reaches a person directly rather than an operator or a receptionist

disability income insurance—insurance that covers lost wages and certain other benefits due to disability that prevents the individual from working; also called disability insurance

discovery rule—legislation that states the statute of limitations begins when an injury was discovered or should have been discovered

discriminating—acting against a person's interest due to a perceived difference in race, gender, economic, or other status

documenting—process of capturing information in the patient's chart

double booking—scheduling more than one patient for the same appointment time

downcode—to assign a code for a lower level of service than was actually performed; done by some insurance companies to save money; done by some physicians to avoid fraud or abuse charges

dual fee schedule—facility or health care provider with two fees for the same service

duress—act of coercing someone into an act

edit—a specific coding or billing criterion that is checked for accuracy based on predetermined rules

elective procedure—a medical procedure that will benefit the patient but does not need to be scheduled immediately

electronic health record—medical record kept via computer; refers to a patient's entire medical history in electronic form

electronic mail—message sent electronically from one person to another; also called e-mail

electronic signature—electronic version of a person's signature to be used in electronic health records

financial information—data on payment record or ledger, health insurance identification numbers, and policy numbers

electronic signature—electronic version of a person's signature to be used in electronic health records

electronic sign-in sheet—computer program that displays the names of those who sign in

eligibility—the process to determine if a patient is qualified to receive coverage/paid benefits according to the insurance policy guidelines

empathy—ability to identify with and understand another person's feelings

Employment Assistance Programs (EAPs)—resources, such as counseling and drug or alcohol rehabilitation, for those in personal crisis

encounter form—document on which the physician indicates procedure and diagnosis codes

endorsement stamp—rubber tool that imprints a receiving agency's banking information

ergonomic—designed for proper body posture

established patient—a patient who has seen the same provider, or another provider of the same specialty or subspecialty, in the same practice within the past three years

ether—anesthetic used in the mid-19th century to alleviate pain during surgical procedures

etiology—cause of a disease or an illness

Evaluation and Management—CPT codes used for billing physician services to evaluate and manage patient care, such as office visits

evaluation—to judge or interpret the value of something (e.g., a patient's progress)

evidence-based medicine—the practice of integrating the best, current clinical evidence from systematic research with individual clinical expertise

examination—a key component of E&M coding that describes the complexity of the physical assessment of the patient

examples—illustrations of concepts or ideas

exclusions—procedures or services not covered under an insurance plan

exclusive provider organization—a managed care contract with a smaller network of providers under which the employer agrees to not use any other networks in return for favorable pricing

expert witness—person deemed by the court to be an authority on a particular subject matter

expiration date—date on which something loses full strength or validity

explanation of benefits—a statement accompanying payment from the insurance company that summarizes how the payment for each billed service was calculated and gives reasons for any items not paid

expressed consent—agreement, either verbally or in writing, from the patient before a procedure is performed

expressed contract—a contract that identifies all the elements are specifically stated

face-to-face time—a contributory factor in E&M coding that measures the amount of time the provider spent in the presence of the patient and/or family, as opposed to time spent documenting the visit or arranging referrals

Fair Debt Collection Practices Act (FDCPA)—law that dictates how debts may be collected

Fair Labor Standards Act (FLSA)—law passed by U.S. Congress in 1938 to address employment issues like federal minimum wage

faith healer—practitioner who uses prayer or faith rather than medicine to heal patients

Family Medical Leave Act (FMLA)—law pertaining to employees' ability to take unpaid leave for medical conditions, birth or adoption of a child, or to care for a family member

Federal Insurance Contributions Act (FICA)—law that addresses Social Security withholding taxes

Federal Unemployment Tax Act (FUTA)—law that addresses federal unemployment tax withholdings

fee schedule—a list of the approved fees that an insurance carrier agrees to pay to participating providers; also refers to the standard set of fees the provider charges to all insurers

feedback—information that is reflected back to an individual in an interpersonal exchange (e.g., during patient–provider communication)

fee-for-service—the payment method in which insurance companies pay providers fees for each service provided to covered patients

felony—a crime considered to be of a serious nature; characterized as any offense punishable by imprisonment for more than one year, or by death

first listed—the diagnosis that is chiefly responsible for the outpatient services provided; formerly called *primary diagnosis*

First Report of Injury or Illness—the initial report of a workers' compensation illness or injury that documents the circumstances of the illness, injury, treatment plan, and prognosis

fixed-appointment scheduling—scheduling system that assigns every patient a specific appointment time

flash drive— small, external data storage device; see also *thumb drive*

flexibility—willingness to change when needed or requested

flowcharts—graphs in patient medical records that track such things as weight gain or newborn growth

focus group—a representative group of individuals brought together and questioned about their ideas on new products or services

font—style of type

Four Ds of Negligence—elements patients must prove in malpractice (i.e., duty, dereliction of duty, direct cause, and damages)

fraud—deceitful act done to conceal the truth

fraud (in billing)—the act of intentionally billing for services that were never given, including billing for a service that has a higher reimbursement than the service provided

front desk—place in a medical office where the receptionist welcomes patients as they enter

garnish—to withhold wages from an employee's paycheck due to a court order

generic message—telephone answering message that fails to identify the receiver specifically

geographic adjustment factor—a numeric multiplier used by Medicare to adjust fees for the varying costs of practicing medicine in different areas of the country

geographical practice cost index (GPCI)—Medicare system of adjusting fees based on the area in which the health care provider practices

global period—the number of days surrounding a surgical procedure during which all services relating to that procedure—preoperative, during the surgery, and postoperative—are considered part of the surgical package

Good Samaritan Act—a law that may protect a person from negligence for voluntarily performing lifesaving care

gross pay—amount earned before taxes or deductions are subtracted

group health insurance—a commercial insurance policy with rates based on a group of people, usually offered by an employer

guidelines—specific instructions at the beginning of each section of the CPT manual that define terms and describe specific information about how to use codes in that section

hands-free telephone device—headset or headphones with a speaker and microphone that allow users to participate in calls without picking up the telephone's receiver

hardship agreement—agreement a patient signs to indicate an inability to pay full health care costs due to financial hardship

hazard—something that is dangerous or possibly dangerous

health insurance exchange—an organization created by the Patient Protection and Affordable Care Act that offers a choice of health insurance plans, certifies the plans that participate, and provides consumer information regarding options

Health Insurance Portability and Accountability Act (HIPAA)—legislation that addresses patient privacy

health maintenance organization—a group of physicians or medical centers that provides comprehensive service to members under a capitated payment plan; members' care is covered only when using these designated providers

Healthcare Common Procedure Coding System—the code set used to code procedures and services in the outpatient health care setting

health-related calculator—computer program that quantifies health-related conditions (e.g., target body weight)

HIPAA compliant—in line with federal patient confidentiality laws

Hippocrates—an ancient Greek physician who is known as the "Father of Medicine"; considered one of the most outstanding figures in the history of medicine

history—a key component of E&M coding that describes the background, onset, and progression of the patient's current condition

hold feature—telephone feature that allows the user to place one call on hold and take another

Human Genome Project—a scientific project designed to study and identify all human genes

immunity—state of being held unaccountable for one's actions

implementation—process of taking action; putting a plan in place

implied consent—agreement through actions only

implied contract—agreement to a contract through actions only

inactive patient files—files for patients who have not seen the physician for extended periods

indecipherable—unreadable

indented code—a CPT code whose description is indented three spaces under another (standalone) code and whose definition includes the portion before the semicolon (;) in the standalone code

Index (CPT)—the alphabetical listing of CPT codes by procedure name, condition, eponym, and acronym

Index to Diseases and Injuries—the portion of the ICD-10-CM manual that lists conditions and diseases in alphabetical order by Main Term

individual health insurance—a commercial health insurance policy with rates based on individual health criteria

individual mandate—the requirement of the Patient Protection and Affordable Care Act that, as of 2014, requires most people to have health insurance and requires them to pay a tax penalty if they do not

infectious waste—any item exposed to bodily fluids or any laboratory cultures or blood products

informed consent—process in which a physician reviews with a patient the risks associated with a procedure, the risks of nontreatment, and accepted treatment alternatives

initiative—energy or aptitude displayed in starting a task without prompting

inpatient—a patient who has been formally admitted to a facility with written admission orders from a physician

instructional notes—directions in the Tabular List, which appear in parentheses before or after a code entry, to point the user to alternative codes for closely related procedures or to codes that must or must not be used together

insurance fraud—illegal act by a health care provider involving an insurance company

insured—person who holds or owns an insurance policy; same as the member or the policyholder

intentional tort—act of purposefully harming another

international law—legislation that relates to the actions that occur between two or more countries

Internet search engine—Web site that searches the Internet for information based on set criteria

interview—meeting, usually face-to-face, between an employer and an applicant

invasion of privacy—the intentional prying or intruding into another person's confidential information or matters

inventory—supplies on hand

Item—the name of a box to be completed on the CMS-1500 claim form

key component—three primary determining criteria in selecting an E&M code; include history, examination, and medical decision making

last number redial—telephone feature that dials the last number dialed from that telephone

letterhead—professional-quality stationery with a business's contact information (e.g., name, address, telephone and fax numbers)

Level I codes—same as Current Procedural Terminology

Level II codes—HCPCS alphanumeric codes created by CMS to bill supplies, drugs, and certain services

liability insurance—the type of insurance that covers injuries that occur on, in, or because of the insured's property; also called *property and casualty insurance*

lifetime maximum benefit—monetary amount allowed by an insurance carrier for a covered member's covered expenses over the member's lifetime

logo—image that represents a business entity or brand

long-term disability—a disability income insurance policy that has a longer waiting period, usually three months to two years, and pays benefits for an extended length of time, which may be several years, to age 65, or the lifetime

loyalty—devotion to another

Main Term (CPT)—words by which procedures and services are alphabetized in the CPT Index; may be a procedure, service, anatomic site, condition, synonym, eponym, or abbreviation

Main Term (ICD-10-CM)—words by which conditions and diseases are alphabetized in the ICD-10-CM Index; may be name of condition, eponym, acronym, or synonym, but not an anatomical site

maintained—kept in good working order

malfeasance—state of performing an incorrect treatment resulting in injury to the patient

malpractice—a breach of duty

malpractice insurance policy—insurance to cover actions that have hurt a patient

malware—computer software that can destroy or disable computer programs

managed care organization—a company that attempts to control the cost of health care while providing better outcomes by transferring financial risk to the provider

marketing budget—the amount of money allocated by a company to promote its products or services

marketing firm—an organization hired to design a marketing plan

marketing plan—a comprehensive plan that outlines a business's overall marketing objectives in a given period

matrix—process of blocking out times in the appointment schedule when the provider is unavailable or out of the office

meaningful use—an incentive program put in place by the Centers for Medicare and Medicaid Services (CMS) to promote the use of electronic health records in medical facilities

Medicaid—a joint federal and state program that helps with medical costs for some people with low incomes and limited resources

medical decision making—a key component of E&M coding that describes the complexity of establishing a diagnosis and/or selecting a management option

medical ethics—the concepts that govern the actions of health care professionals

medical information—information on a patient's medical care and history

medical management software—software medical offices use to perform day-to-day functions (e.g., billing, appointment scheduling)

medical necessity—criteria established by a payer to determine when a service is justified, based on the health care needs of a patient

medical record—legal document consisting of medical information obtained from the patient via consultations, examinations, and tests

medical research program—research conducted to determine the effectiveness or harm of certain medications or medical treatments

Medicare—federal program that covers medical expenses for those age 65 and over, those with end-stage renal disease, and those with long-term disabilities

Medicare Severity Diagnosis Related Groups—a case-based payment method used by Medicare for inpatient hospital stays in which patients with similar conditions and care requirements are classified together and are eligible for the same amount of reimbursement

Medigap—a private insurance policy that supplements Medicare coverage, in order to fill "gaps" in Part A and Part B coverage

member—the person who owns the insurance policy

memo—interoffice note

mentor—person who supervises a practicum in a health care facility; also called a preceptor

misdemeanor—crime of a less serious nature; characterized as any offense punishable by no more than one year in prison

misfeasance—state of performing a procedure incorrectly resulting in injury to the patient

mission statement—summary of an organization's purpose or reason for existing

modified wave scheduling—a scheduling system where two or three patients are scheduled at the beginning of each hour, followed by single patient appointments every 10 to 20 minutes for the rest of that hour

modifier—a two-character alphanumeric code appended to CPT (Level I) or Level II codes to further describe circumstances

modifying term—descriptive words in the Index that appear indented under the Main Term to further describe the service or procedure

morals—codes or guidelines used to determine behavior or a course of action

morbidity—cause of illness or injury

mortality—cause of death

multidisciplinary—combining many fields of study

multiple coding—a diagnosis that requires more than one code to completely describe it; often indicated by a second code in slanted brackets

narrative—type of medical charting in which the health care provider writes a narrative version of patient contact

national conversion factor—number released by Medicare each year that determines fee schedules for all health care services

national standard—point of reference for developing charges for health care services used throughout the United States

negligence—not acting responsibly resulting in patient harm

negotiated fee schedule—a reimbursement method in which the managed care plan develops a fees schedule that participating providers agree to accept

neoplasm—the medical term for an abnormal growth of new tissue; often referred to as a tumor

net pay—amount remaining after deductions and taxes are subtracted

new patient—a patient who has not seen the same provider, or another provider of the same specialty and subspecialty in the same practice, for more than three years

new patient checklist—list of information new patients must provide when calling to schedule appointments

non-covered—services not eligible for reimbursement under any circumstance

nonessential modifiers—words in parentheses after a Main Term in the ICD-10-CM that clarify the Main Term but that need not be present in the medical record

nonfeasance—the act of delaying or failing to perform a treatment

nontherapeutic research—research programs that do not benefit the study's patients

obliterate—to make unreadable or unrecognizable

office brochure—pamphlet outlining an office's staff and services

office policy—agreed-upon standard for handling a situation or procedure in the office

Omnibus Budget Reconciliation Act (OBRA)—legislation passed by Congress in 1989 to calculate health care service fees by formula

open hours—scheduling method that allows patients to seek treatment without appointment times

open-ended question—question that requires more than a "yes" or "no" answer

open-panel—an HMO in which providers treat both HMO patients and non-HMO patients

organizational chart—breakdown of the chain of command in a business

outliers—exceptional circumstances that cost far more or less than the average

outpatient—a patient who has not been formally admitted to a facility, such as one seen for office visits, emergency department visits, and observation status

outsource—to send to another business for completion

overtime—wages paid beyond 40 hours in a workweek, at a rate 1.5 times the normal rate for that employee

packing slip—list of supplies ordered and included in a shipment

panel—a group of laboratory tests ordered together to detect particular diseases or malfunctioning organs

parent code—see *standalone code*

participating provider—a health care provider who has contracted with a particular health insurance carrier

patient billing statements—monthly statements sent to patients who have an outstanding balance

Patient Care Partnership—a list from the American Hospital Association (AHA) of patients' expectations, rights, and responsibilities while under care in the hospital setting

patient information—the information contained within the patient's medical record

Patient Protection and Affordable Care Act—federal legislation passed in 2010 to help decrease the number of uninsured Americans and reduce the overall costs of health care through the use of mandates, subsidies, and tax credits; also referred to as the Affordable Care Act (ACA)

patient status—the classification of patients as new or established

payroll—process of calculating the amounts employees receive for their work

payroll taxes—monies withheld from wages for federal income tax, Social Security, and Medicare obligations

personal digital assistant (PDA)—small, portable device that stores and transmits data

personal information—information such as patient's name, birthdate, gender, marital status, occupation, next of kin, and any other items collected for personal identification

personal injury protection—the portion of automobile insurance that pays for injuries sustained due to an automobile accident

personal space—area around a person deemed the "comfort zone"

personnel file—set of employment-related documents for an employee, including an original application, federal withholding requests, and dates and copies of evaluations

personnel manual—compilation of employment policies for an office; also called an *employee handbook*

pharmaceuticals—drugs, medicines, and chemical compounds

physiology—study of the mechanical, physical, and biochemical functions of living organisms

planning—process of researching the actions or steps needed to implement a plan or project

point of service—an insurance offering in which a patient has access to multiple plans, such as an HMO, PPO, and indemnity and may choose to use any of them for any given service

policy—a rule by which an individual or organization is guided

policyholder—person who holds or owns an insurance policy; same as the *member* or the *insured*

portability—state of being able to move an insurance policy from one employer to another

postage meter—electronic scale used for weighing packages and printing postage labels

post—to add charges or payments to a patient's account

practicum—educational learning opportunity outside the classroom that gives students hands-on experience; final phase of an accredited medical assisting program

preapproval—the process of calling a patient's insurance carrier prior to a service to obtain preapproval or authorization for the service to be performed

preauthorization—approval for treatment or service obtained from an insurance company before the care is provided

precedent—legal decision that sets the standard for subsequent, like cases

preceptor—person who supervises a practicum in a health care facility; also called a mentor

pre-existing condition—condition for which a patient received treatment in a certain period before beginning coverage with a new insurance plan

preferred provider organization—organization that contracts with independent providers to perform services for members at discounted rates

premium—dollar amount paid to the insurance company to have coverage in force; usually paid monthly; employers may pay part or all of the premium as an employee benefit

presenting problem—a contributory factor in E&M coding that consists of a disease, condition, illness, injury, symptom, sign, finding, complaint, or other reason for the encounter, as stated by the patient

preventive care—care a patient receives to maintain good health and screen for potential health risks

primary care provider—person or entity responsible for determining when and if a patient needs specific types of health care

primary diagnosis—patient's chief complaint or reason for visit

private health insurance—health insurance not provided by the government but by an independent not-for-profit or for-profit company; also called *private insurance, commercial health insurance,* or *commercial insurance*

problem-oriented medical record charting—type of medical record charting that focuses on patients' health care problems and addresses those problems at each visit

procedural coding—the process of assigning codes to health care services and procedures

procedure—steps to perform a task or project

procedures—services health care providers perform on or for patients

professional component—the portion of a test or procedure in which a qualified physician interprets the results and writes a report

professional courtesy—to give a patient a discount, or free service, due to the fact that the patient is a health care professional

professional distance—maintaining a professional relationship with patients and coworkers to remain objective and avoid the appearance of impropriety

progress notes—notes in a patient's medical chart outlining the patient's progress or complaints

progress report—with regard to workers' compensation, a report that documents the treatment provided, the worker's current medical status, the expected plan of care, the prognosis, and the expected return-to-work date

proofreader's marks—notations used when reading and reviewing a document for errors

proofreading—process of reading and reviewing a document for errors

property and casualty insurance—insurance on homes, cars, and businesses that protects the policyholder against the loss of or damage to physical property they own and against legal liability for losses caused by injury to others, including medical expenses of those injured; also called *liability insurance*

proprietary school—a private business enterprise that sells vocational/occupational courses (e.g., medical assisting) to the general public for training or employment purposes

protected health information (PHI)—any information about health status, provision of health care, or payment for health care that can be linked to a specific individual

public health—all health services designed to improve and protect community health

purge—to remove closed or inactive patient medical records from the medical office

qualified—diagnosis statement accompanied by terms such as *possible, probable, suspected, rule out* (R/O), or *working diagnosis,* indicating that the physician has not determined the root cause; also called an *uncertain diagnosis*

quarterly payroll reports—documents that specify the taxes withheld from wages quarterly

radioactive waste—any waste contaminated with radioactive material

radiocarbon dating—a radiometric dating procedure that measures a substance's decay of carbon to determine its age

rapport—trust and affection between parties

reception area—waiting area for patients in the medical office

receptionist—medical staff member who greets patients, answers the telephone, and directs office flow

recertification—process of certificate renewal

Red Flags Rule—rule passed in January 2008 by the Federal Trade Commission, along with other governmental agencies, to help prevent identity theft

reference initials—in a professional letter, the all-capital initials of the author followed by the all-lowercase initials of the person who typed the letter (e.g., AJF/cmm)

reflecting—the practice of repeating patient information so that the patient knows he or she has been understood

registered medical assistant (RMA)—credential awarded a medical assistant who has passed the RMA certification examination

regulatory law—legislation that relates to government regulations

rejected—a claim that is returned without processing to the provider due to a technical error

relative value unit (RVU)—numeric value assigned by Medicare to formulate fee schedules for health care providers

relative value unit—unit of measure assigned to medical services based on the resources required to provide it; includes work, practice expense, and liability insurance

relative value unit—unit of measure assigned to medical services based on the resources required to provide it; includes work, practice expense, and liability insurance

res ipsa loquitur—the Latin phrase for, "the thing speaks for itself"

res judicata—the Latin phrase for "the thing has been decided"

resequenced code—a CPT code that appears out of numerical sequence within a subsection in order to group it with similar codes

respect—to hold in high esteem

respondeat superior—Latin phrase for "let the master answer"

résumé—document outlining a job applicant's education and job experience

return on investment—the amount of profit an investment returns after implementation

route—to direct telephone calls to other numbers

salutation—greeting

scanner—device that copies documents or pictures for transfer to computer systems

scope of practice—range of skills and duties a health care professional is expected to have and operate within

screenings—events held to offer free services to individuals, such as blood pressure testing

search engine optimization—the process of affecting the visibility of a Web site or a Web page in a search engine's search

secondary diagnoses—conditions, diseases, or reasons for seeking care in addition to the first-listed diagnosis; they may or may not be related to the first-listed diagnosis

section (CPT)—one of six major divisions of the CPT manual: evaluation and management; anesthesia; surgery; radiology; pathology and laboratory; and medicine

section (ICD-10)—an organizational division of a chapter that groups together multiple categories

security envelope—nontransparent envelope

self-funded—type of insurance in which an employer sets aside a large reserve fund to directly reimburse employees for medical expenses, rather than purchasing a commercial insurance policy

semicolon (;)—a punctuation mark in a standalone code; the part of the definition before the semicolon is used by the indented codes that follow

sentinel event—an occurrence involving death or serious physical or psychological injury, or the risk thereof

sequela—an abnormal condition resulting from a previous injury, condition, or disease

service animal—animal that has been trained to assist a person with a handicap

settled—state in which an offer of money is extended and accepted to drop a lawsuit

sexual harassment—unwanted sexual attention or comments in the workplace

shaman—a religious or spiritual figure that acts as an intermediary between the natural and supernatural worlds; someone who is believed to use magic to cure illness

short-term disability—a disability income insurance policy that has a short waiting period, usually 0 to 14 days, and pays benefits for a limited amount of time, usually anywhere from 3 months to 2 years

sign—a physical sign of a condition that can be observed or measured by a physician

sign-in sheet—paper or electronic document on which patients sign their names upon entering the office

skilled nursing facility—a licensed facility that primarily provides inpatient, skilled nursing care to patients who require medical, nursing, or rehabilitative services but does not provide the level of care or treatment available in a hospital

slack time—an appointment scheduling method of leaving certain times of day open to accommodate situations such as when patients call for same-day appointments or physicians who need to catch up on charting

sliding fee scale—a provider's fee schedule that charges varying fees for a service based on a patient's financial ability to pay

smart phone—cellular phone that has features for browsing the Internet or composing word-processed documents

SOAP note charting—type of charting that considers the patient's subjective and objective findings, the provider's assessment of the patient's condition, and the prescribed plan of action for treatment

social information—information about a patient's social habits, such as tobacco, drug, or alcohol use

social media site—Web site where people can share information, interact, and communicate with each other

Social Security Act—law passed by the U.S. Congress in 1935 to provide workers and their families financial security postretirement

Social Security Disability Insurance—a federal government program that provides health care coverage to people with low income who are disabled and who do not meet the work requirements of SSI

solid waste—paper, cans, cups, and other garbage from nonclinical areas

source-oriented medical record—type of charting that groups similar sections together

speaker phone—telephone feature that broadcasts the speaker's voice

special instructions (CPT)—directions within each section describing specific rules and definitions for use of codes within a particular category or subcategory

speed dial—telephone feature that dials numbers programmed into the system using codes; see also *automatic dialer*

spell check—software that verifies word spellings

standalone code—a CPT code that contains a full description and is not dependent on another code for complete meaning

standard of care—legal term that describes the type of care a reasonable health care provider is expected to provide under the same situation

standard precautions—infection control techniques used by health care professionals that include proper hand hygiene, personal protective equipment, respiratory hygiene and cough etiquette, safe injection practices, and proper handling of potentially hazardous and contaminated materials

standardized—uniform practice

statute of limitations—period after an injury happens within which a patient may file a malpractice lawsuit

stereotyping—to falsely believe that all individuals with particular characteristics (e.g., race, gender, economic status) are the same; judging individuals based on your own opinions

stop loss—a provision in a health insurance policy that limits the maximum amount the patient must pay out-of-pocket for deductibles, copayments, and coinsurance

subcategory (CPT)—a division of a category within the CPT Tabular List

subcategory (ICD-10-CM)—a four- or five-character entry in ICD-10-CM Tabular List that is not a final code

subheading—a division of a subsection within the CPT Tabular List

subject line—in a professional letter, the subject of the letter

subpoena—a formal written document that legally requires a person or persons, via court order, to appear in court

subpoena duces tecum—a formal written document that requires a person or persons to produce records or documents in court, via court order

subscriber—person who holds or owns an insurance policy; same as the *member* or the *insured*

subsection—subdivisions within a section of the CPT Tabular List

subterm—a word indented two spaces under the boldfaced Main Term in the ICD-10-CM, which further describes the Main Term in terms of etiology, coexisting conditions, anatomic site, episode, or similar descriptor

Supplemental Security Income—a federal government program that provides Medicare coverage to disabled workers who have met Social Security requirements for quarters worked and whose disability is not work related

surgical package—the group of services included in the CPT code for a surgical procedure, as defined in the CPT Surgery Section guidelines

sympathy—feelings of pity for someone else's trouble or misfortune

symptom—indication of a condition reported by the patient that the physician cannot observe or measure

syncope—fainting; the sudden loss of consciousness

Tabular List (CPT)—the numerical listing of all CPT codes, accompanied by guidelines and notes

Tabular List (ICD-10-CM)—the portion of the ICD-10-CM manual that lists diagnostic codes in alphanumeric order

technical component—the portion of a test or procedure that involves administering the procedure and providing the necessary personnel and equipment

technical educational program—program designed to give students skills without higher education; also called vocational program

therapeutic communication—face-to-face process of interacting with the patient that focuses on the patient's physical and emotional well-being

thesaurus—resource for locating alternate words with similar meanings

third-party administrator—a company that processes paperwork for claims for a self-insured employer

third-party payer—an organization that pays for health care services on behalf of the patient

thumb drive—small, external data storage device; see also *flash drive*

tickler file—tool for tracking future events, such as patient appointments

time clock—piece of equipment that records employees' arrival and departure times for payroll purposes

tort law—legislation that relates to one party injuring another

transcribe—to type words as they are spoken

transcription machine—piece of equipment that allows the user to listen to and type recorded words

triage notebook—notebook kept near the administrative medical assistant answering incoming telephone calls that outlines questions and steps to follow in the event a caller has a potentially life-threatening condition

triaging—process of prioritizing patients based on need

TRICARE—health insurance administered by the U.S. Department of Defense for active duty military personnel, retired service personnel, and their eligible dependents; formerly known as Civilian Health and Medical Program (CHAMPUS)

ultrasound—method of using sound waves to create three-dimensional images for diagnostic or therapeutic purposes

unbundling—the illegal act of billing multiple services with separate CPT codes and separate charges that should be combined under a single CPT code and one charge

uncollectible—account believed never to be paid

undue influence—to persuade someone to do something they do not want to do

unemployment insurance—program that pays employees who have lost their jobs

unintentional tort—to harm another person accidentally

upcode—to illegally code and bill for a higher level of service than was actually provided

user manual—document that describes how something (e.g., equipment) is used

usual, customary, and reasonable—a method third-party payers use to reimburse providers based on the provider's normal or usual fee; the customary or range of fees charged by providers of the same specialty in the same geographic area; and other factors to determine appropriate or reasonable fees in unusual situations

values—internal points of reference used to differentiate between what is good and what is bad

verify—the process of consulting the Tabular List to read detailed code descriptions, conventions, and instructional notes, and to assign additional specificity

virtual appointment—a medical appointment conducted via e-mail, telephone, or video, rather than in person

vocational program—program designed to give students skills without higher education; also called *technical educational program*

W-2 form—U.S. federal form that annually documents the wages employees drew the previous year

W-4 form—U.S. federal form that indicates employees' marital status and federal tax exemptions

wages—monies paid for work performed

waiting period—period after a new health insurance plan begins and during which certain services are not covered

warranty—a guarantee from a vendor stating that certain defects or problems will be repaired for a predetermined period

wave scheduling—a scheduling system where patients are scheduled only during the first half of each hour

web chat—a system that allows users to communicate in real time using an Internet interface

withholding allowances—number of exemptions on federal tax forms

workers' compensation—insurance coverage provided by employers for job-related illness or injury

write off—to remove a balance from a patient account

References

Books and Manuals

Abreu, Laurinda, and Sheard, Sally (2013). *Hospital Life: Theory and Practice from the Medieval to the Modern.* New York: Peter Lang International Academic Publishers.

Halley, Marc D., and Ferry, Michael J. (2008). *The Medical Practice Start-Up Guide.* Phoenix, Maryland: Greenbranch Publishing.

Harris, Philip R., and Moran, Robert T. (2011). *Managing Cultural Differences.* New York: Routledge Publishing.

Holland, Alex (2000). *Voices of Qi: An Introductory Guide to Traditional Chinese Medicine.* Northwest Institute of Acupuncture and Oriental Medicine. New York: North Atlantic Books.

Konar, Oguz (2013). *10 Ways to Grow Your Medical Practice in the New Age of Marketing: Proven Techniques to Help Your Practice Prosper with Online and Office Marketing.* New York: CreateSpace Independent Publishing Platform.

Maciocia, Giovanni (2005). *The Foundations of Chinese Medicine: A Comprehensive Text for Acupuncturists and Herbalists.* London: Churchill Livingstone.

Porter, R. (1999). *The Greatest Benefit to Mankind: A Medical History of Humanity from Antiquity to the Present.* New York: W.W. Norton and Company.

Wells, Susan (2001). *Out of the Dead House: Nineteenth-Century Women Physicians and the Writing of Medicine.* Madison, WI: University of Wisconsin Press.

Internet-Based References

www.alsa.org: ALS Association

www.alz.org: Alzheimer's Association

www.amrad.org: Amateur Radio Research and Development Corporation Telecommunications for the Deaf

www.aapc.com: American Academy of Professional Coders

www.aama-ntl.org: American Association of Medical Assistants

www.diabetes.org: American Diabetes Association

www.ahima.org: American Health Information Management Association

www.americanheart.org: American Heart Association

www.americanhospice.org: American Hospice Foundation

www.aha.org/aha_app/index.jsp: American Hospital Association

www.lungusa.org: American Lung Association

www.ama-assn.org: American Medical Association

www.amt1.com: American Medical Technologists

www.apdaparkinson.org: American Parkinson Disease Association

www.ahdionline.org: Association for Healthcare Documentation Integrity

www.cdc.gov/: Centers for Disease Control and Prevention

www.cms.hhs.gov/: Centers for Medicare and Medicaid Services

www.cebm.net/: Centre for Evidence-Based Medicine

www.cfhi.org: Child Family Health International

www.epic.com: Epic

www.ftc.gov: Federal Trade Commission

www.hpso.com: Health Care Providers Service Organization

www.ornl.gov/sci/techresources/Human_Genome/home.shtml: Human Genome Project Information Archive 1990–2003

http://www.iom.edu: Institute of Medicine

www.nlm.nih.gov/medlineplus: Medline Plus®

http://nccam.nih.gov/: National Center for Complementary and Alternative Medicine

www.optuminsight.com/: OptumInsight

www.payroll-taxes.com: Payroll Taxes Payroll Research

www.pbs.org/healthcarecrisis/history.htm: PBS's Health Care Crisis: Health Care Timeline

www.powermed.com/: PowerMed

www.citizen.org: Public Citizen

www.shrinershospitalsforchildren.org/: Shriners Hospital for Children

www.skillpath.com: SkillPath Training

www.sorryworks.net/: Sorry Works!

www.jointcommission.org/: The Joint Commission

www.usdoj.gov/: The United States Department of Justice

www.tricare.org/: TRICARE Online.com

http://www.hhs.gov/ocr/hipaa/: U.S. Department of Health & Human Services—Health Insurance Portability and Accountability Act

www.dol.gov: United States Department of Labor

www.bls.gov/: United States Department of Labor—Bureau of Labor Statistics

www.dot.gov: United States Department of Transportation

www.who.org: World Health Organization

Index

A

AAMA. *See* American Association of Medical Assistants
AAPC (American Academy of Professional Coders), 28, 374
Abbreviations
   to avoid, 136
   in charting, 206, 208–209
   common medical, 133–134, 208–209
   state, 128
   USPS, 139, 140
ABHES. *See* Accrediting Bureau of Health Education Schools
ABN. *See* Advance Beneficiary Notice
Abortion, 87
Abuse
   coding and, 383
   reporting cases of, 61, 87
   types of, 87–88
Accept assignment, 313
Accidental injury files, 183
Accidents and injuries, preventing, 270
Accounts payable (AP)
   checkbook register, 441
   deposit slips, preparing, 442–443
   endorsement stamps, 443
   ordering and receiving supplies, 441–442
Accounts receivable (AR), managing, 414–415
Accreditation, 21
Accreditation Council for Pharmacy Education (ACPE), 41
Accrediting Bureau of Health Education Schools (ABHES), 21
Acquired immune deficiency syndrome. *See* AIDS
ACPE. *See* Accreditation Council for Pharmacy Education
ACS. *See* American Cancer Society
Active listening, 100–101
Active patient files, 214
ADA. *See* Americans with Disabilities Act
Adding machines, 249–250
Add-on codes, 393
ADEA. *See* Age Discrimination in Employment Act
Administrative law, 51
Administrative procedures, outlining, 261–262
Administrative skills, 21, 22, 35
ADN. *See* Associate degree in nursing
Advance Beneficiary Notice (ABN), 313, 314
Advance directives, 71–73, 202
Adverse outcomes, 462–463
Advertising. *See* Marketing
Advocate, 35, 484
AEDs. *See* Automated external defibrillator units
Affordable Care Act (ACA), 15, 301
Age Discrimination in Employment Act (ADEA), 454
Agendas, 451
Aging reports, 415
AHA. *See* American Heart Association; American Hospital Association
AHDI. *See* Association for Healthcare Documentation Integrity
AHIMA. *See* American Health Information Management Association

AI. *See* Artificial insemination
AIDS, treating patients with, 12, 91
Airway obstructions, 281–282, 283
Allowed amounts, 302, 305
Alphabetic filing, 211–212
AMA. *See* American Medical Association
Ambulatory care centers, 34
Ambulatory care issues, 77
American Academy of Professional Coders. *See* AAPC
American Association of Medical Assistants (AAMA)
   code of ethics, 84–85
   CPR certification, 270
   history of, 16
   Occupational Analysis Grid, 21, 22
American Cancer Society (ACS), 116
American Health Information Management Association (AHIMA), 28–29, 66, 374
American Heart Association (AHA), 12, 270, 275
American Hospital Association (AHA), 12, 76
American Medical Association (AMA), 300
   coding, 381
   ethical issues, 86–87
   history of, 12–13
American Medical Technologists (AMT), 24, 25, 28
American Public Health Association (APHA), 355
American Red Cross, 13, 270
Americans with Disabilities Act (ADA), 74, 103, 161, 175–176, 454
Amputations, anesthesia for, 8
AMT. *See* American Medical Technologists
Anaphylaxis, 271
Anatomy, 6
Ancient Medicine (Hippocrates), 5
Anesthesia
   chloroform, 8
   ether, 7–8
Angry patients, communicating with, 105, 156
Animals, service, 103–104, 176
Annotation, 141, 142
Answering services, 150
Answering telephones, 151–157
Antisepsis, 9
Antiseptic, 9
AP. *See* Accounts payable
APHA. *See* American Public Health Association
Appeal, 77
Appointments
   allowing adequate time for, 183
   automated telephone reminders, 188
   balancing patient and office needs, 184
   books and HIPAA regulations, 185
   chronically late patients, handling, 188
   cluster scheduling, 185
   double booking, 185
   electronic, 184–185
   emergency (triage), 188
   fixed appointment scheduling, 185, 187

Health unit coordinators (HUCs)
  educational requirements, 43
  role of, 42–43
Hearing-impaired patients, communicating with, 103, 104
Heart attack, signs and symptoms of, 279
Heart disease, 12
Heart transplants, 11
Herbal use, early, 4–5
Hierarchy of needs, 113
Hill-Burton Act, 415
HIPAA. *See* Health Insurance and Portability and Accountability
    Act
Hippocrates, 5, 84
Hippocratic Oath, 5, 84
Hiring employees, 456
History (H, HX), 396
HITECH (Health Information Technology for Economic and
    Clinical Health) Act (2009), 226–227
HIV, 91, 372
HMOs. *See* Health maintenance organizations
Hold (telephone), placing callers on, 149–150
Hopps, J., 11
Hospitals
  history of, 7, 12
  types of, 12
Hospital services and admissions, scheduling, 191, 193
HUCs. *See* Health unit coordinators
Human Genome Project, 11–12
Human immunodeficiency virus. *See* HIV
Hunter, J., 7
Hypertension, coding for, 369

I

Ibn-Sina, 7
ICD-9-CM coding, 355, 356
ICD-10-CM coding, 324
  assigning diagnosis codes, 360–369
  for burns, 372
  combination codes, 369
  compared to ICD-9-CM, 356
  conventions, 357–360
  development of, 355
  for diabetes, 374
  external cause codes, 371
  for fractures, 370–371
  for HIV, 372
  for hypertension, 369
  Index to Diseases and Injuries, 360
  for influenza, 372–373
  for neoplasms, 369–370
  for obstetrics, 373–374
  organization of, 357–360
  for poisonings and adverse effects, 371–372
  Tabular List, 360, 361
  transition to, 356
  Z-codes, 370
Imhotep, 4, 5
Immunizations
  See also Vaccines
  coding for, 402
  employer-mandated, 92

Implementing, patient education and, 112
Implied consent, 53
Implied contracts, 63
Inactive patient files, 214
Incidents, reporting, 462–463
Indecipherable handwriting, 228
Indemnity plans, 306
Indented code, 390, 391
Indirect questions, 102
Individual health insurance, 309, 311
Infants
  airway obstruction in, 283
  choking, 279–280, 281
  CPR for, 272–273
Infection control procedures, documenting, 262
Infectious waste, 464
Infertility treatments, 89
Influenza, coding for, 372–373
Information contained in medical records, type of, 200
Information technology, use of, 12
Informed consent, 54, 55
Inpatient versus outpatient, 396
Institute of Medicine, 12, 228
Insurance fraud, 415
  See also Health insurance
Insured, 302
Intentional tort, 52
Internal Revenue Service (IRS), 51, 430, 433
International Classification of Diseases (ICD), 355
  See also ICD-9-CM coding; ICD-10-CM coding
International law, 52
International Red Cross, 13
Internet
  accessing bank accounts via, 443
  buying medications, 241
  marketing and using the, 472
  medical records and use of, 229
  patient education and the use of the, 118–119, 240
  search engines, 240–241
  web chat, 150
Interpreters, use of, 104, 106, 192
Interviewing for a job
  arranging for, 489, 492
  common questions asked, 493
  dressing for, 492–493
  follow-up after, 493–494
  preparing for, 492
Interviewing patients, techniques for, 101–102
Inventorying supplies, 251–252
In vitro fertilization, 89
IRS. *See* Internal Revenue Service

J

JAMA *(Journal of the American Medical Association)*, 13
Jenner, E., 7
Job, applying for a
  application, completing, 489, 490–491
  cover letter, preparing a, 488–489
  interview, preparing for an, 489, 492–494
  recommendation letters, 494
  résumé, writing an effective, 484–488